DIET *and* NUTRITION *in* PALLIATIVE CARE

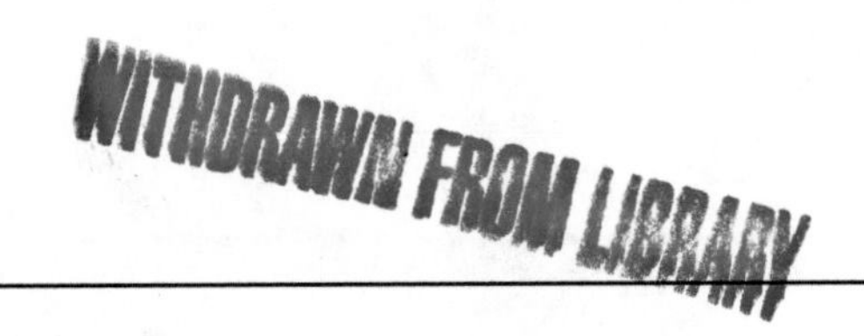

DIET *and* NUTRITION *in* PALLIATIVE CARE

Edited by
Victor R. Preedy

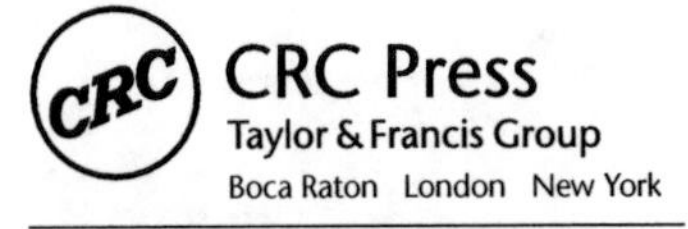
CRC Press
Taylor & Francis Group
Boca Raton London New York

CRC Press is an imprint of the
Taylor & Francis Group, an **informa** business

CRC Press
Taylor & Francis Group
6000 Broken Sound Parkway NW, Suite 300
Boca Raton, FL 33487-2742

Printed in the United States of America on acid-free paper

International Standard Book Number: 978-1-4398-1932-6 (Hardback)

Visit the Taylor & Francis Web site at
http://www.taylorandfrancis.com

and the CRC Press Web site at
http://www.crcpress.com

Contents

SECTION I Setting the Scene

SECTION II Cultural Aspects

SECTION IV Cancer

SECTION V Other Conditions

SECTION VI Pharmacological Aspects

Preface

Optimal terminal and palliative care requires consideration of the patient and family unit as well as cultural and religious sensitivities. The patient's well-being in terms of mobility, anxiety, stress, social interaction and pain control needs expert focus and attention. This is particularly relevant as the population ages and life can be prolonged. However, there is an increasing awareness that diet and nutritional support play an integral part in the patient's holistic well-being. Most nutritional textbooks or handbooks will have material aimed at prolonging life or improving the quality of life of an individual and alleviating symptoms with a long-term view of complete rehabilitation. Occasionally, such books are directed toward subgroups such as infants or the old. However, there are no comprehensive books on nutrition in terminal or palliative care that simultaneously cover physical, cultural and ethical aspects, and bridge the intellectual divide in being suitable for novices and experts alike. This book addresses such a deficiency.

The *Diet and Nutrition in Palliative Care* is divided into six sections:

1. Setting the Scene
2. Cultural Aspects
3. General Aspects
4. Cancer
5. Other Conditions
6. Pharmacological Aspects

Coverage in the *Diet and Nutrition in Palliative Care* includes the need for a specialized interest that combines palliative care and nutrition; concepts; personal perspective; quality of life in the young and adults; Japanese, Chinese and Indian perspectives; forgoing of tube feeding; artificial nutrition including total parenteral nutrition, gastrointestinal side effects and symptoms; gastrojejunostomy; withholding or withdrawing nutritional support; vitamin deficiency; hydration; dysphagia; appetite; fatigue; taste and smell alterations; nausea; refractory cancer cachexia and cachexia-related suffering; head and neck cancer; the vegetative state; renal failure; end-stage liver disease; amyotrophic lateral sclerosis; motor disease; effects of steroids; appetite stimulants and warfarin.

Unique features of each chapter include relevant sections on

- Applications to other areas of terminal or palliative care
- Practical methods and techniques or guidelines
- Key points or features that highlight important areas within chapters
- Ethical issues
- Summary points

The *Diet and Nutrition in Palliative Care* is for doctors, nurses and carers and those interested or working in the palliative or end-of-life domain. This will, of course, include nutritionists and dietitians, health workers and practitioners, hospice or palliative centre managers, college and university teachers and lecturers, and undergraduates and graduates. The chapters are written by either national or international experts or specialists in their field. The material is well illustrated with numerous figures and tables.

Professor Victor R. Preedy

Editor

Professor Victor R. Preedy (BSc, PhD, DSc, FIBiol, FRCPath, FRSPH) is currently professor of nutritional biochemistry in the Department of Nutrition and Dietetics, King's College London, and honorary professor of clinical biochemistry in the Department of Clinical Biochemistry, King's College Hospital. He is also director of the Genomics Centre, King's College London. Professor Preedy gained his PhD in 1981 and in 1992 he received his Membership of the Royal College of Pathologists, based on his published works. He was elected a Fellow of the Royal College of Pathologists in 2000. In 1993 he gained a DSc degree for his outstanding contribution to protein metabolism. Professor Preedy was elected as a fellow to the Royal Society for the Promotion of Health (2004) and The Royal Institute of Public Health (2004). In 2009 he was elected as a fellow of the Royal Society for Public Health (RSPH). The RSPH is governed by Royal Charter and Her Majesty the Queen is its patron. Professor Preedy has written or edited over 550 articles, including over 160 peer-reviewed manuscripts based on original research, 85 reviews, and numerous books. His interests pertain to matters concerning nutrition and health at the individual and societal levels.

Contributors

Amy P. Abernethy
Division of Medical Oncology
Duke University Medical Center
Durham, North Carolina

N. Ananthakrishnan
Department of Surgery
Mahatma Gandhi Medical College and Research Institute
Pondicherry, India

Michaela Bercovici
Oncological Hospice
The Chaim Sheba Medical Center
Tel-Hashomer, Israel

Johan Bilsen
Department of Medical Sociology and Health Sciences
Vrije Universiteit Brussel
Brussels, Belgium

D. Blum
Department of Internal Medicine and Palliative Care Centre
Cantonal Hospital
St. Gallen, Switzerland

Giacomo Bovio
Metabolic–Nutritional Unit and Palliative Care Unit
Salvatore Maugeri Foundation
Pavia, Italy

Hilde M. Buiting
Department of Public Health
Erasmus MC, University Medical Center Rotterdam
Rotterdam, the Netherlands

Hans-Henrik Bülow
Intensive Care Unit
Holbaek Hospital
Holbaek, Denmark

Francesco Caporusso
Department of Radiation Oncology
Sunnybrook Health Sciences Centre
Toronto, Ontario, Canada

Paola Cassolino
Department of Emergency
San Giovanni Battista Hospital
Via Genova, Torino, Italy

Helen Yue-lai Chan
The Nethersole School of Nursing
The Chinese University of Hong Kong
Shatin, Hong Kong

Ching-Yu Chen
Department of Family Medicine
National Taiwan University Hospital
Taipei City, Taiwan, ROC

Michele Chiaverina
Department of Internal Medicine
San Giovanni Battista Hospital
Torino, Italy

Tai-Yuan Chiu
Department of Family Medicine
National Taiwan University Hospital
Taipei City, Taiwan, ROC

Edward Chow
Department of Radiation Oncology
Sunnybrook Health Sciences Centre
Toronto, Ontario, Canada

Fabio Cisarò
Department of Internal Medicine
San Giovanni Battista Hospital
Torino, Italy

Finella Craig
Department of Palliative Care
Great Ormond Street Hospital for Children
London, United Kingdom

Reinhard Dengler
Department of Neurology
Hannover Medical School
Hannover, Germany

Jörg Dötsch
Department of Pediatrics
University of Erlangen-Nuremberg
Erlangen, Germany

Luca Dughera
Department of Internal Medicine
San Giovanni Battista Hospital
Torino, Italy

Geoffrey P. Dunn
Department of Surgery
Hamot Medical Center
Erie, Pennsylvania

Robin L. Fainsinger
Department of Oncology
University of Alberta
Edmonton, Alberta, Canada

Jeffrey M. Farma
Department of Surgical Oncology
Fox Chase Cancer Center
Philadelphia, Pennsylvania

Susanne Fischer
Department of Sociology
Institute of Social and Preventive Medicine
University of Zurich
Zurich, Switzerland

Mick Fleming
School of Health, Nursing and Midwifery
University of the West of Scotland
Ayr, United Kingdom

Renata Gorska
The Nutristasis Unit
Centre for Haemostasis and Thrombosis
Guy's and St. Thomas' Hospital (GSTS Pathology)
London, United Kingdom

Dominic J. Harrington
The Nutristasis Unit
Centre for Haemostasis and Thrombosis
Guy's and St. Thomas' Hospital (GSTS Pathology)
London, United Kingdom

Jeroen G. J. Hasselaar
Department of Anaesthesiology, Pain and Palliative Medicine
Radboud University Nijmegen Medical Centre
Nijmegen, The Netherlands

Ryuichi Hayashi
Division of Head and Neck Surgery
National Cancer Center Hospital East
Kashiwa, Chiba, Japan

Agnes van der Heide
Department of Public Health
Erasmus MC, University Medical Center Rotterdam
Rotterdam, the Netherlands

Lori Holden
Department of Radiation Therapy
Sunnybrook Health Sciences Centre
Toronto, Ontario, Canada

Meng-Yun Hsieh
Department of Family Medicine
National Taiwan University Hospital
Taipei City, Taiwan, ROC

Kuo-Chin Huang
Department of Family Medicine
National Taiwan University Hospital
Taipei City, Taiwan, ROC

Vikram Kate
Department of Surgery
Jawaharlal Institute of Postgraduate Medical Education and Research
Pondicherry, India

Takumi Kawaguchi
Department of Digestive Disease Information & Research and Department of Medicine
Kurume University School of Medicine
Kurume, Japan

Michelle Koh
Department of Palliative Care
Great Ormond Street Hospital for Children
London, United Kingdom

Katja Kollewe
Department of Neurology
Hannover Medical School
Hannover, Germany

Sonja Körner
Department of Neurology
Hannover Medical School
Hannover, Germany

Yeur-Hur Lai
College of Medicine
National Taiwan University
Taipei, Taiwan

Martin Leung
Department of Radiation Oncology
Sunnybrook Health Sciences Centre
Toronto, Ontario, Canada

Rurik Löfmark
Centre for Bioethics
Karolinska Institutet and Uppsala University
Stockholm, Sweden

Marco Luchetti
Department of Anesthesia and Intensive Care 1
"A. Manzoni" General Hospital
Lecco, Italy

Iruru Maetani
Department of Internal Medicine
Toho University Ohashi Medical Center
Tokyo, Japan

Nanda Kishore Maroju
Department of Surgery
Jawaharlal Institute of Postgraduate Medical Education and Research
Pondicherry, India

Caroline J. Hollins Martin
Department of Community, Women and Children's Health
Glasgow Caledonian University
Glasgow, United Kingdom

Colin R. Martin
School of Health, Nursing and Midwifery
University of the West of Scotland
Ayr, United Kingdom

Frank Mayer
Department of Oncology, Hematology, Immunology, Rheumatology and Pneumology
University of Tuebingen Medical Center II
Tuebingen, Germany

Valentina Medici
Department of Internal Medicine
University of California Davis
Sacramento, California

Guido Miccinesi
Epidemiology Unit
Centre for Study and Prevention of Cancer
Florence, Italy

Cheryl Ann Monturo
Department of Nursing
West Chester University of Pennsylvania
West Chester, Pennsylvania

Tatsuya Morita
Department of Palliative and Supportive Care
Seirei Mikatahara General Hospital
Hamamatsu, Japan

Yumiko Nagao
Department of Digestive Disease Information and Research
Kurume University School of Medicine
Kurume, Japan

Samya Z. Nasr
Department of Pediatric Pulmonology
University of Michigan Health System
Ann Arbor, Michigan

Giuseppe Nattino
Department of Anesthesia and Intensive Care 1
"A. Manzoni" General Hospital
Lecco, Italy

Janet Nguyen
Department of Radiation Oncology
Sunnybrook Health Sciences Centre
Toronto, Ontario, Canada

Michael Norup
Department of Medical Philosophy and Clinical Theory
University of Copenhagen
Copenhagen, Denmark

Kai-Dietrich Nüsken
Department of Pediatrics
University of Erlangen-Nuremberg
Erlangen, Germany

R. Oberholzer
Department of Internal Medicine and Palliative Care Centre
Cantonal Hospital
St. Gallen, Switzerland

Bregje D. Onwuteaka-Philipsen
Department of Public and Occupational Health and Institute for Research in Extramural Medicine
Vrije University Medical Center
the Netherlands

Samantha Mei-che Pang
School of Nursing
The Hong Kong Polytechnic University
Kowloon, Hong Kong

Susanne Petri
Department of Neurology
Hannover Medical School
Hannover, Germany

Jana Pilkey
Department of Family Medicine
University of Manitoba
Winnipeg, Manitoba, Canada

Roseanna Presutti
Department of Radiation Oncology
Sunnybrook Health Sciences Centre
Toronto, Ontario, Canada

Poornima B. Rao
Department of Surgical Oncology
Fox Chase Cancer Center
Philadelphia, Pennsylvania

Sebastian Renger
Institute of Biological Chemistry and Nutrition
University of Hohenheim
Stuttgart, Germany

Judith A. C. Rietjens
Department of Public Health
Erasmus MC, University Medical Center Rotterdam
Rotterdam, the Netherlands

Tiziana Sappia
Registered Dietician
Pavia, Italy

Michio Sata
Department of Digestive Disease Information & Research and Department of Medicine
Kurume University School of Medicine
Kurume, Japan

Christian Selinger
Department of Gastroenterology
Salford Royal Hospital
Salford, United Kingdom

Takeshi Shinozaki
Division of Head and Neck Surgery
National Cancer Center Hospital East
Kashiwa, Japan

Shiow-Ching Shun
College of Medicine
National Taiwan University
Taipei City, Taiwan, ROC

Jeffrey L. Spiess
Hospice of the Western Reserve
Cleveland, Ohio

F. Strasser
Department of Internal Medicine and Palliative Care Centre
Cantonal Hospital
St. Gallen, Switzerland

Darcie D. Streetman
Department of Pediatric Pulmonology
University of Michigan Health System
Ann Arbor, Michigan

Yoav P. Talmi
Department of Otolaryngology—Head and Neck Surgery
The Chaim Sheba Medical Center
Tel-Hashomer, Israel

Eleni Tsiompanou
Department of Palliative Medicine
Kingston Hospital NHS Trust
Surrey, United Kingdom

Johannes J. M. van Delden
Julius Center for Health Sciences
University Medical Center Utrecht
Utrecht, the Netherlands

Constans A. Verhagen
Department of Anaesthesiology, Pain and Palliative Medicine
Radboud University Nijmegen Medical Centre
Nijmegen, the Netherlands

Kris C. P. Vissers
Department of Anaesthesiology, Pain and Palliative Medicine
Radboud University Nijmegen Medical Centre
Nijmegen, the Netherlands

Catherine Walshe
School of Nursing, Midwifery and Social Work
The University of Manchester
Manchester, United Kingdom

Jane L. Wheeler
Division of Medical Oncology
Duke University Medical Center
Durham, North Carolina

Arkadi Yakirevitch
Department of Otolaryngology—Head and Neck Surgery
The Chaim Sheba Medical Center
Tel-Hashomer, Israel

Section I

Setting the Scene

1 Need for a Specialized Interest in Food and Nutrition in Palliative Care

Eleni Tsiompanou

CONTENTS

1.1 INTRODUCTION

Since antiquity, it has been known that food, exercise, and lifestyle, as well as our external environment, have an influence on our health. The father of medicine, Hippocrates, advocated the treatment of illnesses through modification of diet (δίαιτα), which in ancient Greek meant 'way of life' and encompassed food, exercise, massage, baths, and other aspects of everyday activities. Food was a subject of interest for laypeople, writers, and philosophers. In the 'Deipnosophists' ('the Banquet of the Philosophers'), written by Athenaeus in the early third century AD, we read the story of Democritus of Abdera, the 'Laughing Philosopher' (Athenaeus 1927). At the age of 104, approaching the end of his life, his food intake had gradually reduced and he was expecting to die. It was the time of the important Thesmophorian festival (a women's festival in honor of goddesses Demeter and Persephone) and his centenarian sister, who looked after him at his home, asked him not to die during the festivities so that she could take part in them. Wanting to grant her request, he asked for a pot of honey to be brought to him. He was kept alive for 3 days by inhaling the fumes from the honey. When the festival finished, the pot of honey was taken away and he passed away without any suffering. This story from Ancient Greece graphically depicts many elements of nutritional care we categorize as physical, cultural, social, ethical, and emotional, which we encounter in our modern palliative care practice.

1.2 NUTRITION IS A SCIENCE AND AN ART

Nutrition, like medicine, is both a science and an art. As a science, it provides us with evidence to forge a better understanding of how various foods influence the human body on macro and a micro (cellular) levels. As an art, it asks us to appreciate the magnificent complexity of the human body and the uniqueness of each individual and their needs. More importantly, it challenges us to develop experience to recognise the right thing to do, often in the face of considerable uncertainty.

Despite the complexity of the correlation between diet and disease, there is now a sufficient body of evidence to start applying nutritional science in everyday clinical practice. Increasingly, a strong interest in and up-to-date knowledge and understanding of scientific studies on nutrition can enable us, as clinicians, to help our patients more effectively at every stage of their illness.

1.3 NUTRITION AS AN IMPORTANT SUBJECT FOR PATIENTS AND THEIR CARERS

Every healthcare professional would agree that our duty is to take an active interest in what matters most to patients. Primarily this is about relieving suffering, pain, and other debilitating symptoms.

In palliative care there is a critical interlinking of nutrition, symptoms, and patient experience. Symptoms can not only adversely affect food and fluid intake but also, importantly, a patient's nutritional intake can influence their symptoms and general state of being. Research has again confirmed that appetite and the ability to eat are very important physical aspects of a patient's quality of life. These are affected as the disease progresses and the patient experiences a series of losses: loss of weight and the desire to eat; loss of the ability to smell, taste, chew, and swallow food; and loss of the ability to digest and absorb nutrients, and eliminate waste products independently.

Good nutrition can enhance recovery when healing is possible. Conversely, poor nutrition can result in poor resistance to infections, impaired wound healing, increased susceptibility to pressure ulcers, and fatigue. Good, nutritious food contributes to the patient's overall sense of well-being. A drop in essential amino acids, glucose, or vitamins and minerals in the body tends to affect the nervous system and behaviour adversely (Table 1.1).

Nutrition is important because it is an avenue of empowerment for patients; it offers them the possibility to do something for themselves. Once a patient has been diagnosed with a serious illness, they become more aware of the impact their lifestyle has on their body. So they often initiate changes hoping this will help relieve their suffering and increase their chances of survival. They seek to improve their diet, physical activity, and daily routine in general. Their carers want to show their love and care by providing good food and drink. Patients and carers alike often turn to healthcare professionals for information and advice. We need to assist them to appreciate the importance and relevance of nutrition and discuss with them what can help and what can harm them.

As we meet people at different stages of their illnesses we can help them understand how their nutritional needs change as their disease progresses. We can support them and those caring for them, to accept the inevitable changes in their body and the nutritional decline prior to death.

TABLE 1.1
New Definitions in Science

Nutrigenomics: a new science looking at the relationship between nutrition, genetics, and health
Epigenetics: the study of mechanisms that cause changes in gene activity, without modifying the DNA sequence, which are maintained during cell division
Telomere: the end region of the chromosome that protects it from alteration during replication. Its length controls how long cells live
Telomerase: the enzyme that sustains the length of telomere

1.4 RECENT ADVANCES IN THE SCIENCE OF NUTRITION: GENES AND THE ENVIRONMENT

Over the last few decades, great advances in food and nutrition research have increased our understanding of the way foods affect people's health. Following the evidence that tobacco is, beyond doubt, a carcinogen and contributes to a number of other diseases, diet has emerged from the shadows of ancient history as a major environmental, external factor that influences health and well-being.

Palliative care organisations are generally very good at providing the right environment for patients and families. It is not unusual for patients to improve, even if temporarily, after they are admitted to a hospice. This is, of course, due to good symptom control, but it is also due to the supportive healing environment provided for patients. If the right environment and support are given to sick people, they revitalise. When it is less than optimal, they weaken.

The important influence of the environment can now be strikingly observed at a cellular level. Diet, exercise, stress, and many other lifestyle factors have a profound effect on our body chemistry, our internal environment, as current research is showing in greater detail.

1.4.1 Nutrigenomics and Epigenetics: How Diet Affects Our 'Internal Environment'

Knowledge of nutrition has progressed from simple data about macronutrients (fat, proteins, and carbohydrates) and micronutrients (minerals and vitamins) to the more complex world of phytochemicals and bioactive food components, which can alter our cells' phenotype and, ultimately, influence how a disease progresses. The combination of a key number of nutrients working together can alter our cells' protein expression and metabolite production and, in some cases, switch certain genes on or off. As a result, a new branch of science, *nutrigenomics*, has emerged, which studies the relationship between nutrition, genetics, and health (Table 1.1).

Furthermore, our developing understanding of the effect environmental factors have at a cellular level has led to *epigenetics*, another new field of research which looks at the mechanisms that cause changes in gene activity, without modifying the DNA sequence, which are maintained after cell division. Epigenetics is attracting intense research activity around the world. Different environmental factors, such as a poor diet, can initiate epigenetic changes: DNA methylation and histone modification. In turn, these translate into abnormal gene expression, which encourages the initiation and progression of cancer (Tollefsbol 2009). Such gene changes were examined closely in a recent study of patients with early prostate cancer who received no anti-cancer treatment and who enrolled on a programme of lifestyle improvement (Ornish, Magbanua et al. 2008). This included a healthy diet, regular exercise, and stress management. In just 3 months, a number of biological changes in their prostate tissue were seen which meant that prostate cancer promoter genes were deactivated, while anti-cancer genes were switched on. Is it then possible that lifestyle changes can reverse the progression of chronic diseases, such as cancer? Further research will help us understand better the impact of diet and behaviour on the development and progression of chronic diseases.

What makes the study of epigenetic changes so important and exciting is that they can be reversed with even simple lifestyle changes, including the right diet (Feinberg 2008). For example, garlic, turmeric, broccoli, tomatoes, and green tea contain a variety of active dietary photochemicals that influence the release of nuclear factor erythroid-derived 2-related factor 2 (Nrf2). Nrf2 is a "master gene" product that coordinates the activation of a number of antioxidant genes that maintain or restore the activity of normal cells and promote apoptosis of malignant cells (Gopalakrishnan & Tong-Kong 2008). The activation of Nrf2 by these nutrients promises to result in powerful beneficial effects that invite further study. This limited description, hopefully, provides an indication as to why some investigators think that epigenetics may, in the future, play a greater role in health and disease than genetics currently does.

1.4.2 Telomeres

The telomere (derived from the Greek tells (τέλος) "end" and meros (μέρος) "part") is the end region of the chromosome that protects it from alteration during replication. The length of a telomere diminishes with each cell division and so shortens, as we grow older, essentially controlling how long we live. The discovery of the enzyme that sustains the length of telomeres, called telomerase, led to the award of the 2009 Nobel Prize in Physiology and Medicine to three scientists, one of whom was Professor Elizabeth Blackburn. Her research focuses on the effects of stress and diet on telomeres and telomerase. In a landmark study published in 2008, she and her co-investigators showed, for the first time, that telomerase can be activated in the normal white cells of men with low-risk prostate cancer by adopting certain lifestyle changes. These included following a healthy diet, doing regular physical exercise, and undergoing stress management for a short period of just 3 months (Ornish, Lin et al. 2008). In a later study they examine evidence that practices like meditation have a positive effect on the length of telomeres (Epel et al. 2009).

This area of current interest is shedding new light on our understanding of the impact dietary and lifestyle habits have on chronic and degenerative diseases.

1.4.3 The Importance of Micronutrients on Symptom Control

The complexity and importance of nutritional care becomes apparent when we consider the powerful effects of micronutrients: vitamins, minerals, phytochemicals, and others. Dieticians and nutritionists study these in detail during their training, whilst the study of micronutrients does not as yet form a major part in the training of many other healthcare professionals.

This is an additional specialist field that can have a profound effect on care. The reason why it matters is because a steady supply of a combination of nutrients determines the functioning of various organs and systems in the body. If the vitamins and minerals that may be missing in a particular case are identified and if they are replenished, then the healing effect can be dramatic and function can improve. Conversely, if an undiscovered deficiency persists, it may not be clear why there is no real improvement as expected and hoped for.

For example:

- Vitamin D, magnesium, and phosphate deficiencies can contribute to symptoms of weakness, myalgia, and pain (Fabbriciani et al. 2010). It is still unclear to what extent vitamin D supplements are helpful in chronic pain conditions (Straube, Moore et al. 2010; Straube, Derry et al. 2010). As many palliative care patients experience pain and occasionally this is difficult to control, more research is needed to establish how much the correction of deficiencies of micronutrients, such as vitamin D and minerals, for example magnesium and phosphate, could help patients achieve better analgesia (van Veldhuizen et al. 2000; Khan et al. 2010).
- Hypomagnesemia can be the result of a number of pharmacological treatments (Atsmon and Dole 2005): platinum-based chemotherapy (Hodgkinson, Neville-Webbe and Coleman

TABLE 1.2
Key Nutrients Needed for the Optimal Functioning of the Nervous System

- Glucose
- Fatty acids
- Amino acids
- B-vitamins (vitamin B12, thiamine, niacin, pyridoxine)
- Folic acid
- Vitamins A, D and E
- Iron
- Copper

2006) and proton pump inhibitors (Broeren et al. 2009). Such treatments are used commonly in palliative care and can add significant morbidity.

- A combination of nutrients is necessary for the optimal function of the nervous system (Kumar 2010) (Table 1.2). B vitamins and folic acid are especially important. Understanding their effect on the nervous system will allow professionals to offer better help to palliative care patients, who are often malnourished.

1.4.4 Cancer Survivors

'Cancer survivors' is a term encompassing all people who have had a diagnosis of cancer and have recovered from it following treatment, or continue to live with residual or recurrent disease. In this group are included those patients with metastatic and terminal cancer. Cancer survivors can have a number of special medical and psychosocial needs. Palliative care professionals, who often provide care for them, need to have the knowledge base to support them, which unfortunately in many cases at present is insufficient.

However, a number of programs are being developed to assist cancer survivors make the right lifestyle choices, as it is increasingly obvious that these can influence morbidity and mortality (Demark-Wahnefried and Jones 2008). The World Cancer Research Fund (WCRF) and American Institute for Cancer Research (AICR) in their report on 'Food, Nutrition, Physical Activity and the Prevention of Cancer' make a number of recommendations, based on current evidence, to promote cancer prevention through changes in diet (WCRF/AICR 2007). They recommend cancer survivors also observe the same advice (Table 1.3).

TABLE 1.3
WCRF/AICR Recommendations for Cancer Survivors

1. Avoid smoking and exposure to tobacco
2. Aim to be slim without being underweight
3. Maintain regular physical activity
4. Avoid drinks full of sugar
5. Include in your diet a variety of vegetables, fruits, whole grains, and legumes
6. Reduce red meats and processed meats in your diet
7. Limit consumption of alcohol
8. Limit consumption of salt
9. Avoid the use of supplements for protection against cancer

Source: Adapted from World Cancer Research Fund/American Institute for Cancer Research, *Food, nutrition, and physical activity, and the prevention of cancer: A global perspective*. Washington, DC, AICR, 2007.

1.5 MULTISTEP APPROACH TO NUTRITIONAL CARE

Patients who are referred to palliative care services have a range of cancer and non-cancer diagnoses and are at different stages along their disease trajectory. Some of them present with a longer prognosis of many months to a few years whilst others are at the end of their life. This means that patients can have a wide spectrum of nutritional needs, which change during the transition from an earlier to a later stage. Their care will vary from advice on foods and special diets to enteral and, occasionally, parenteral feeding.

Nutritional care is complex because of its many aspects: physical, emotional, social, and cultural. This has been captured in the well-known phrase: 'we are what we eat.' A multistep approach is required to recognize the patient's needs and what is needed to help them (Table 1.4).

Step 1: Nutrition Screening and Assessment

Patients with palliative care needs are nutritionally 'at-risk' for many reasons. The first step in the provision of nutritional care is to perform nutrition screening to recognize those patients who require special attention and care. They will then have to go through a careful assessment to identify nutrition issues and whether they are reversible and treatable. The nutrition assessment should lead to an individualised nutritional care plan (Food and Nutrition Group at Help the Hospices 2009) (Table 1.5). As Professor Lennard-Jones said two decades ago: 'only when the assessment of every patient's nutritional status has become routine will the full benefits of nutrition treatment be realised' (Lennard-Jones 1992).

Step 2: Developing a Care Plan

Nutritional treatment will vary considerably from patient to patient. A cachectic patient with esophageal cancer and dysphagia needs a certain nutrition intervention, food consistency, and diet distinct from that of a cachectic patient with lung cancer and no swallowing difficulties. An overweight patient with metastatic breast carcinoma and a prognosis of months to years requires a different dietary approach to that of an overweight bedridden patient with a brain tumour and a prognosis of a few weeks. Furthermore, the needs of patients with end-stage dementia, amyotrophic lateral sclerosis, congestive heart failure, chronic obstructive pulmonary disease, chronic renal failure, and chronic hepatic failure are also quite variable and complex.

Step 3: Recognizing Changes in Nutritional Needs

Nutritional needs often change when the patient approaches the end of their life. The primary focus of nutritional intervention can shift at this point towards maintenance of optimal quality of life and general support of patients and carers to help them recognise and accept this transition. Carers often say 'food and love' are the last precious gifts we can offer our loved one at the end of their life. Who are we to argue? Perhaps one could say that at the end-of-life food is not the only important aspect of care. The total comfort and peace of mind of the patient at this time is paramount.

TABLE 1.4
Multistep Approach to Nutritional Care of Palliative Care Patients

Step 1: Nutrition screening and assessment
Step 2: Developing a care plan
Step 3: Recognising changes in nutritional needs

TABLE 1.5
Professional Consensus Statement on Nutritional Care in Palliative Care Patients

1. Nutritional care
   - is an essential aspect of palliative care
   - needs to be individualized
   - may change for people at the end-of-life
   - needs to be delivered safely and with compassion and dignity
   - can have physical, social, cultural, and emotional aspects
   - is a matter for all palliative care professionals
2. All staff and volunteers should receive regular training on nutrition
3. Healthcare organisations are responsible for delivering nutritional care

Source: Adapted from the Food and Nutrition Group at Help the Hospices. 2009. Professional consensus statement of nutritional care in palliative care patients. http://www.helpthehospices.org.uk/our-services/running-your-hospice/food-and-nutrition/consensus-statement/ (Accessed February 2010).

1.6 THE DIET OF PEOPLE IN ILLNESS SHOULD BE DIFFERENT TO THEIR DIET IN HEALTH

In his book Ancient Medicine (*Αρχαία* Ιητρική), Hippocrates traces the origins of dietetics and explains how cooking methods influenced human evolution. He wrote, 2500 years ago, how primitive people suffered many illnesses as a result of eating unprocessed raw foods, which led them to seek and discover cooking methods. It is remarkable that there was an appreciation, even millennia ago, that certain foods had harmful constituents, which needed to be avoided or modified. The search/re-search for the impact of diet and lifestyle modification on people's health is what the ancients first called medicine. The practice of medicine developed as doctors observed that men in illness benefited from a diet that was different from that of healthy men.

1.6.1 Alteration of Diet in Palliative Care Patients

It is important for the public to recognize that the dietary guidelines followed by people in health could be inappropriate for them when they become ill. This is equally vital for palliative care patients. For example:

- The advice to have three meals a day and to consume a certain number of calories when healthy would need to be modified for a cancer patient with anorexia-cachexia syndrome (ACS) to many snacks a day and to energy-dense and nutrient-dense foods that are easily digestible.
- Lactose intolerance can contribute to gastrointestinal symptoms in a number of patients. People belonging to certain ethnic groups (Chinese, Japanese, Africans, Southern Europeans, Jews, etc.) often become lactose intolerant as they grow older (Johnson 1981). Others (up to 70% of the population) can develop temporary hypolactasia for a variety of reasons (Matthews et al. 2005), while a few can become lactose intolerant after radiotherapy (Wedlake et al. 2008), gastrointestinal infection, or complex antibiotic treatment (Noble, Rawlinson, and Byrne 2002). Taking into account the underlying condition and changing the patient's diet and pharmacological treatment to avoid foods, drugs, and supplements that contain lactose can make a huge difference to quality of life (Vaillancourt et al. 2009).

- A number of dietary challenges are common in patients with other advanced non-cancer diseases, such as dementia. This is particularly relevant to palliative care services, as in the last few years they have been looking after more patients with advanced dementia. Health professionals then have to assist them with a variety of nutrition and feeding issues. People with dementia often need their diet to be adapted to their reduced appetite, have diminished ability to feed themselves, and experience swallowing difficulties. Such patients may benefit from increasing meal frequency, a texture-modified diet, assistance with feeding, flexibility with mealtimes, and the use of nutritional supplements. Existing evidence shows there are only a few selected cases of patients with dementia where artificial nutrition via a nasogastric or PEG tube could be of help (Royal College of Physicians and British Society of Gastroenterology 2010).

1.6.2 Food as Medicine

Food has important psychological and social significance and shapes many aspects of our culture. Although eating is customarily seen as concerning sensory pleasure, it is about much more than that. It is about the energy and nutrients that we acquire through our diet which influence our whole being. So which foods are beneficial and which are not? (Table 1.6)

Each day new data emerge that show the link between diet and health. For example, a number of dietary phytochemicals have been shown to exhibit anti-cancer potential: sulforaphane in broccoli, indole 3-carbinol in cabbage, diallyl sulphide in onions, and quercetin in oranges and apples, to name a few. Polyphenols found in green tea exhibit activities that promote cancer cell death, suppress cancer cell growth, and inhibit the formation of new blood vessels in the tumours, thereby delaying cancer progression (Yang et al. 2009). A diet rich in phytochemicals has also been shown to be beneficial by reducing the risk of a number of diseases, such as cardiovascular disease, Alzheimer's disease, and a number of metabolic and inflammatory diseases.

Although the above data are impressive, we need to be careful not to make exaggerated claims suggesting that certain nutrients are the answer to disease processes. Instead we must proceed with carefully designed studies to examine the effects of specific diets and combinations of nutrients on patients' conditions.

Foods have been shown to influence the human body in a variety of ways:

- **Inflammatory Processes**
  Chronic inflammation is especially relevant to palliative care patients, not least because it is a well-recognised major component of ACS that is seen in many patients with advanced disease. A plethora of scientific evidence points to diet, cooking methods, and physical activity as having a significant pro-inflammatory or anti-inflammatory effect (O'Connor and Irvin 2010; Warnberg et al. 2009) (Table 1.7). A number of nutrients such as omega-3 fatty acids have been shown to

TABLE 1.6
How to Recognise What Food is Right for the Patient

Food as Medicine
• Source of energy
• Source of nutrients for cells and organs
• Easily digested
• Helpful to the patient's condition
• Not harmful

TABLE 1.7
Diet, Lifestyle and Inflammatory Process

Pro-inflammatory Factors	Anti-inflammatory Factors
• Foods containing trans-fats and omega-6 fatty acids • Meats cooked at high temperature • Barbecued meats • Fried foods • Smoking • Sedentary lifestyle • Overweight/obesity	• Mediterranean diet (seasonal fruit and vegetables, pulses, little meat, more fish, olive oil, herbs) and outdoor lifestyle • Higher intake of whole grains • Higher intake of omega-3 fatty acids • Weight loss • Physical activity

have an anti-inflammatory effect and help cancer patients with ACS stabilise their weight (August and Huhmann 2009). Increased consumption of lean and oily fish can also lead to a reduction in serum C-reactive protein (Pot et al. 2010).

Incorporation of these findings into the care of patients with advanced illnesses could complement their treatment by enhancing the anti-inflammatory effect of drugs. This needs to be further investigated as it can potentially have a positive impact on their quality of life.

- **Hyperglycemia – Insulin Resistance**

  Prospective studies have confirmed epidemiological findings that high blood glucose levels increase the incidence of many cancers and the risk of many fatal cancers (Stocks et al. 2009; Barone et al. 2008). Other studies have shown an increased risk of cardiovascular disease and all-cause mortality in association with increased blood glucose levels and insulin resistance (Barr et al. 2007). More recently, it has been shown that diabetic women with breast cancer who are treated with metformin and chemotherapy have a better prognosis (Jiralerspong et al. 2009). This has been attributed to a number of cellular processes, including reduced levels of circulating glucose and increased insulin sensitivity. A number of research groups around the world are investigating this further.

  Such research findings can be used for the benefit of palliative care patients. As insulin resistance is a key component of ACS, the question of the effect of hyperglycemias and insulin resistance induced by dietary and lifestyle factors needs to be further explored.

- **Mood**

  Another interesting area of research is the effect of different foods and nutrients on mood. In many studies, carbohydrate-rich meals have been shown to result cumulatively in better mood, possibly through an increase in serotonin in the brain. The glycaemic index and glycaemic load of a meal especially, appear to play an important role in mood regulation, by influencing the pattern of glucose supply. Could this really mean that a breakfast of muesli and porridge can give an 'anti-depressant' start to a patient's day?—an interesting thought. Caffeine and alcohol have clearly observable effects on mood and behaviour, while dark chocolate has been shown to improve energy and reduce stress levels, amongst other effects (McShea, Leissle, and Smith 2009). The role of fatty acids in mood disorders is another area of interesting research work. It appears that a diet containing a lot of oily fish may contribute to improvement in mood and also to better pain control.

1.6.3 Nutrition as a Safety Issue

When caring for people, one always has to consider safety matters regarding nutrition (National Patient Safety Agency 2009) (Table 1.8). This becomes especially critical when these are vulnerable

TABLE 1.8
Safety Issues Surrounding Nutrition

1. Lack of nutrition screening and assessment
2. Inappropriate diet
3. Inappropriate fluid provision: dehydration, overhydration
4. Food allergies and intolerances
5. Choking
6. Nil by mouth
7. Artificial nutrition
8. Re-feeding syndrome
9. Missed meals
10. Lack of assistance with eating and drinking
11. Catering issues

patients with advanced illness. In modern palliative care, understanding of the most important safety issues surrounding nutrition will help professionals provide better care for an increasing variety of conditions, minimising risk for patients.

1.6.4 Nutritional Care at the End-of-Life

Nutritional care at the end-of-life calls for a sensible, informed, and personalised approach. There is a prevailing opinion that it is too late to employ meaningful changes in diet when a person is approaching the end of their life. While this certainly is a time when the priority is comfort and quality of life, it is also a time when we need to minimise any harm to the patient so that they are allowed to face their approaching end in peace. Giving the right food and removing anxieties about food and fluid intake may not only give valuable relief and increased comfort for patients but may also provide some precious time.

Healthcare professionals working in palliative care, when asked to express an opinion on a variety of complex psychosocial and ethical issues in relation to nutritional care and support at the end-of-life, need to use a flexible and compassionate approach to be reassuring and supportive for the patient and the relatives.

1.7 DEVELOPMENT OF SPECIALISTS: THE NEED FOR NUTRITION EDUCATION

In the United Kingdom, the Royal College of Nursing launched the Nutrition Now campaign in 2007. It stated that: "Nutrition and hydration are essential to care, as vital as medication and other types of treatment… it is the responsibility of the multidisciplinary team to ensure that patients have the right type of nutrition and hydration at the right time." This message is slowly spreading to reach all healthcare disciplines. As a result, there is a growth in interest from healthcare professionals who want to acquire an adequate scientific and research background to appreciate the enormous advances in nutritional knowledge and be able to translate them into clinical practice.

Our current education system urgently needs to incorporate the new findings and include upgraded and expanded nutrition education for healthcare professionals. Palliative care centres need to become aware of the importance of providing advanced nutrition education and be encouraged to participate in research projects that will increase the understanding of the numerous nutritional issues. A training program is needed to provide palliative care professionals with the nutritional knowledge to help patients and carers. This will lead to a better experience for patients, as doctors, nurses, dieticians, and other palliative care professionals who have an advanced understanding of nutrition will then care them for.

The vast amount of new data in nutrition means that it is difficult for the individual healthcare professional to find, assimilate, and interpret all the information. Professionals would benefit from guidelines and recommendations to help them in their practice. We need specialists within palliative care with a particular interest and expertise in nutrition, capable of translating scientific findings into practical help and advice for patients and carers.

1.8 CONCLUSION

In the last few years the subject of nutrition has increasingly come to the forefront of patient care and media interest. The public, healthcare professionals, and organisations are beginning to acknowledge the contribution of appropriate nutritional care and treatment in the therapeutic process. Research findings are beginning to influence our clinical practice. Although it will require a comprehensive effort to raise awareness, overcome prejudices, and advance its status, nutrition has now matured enough to become a potent tool for better patient care.

SUMMARY POINTS

- Recent advances in scientific and nutritional knowledge have paved the way to a deeper understanding of the interaction between nutrition, health, and disease.
- Diet affects our 'internal environment' in profound ways.
- The study of the effect of micronutrients on cell and organ function has revealed their importance in improving symptom control.
- Cancer survivors have special nutritional considerations that palliative care professionals are often asked to address.
- A multistep approach to nutritional care is needed.
- The diet of people in illness should be different to their diet in health.
- The incorporation of advanced nutritional knowledge in palliative care practice will result in better patient care and experience.

ACKNOWLEDGMENTS

I am grateful to Professor Joe Millard for his ever-helpful guidance and breadth of knowledge that provided me with a scientific basis for my studies in nutritional medicine.

LIST OF ABBREVIATIONS

ACS Anorexia-Cachexia Syndrome
AICR American Institute for Cancer Research
Nrf2 Nuclear factor erythroid-derived 2-related factor 2
PEG Percutaneous Endoscopic Gastrostomy
WCRF World Cancer Research Fund

REFERENCES

Athenaeus. 1927. *The Deipnosophists* ed. and tr. C. B. Gulick, 1927–41 (7 vols). Cambridge, MA: Harvard University Press.

Atsmon, J., and E. Dole. 2005. Drug-induced hypomagnesaemia: Scope and management. *Drug Safety: An International Journal of Medical Toxicology and Drug Experience* 28:763–88.

August, D. A., and M. B. Huhmann, and American Society for Parenteral and Enteral Nutrition (A.S.P.E.N.) Board of Directors. 2009. A.S.P.E.N. clinical guidelines: Nutrition support therapy during anticancer treatment and in hematopoietic cell transplantation. *Journal of Parenteral and Enteral Nutrition* 33:472–500.

Barone, B. B., H. C. Yen, C. F. Snyder, K. S. Pairs, K. B. Stein, R. L. Derr, A. C. Wolff, and F. L. Brancusi. 2008. Long term all-cause mortality in cancer patients with preexisting diabetes mellitus: A systematic review and meta-analysis. *Journal of the American Medical Association* 300:2754–64.

Barr, E. L., P. Z. Zimmer, T. A. Welborn, D. Jolly, D. J. Magliano, D. W. Dunstan, A. J. Cameron et al. 2007. Risk of cardiovascular and all-cause mortality in individuals with diabetes mellitus, impaired fasting glucose, and impaired glucose tolerance: The Australian Diabetes, Obesity, and Lifestyle Study (AusDiab). *Circulation* 116:151–57.

Broeren, M. A. C., E. A. M. Geerdink, H. L. Vader, and A. W. L. van den Wall Bake. 2009. Hypomagnesaemia induced by several proton-pump inhibitors. *Annals of Internal Medicine* 151:755–56.

Demark-Wahnefried, W., and L. W. Jones. 2008. Promoting a healthy lifestyle among cancer survivors. *Hematology/Oncology Clinics of North America* 22:319–42.

Epel, E., J. Daubenmier, J. T. Moskowitz, S. Folkman, and E. Blackburn. 2009. Can meditation slow rate of cellular aging? Cognitive stress, mindfulness and telomeres. *Annals of the New York Academy of Sciences* 1172:34–53.

Fabbriciani, G., M. Prior, C. Leli, A. Cecchetti, L. Callarelli, G. Rinonapoli, A. M. Scorpion, and E. Mannering. 2010. Diffuse musculoskeletal pain and proximal myopathy: Do not forget hypovitaminosis D. *Journal of Clinical Rheumatology* 16:34–37.

Feinberg, A. P. 2008. Epigenetics as the epicenter of modern medicine. *Journal of the American Medical Association* 299:1345–50.

Food and Nutrition Group at Help the Hospices. 2009. Professional consensus statement of nutritional care in palliative care patients. http://www.helpthehospices.org.uk/our-services/running-your-hospice/food-and-nutrition/consensus-statement/ (Accessed February 2010).

Gopalakrishnan, A., and A. N. Tong-Kong. 2005. Anticarcinogenesis by dietary phytochemical: Cytoprotection by Nrf2 in normal cells and cytotoxicity by modulation of transcription factors NF-κB and AP-1 in abnormal cancer cells. *Food & Chemical Toxicology* 46:1257–70.

Hodgkinson, E., H. L. Neville-Webbe, and R. E. Coleman. 2006. Magnesium depletion in patients receiving cisplatin-based chemotherapy. *Clinical Oncology (Royal College of Radiologists (Great Britain))* 18:710–18.

Jiralerspong, S., S. L. Palla, S. H. Giordano, F. Meric-Bernstam, C. Liedtke, C. M. Barnett, L. Hsu, M. C. Hung, G. N. Hortobagyi, and A. M. Gonzalez-Angelo. 2009. Metformin and pathological complete responses to neoadjuvant chemotherapy in diabetic patients with breast cancer. *Journal of Clinical Oncology* 27:3297–302.

Johnson, J. D. 1981. The regional and ethnic distribution of lactose malabsorption. Adaptive and genetic hypotheses. In *Lactose digestion. Clinical and nutritional implications,* eds. D. M. Paige and T. M. Bayless, 11–22. Baltimore: John Hopkins University Press.

Khan, Q. J., P. S. Reddy, B. F. Kilmer, P. Sharma, S. E. Baca, A. P. O'Dea, J. R. Kemp, and C. J. Fabian. 2010. Effect of vitamin D supplementation on serum 25-hydroxy vitamin D levels, joint pain, and fatigue in women starting adjuvant letrozole treatment for breast cancer. *Breast Cancer Research and Treatment* 119:111–18.

Kumar, N. 2010. Neurological presentations of nutritional deficiencies. *Neurologic Clinics* 28:107–70.

Lennard-Jones, J. E., ed. 1992. *A positive approach to nutrition as treatment.* London: King's Fund Centre.

Matthews, S. B., J. P. Wad, A. G. Roberts, and A. K. Campbell. 2005. Systemic lactose intolerance: A new perspective of an old problem. *Postgraduate Medical Journal* 81:176–73.

McShea, A., K. Leissle, and M. A. Smith. 2009. The essence of chocolate: A rich, dark, and well kept secret. *Nutrition* 25:1104–5.

National Patient Safety Agency: Nutrition factsheets. 2009. 10 key characteristics of good nutritional care 01-food and nutritional care is delivered safely. http://www.nrls.npsa.nhs.uk/resources/?entryid45=59865 (Accessed February 2010).

Noble, S., F. Rawlinson, and A. Byrne. 2002. Acquired lactose intolerance: A seldom considered cause of diarrhoea in the palliative care setting. *Journal of Pain and Symptom Management* 23:449–50.

O'Connor, M. F., and M. R. Irvin. 2010. Links between behavioral factors and inflammation. *Clinical Pharmacology and Therapeutics* 87:479–82.

Ornish, D., J. Lin, J. Daubenmier, G. Weidner, E. Epel, C. Kemp, M. J. Magbanua et al. 2008. Increased telomerase activity and comprehensive lifestyle changes: A pilot study. *Lancet Oncology* 9:1048–57.

Ornish, D., M. J. Magbanua, G. Weidner, V. Weinberg, C. Kemp, C. Green, M. D. Mattie et al. 2008. Changes in prostate gene expression in men undergoing an intensive nutrition and lifestyle intervention. *Proceedings of the National Academy of Sciences USA* 105:8369–74.

Pot, G. K., A. Geelen, G. Majsak-Newman, L. J. Harvey, F. M. Nagengast, B. J. Witteman, P. C. van de Meeberg et al. 2010. Increased consumption of fatty and lean fish reduces serum C-reactive protein concentrations but not inflammation markers in feces and colonic biopsies. *Journal of Nutrition* 140:371–76.

Royal College of Physicians and British Society of Gastroenterology. 2010. *Oral feeding difficulties and dilemmas: A guide to practical care, particularly towards the end-of-life.* London: Royal College of Physicians.

Stocks, T., K. Rapp, T. Bjørge, J. Manjer, H. Ulmer, R. Selmer, A. Lukanova et al. 2009. Blood glucose and risk of incident and fatal cancer in the metabolic syndrome and cancer project (me-can): Analysis of six prospective cohorts. *PLoS Medicine* 6 (12): e1000201, doi:101371/journal.pmed.1000201.

Straube, S., S. Derry, R. A. Moore, and H. J. McQuay. 2010. Vitamin D for the treatment of chronic painful conditions in adults. *Cochrane Database of Systematic Reviews* 20:CD007771.

Straube, S., R. A. Moore, S. Derry, E. Hallier, and H. J. McQuay. 2010. Vitamin D and chronic pain in immigrant and ethnic minority patients—investigation of the relationship and comparison with native western populations. *International Journal of Endocrinology*, doi:10.1155/2010/753075.

Tollefsbol, T. O. 2009. Role of epigenetics in cancer. In *Cancer Epigenetics*, ed. T. O. Tollefsbol, 1–4. Boca Raton: CRC Press.

Vaillancourt, R., R. Siddiqui, C. Vadeboncoeur, M. Rattrap, and D. Lariviere. 2009. Treatment of medication intolerance with lactase in a complex palliative care patient. *Journal of Palliative Care* 25:142–44.

Van Veldhuizen, P. J., S. A. Taylor, S. Williamson, and B. M. Dries. 2000. Treatment of vitamin D deficiency in patients with metastatic prostate cancer may improve bone pain and muscle strength. *Journal of Urology* 163:187–90.

Warnberg, L., S. Gomez-Martinez, J. Romeo, L. E. Diaz, and A. Marcos. 2009. Nutrition, inflammation and cognitive function. *Annals of the New York Academy of Sciences* 1153:164–75.

Wedlake, L., K. Thomas, C. Cough, and H. J. Andreyev. 2008. Small bowel bacterial overgrowth and lactose intolerance during radical pelvic radiotherapy: An observational study. *European Journal of Cancer* 44:2212–17.

World Cancer Research Fund/American Institute for Cancer Research. 2007. *Food, nutrition, and physical activity, and the prevention of cancer: A global perspective.* Washington, DC: AICR.

Yang, C. S., X. Wang, G. Lu, and S. C. Picnic. 2009. Cancer prevention by tea: Animal studies, molecular mechanisms and human relevance. *Nature Reviews Cancer* 9:429–39.

2 What Do We Mean by Palliative Care?

Catherine Walshe

CONTENTS

2.1 INTRODUCTION: WHY IS IT IMPORTANT TO DEFINE PALLIATIVE CARE?

> "Definitions are important. They can serve as an impetus for changing practice, for introducing new programs and for working toward the allocation of more resources for palliative care. Moreover, the understanding of these concepts influences how medicine is practiced." (Kaasa 2001, 413)

> "As new understandings of the needs of people at the end-of-life emerge it is becoming apparent that we need to communicate clearly and unambiguously with groups of people with different perspectives and needs … The lack of consistency in our use of terminology has created and will continue to create confusion as we seek to communicate and understand the needs of different cohorts of people facing the challenges of providing or needing end-of-life care, including palliative care." (Palliative Care Australia 2008, 3)

Defining what we mean by a term is important. In this chapter definitions such as palliative care, terminal care* and end-of-life care will be explored and discussed. This should enable subsequent chapters to be put in context with reference to the practice of palliative care, the professionals involved in such care* and the patient groups receiving palliative care.

Defining what we mean by palliative care is particularly important because of the confusions referred to above. There seems to be an acknowledged lack of consistency because defining terms in this practice area appears to be difficult to do. Three broad reasons for these difficulties can be identified:

a. The terms used have changed over time.
b. Our interpretations are value laden.
c. Defining palliative care itself seems difficult.

Each of these reasons will now be explored in turn, which will give a context and background to the definitions then presented and the implications for operationalising these definitions.

2.1.1 Changing Terms and Their Usage

There are many terms in current and past usage that refer to the care of people before and around the time of an anticipatable death. Terms such as hospice care, palliative care, and end-of-life care are in current usage, whereas terms such as continuing care and terminal care seem to have fallen out of favour.

Chronologically, hospice appears to be one of the earliest terms used. It is derived from the words "hospes" and "hospitium", which were used to denote not only a relationship between individuals, but also the place in which the relationship developed. Later, hospice, derived from these words, described a place of refuge for weary or sick travellers seeking rest on life's journey (Hawthorne and Yurkovich 2004). The term was adopted by those building the earliest physical spaces for the provision of palliative care, primarily to cancer patients whose curative treatment had ended. The first "modern" hospice is identified as St Christopher's Hospice, opened in the UK in 1967 (Clark 2007). Whilst in some countries the term "hospice" is still used primarily to denote a building or physical space within which care is delivered, in other countries it describes the approach to care, such as home hospice provision in the USA.

The term "terminal care" was also in wide usage at the time the first "modern" hospices were being built, describing much of the care they provided. Terms started to change when the philosophies of care promoted by these hospices started to move into other settings. For example, the team at St Thomas' Hospital, established in 1976, were called the "hospital support team for terminal care" (Clark 2007) and the unit at the Royal Marsden Hospital (opened in 1964) called the "Continuing Care Unit" (Hanks 2008).

The term "palliative care" was coined by Balfour Mount around 1973 to describe a new programme in Canada, based on St Christopher's Hospice (Billings 1998). In French the term hospice had negative connotations, and so he wished to use a different term when embracing the hospice philosophy of care and bringing the approach to a wider group of patients (Meghani 2004). Palliative care rapidly became a widely adopted term, especially as it became the chosen term to describe medical care with the recognition of palliative medicine as a medical speciality in the UK and elsewhere (Doyle 2005).

The literal, dictionary definition of palliation does not easily assist a clinical definition of care. Palliate is normally described as derived from the Latin palla (garment) and pallium, meaning "to cloak", seen as "covering up problems" (Billings 1998). It is also suggested that the understanding could be from an Indo-European linguistic tradition, derived from "pelte", which means to shield. This has been related to palliative care as the shielding of patients from the assault of symptoms. Palliate has been described as a transitory verb, "to make disease less severe, without removing its cause" (Meghani 2004).

More recently, end-of-life care appears to be a favoured term, used perhaps primarily because palliative care has become associated for some with cancer care. In the UK it has become widely used, particularly strategically, as in the eponymous "end-of-life care strategy" (Department of Health 2008).

A problem with definitions therefore seems to be the varied terms used to describe care around the time of an anticipatable death and the way that the use of such terms has changed over time.

2.1.2 Value-Laden Interpretations

One possible explanation for the many terms used to describe care around the time of an anticipatable death is that some terms have or have acquired value-laden interpretations.

Healthcare professionals describing a service or their role to patients often don't wish to be explicit about death and dying. Different definitions have emerged because people want to be clear about their service, not use euphemisms, but not be too blunt or too vague. It appears that as one term becomes overly associated with care around death, then people move on to another. Partly this is because professionals want to offer care earlier in the disease trajectory, when patients may not be thinking actively about death and dying, and as particular terms become associated with such care they fall out of favour.

For example, there are recent studies that demonstrate that the term "palliative care" has more negative connotations than "supportive care" (Boldt, Yusaf, and Himelstein 2006). Boldt et al.'s (2006) study found that professionals were more likely to refer patients to a service with the name "supportive care" when they were still undergoing active primary cancer treatment, were in remission or had no evidence of disease, or were undergoing treatment for advanced cancer. The term "palliative care" was only acceptable when all active therapies had ceased, much later in the trajectory of illness. In a later study, 57% of respondents preferred the term supportive care when discussing care with patients and relatives, because of the potential for distress associated with the term "palliative" (Fadul et al. 2009). We do know that patients can be distressed by an early referral to specialist palliative care (Chapple, Ziebland, and McPherson 2006). It appears that palliative care as a term is a barrier to early referrals, but not to referrals at the very end-of-life.

Cherny (2009) argues that this is because there is dissonance between the defined meanings of terms such as palliative care (i.e., to improve quality of life of patients and families at all stages of a life-threatening illness) and the meaning derived from common association (i.e., care in the last days of life). Supportive care is more acceptable because although it is often used as a euphemism for palliative care, it also has a wider, definition that includes toxicity minimisation and survivorship (Cherny 2009).

It seems that people are keen to use terms that are interpreted by patients in more positive ways, which may explain some of the changes in terminology from, for example, hospice care to palliative care, and from palliative care to supportive care.

2.1.3 Defining Palliative Care is Difficult

Defining what we mean by palliative care, or indeed any other term referring to care around the time of an anticipatable death, appears to be difficult because it is not a "neat" definition.

a. Palliative care is not neatly delineated, as other specialities are, by reference to organs (such as the kidney and renal services), by reference to systems (such as the gastrointestinal system and gastroenterologists), or reference to age (such as children and paediatricians) (Billings 1998). Whilst the term was initially associated with cancer services, developments in the definition have widened this focus (Sepúlveda et al. 2002).
b. Palliative care is not limited to a particular healthcare setting. Palliative care's reference point is the patient, not the setting (Pastrana et al. 2008).
c. Palliative care can be seen as a function (the direct provision of care to patients), a structure (such as a specialist palliative care service) or as a philosophy of care (an underlying approach to care) (Pastrana et al. 2008).

These complexities mean that agreeing a definition of palliative care is especially important so that confusion is avoided between healthcare professionals and patients about when, how, why and by whom such care should and could be provided.

Introduction: Key Facts

- There are many terms used to describe care around the time of an anticipatable death.
- Terms can be interpreted by patients and professionals in negative ways, which constrains their use.
- Palliative care is difficult to define because it describes care that is not neatly delineated, occurs in all healthcare settings, and can be used to describe direct care provision, structures of care or philosophies of care.

2.2 CURRENT DEFINITIONS OF PALLIATIVE CARE AND ITS ASSOCIATED TERMS

Because of these complexities in definition, there are, and have been, a multiplicity of definitions. The first widely cited definition of palliative care was constructed by the World Health Organization:

> "Palliative care is the active total care of patients whose disease is not responsive to curative treatment. Control of pain, of other symptoms, and of psychological, social and spiritual problems is paramount. The goal of palliative care is achievement of the best possible quality of life for patients and their families. Many aspects of palliative care are also applicable earlier in the course of the illness, in conjunction with anti-cancer treatment." (World Health Organization Expert Committee 1990.)

This definition was not without its critics. Criticisms centred on some of the terms such as "active" and "total" (and whether this means other care is inactive or partial), and the use of euphemisms such as "not responsive to curative treatment" rather than a focus on death and dying. It was also argued that palliative care does not have a special claim on particular virtues such as quality of care, compassion, etc. (Billings 1998).

Following on from this, many definitions of palliative care and associated terms have been developed. Recently, searches revealed 37 English language definitions of palliative care from web pages and textbooks (Pastrana et al. 2008). Some examples of current definitions of palliative care, supportive care and end-of-life care are displayed in Box 2.1, including the updated World Health Organization definition of palliative care. These definitions appear to be most widely used, or represent definitions used in major policies or from significant national associations. It seems that many different international and national organisations have developed definitions of supportive and palliative care. These different definitions may lead to different interpretations of terms in different situations and settings, and mean that it is important to clarify meanings when communicating with others.

BOX 2.1 SELECTED CURRENT DEFINITIONS OF PALLIATIVE CARE, END-OF-LIFE CARE AND SUPPORTIVE CARE

WHO Definition of Palliative Care

Palliative care is an approach that improves the quality of life of patients and their families facing the problems associated with life-threatening illness, through the prevention and relief of suffering by means of early identification, impeccable assessment and treatment of pain and other problems, physical, psychosocial and spiritual. Palliative care:

- provides relief from pain and other distressing symptoms;
- affirms life and regards dying as a normal process;
- intends neither to hasten nor postpone death;
- integrates the psychological and spiritual aspects of patient care;
- offers a support system to help patients live as actively as possible until death;
- offers a support system to help the family cope during the patient's illness and in their own bereavement;
- uses a team approach to address the needs of patients and their families, including bereavement counselling, if indicated;

- will enhance quality of life, and may also positively influence the course of illness;
- is applicable early in the course of illness, in conjunction with other therapies that are intended to prolong life, such as chemotherapy or radiation therapy, and includes those investigations needed to better understand and manage distressing clinical complications.

(Sepúlveda et al. 2002) Also available at http://www.who.int/cancer/palliative/definition/en/ [accessed 04.01.10]

European Association of Palliative Care Definition of Palliative Care

Palliative care is the active, total care of the patients whose disease is not responsive to curative treatment. Control of pain, of other symptoms, and of social, psychological and spiritual problems is paramount.

Palliative care is interdisciplinary in its approach and encompasses the patient, the family and the community in its scope. In a sense, palliative care is to offer the most basic concept of care – that of providing for the needs of the patient wherever he or she is cared for, either at home or in the hospital.

Palliative care affirms life and regards dying as a normal process; it neither hastens nor postpones death. It sets out to preserve the best possible quality of life until death.

Available at: http://www.eapcnet.org/about/definition.html [accessed 04.01.10]

American Academy of Hospice and Palliative Medicine Definition of Palliative Care

The goal of palliative care is to prevent and relieve suffering and to support the best possible quality of life for patients and their families, regardless of the stage of the disease or the need for other therapies. Palliative care is both a philosophy of care and an organized, highly structured system for delivering care. Palliative care expands traditional disease-model medical treatments to include the goals of enhancing quality of life for patient and family, optimizing function, helping with decision-making and providing opportunities for personal growth. As such, it can be delivered concurrently with life-prolonging care or as the main focus of care.

Palliative care is operationalized through effective management of pain and other distressing symptoms, while incorporating psychosocial and spiritual care according to patient/family needs, values, beliefs and culture(s). Evaluation and treatment should be comprehensive and patient-centered, with a focus on the central role of the family unit in decision-making.

Palliative care affirms life by supporting the patient and family's goals for the future, including their hopes for cure or life-prolongation, as well as their hopes for peace and dignity throughout the course of illness, the dying process and death. Palliative care aims to guide and assist the patient and family in making decisions that enable them to work toward their goals during whatever time they have remaining.

National Consensus Project for Quality Palliative Care (2009) available at http://www.nationalconsensusproject.org/guideline.pdf and http://www.aahpm.org/positions/definition.html [accessed 04.01.10]

Terminal Care Definition

Terminal care is an important part of palliative care and usually refers to the management of patients during the last few days or weeks or even months of life from a point at which it becomes clear that the patient is in a progressive state of decline (National Council for Hospice and Specialist Palliative Care Services 1995).

A Working Definition of End-of-life Care

End-of-life care is care that: helps all those with advanced, progressive, incurable illness to live as well as possible until they die. It enables the supportive and palliative care needs of both patient and family to be identified and met throughout the last phase of life and into bereavement. It includes management of pain and other symptoms and provision of psychological, social, spiritual and practical support (Department of Health 2007).

NCHSPCS Definition of Supportive Care

Supportive care is provided to people with cancer and their carers throughout the patient pathway, from pre-diagnosis onwards. It should be given equal priority with other aspects of care and be fully integrated with diagnosis and treatment. It encompasses: self help and support; user involvement; information giving; psychological support; symptom control; social support; rehabilitation; complementary therapies; spiritual support; palliative care; end-of-life and bereavement care (National Council for Hospice and Specialist Palliative Care Services, 2002).

Canadian Definition of Supportive Care

Supportive care is the provision of the necessary services, as defined by those living with or affected by cancer, to meet their physical, informational, emotional, psychological, social, spiritual, and practical needs during the pre-diagnostic, diagnostic, treatment and follow-up phases.

http://www.cancercare.on.ca/pdf/GTA2014Chapter12.pdf [accessed 04.01.10].

It appears from these definitions that they range from the broadest (supportive care) to the narrowest (terminal care), such that it could be argued that all terminal care is palliative care, but not all palliative care is terminal care. All palliative care could be described as supportive care, but not all supportive care is palliative care. The relationships between these definitions are represented in Figure 2.1.

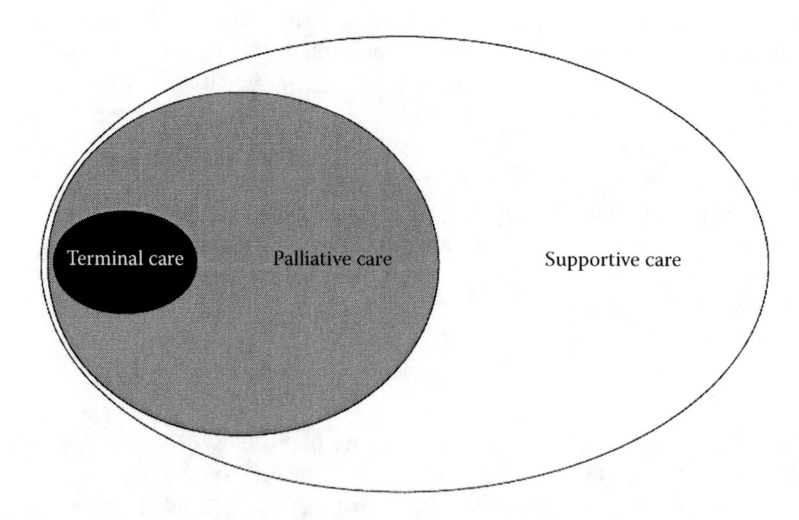

FIGURE 2.1 The interrelationship of supportive, palliative and terminal care. This figure illustrates the increasing breadth of definition of the terms supportive, palliative and terminal care.

Current Definitions: Key Facts

- Supportive care, end-of-life care, palliative care and terminal care are currently used terms, but which have overlapping meanings.
- Many different international and national organisations have developed definitions, which may lead to different interpretations of terms in different situations and settings.

2.3 KEY ELEMENTS OF DEFINITIONS

Even with the wide range of definitions of palliative, supportive, end-of-life and terminal care in Box 2.1, it can be seen that there are certain key features common to many definitions. There have been recent attempts to capture the key elements of palliative care from these definitions and Figures 2.2 and 2.3 display approaches to this work.

2.3.1 Patient Population

Palliative care was originally a disease-specific approach, associated very clearly with cancer care in the original WHO definition (World Health Organization Expert Committee 1990). Developments in the definition have widened this approach. Most definitions do include reference to the target population for palliative care, with reference to issues such as "life-threatening illness" (Sepúlveda et al. 2002) or "disease not responsive to curative treatment" (EAPC). These mainly refer to attributes of the illness, such as its progressive, far advanced, life-threatening and active nature (Pastrana et al. 2008). The widening of these definitions is argued to reflect demographic and technological advances such as an ageing population, longer life expectancies, changing illness trajectories, and advances in pharmacological and surgical techniques (Meghani 2004).

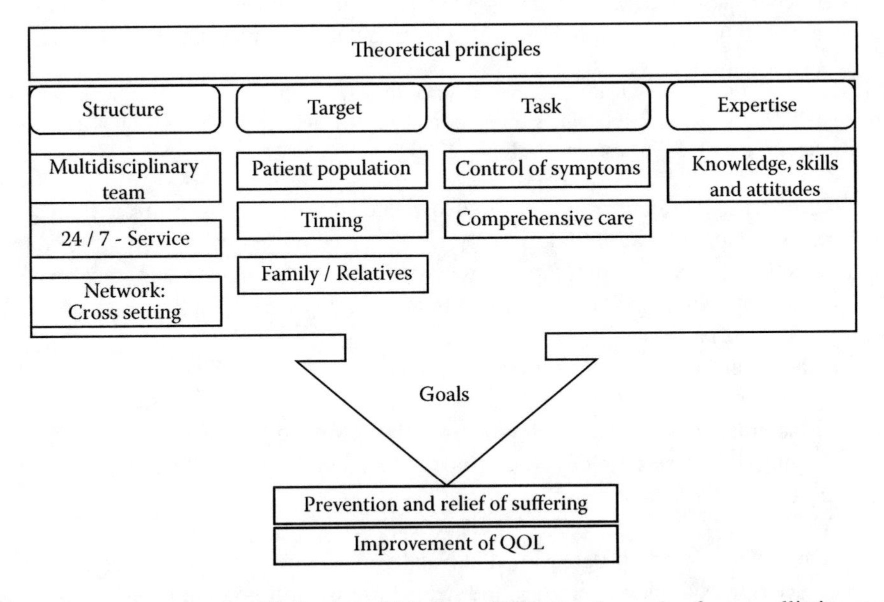

FIGURE 2.2 Key elements of palliative care. This figure illustrates the range of ways palliative care is provided, the core tasks of palliative care and some desired outcomes of such care. (Reprinted from Pastrana, T. et al., *Palliat. Med.*, 22, 224, 2008. With permission of SAGE publishers.)

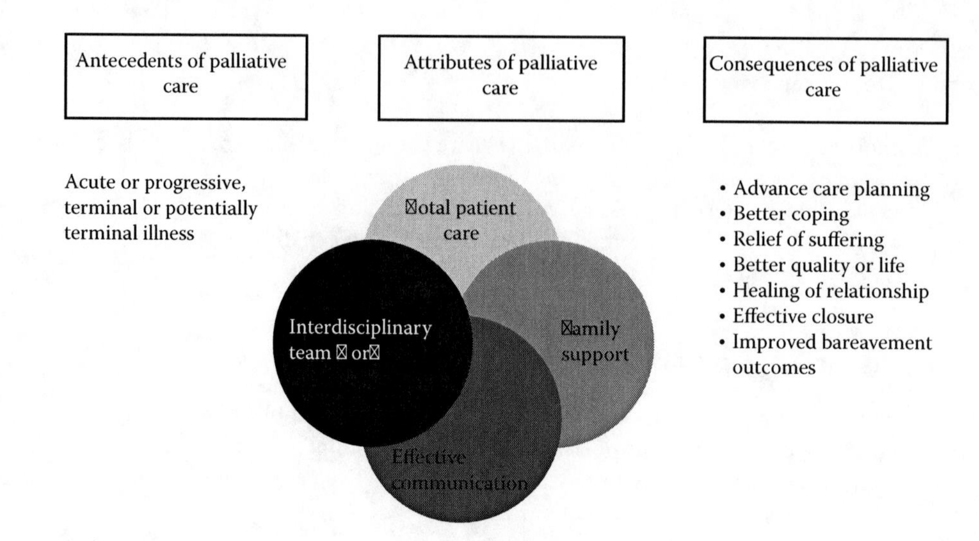

FIGURE 2.3 The antecedents, attributes and consequences of palliative care. This figure illustrates what precedes palliative care, what the essence of palliative care provision is and the outcomes of palliative care. (Meghani, S. H.: A concept analysis of palliative care in the United States. *J. Adv. Nurs.* 2004, 46, 157. Copyright Wiley-VCH Verlag GmbH & Co. KGaA. Reproduced with permission.)

2.3.2 Timing

The timing of the provision of palliative care has always been problematic. This is clearly related to the difficulties in defining the patient population. Whilst it is apparent that palliative care should be provided in the last days and weeks of life, there is now wide recognition that the principles of palliative care should be applied as early as possible in the course of any chronic, ultimately fatal illness (Sepúlveda et al. 2002). This recognises that problems at the end-of-life frequently have their origins earlier in the trajectory of the disease. Other advantages of earlier inception of palliative care are seen as an increase in patients accessing symptom relief and support, and a smoother transition from care to cure (Pastrana et al. 2008). An emphasis on the provision of palliative care throughout the course of a serious illness means that every heath-care professional needs to understand the concepts of palliative care:

> "It is the responsibility of every healthcare professional to practice the palliative care approach, and to call in specialist palliative care colleagues if the need arises, as an integral component of good clinical practice, whatever the illness or its stage." (Tebbit 1999, 9)

The timing of palliative care provision is also related, in some healthcare systems, to funding issues. For example, to be admitted to many US "hospice programs" the patient has to have a prognosis of less than 6 months, often foregoing active treatments such as chemotherapy (Meghani 2004). Prognosis is frequently explicit or implied in many definitions of palliative care, and this can make the timing of palliative care particularly difficult.

Patients with cancer follow a typical trajectory including a short decline before death. However, offering palliative care to those with other illnesses may be more difficult, as their typical trajectories may not be so amenable to our current models of palliative care provision (Murray et al. 2005). Three typical dying trajectories are often described (Lynn and Adamson 2003; Murray et al. 2005) and are illustrated in Figure 2.4.

1. A trajectory with a steady progression and usually a clear terminal phase, mostly cancer.
2. A trajectory (for example respiratory and heart failure) with gradual decline, punctuated by episodes of acute deterioration and some recovery, with a more sudden, seemingly unexpected, death.

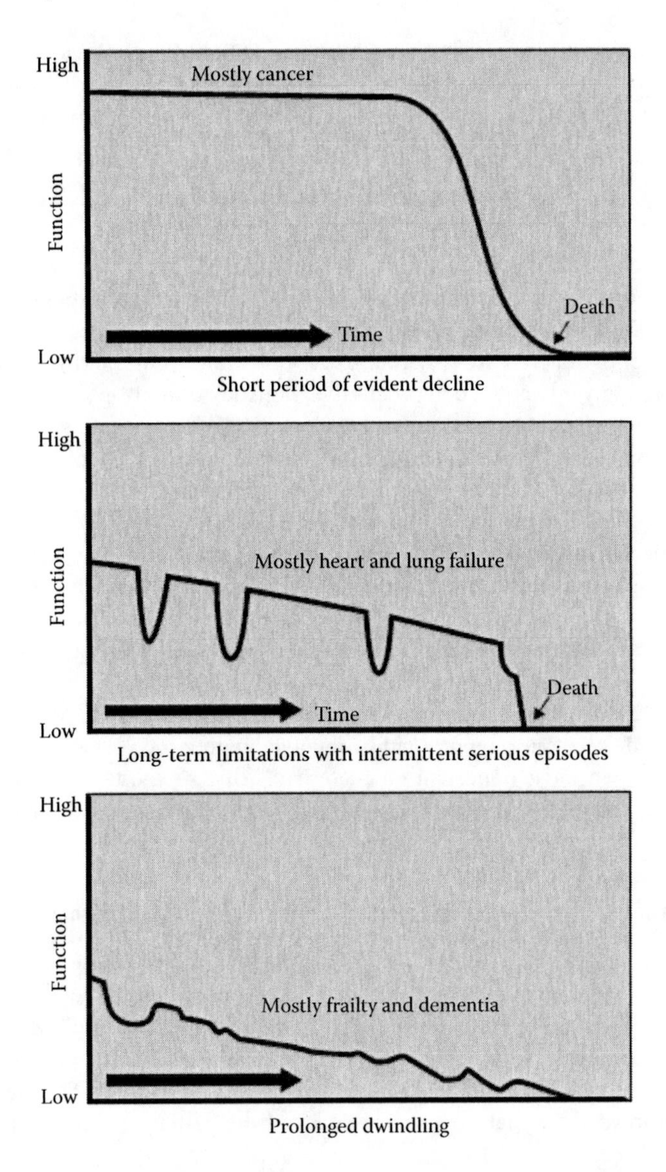

FIGURE 2.4 Typical illness trajectories for people with chronic illness. This figure illustrates the different changes in physical function and decline that people dying from different illnesses may experience. (Reprinted from Lynn, J., Adamson, D. M., *Living well at the end-of-life*, Rand Health, Santa Monica, 2003. With permission of RAND corporation.)

3. A trajectory with prolonged gradual decline (typical of frail elderly people or people with dementia).

Palliative care providers have typically focused on the first trajectory (cancer), although even that is problematical when the timing of the introduction of palliative care is concerned, as prognostication is known to be difficult. (Vigano et al. 2000; Glare et al. 2003). These difficulties have led to a typically short period (days or months) when palliative care services are involved with patients (Walshe et al. 2009). Prognostication is even harder in the other two typical trajectories, leading Murray et al. (2005) to argue that uncertainty about prognosis should not result in patients being neglected by (palliative) health services.

These difficulties have led many to argue that there should be an integrated approach to palliative care, where palliative and curative care are not sequential but coexist. Palliative care is not just for the very end-of-life, but is appropriate over the continuum of any progressive, life-limiting illness.

2.3.3 Holistic Care (Total, Active, and Individualised Patient Care)

The "care" part of definitions is of fundamental significance to those who provide palliative care. The physical, emotional, social, cultural and spiritual needs of the patient are all considered important concerns in palliative care (Sepúlveda et al. 2002) and these emerge as a central attribute of the concept of palliative care (Meghani 2004; Pastrana et al. 2008).

Perhaps unsurprisingly, given the comprehensive, holistic nature of palliative care, many argue that providing this type of care demands a certain level of healthcare professional expertise. This is a complex issue when it is also argued that palliative care does not just encompass provision by specialists, but should be the responsibility of all healthcare professionals (Tebbit 1999). We'll examine this issue further when discussing the multidisciplinary team.

Certainly for specialists, there is a strong argument that providing this type of care demands a certain level of expertise: particular knowledge, skills and attitudes which should be acquired by specific education and training (Pastrana et al. 2008). Research has demonstrated that some professional and personal attributes are linked with the provision of excellent palliative care. For example, palliative care nurses are expected to have professional attributes which enable them to deal with death, make connections, make contracts, act as an advocate, build interpersonal relationships, give family and colleague support, and be involved with issues (Taylor et al. 2001). Another study found that the two most important characteristics of an expert palliative care nurse were interpersonal skills and qualities such as kindness, warmth, compassion and genuineness (Johnston and Smith 2006).

2.3.4 Patient, Family and Carers (Support for the Family), and Bereavement Care

It is clear from the definitions of palliative care that both the patient and the family/informal carers are seen as recipients of care. Family are seen as part of the patients' social context, as decision makers, as part of the team, as team partners and as part of the "unit of care" (Pastrana et al. 2008). Family/informal carers therefore have a double role: they are both recipients of care given by the palliative care team, but also frequently givers of care to their loved one. This has the potential to lead to tension, but most agree that the primary focus of the palliative care team should be on the patient.

It is argued that the need for family support becomes more critical as patients progress towards the end of their lives. It is at this stage that families can encounter many problems, and the provision of palliative care can offer opportunities to reconcile conflicts, heal relationships, provide counselling and commence bereavement support (Meghani 2004).

Bereavement support is an integral part of palliative care and it is argued that this should start early, assessing family/informal carers for the likelihood of adverse grief reactions, and then assessing and providing bereavement support after the death of the patient (Walshe 1997).

2.3.5 Multidisciplinary/Multiprofessional Team

Whilst it is argued that any health care provider can subscribe to the palliative philosophy of care, the organisation of palliative care services is often multidisciplinary and multiprofessional. Within multiprofessional and multidisciplinary systems of palliative care delivery there are usually two distinct categories of health and social care professionals: the patient and family's usual carers and those specialising in palliative care provision. These are often referred to as "general" palliative care services (who may specialise in another field such as primary care) and "specialist" palliative care services. These generalists and specialist providers of palliative care have been defined thus:

> "General palliative care services are provided by the usual professional carers of the patient and family with low to moderate complexity of palliative care need. Usual professional carers provide palliative care as a vital and integral part of their routine clinical practice.
>
> Specialist palliative care services are provided for patients and their families with moderate to high complexity of palliative care need. They are defined in terms of their core service components, their functions and the composition of the multiprofessional teams that are required to deliver them." (National Council for Hospice and Specialist Palliative Care Services 2002.)

Specialist palliative care services are normally provided by people from many different professional backgrounds, whose substantive work is with patients who have an eventually fatal condition. They work in all care settings. Specialist palliative care services work in three key ways:

a. Providing direct care to referred patients with complex needs.
b. Providing consultation-based services to patients being cared for by general/usual care providers.
c. Providing support and education to services providing end-of-life care (Palliative Care Australia 2008).

Such an approach has been described as a "complex web of care", and demands co-ordination, cooperation and communication (Corner 2003). Effective communication is another cornerstone of many conceptualisations of palliative care and includes communication between patients, families and the professional team(s) providing care.

Key Elements of Definitions: Key Facts

- Patient population: the target population for palliative care is wide, and not constrained by diagnosis.
- Timing: palliative care should be provided as early as possible.
- Holistic care: palliative care should encompass physical, psychological and social aspects.
- Patient, family and carers: palliative care is not just focused on the patient, but on their family and informal carers and through to bereavement care.
- Multi-disciplinary and multi-professional teams: all professionals should provide palliative care, but some may have particular expertise in this area. Effective communication between professionals, patient and carer is essential.

SUMMARY POINTS

- Palliative care is not straightforward to define.
- Terms associated with care at the time of an anticipatable death have had a complex history and are value laden.
- There are multiple definitions of palliative care, although many have similar, core features.
- Professionals need to be clear and unambiguous about the definition of palliative care they subscribe to.

- Definitions should be explicitly shared so that all those working with particular patients or within or across organisations are working with the same definition so there is clarity about role and function.
- Such clarity should both facilitate excellence in current care to those at the end of their lives and stimulate debate about how to improve care in the future.

LIST OF ABBREVIATIONS

EAPC European Association of Palliative Care
WHO World Health Organisation

REFERENCES

Billings, J. A. 1998. What is palliative care? *Journal of Palliative Medicine* 1:73–81.

Boldt, A. M., F. Yusuf, and B. P. Himelstein. 2006. Perceptions of the term palliative care. *Journal of Palliative Medicine* 9:1128–36.

Chapple, A., S. Ziebland, and A. McPherson. 2006. The specialist palliative care nurse: A qualitative study of the patients' perspective. *International Journal of Nursing Studies* 43 (8): 1011–22.

Cherny, N. 2009. Stigma associated with "palliative care". Getting around it or getting over it. *Cancer* 115:1812.

Clark, D. 2007. From margins to centre: A review of the history of palliative care in cancer. *The Lancet Oncology* 8:430–38.

Corner, J. 2003. The multidisciplinary team - fact or fiction? *European Journal of Palliative Care* 10:10–12.

Department of Health. 2007. *Operating Framework 2007/08: PCT Baseline Review of Services for End-of-Life Care.* http://www.dh.gov.uk/prod_consum_dh/groups/dh_digitalassets/@dh/@en/documents/digitalasset/dh_074107.pdf. Accessed January 4, 2010.

Department of Health. 2008. *End-of-life care strategy. Promoting high quality care for all adults at the end-of-life.* London: The Stationery Office.

Doyle, D. 2005. Palliative medicine: The first 18 years of a new sub-specialty of General Medicine. *Journal of the Royal College of Physicians of Edinburgh* 35:199–205.

Fadul, N., A. Elasayem, L. Palmer, E. Del Fabbro, K. Swint, Z. Li, V. Poulter, and E. Bruera. 2009. Supportive versus palliative care: What's in a name. *Cancer* 1st May:2013–21.

Glare, P., K. Virik, M. Jones, M. Hudson, S. Eychmuller, J. Simes, and N. A. Christakis. 2003. A systematic review of physicians survival predictions in terminally ill cancer patients. *British Medical Journal* 327:195–201.

Hanks, G. 2008. Palliative care: Careless use of language undermines our identity. *Palliative Medicine* 22:109–10.

Hawthorne, D. L., and N. J. Yurkovich. 2004. Hope at the end-of-life: Making a case for hospice. *Palliative & Supportive Care* 2:415–17.

Johnston, B., and L. N. Smith. 2006. Nurses' and patients' perceptions of expert palliative nursing care. *Journal of Advanced Nursing* 54:700–9.

Kaasa, S. 2001. Assessment of quality of life in palliative care. *Journal of Palliative Medicine* 4:413–16.

Lynn, J., and D. M. Adamson. 2003. *Living well at the end-of-life. Adapting healthcare to serious chronic illness in old age.* Santa Monica: Rand Health.

Meghani, S. H. 2004. A concept analysis of palliative care in the United States. *Journal of Advanced Nursing* 46:152–61.

Murray, S. A., M. Kendall, K. Boyd, and F. Sheldon. 2005. Illness trajectories and palliative care. *British Medical Journal* 330:1107–11.

National Council for Hospice and Specialist Palliative Care Services. 1995. Occasional paper 8. *Specialist palliative care: A statement of definitions.* London: National Council for Hospice and Specialist Palliative Care Services.

National Council for Hospice and Specialist Palliative Care Services. 2002. *Definitions of supportive and palliative care.* Briefing number 11 edn. London: National Council for Hospice and Specialist Palliative Care Services.

Palliative Care Australia. 2008. *Palliative and end-of-life care glossary of terms.* http://www.palliativecare.org.au/Portals/46/docs/publications/PCA%20Glossary.pdf.

Pastrana, T., S. Junger, C. Ostgathe, F. Elsner, and L. Radbruch. 2008. A matter of definition - key elements identified in a discourse analysis of definitions of palliative care. *Palliative Medicine* 22:222–32.

Sepúlveda, C., A. Marlin, T. Yoshida, and A. Ullrich. 2002. Palliative care: The World Health Organisation's global perspective. *Journal of Pain and Symptom Management* 24:91.

Taylor, B., N. Glass, J. McFarlane, and K. Stirling. 2001. Views of nurses, patients and patients' families regarding palliative nursing care. *International Journal of Palliative Nursing* 7:186–91.

Tebbit, P. 1999. *Palliative care 2000: Commissioning through partnership.* London: The National Council for Hospice and Palliative Care Services.

Vigano, A., M. Dorgan, J. Buckingham, E. Bruera, and M. E. Suarez-Almazor. 2000. Survival prediction in terminal cancer patients: A systematic review of the medical literature. *Palliative Medicine* 14:363–74.

Walshe, C. 1997. Whom to help? An exploration of the assessment of grief. *International Journal of Palliative Nursing* 3:132–37.

Walshe, C., C. Todd, A. Caress, and C. Chew-Graham. 2009. Patterns of access to community palliative care services: A literature review. *Journal of Pain and Symptom Management* 37 (5): 884–912.

World Health Organization Expert Committee. 1990. *Cancer pain relief and palliative care.* Technical Report Series. No.804. Geneva: World Health Organization.

3 The World's Major Religions' Views on End-of-Life Issues

Hans-Henrik Bülow

CONTENTS

3.1 INTRODUCTION

This chapter presents the rules and points of view of the major religions in the world regarding end-of-life decisions. Many of the references are from intensive care unit (ICU) studies, because that branch of medical science frequently deals with the ethics of withholding or withdrawing life-sustaining therapy, alleviation of pain, treatment of patients in a persistent vegetative state and whether further therapy will be futile.

This review is primarily based on a paper from *Intensive Care Medicine* with a considerably longer list of references than that given here (Bülow et al. 2008). Table 3.1 summarises the various religions' attitudes and rulings with regard to end-of-life decisions, but not all religions have a ruling/point of view on all the above-mentioned issues.

3.2 DEMOGRAPHIC CHALLENGES

In the future, healthcare systems and individuals will have to acknowledge and cope with the religious attitudes and beliefs of patients and physicians from other ethnic and religious groups, because increasing globalisation is changing the world so that it no longer consists of homogeneous religious and cultural entities.

Islam is *the* example of a worldwide religion. There are 1.1 billion Muslims, but only 18% live in the Arab world. In Indonesia Muslims constitute 88% of its citizens and in India 12.4% of the population. The prediction is that by 2050, one in five Europeans will likely be Muslim. Likewise North America

TABLE 3.1
The Various Religions' Views on End-of-Life Decisions

	Withhold	Withdraw	Withdraw Artificial Nutrition	Double Effect[a]	Euthanasia
Catholics	Yes	Yes	No	Yes	No
Protestants	Yes	Yes	Yes	Yes	Some
Greek Orthodox	No	No	No	No[b]	No
Muslims	Yes	Yes	No	Yes	No
Jewish Orthodox	Yes	No	No	Yes	No
Buddhism	Yes	Yes	Yes	Yes	No
Hinduism & Sikh	Yes	Yes	?	?	Some
Taoism	Most	Most	?	?	?
Confucianism	No	No	?	?	No

Source: Reproduced with kind permission from Springer Science+Business Media: *Intensive Care Med.*, The world's major religions' point of view on end-of-life decisions in the intensive care unit, 34, 2008, 423, Bülow, H.H., Sprung, C.L., Reinhart, K. et al.

Note: Shows which end-of-life decisions and acts are allowed by the world's major religions. Question marks show that the religion has no official stance on that question.

[a] Double effect (see Table 3.2).

[b] Alleviation of pain is allowable, if it will in no way lead to the patient's death.

will change. Within the next 50 years, the majority of US citizens will be of non-European descent, with Latinos representing the nation's largest racial/ethnic group. In Ontario, Canada, the number of Muslims increased 142% from 1991 to 2001 and the number of Sikh increased 110%, while the Christian community only increased 3%.

The challenge in the forthcoming years is that patients and medical teams with different religious, cultural and ethical backgrounds will adopt different approaches, even within the same religion (Sprung et al. 2007; Daar and Khitamy 2001; Pauls and Hutchinson 2002; Prendergast 2001).

3.3 THE VARIOUS RELIGIONS

3.3.1 Christianity

Christianity encompasses such diverse groups as Mormons, Jehovah's Witnesses, Lutherans, Roman Catholics and Orthodox Christians.

3.3.1.1 Roman Catholic Perspective

The Church's official attitude was published in 1997 during the reign of Pope John Paul II (Cathechismus Catholicae ecclesiae 1997). If futile therapy is burdensome or disproportionate to the expected outcome, then withholding or withdrawing is allowed. Despite allowing withdrawal of futile therapy, Pope John Paul II, shortly before his death, expressed a firm stand against withdrawing artificial nutrition from patients in a persistent vegetative state—a statement which has raised controversy (Shannon 2006).

In 1980 the "Declaration on Euthanasia" allowed alleviation of pain in the dying, even with life shortening as a non-intended side effect, also known as "the double effect" (McIntyre 2009) (Table 3.2), but active euthanasia is never allowed and palliative care is to be offered (Cathechismus Catholicae 1997).

TABLE 3.2
The Doctrine of Double Effect

- Definition: Nothing hinders one act from having two effects, only one of which is intended, while the other is beside the intention
- In this context: to relieve pain and suffering with the unintended side effect that the medication can lead to a prior death

A variety of substantive medical and ethical judgements provide the justification:

- The patient is terminally ill
- There is an urgent need to relieve pain and suffering
- Death is imminent
- The patient and/or the patient's proxy consents

Source: From McIntyre, A., In *The Stanford encyclopedia of philosophy*, The Metaphysics Research Lab, Stanford, CA, 2009.
Note: Explains the term "double effect" where provision of pain relief may lead to a somewhat hastened death and the table also explains under which circumstances such an act is acceptable/allowed.

3.3.1.2 Protestantism

Most Protestants will, if there is little hope of recovery, understand and accept the withholding or withdrawal of therapy (Pauls and Hutchinson 2002). But one example of the diversity within Protestantism is the question of euthanasia. The Evangelical Lutheran Church in Germany has developed advance directives for end-of-life choices but rejects active euthanasia (May 2003), whereas theologians in the reformed tradition, e.g., in the Netherlands, defend active euthanasia.

3.3.1.3 Greek Orthodox

The Greek Orthodox Church has no position on end-of-life decisions, since the task of Christians is to pray and not to decide about life and death. The church does not allow human decisions on such matters and condemns as unethical every medical act which does not contribute to the prolongation of life. The bioethics committee of the Church of Greece has stated: "… There is always the possibility of an erroneous medical appraisal or of an unforeseen outcome of the disease, or even a miracle" (The Holy Synod of the Church of Greece Bioethics Committee 2000). Therefore, it is not surprising that withholding or withdrawing of artificial nutrition is not allowable even if there is no prospect of recovery.

The church also states that should a fully conscious patient request an omission of treatment (that might save him) it is the moral obligation of the physician to try to persuade him to consent to that treatment.

Alleviation of pain is allowable if medication is provided in doses that are certain not to lead to death. This is somewhat surprising as "euthanasia" is actually the Greek word for "good death", which is defined as "a peaceful death with dignity and without pain."

The actual international meaning of "active euthanasia" is perceived as "mercy killing" and is under no circumstances allowed by the Greek Church.

3.3.2 Judaism

There are three Jewish denominations: reform, conservative and religious orthodox.

The Jewish legal system (*Halacha*) was developed from the Bible (Tanach), Talmud and rabbinic responsa (Steinberg and Sprung 2006). Israeli law was updated in 2006 in order to balance between the sanctity of life and the principle of autonomy. Withdrawal of a continuous life-sustaining therapy is still not allowed, but withholding further treatment is allowed as part of the dying process if it is an intermittent life-sustaining treatment—and if it was the clear wish of the patient (Steinberg and Sprung 2006). This is based on the assumption that each unit of treatment is an independent and new decision, hence it is permissible to withhold it. Thereby you can withhold chemotherapy or dialysis, even after initiation, because such treatment is viewed as omitting the next treatment rather than committing an act of withdrawal.

Food and fluid are regarded as basic needs and not treatment. Withholding food and fluid from a dying patient (or patients with other disorders) is unrelated to the dying process and therefore is prohibited and regarded as a form of euthanasia (Steinberg and Sprung 2006). If a dying patient is competent and refuses treatment, including food and fluids, he/she should be encouraged to change his/her mind regarding food and fluid, but should not be forced against his/her wishes (Steinberg and Sprung 2006). The situation changes however when the patient approaches the final days of life, when food and even fluids may cause suffering and complications. In such an event, it is permissible to withhold food and fluid if this was the patient's expressed wish.

Based on the moral requirement to alleviate pain and suffering, the law and *Halacha* require providing palliative care to the patient and to his/her family. Treatments include palliative therapy that might unintentionally shorten life, based on the principle of double effect (McIntyre 2009; Steinberg and Sprung 2006).

However, active euthanasia or physician-assisted suicide is prohibited, even at the patient's request (Steinberg and Sprung 2006).

3.3.3 Islam

Islamic bioethics is an extension of Shariah (Islamic law) based on the Qur'an (the holy book of all Muslims) and the Sunna (Islamic law based on the Prophet Muhammad's words and acts) (Daar and Khitamy 2001), and the primary goal is: "*la darar wa la dirar*" (no harm and no harassment).

For Muslims, premature death should be prevented, but not at any cost, and treatments can be withheld or withdrawn in terminally ill Muslim patients when the physicians are certain about the inevitability of death, and that treatment *in no way* will improve the condition or quality of life (Ebrahim 2000). The intention must never be to hasten death, only to abstain from overzealous treatment.

According to Islamic faith, it would be a crime to withdraw basic nutrition (Ebrahim 2000; da Costa et al. 2002) because such a withdrawal would in effect starve the patient to death.

The Qur'an states that "Allah does not tax any soul beyond that which he can bear" and pain and suffering is a "*kaffarah*" (expiation) for one's sins. But relieving a patient with painkillers or a sedative drug is allowed even if death is hastened (double effect) (McIntyre 2009), if death was definitely not intended by the physician (da Costa et al. 2002).

The two major branches of Islamic faith, the Shia and the Sunni branches, may differ somewhat, but not fundamentally in bioethical rulings. But the majority of Islamic communities will seek advice from their own religious scholars because the Islamic faith is not monolithic but rather a diversity of opinions (Daar and Khitamy 2001).

The Qur'an emphasises that "it is the sole prerogative of Allah to bestow life and to cause death" and consequently euthanasia is not allowable (Ebrahim 2000).

3.3.4 Hindu and Sikh

Hindu and Sikh religions are different, but both are duty-based rather than rights-based and they both believe in *karma*, a causal law where all acts and human thoughts have consequences; good *karma* leads to a good rebirth and vice versa. Since Hindu religion does not have a single central authority to secure enforcement in Hinduism (Desai 1988), diverse interpretations, opinions and followings are possible.

Death is denied—death is merely a passage to a new life, but untimely death is seriously mourned (Desai 1988). The way you die is important. A good death is when you are old, have said your goodbyes and all dues are settled. Bad death is violent, premature, in the wrong place (not at home or at the river of Ganges) and signified by vomit, faeces, urine and an unpleasant expression.

A do-not-resuscitate order is usually accepted or desired because death should be peaceful (Desai 1988).

Little is taught in Indian medical schools on palliative care and management of death.

The Indian Penal Code from 1860 British India prohibits euthanasia, but there is a longstanding tradition of suicide in certain defined circumstances—exemplified by the rule that a terminally ill person may hasten death—as a spiritual purification and to ensure no signs of bad death (faeces, vomit or urine).

3.3.5 Confucian and Taoism

Bioethics does not formally exist within traditional Chinese culture. The predominant religion in the elderly Chinese population is Buddhism/Taoism, whereas almost 60% of the younger generation claim to have no religion, because Confucianism is not generally considered as a religion by most Chinese people. The moral perspective is influenced primarily by Confucianism but also by Taoism and Buddhism (Bowmann and Hui 2000). Consequently, with this mixture of different religions and philosophies in one population, very diverse opinions and dilemmas can be encountered:

According to Confucian teaching, death is good if one has fulfilled one's moral duties in life, and resistance to accepting terminal illness or insisting on futile treatment may reflect the patient's perception of unfinished business (Bowmann and Hui 2000).

Taoism is divided into philosophical and religious Taoism. In philosophical Taoism acceptance is the only appropriate response when facing death and artificial measures contradict the natural events. In religious Taoism death may lead to an afterlife in torture in endless hell—where a Taoist might cling to any means of extending life to postpone that possibility (Bowmann and Hui 2000).

One thing is common in Chinese culture: The maintenance of hope is considered very important in the care of the dying, as hope prevents suffering by avoiding despair. Face-to-face interviews with 40 Chinese seniors 65 years of age or older showed that all respondents rejected advance directives (Bowman and Singer 2001). This is problematic seen from a Western (autonomous) point of view because it prohibits the physicians from discussing death in much detail with the patient or the patient's family.

The Chinese are more likely to prefer family-centred decision making than other racial or ethnic groups. For example, do-not-resuscitate orders in dying Chinese cancer patients were seldom signed by the patient personally (Liu et al. 1999). Moreover, even if a Chinese patient is resigned to death, the children may strongly advocate for (even) futile therapy, because filial piety can only be shown when a parent is alive and accepting impending death is equalled with removing the opportunity to show piety (Bowmann and Hui 2000). Some Chinese patients may think differently. A study in Taiwan showed that cancer patients strongly proclaimed their superior rights to be informed about their disease before their family was informed (Tang et al. 2006).

Euthanasia is illegal in Hong Kong and on mainland China. The first reported case of euthanasia in China caused great debate because the Supreme Court announced the accused physician innocent of a crime, but the topic is seldom discussed in medicine and the law.

3.3.6 Buddhism

As with Hinduism, there is no central authority to pronounce on doctrine and ethics. Buddhism is a flexible and moderate religion and, in practice, local customs will often be more important in the relationship between physician and patient than Buddhist doctrine (Keown 2005).

Classically, attitudes towards illness and death may be different for Tibetan, Indian, Thai, Japanese and Western Buddhists, because they are more culturally than religiously based. Hence, it is extremely important to inquire about specific attitudes that may be deeply held by a Buddhist patient and family who come from a particular culture.

But there are basic values shared by most Buddhists. The primary point is that there is no mandate or moral obligation to preserve life at all costs in Buddhism—this would be a denial of human mortality. There are no specific Buddhist teachings on patients in a persistent vegetative state, but maintaining artificial nutrition is a way to keep the patient alive artificially, which is not mandatory in Buddhism. Alleviation of pain, and the principle of double effect (McIntyre 2009), is accepted, but Buddhists strive to meet death with mental clarity. Therefore, some may abstain from analgesia or sedation. Terminal care should be available and Buddhism supports the hospice movement (Keown 2005).

Euthanasia or mercy killing is not acceptable (Keown 2005).

3.4 GUIDELINES

In palliative therapy, there are questions that will almost inevitably rise: What should our level of information to the patient and relatives be? Is euthanasia an issue? What are the final wishes with regard to death and burial?

The level of information is in Western Europe tightly connected to the question of patient autonomy. One of the main themes of the Protestant Reformation was that earthly authorities are not infallible. This emphasis on personal freedom promoted the concept that patients have a right to be truthfully informed, which today is so widely accepted in Western countries that it is no longer considered a unique feature of Protestant (religious) bioethics (Pauls and Hutchinson 2002). Greece, however, is an example of a Western country with a different view on patient autonomy. Ninety-six percent of the Greek Orthodox community believe that communication is important in the final stage of a disease, but only 23% agree that the patient should be informed of the prognosis (Mystakidou et al. 2005). This must be due to culture, because the Orthodox Church has not issued such a statement.

Likewise, in many Asian cultures patient autonomy is not an agenda (Bowmann and Hui 2000), here based not on culture, but on religious principles or thinking. In the Confucian concept of relational personhood, the family or community should be informed, coordinate the patient's care (Bowmann and Hui 2000) and protect the patient from the burden of knowledge. Also in the Hindu ethos, where death is a concern not only for the dying, but also for those close to him, it is the physician's task not to inform of imminent death, but to nurture the will to live in the dying (Desai 1988).

Therefore, medical teams are well advised early on to establish their patient's cultural background and religious affiliations before deciding on the level of information e.g., by following the check list proposed in Table 3.3 (Klessig 1992), and it may be universally advisable to involve the clergy of the patient's religion (Daar and Khitamy 2001; Pauls and Hutchinson 2002).

The question of euthanasia is the least complicated when you investigate the religions' points of view. In Table 3.1 it is evident that euthanasia is almost universally not accepted.

TABLE 3.3
Checklist to Establish Religious Beliefs, Cultural Affiliation and Family Background When End-of-Life Decisions Are Necessary

- What do they think of the sanctity of life?
- What is their definition of death?
- What is their religious background and how active are they presently?
- What do they believe are the causal agents in illness and how do these relate to the dying process?
- What is the patient's social support system?
- Who makes decisions about matters of importance in the family?

Source: From Klessig, J., *West J. Med.*, 157, 316, 1992.
Note: Examples of questions that are suitable to ask when trying to explore patients' and relatives' cultural and religious background.

When death is imminent, the question of tending to the dead and burial arrangements will arise. Again it is important to adhere to the wishes of the patient and the family, because each person may have specific rules based on culture and religion (Cheraghi, Payne, and Salsali 2005).

Physicians and nurses can prevent or at least minimise the potential religious conflicts and discussions among patients, families and medical professionals by becoming knowledgeable and respecting their patients' faiths and beliefs. But you should also be aware that people who classify themselves as belonging to a religion do not necessarily attend their Church or follow any of the religion's rulings. It is not enough, however, to look at religious issues alone, because many laws and public policies on end-of-life decisions are based not only on religion, but also on secular law and cultural development.

Reaching consensus is a key to success, but is not always possible. In those (hopefully few) instances where consensus cannot be accomplished, it is my point of view that you should then act according to the local rules and ethics of your workplace. The climate of cooperation and working conditions among colleagues can be put in jeopardy if you change your way of dealing with end-of-life issues for each new patient.

ETHICAL ISSUES

Until now, critical care medicine, and other advanced medical measures to keep patients alive, has essentially been a discipline of Western medicine because it demands a highly developed medical and economic system. Consequently, Far Eastern countries have not had the same need to develop distinct attitudes on advanced therapy and life-supporting systems. With increasing economic growth, it is more than likely that these countries will also have to develop local guidelines covering advanced medical therapy. However, they will run into the problem that there are no established heads of the various Far Eastern religions who can adjust and express the religious rulings on these issues in the twenty-first century.

But even when there is a clear-cut statement from church leaders, it may be difficult to incorporate the religious perspectives into modern medical decision making. The Catholic Church allows withholding or withdrawing of "extraordinary" therapy, but what is extraordinary? Mechanical ventilation could be ordinary at one stage in an illness and extraordinary at a later stage of the same illness.

Strict ethnic and religious background is not the only factor that one must take into account when dealing with end-of-life decisions. Recent immigrants will generally adhere rather strictly to the rules of the religion and culture in their native country (Bowmann and Hui 2000), whereas second- or third-generation immigrants will often have adopted the dominant bioethics of their new country (this is known as acculturation) (Matsumura et al. 2002). However, when facing death, many individuals tend to fall back on their traditional cultural or religious background (Klessig 1992).

Not only are patients changing their behavioural pattern when they move to other parts of the world. Although religion is an important part in decision-making, regional differences among physicians of the same religion have been documented too, and these differences are most probably due to acculturation (Sprung et al. 2007; Matsumura et al. 2002). Even a straight religious statement is not necessarily adopted. According to Islamic Law one is allowed to abstain from futile treatment, but withdrawal of treatment (Yazigi, Riachi, and Dabbar 2005) or do-not-resuscitate orders (da Costa et al. 2002) are not as frequent as in Western Europe—and this is primarily explained by cultural differences.

To make matters even more complicated, when secular law is adjusted to adhere to religious rulings (Steinberg and Sprung 2006) the actual attitudes of physicians may still differ. In a study, 443 Jewish doctors in four Israeli hospitals were asked the following questions: Can life support be stopped? Would you administer medication with the risk of double effect? Do you accept euthanasia? The most religious physicians were significantly less likely to answer yes to any of these questions (Wenger and Carmel 2004).

SUMMARY POINTS

- Increasing globalisation is changing the world, so that it no longer consists of homogeneous religious and cultural entities. These demographic changes create the challenge that medical staff will have to acknowledge and cope with the religious attitudes and beliefs of patients from many ethnic and religious groups.
- It is also a challenge in a globalised world that religion and culture have an impact not only on how patients want to be treated, but also on the way physicians and nursing staff from different parts of the world act and decide.
- Both religion and culture play an important role when end-of-life issues are at stake, but most physicians do not know their patients' religious affiliation and authors have used strong words to characterise the consequences if religion and culture are not taken into account, e.g., "it can lead to a complete break-down in communication".
- It is paramount to explore and understand religious and cultural differences. Both regarding treatment, and with regard to questions concerning death and burial rituals. To avoid pitfalls it has been recommended to involve the clergy of the patient's religion early on and to follow the checklist in Table 3.3.
- Preferences for care emerge in a clinical context by discussion and feedback within the network of the patient's most important relationships. The approach should emphasise communication, building trust over time and working within the patient's most important relationships.
- By exploring these issues, it is usually possible to reach consensus, but if that is impossible, then the staff must apply the local ruling laws and ethical guidelines.
- In the context of a globalised world the statement of the ethics committee at Stanford University is important: "The key to resolving ethical problems lies in clarifying the patient's interests".

REFERENCES

Bowman, K. W., and E. C. Hui. 2000. Bioethics for clinicians: Chinese bioethics. *CMAJ* 163:1481–85.

Bowman, K. W., and P. A. Singer. 2001. Chinese seniors' perspectives on end-of-life decisions. *Soc Sci & Med* 53:455–64.

Bülow, H. H., C. L. Sprung, K. Reinhart, S. Prayag, B. Du, A. Armaganidis, F. Abroug, and M. M. Levy. 2008. The world's major religions' point of view on end-of-life decisions in the intensive care unit. *Intensive Care Med* 34:423–30.

Catechismus Catholicae Ecclesiae. 1997. Section 2278 and 2279. *Libreria Editrice Vaticana*. ISBN 88-209-2428-5.

Cheraghi, M. A., S. Payne, and M. Salsali. 2005. Spiritual aspects of end-of-life care for Muslim patients: Experiences from Iran. *Int J Palliat Nurse* 11:468–74.

Daar, A. S., and A. B. Khitamy. 2001. Bioethics for clinicians: 21. Islamic bioethics. *CMAJ* 164:60–63.

da Costa, D. E., H. Ghazal, S. A. Khusaiby, and A. R. Gatrad. 2002. Do not resuscitate orders in a neonatal ICU in a Muslim community. *Arch Dis Child Fetal Neonatal Ed* 86:F115–19.

Desai, P. N. 1988. Medical ethics in India. *J Med Phil* 13:231–55.

Ebrahim, A. F. H. 2000. The living will (Wasiyat Al-Hayy): A study of its legality in the light of Islamic jurisprudence. *Med Law* 19:147–60.

Keown, D. 2005. End-of-life: The Buddhist view. *Lancet* 366:952–55.

Klessig, J. 1992. Cross-cultural medicine. The effect of values and culture on life support decisions. *West J Med* 157:316–22.

Liu, J. M., W. C. Lin, Y. M. Chen, H. W. Wu, N. S. Yao, L. T. Chen, and J. Whang-Peng. 1999. The status of the do-not-resuscitate order in Chinese clinical trial patients in a cancer centre. *J Med Ethics* 25:309–14.

Matsumura, S., S. Bito, H. Liu, K. Kahn, S. Fukuhara, and M. I. Kagawa-Singer. 2002. Acculturation of attitudes toward end-of-life care. *J Gen Intern Med* 17:531–39.

May, A. T. 2003. Physician assisted suicide, euthanasia, and Christian bioethics: Moral controversy in Germany. *Christ Bioeth* 9:273–83.

McIntyre, A. 2009. Doctrine of double effect. In *The Stanford encyclopedia of philosophy,* ed. Edward N. Zalta (Accessed from http://plato.stanford.edu/archives/fall2009/entries/double-effect/).

Mystakidou, K., E. Parpa, E. Tsilika, E. Katsouda, and L. Vlahos. 2005. The evolution of euthanasia and its perceptions in Greek culture and civilization. *Perspect Biol Med* 48:95–104.

Pauls, M., and R. C. Hutchinson. 2002. Bioethics for clinicians: Protestant bioethics. *CMAJ* 166: 339–44.

Prendergast, T. J. 2001. Advance care planning: Pitfalls, progress, promise. *Crit Care Med* 29 (2 suppl): N34–39.

Shannon, T. A. 2006. Nutrition and hydration: An analysis of the recent Papal statement in the light of the Roman Catholic bioethical tradition. *Christ Bioeth* 12:29–41.

Sprung, C. L., P. Maia, H. H. Bülow, B. Ricou, A. Armaginidis, M. Baras, E. Wennberg et al. 2007. The impact of religion on end-of-life decisions in European intensive care units. *Intensive Care Med* 33:1732–39.

Steinberg, A., and C. L. Sprung. 2006. The dying patient: New Israeli legislation. *Intensive Care Med* 32:1234–37.

Tang, S. T., T. W. Liu, M. S. Lai, L. N. Liu, C. H. Chen, and S. L. Koong. 2006. Congruence of knowledge, experiences, and preferences for disclosure of diagnosis and prognosis between terminally-ill cancer patients and their family caregivers in Taiwan. *Cancer Invest* 24:360–66.

The Holy Synod of the Church of Greece Bioethics Committee. 2000. Press Release on 17th of August. Basic positions on the ethics of transplantation and euthanasia. www.bioethics.org.gr.

Wenger, N. S., and S. Carmel. 2004. Physicians' religiosity and end-of-life care attitudes and behaviours. *Mt. Sinai J Med* 71:335–43.

Yazigi, A., M. Riachi, and G. Dabbar. 2005. Withholding and withdrawal of life-sustaining treatment in a Lebanese intensive care unit. *Intensive Care Med* 31:562–67.

4 Why Surgeons Are Ambivalent about Palliative Treatments: A Personal Perspective

Geoffrey P. Dunn

CONTENTS

4.1 INTRODUCTION

The ever-widening clinical spectrum of palliative care requires the inclusion of surgery and surgeons to assure informed decision-making, symptom control, and improvement of quality of life (QOL). Few surgeons would dispute the relevance of these tasks to their practices though considerable ambivalence remains for many about pursuing these as primary goals of care. Adding to their reluctance to endorse palliative care is the stunning progress that has been made in the amelioration or eradication of many chronic and fatal illnesses. This ambivalence can be understood as the expression of multiple barriers to the acceptance of palliative care as a clinical framework of care that replaces the disease-directed or "cure"-based model of care. The barriers can be classified as cognitive, psychological, socioeconomic, and spiritual, which roughly align them with the four principal domains of "total pain" described by Dame Cicely Saunders.

All of these barriers are surmountable, but not by surgeons alone or even through the assistance of palliative medicine consultants. A collective commitment by surgeons, surgical educators, palliative medicine practitioners, other health care professionals, and the public will be required to guide the surgeon over the reef from cure to care. No clinical issue has the capacity to highlight the conflict of the two models of care within the surgeon's heart and mind more than nutritional support.

4.2 BACKGROUND: THE CONVERGENT EVOLUTION OF THE PALLIATIVE MODEL WITHIN AND OUTSIDE OF THE FIELD OF SURGERY

My surgical practice commenced in the mid-1980s, ten years after the hospice philosophy of care had been introduced to the United States. At that time, physicians in that country had only a vague acquaintance with the concept, although the public's perception of hospice was already positive. There was virtually no reference to hospice or palliative care in the mainstream medical literature or textbooks at that time, especially those related to surgery. I heard of hospice only because my father, a surgeon, had been a founder of a hospice program in our community in 1980. He had heard of it only because a family member of a terminally ill patient of his had told him of this innovative approach that had just become available near New York City.

My father, a third-generation surgeon, believed the hospice approach was a welcome and badly needed humane solution to problems and situations far beyond the reach of surgery and "standard medical care." In addition to a wide-ranging and busy practice, he had experience as a commanding officer of a field hospital that was charged with resuscitating survivors of a concentration camp following the Second World War, so he had seen more than enough to welcome a more effective approach to care for the irredeemably ill. Twenty years after co-founding a hospice, when he had the good fortune of having Dame Cicely Saunders as a houseguest, she mentioned how profoundly influenced the modern hospice movement was by two survivors of the Holocaust, Victor Frankl and David Tasma. She also pointed out several intriguing connections between the worlds of surgery and hospice: she had been encouraged to read medicine by a surgeon, Howard Barrett, in order to enhance her expertise and the credibility of her ideas within the medical establishment. Balfour Mount, a Canadian oncologic surgeon, had spent time at St. Christopher's Hospice and subsequently was among those who introduced the hospice concept to Canada. Additionally, he coined the term "palliative care" when he opened the first palliative care unit in an acute care hospital in North America in 1975.

During my first ten years of surgical practice, as a trauma and burn surgeon, I frequently encountered patients with end-stage or critical illness in addition to geriatric referrals from my father's contemporaries. This patient mix presented me with all of the salient problems seen in palliative care practice without any previous guidance or formal training about even the most rudimentary techniques for communication, symptom control, or self-conduct. It was not until 1988 that a formal medical society, the Academy of Hospice Physicians, was formed for US physicians active in hospice or palliative care. Among the Academy's early membership, less than half a dozen surgeons could be counted.

Despite surgery's low profile in the establishment of hospice and palliative care in the United States, isolated striking examples of surgeons taking initiative in promoting hospice care can be found during this time. In 1976, a leading surgical researcher and educator, J. Englebert Dunphey, who was dying from prostate cancer at the time, in the Annual Oration to the Massachusetts Medical Society, titled "On Caring for the Patient with Cancer" (Dunphey 1976), stressed the importance of non-abandonment of the dying patient. He challenged the deep-seated belief of surgeons that death is failure with his words, "Death holds no fearful threat. Living without life is hell. Death is natural; it may be just; it is often easeful and merciful; it always to be dignified." At that time, the field of surgery seemed to be going in a very different direction with the expansion of surgical intensive care units and the proliferation of new technologies, such as total parenteral nutrition, often inappropriately initiated in patients with far advanced and incurable illness. It was not until 1998 that the American College of Surgeons formally ratified a statement of principles of care (American College of Surgeons, Committee on Ethics 1998) consistent with Dr. Dunphey's affirmative vision of dying.

Other noteworthy surgical pioneers of hospice and palliative care include Robert Milch, who in 1978 founded what has for years been a highly regarded hospice program in Buffalo, New York, and Jack Zimmerman at Johns Hopkins University, who published a book in 1982, *Hospice: Complete Care of the Terminally Ill* (Zimmerman 1981), and one of the first references to hospice care integrated with acute hospital care (Zimmerman 1979) in the surgical literature.

In contrast to the practical and clinical focus of the above pioneers, the prevailing view about end-of-life care for most surgeons was established by ethical debate and court rulings during the 1970s and 1980s centering on the principle of individual autonomy. Unfortunately, the abstract and intellectual exercises of ethical and legal debate about care of patients in vegetative states seemed distant from the day-to-day hurried reality of surgical practice. Indicative of this gap was a poll in 1992 that found a third of attending physicians (surgeons among them), residents, and students believed that withdrawing life support was active euthanasia (Caralis and Hammond 1992). A poll at that time of the membership of the Society of Critical Care Medicine, which includes surgeons, found that only half of the respondents equated withholding with withdrawing life support (Society of Critical Care Medicine Ethics Committee 1992). A very typical response from surgeons with whom I have broached the subject of palliative care is, "It's really important… I have a partner who is interested in ethics." This implies that surgeons have until recently seen end-of-life care as an "ethical issue," (even though the ethics of caring for those at end-of-life are fundamentally no different than for any other group) and therefore something for ethicists and others to worry about.

When the historical contributions by surgeons to the mitigation of suffering and improvement of QOL are pointed out to them, then surgeons are able to see themselves in the mirror of palliative caring. Surgeons have always been trained in a hierarchical system where the locus of authority has been the past, whether through accumulated evidence or the personal impact of a recognized leader. Once a surgeon can recognize the salient principles of palliative care in the history of surgery, then the concept can be accepted as a natural and integral part of the surgeon's practice. Several noteworthy examples of this are readily apparent to all surgeons and come from a time when the field of surgery was in its transition from palliating most conditions to cure for many, the late nineteenth to the mid-twentieth century. In each instance, the procedure was effective for immediate relief of symptoms and subsequently proved to be curable in some cases. In 1894, Halsted reported on a series of patients who had undergone his radical treatment for cancer of the breast (Halsted 1894). The treatment later proved to be curative for some, but it was initially effective for the relief of highly symptomatic or disfiguring disease. Billroth's first successful gastrectomy for carcinoma of the pylorus relieved his patient of a rapid and undignified death from gastric outlet obstruction, allowing her a more peaceful death months later from liver metastases. In his report he described the prerequisites and goals of palliative surgery: "Our next care…must be to determine the indications, and to develop the technique to suit all kinds of cases. I hope we have taken another good step towards securing unfortunate people hitherto regarded as incurable or, if there should be recurrences of cancer, at least alleviating their suffering for a time." (Billroth 1881). When Whipple reported on his eponymous operation for the treatment of pancreatic cancer in 1942, he wrote, " the considerable risk (i.e., operative mortality) of 30% to 35% is justified if they (the patients) can be made comfortable for a year or two" (Whipple 1942).

4.3 WHAT BURN CARE HAS TAUGHT SURGEONS ABOUT PALLIATIVE CARE

The delivery method of palliative care, the team approach, has a precedent in surgical experience. Without knowledge of hospice and palliative medicine, burn surgeons discovered a model of care very similar to the interdisciplinary model that is associated with palliative care. The Coconut Grove fire disaster in 1942 and burn casualties during the Second World War provided the impetus for this. The Coconut Grove fire drew attention to the importance of recognizing and treating not only pain but also the non-physical distress of critically ill surgical patients. A landmark paper by Lindemann (1944), based on his experience providing psychiatric care for the Coconut Grove fire victims at Massachusetts General Hospital, became the foundation of the study of grief and bereavement. In his paper he presciently recommended the now routine inclusion of psychiatric support in interdisciplinary efforts responding to disaster.

The team approach to burn care initiated by the US military at the end of the Second World War dramatically improved survival.

The emergence of the team approach from burn care experience is not at all surprising given the profound physical, psychologic, socioeconomic, and spiritual impact wrought by major burns. Unlike chronic, life-limiting illness, major burns present the additional burdens of suddenness and reliance upon sophisticated in-patient settings. Given the extreme metabolic rate of the major burn patient, the connections between nutritional support, function, and survival are quite plain to see for all involved, with implications that invariably call for a wide range of expertise. The salvage of the major burn patient begins with analgesia and concludes with restoration of function, just as the "salvage" of the terminally ill cancer patient begins with relief from the physical distractions of pain and other symptoms and concludes with whatever restoration of function the patient deems relevant to meet his personal goals.

My personal interest in palliative care as a surgeon had its roots in my experience with a burn unit in a very poor and under-resourced setting in which the grim statistics for major burns virtually guaranteed demise. Though the prospects for survival were dismal for these patients, the need for pain relief, psychological and social support, and spiritual succor was undeniable and achievable. I was working in a burn "hospice" and didn't realize it. Five years later when participating in a hospice interdisciplinary team meeting, I was suddenly struck by the similarity of burn care and hospice care. I believed from that point on that the two worlds of palliative care and surgery should be as one.

4.4 BARRIERS TO THE ASSIMILATION OF PALLIATIVE PRINCIPLES IN SURGICAL PRACTICE

Shortly after my epiphany, in 1996, I began to give grand rounds presentations about palliative care to surgeons in the United States, and later in Canada, the UK, and Hong Kong. I noted a consistent response—respect for the concept of palliative care, agreement that it would benefit surgery, and some degree of personal uneasiness with the topic. Allied health personnel attending these presentations were always very enthusiastic and overwhelmingly female. For purposes of planning future initiatives for surgeon education and research, I identified what I believe are the four categories of barriers to the assimilation of a palliative care practice model into surgical practice (Table 4.1). They are roughly aligned with Cicely Saunders's four dimensions of pain, which in aggregate represent "Total Pain" (Saunders and Sykes 1993): (1) physical (in this instance the cognitive aspects of surgery), (2) the psychologic, (3) the social, and (4) the spiritual.

4.4.1 Cognitive Barriers

Several reviews (Rabow and McPhee 2002, Easson 2001, Milch and Dunn 1997) of surgical textbooks and the surgical literature have documented a paucity of information about hospice, palliative care, and the dying process as a clinical phenomenon despite the number of individuals under surgical care for whom these entities would be appropriate or relevant. Until the last few years, there have been no surgical textbook chapters specifically addressing palliative care as a primary framework for surgical care for patients such as the intensive care unit patient with multiple organ system failure or the patient presenting with malignant bowel obstruction and widely disseminated metastases.

When palliation has been addressed in the surgical literature it has traditionally been confined to discussion of operative procedures, not as an approach to care that may or may not include operative intervention. The term "palliative surgery" has not been consistently defined and at least one common definition in the older literature has directly contributed to the perception that palliative surgery indicates failure. Palliative surgery has been variably defined as (1) an operation that has residual micro- or macroscopic disease at its conclusion, (2) an operation for cancer recurrence for a failed cancer operation, and (3) an operation primarily for the relief of symptoms. Of these three, the third definition is emerging as the consensus definition by surgeons. Miner (2005) defines palliative surgery for cancer

TABLE 4.1
Barriers to the Assimilation of Palliative Principles in Surgical Practice

Cognitive	• Lack of information about the dying process, hospice, and palliative care in surgical textbooks • No formal palliative care training in surgical residency and fellowship programs • Conflicting definitions of "palliative surgery" in the surgical literature • Lack of quality and quantity of quality of life (QOL) data and research in surgical specialties • Lack of standard approaches to common end-of-life surgical problems
Psychologic	• Belief that palliative treatments represent "failure" • Fear of rejection if disease isn't "fixed" • Fear related to loss of control and personal fear of death • Fear of own and patient/family's emotional response
Social and economic	• Physical isolation from others in hospital • Unique identity of surgical culture • Surgeon's belief in the "captain of the ship" model of leadership • Emphasis on mortality and morbidity only in surgical rounds • Poor reimbursement for patient/family meeting time • Conflict of goals with referring physicians or families leading to loss of referrals • Fear of increased mortality and morbidity statistics stemming from treating patients at end-of-life
Spiritual	• Deconstruction of illness by surgeons focused on procedures and technology • Difficulty differentiating spirituality from religion • Reluctance of surgeons to acknowledge importance of spiritual needs in clinical decision making • Surgeons' and patients' mutual denial of death

as "a procedure used with the primary intention of improving QOL or relieving symptoms caused by the advanced malignancy. The effectiveness of a palliative intervention should be judged by the presence and durability of patient-acknowledged symptom resolution." A more consistent and affirmative definition of palliative surgery will likely encourage surgeons to expand their role in the overall palliative care for their patients. Rosenberg et al. (1982) presciently observed in their groundbreaking paper on QOL outcomes for extremity sarcoma trials that doing QOL research had a humanizing effect upon the researchers because of their attention to their patients' personal experience with illness.

Until the last decade, the lack of QOL research and the poor quality of research that had been done hindered the acceptance of improved QOL as a legitimate primary goal for surgical care. A review (Miner et al. 1999) of palliation in the surgical literature prior to 1997 revealed that studies were retrospective; they were focused on risks, mortality, and morbidity; and established methods for QOL measurement were not being adequately utilized. Until very recently the only generally accepted measures of successful palliative intervention by surgeons were lack of post-operative mortality and morbidity. Clearly, this would pose difficulties in advocating invasive procedures for palliation for patients with very limited or uncertain prognosis and at high nutritional risk for post-operative complications. Koller, Nies, and Lorenz (2004) pointed out that QOL outcomes measurement may suffer from the perception by investigators that it is "soft" compared to the hard data of mortality and morbidity outcomes and thus would not attract clinical researchers.

Several surveys have documented a lack of formal training in palliative care for a majority of surgeons (Galante et al. 2005) and surgical oncologists (McCahill et al. 2002). In a survey (Galante et al. 2005) of general surgeons given four vignettes portraying patients with advanced illness and limited prognosis, no consensus was reached on treatment recommendations in three out of four of the vignettes. It was noted that surgeons with less palliative care training were more likely to recommend a major operative intervention in a patient with far advanced disease while less likely to recommend repair of a symptomatic inguinal hernia in a patient with Stage IV prostate cancer with no evidence of disease.

4.4.2 Psychologic Barriers

The fact that the world of surgery has been, at best, slow to respond to the shortcomings in care of patients known to be at the end-of-life, the SUPPORT study (The SUPPORT Clinical Investigators 1995) suggests other more profound impediments may exist preventing surgeons' endorsement of timely palliative care. The most charitable reason that can be given for this is the surgeon's psychological barrier to acknowledging that even in the twenty-first century there comes a point in the course of an illness when the disease is no longer under his control. Why is lack of control over an advanced and progressing disease so often interpreted by the surgeon as failure? Often I have heard a surgeon describe a well-advised procedure for relief of intractable symptoms as "just a palliative procedure" as if it had less merit than one that would cure.

Sherwin Nuland, noted surgeon and author of the best-selling book *How We Die* (Nuland 1994), identified two fundamental psychological barriers to surgeons fulfilling an effective, empathic role in providing palliative care (Nuland 2001). Both of these barriers are evidenced by the surgeon's fear of reflection and introspection, an unwillingness to look into his own heart. Because of the frequent call for surgeons' sudden and often dramatic intervention, the surgeon's avoidance of self-doubt brought on by introspection or reflection has been excused as necessary to "act" effectively. This was undoubtedly true when amputating a mangled extremity was more traumatic than the initial injury itself. The world of surgery at those times had no invisible domains – no knowledge of micro-organisms, cellular structure, or metabolic processes. Now that the landscape of surgery has so vastly changed and includes so much that is invisible, new coping mechanisms are required. Nuland argues that the old coping mechanisms, aloofness and coldness, have become internalized and the surgeon is prone to psychologically abandon the patient he cannot "fix" because of the threat to his narcissism. The surgeon's self-esteem and the esteem of surgeons by others have been based on his success as a "man of action."

The other, more profound, psychological barrier for surgeons is their unconscious fear of their own mortality. It was suggested long ago that the choice of a medical career reflects a deep-seated fear of death and the wish to avoid it by acquiring an extra measure of control over health (Feifel 1967). If this is true, then it could be postulated that those who seek the most control (surgery) over life processes have a greater underlying fear of death.

Nuland proposes that surgeons do more to acknowledge and cultivate their "pastoral" role, to unburden the anxieties of their patients, and to reduce their own anxiety by closing the gap between what is seen on the surface and what lurks within. He challenges surgeons to fear not and be willing to remove their masks.

4.4.3 Socioeconomic Barriers

Surgery is a culture. Surgery possesses a set of shared attitudes, values, goals, and practices that gives it a unique identity. The most unique experience for surgeons, surgery itself, occurs in a sanctuary in which specific vestments are worn while performing duties according to set rules of decorum learned in a long apprenticeship. This is exotic or alien for much of the rest of the healthcare system, creating a potential conflict of social, economic, and spiritual interests.

Surgery is a hierarchical culture that strongly adheres to the concept of the surgeon as "captain of the ship." The dangers of paternalism and hubris of surgeons undermining ethical decisions about palliative surgery have been identified by Norwegian surgical researchers (Hofmann, Håheim, and Søreide 2005). The "captain of the ship" mindset is also problematic for the patient-centered palliative care delivery model, the interdisciplinary team which defers primary authority in decision making to the patient or his surrogate.

One of the hallowed rituals of surgical culture has been mortality and morbidity rounds, when surgeons periodically review cases in which a patient dies or has sustained a complication during their hospitalization or during the post-operative period. It is an occasion for scientific, ethical, and moral instruction for house staff and attending surgeons. Accountability is determined and ultimately absolution is granted, when possible, for adverse events. QOL considerations have not traditionally factored into these discussions unless related to a complication. The format of mortality and morbidity rounds does not easily make an exception for the patient who undergoes a palliative surgical procedure who then succumbs soon to their underlying disease. Furthermore, as hospitals are ranked, as they are in the United States, by their mortality and morbidity statistics, what would be the incentive to surgically treat high-risk patients with advanced disease?

The remaining potential socioeconomic barriers to surgical palliative care are referral patterns. Referral patterns may be directed by a surgeon's proclivity to "take action" even if the desired intervention is of questionable benefit. A referring physician promises a family, "The surgeon will put in a feeding tube." What if the surgeon believes this would not serve a patient with advanced dementia? Or, the surgeon believes an operation for malignant obstruction will benefit a particular patient, but the referring physician mistakenly believes "terminal" patients should not have surgery? An additional socioeconomic disincentive for adherence to palliative care principles is the lack of reimbursement and time in some healthcare systems for patient/family conferencing.

4.4.4 Spiritual Barriers

Recently, several papers (Tarpley and Tarpley 2002; Hinshaw 2005) about spirituality in surgical practice have appeared, while public opinion polls and hospital surveys indicate that a majority of patients want their physicians to discuss spiritual issues with them. In my own practice I have noted a wide range of responses from patients when inquiring about spiritual beliefs—delight by some and fear by a few because of their belief that attention to spiritual matters will distract the surgeon from technical considerations.

A well-known surgical authority on medical ethics, when writing about the spiritual dimensions of surgical palliative care, stated, "Surgeons are technicians for whom the spirituality of death and the dying process is terrifying." (Krizek 2001).

By contrast, several visionary surgeons set a commendable example for all physicians by their willingness to incorporate psychological and spiritual considerations into practice. Barney Brooks, chairman of surgery at Vanderbilt University, spoke about the importance of the psychologic nature of the surgeon in the patient-physician relationship (Brooks 1944). He explicitly stated that technically skilled but socially deficient surgeons were unworthy of the profession. Another chairman of surgery, Matthew Walker, insisted that medical students and physicians needed to be in touch with their own mortality if they were to assist patients and their families in dealing with end-of-life issues (Organ and Kosiba 1987).

4.5 OVERCOMING SURGEONS' AMBIVALENCE ABOUT PALLIATIVE TREATMENTS: THE WAY FORWARD

Despite the numerous reasons given for surgeons' ambivalence about palliative treatments, many of them apply to non-surgeons and patients. The surgeon's reluctance to consider a palliative course of action is occasionally the conscious or unconscious response to pressure from unrealistic patients and family members. The denial of death so prevalent in Western societies provides the background for this conflict of goals. Surgical institutions and societies can do much to validate the standing of palliative care as an orthodox treatment strategy for a wide range of clinical problems. This will be particularly important in the field of nutritional support because of surgeons' credibility and interventions related to nutrition.

Currently, many surgeons would be uncomfortable responding to a question frequently asked on behalf of a cachectic patient with advanced cancer: "Doctor, is my husband going to starve to death?" The temptation for the surgeon would be to deconstruct this question and render it to a physical or technical problem to be solved.

The self-knowledge and skills a surgeon needs to respond to this type of question go far beyond knowing the pathophysiology of cachexia or presenting a menu of treatments. The surgeon achieved his current status by the ever-narrowing focusing of his technical skills based on increasing application of scientific methodology. This has paid off handsomely for problems that are straightforward and solvable, just as Newtonian mechanics landed us on the moon but cannot explain the extremes of reality—the subatomic or galactic worlds. The world of surgery has become so dynamic during the past quarter century that the perfect opportunity for an ancient and yet radically new vision now exists. A new vision will require surgeons to look at things they haven't looked at closely before, as well as require them to discover things about ourselves.

Within the past 150 years the field of surgery has radically changed. During the 1920s my grandfather, a residency trained surgeon, often gave his patients their anesthetics, performed their surgery, did the microscopy of tissue taken in order to make diagnoses, made some of the medications, and did the billing for his services himself in addition to serving as the family doctor and obstetrician. This was not unusual at the time. This was certainly commendable then, but probably criminal now.

Then, the idea of a surgeon assuming parity with other non-physician professionals at a conference table planning a patient's care would have been unthinkable. Now, it should be equally unthinkable if the surgeon didn't assume parity with other professionals when seated at the interdisciplinary table. This redistribution of power and the acceptance of an evidence-based framework for treatments represent the most profound changes that have occurred in the field of surgery over the past thirty years.

The implications of these changes bode well for the future of palliative care, especially given the recent initiatives made by surgical institutions. Since the 1990s, the Royal College of Surgeons has required a degree of competency in palliative and end-of-life care for its fellowship candidates (Kirk, Mansfield, and Cochrane 1999). As of 2008, the American Board of Surgery along with ten other American Board of Medical Specialties (ABMS) boards has authorized a specialty certificate in Hospice and Palliative Medicine (American Board of Surgery 2010). The American College of Surgeons has consistently supported palliative care initiatives since the late 1990s, including the formation of a surgical palliative care task force, presenting symposia and courses about palliative care annually, issuance of two statements (American College of Surgeons, Committee on Ethics 1998; American College of Surgeons, Committee on Ethics and Task Force on Palliative Care 2005) with guidelines for end-of-life and palliative care (Table 4.2), and the recent publication of a guide (Dunn, Martensen, and Weissman 2009) for surgical residents' training in palliative care.

TABLE 4.2
Statement of Principles of Palliative Care

- Respect the dignity and autonomy of patients, patients' surrogates, and caregivers
- Honor the right of the competent patient or surrogate to choose among treatments, including those that may or may not prolong life
- Communicate effectively and empathically with patients, their families, and caregivers
- Identify the primary goals of care from the patient's perspective and address how the surgeon's care can achieve the patient's objectives
- Strive to alleviate pain and other burdensome physical and non-physical symptoms
- Recognize, assess, discuss, and offer access to services for psychological, social, and spiritual issues
- Provide access to therapeutic support, encompassing the spectrum from life-prolonging treatments through hospice care, when they can realistically be expected to improve the quality of life as perceived by the patient
- Recognize the physician's responsibility to discourage treatments that are unlikely to achieve the patient's goals, and encourage patients and families to consider hospice care when the prognosis for survival is likely to be less than half a year
- Arrange for continuity of care by the patient's primary and/or specialist physician, alleviating the sense of abandonment patients may feel when "curative" therapies are no longer useful
- Maintain a collegial and supportive attitude toward others entrusted with care of the patient

Source: Reprinted with permission from American College of Surgeons, Committee on Ethics and Surgical Palliative Care Task Force, *Bull. Am. Coll. Surg.*, 90, 34. Copyright [2005] American Chemical Society.

4.6 SUMMARY

Although numerous barriers prevent the surgeon from accepting the place of palliative treatments, many of them are not unique to surgeons, and all of the barriers that have been identified are surmountable. History has shown repeatedly that surgeons are innovators and capable of responding to the challenges of each era. Surgery has a much richer background for a palliative philosophy than many surgeons and others have recognized. Currently, the fields of surgery and palliative medicine are showing promising signs of resonance. The greatest clinical challenges for all practitioners are almost always related to nutrition. Collaboration among surgeons, specialists in nutrition, and palliative care professionals is long overdue and will ultimately enrich each of these disciplines.

KEY FACTS

- The term, "palliative care", was coined by a Canadian surgeon, Balfour Mount.
- Historically, surgeons have advocated surgery to relieve suffering even if surgery had minimal impact on survival.
- Since the 1990s, surgical institutions in the USA and UK have officially acknowledged palliative care as a legitimate clinical approach to the care of patients with life-limiting illness.
- Since 2008, the American Board of Surgery has issued certification in Hospice and Palliative Medicine for surgeons meeting the eligibility criteria and passing a certification exam.
- Palliative intervention is an active area of surgical education and research.

FACTS ABOUT SURGEONS

- Training of surgeons typically takes 5 years or more additional training after medical school.
- Surgeons are required by their certifying boards to be knowledgeable in the physiology of nutrition and it's implications for clinical management.
- Surgeons are required by their certifying boards to be knowledgeable about the ethical and clinical aspects of care for the seriously and terminally ill patient.
- Surgeons have been involved in much of the basic research for nutritional support.

SUMMARY POINTS

- The history of surgery was rich with examples of innovation in palliative care even before hospice
- and palliative care became cohesive philosophies of patient care.
- There are multiple, but surmountable, barriers for surgeons to effectively participate in palliative care.
- The future of palliative care research by surgeons is promising and will be enriched by their participation.

LIST OF ABBREVIATIONS

ABMS American Board of Medical Specialties
ABS American board of Surgery
QOL Quality of life

REFERENCES

American Board of Surgery. 2010. www.home.absurgery.org/default.jsp?certhpm. Accessed 2 March 2010.

American College of Surgeons, Committee on Ethics. 1998. Statement on principles guiding care at the end-of-life. *Bull Am Coll Surg* 83:46.

American College of Surgeons, Committee on Ethics and Surgical Palliative Care Task Force. 2005. Principles of palliative care. *Bull Am Coll Surg* 90:34–35.

Billroth, T. 1881. Open letter to Dr. L. Wittelshofer. *Wiener Medizinische Wochenschrift* 31 (1): 162–66.

Brooks, B. 1944. Psychosomatic surgery. *Ann Surg* 119:289–99.

Caralis, P. V., and J. S. Hammond. 1992. Attitudes of medical students, house staff, and faculty physicians toward euthanasia and termination of life-sustaining treatment. *Critical Care Medicine* 20 (5): 683–90.

Dunn, G. P., R. Martensen, and D. Weissman, eds. 2009. *Surgical palliative care: A resident's guide.* Chicago: American College of Surgeons.

Dunphey, J. E. 1976. Annual Oration: On caring for the patient with cancer. *N Engl J of Med* 295:313–19.

Easson, A. M., J. A. Crosby, and S. L. Librach. 2001. Discussion of death and dying in surgical textbooks. *Am J Surg* 182 (1): 34–39.

Feifel, H., S. Hanson, R. James et al. 1967. Physicians consider death. *Proceedings of the American Psychological Association* 201:201–2.

Galante, J. M., T. L. Bowles, V. P. Khatri, P. D. Schneider, J. E. Goodnight, R. J. Bold Jr. 2005. Experience and attitudes of surgeons toward palliation in cancer. *Arch Surg* 140 (9): 873–80.

Halsted, W. S. 1894–95. The results of operations for the cure of cancer of the breast performed at the Johns Hopkins Hospital from June, 1899, to January, 1894. *Johns Hopkins Hospital Reports* 4:297.

Hinshaw, D. 2005. Spiritual issues in surgical palliative care. *Surg Clin N Am* 85 (2): 257–72.

Hofmann, B., L. L. Håheim, and J. A. Søreide. 2005. Ethics of palliative surgery in patients with cancer. *Br J Surg* 92:802–9.

Kirk, R. M., A. O. Mansfield, and J. P. S. Cochrane, eds. 1999. *Clinical surgery in general. Royal College of Surgeons,* 3rd edn. London: Churchill-Livingstone.

Koller, M., C. Nies, and W. Lorenz. 2004. Quality of life issues in palliative surgery. In *Surgical Palliative Care*, eds. G. P. Dunn and A. G. Johnson, 94–111. Oxford: Oxford University Press.

Krizek, T. 2001. Spiritual dimensions of surgical palliative care. *Surg Onc Clin N Am* 10 (1): 39–56.

Lindemann, E. 1944. Symptomatology and management of acute grief. *American Journal of Psychiatry* 101 (2): 141–48.

McCahill, L. E., R. Krouse, D. Chu, G. Juarez, G. C. Uman, B. Ferrell, L.D. Wagman. 2002. Indications and use of palliative surgery- results of Society of Surgical Oncology survey. *Ann Surg Oncol* 9 (1): 104–12.

Milch, R. A., and G. P. Dunn. 1997. The surgeon and palliative care. *Bull Am Coll Surg* 82:15–18.

Miner, T. 2005. Palliative surgery for advanced cancer. Lessons learned in patient selection and outcome assessment. *Am J Clin Onc* 28 (4): 411–14.

Miner, T. J., D. P. Jaques, H. Tavaf-Motamen, C. D. Shriver. 1999. Decision making on surgical palliation based on patient outcome data. *Am J Surg* 177:150–54.

Nuland, S. B. 1994. *How we die: Reflections on life's final chapter*. New York: Alfred A. Knopf.

Nuland, S. B. 2001. A surgeon's reflections on the care of the dying. *Surg Onc Clin N Am* 10:1–6.

Organ, C., Jr., and M. M. Kosiba. 1987. *A century of black surgeons: The USA experience*, vol. 1. Norman, Oklahoma: Transcript Press.

Rabow, M. W., and S. J. McPhee. 2002. Deficiencies in end-of-life care content in medical textbooks. *J Am Geriatr Soc* 50 (2): 397.

Saunders, C., and N. Sykes. 1993. *The management of terminal malignant disease,* edn. 3. London: Edward Arnold.

Society of Critical Care Medicine Ethics Committee. 1992. Attitudes of critical care professionals concerning foregoing life sustaining treatments. *Critical Care Medicine* 20:320.

Rosenberg S. A., J. Tepper, E. Glatstein, J. Costa, A. Baker, M. Brennan, E. V. DeMoss, et al. 1982. Quality of life assessment in extremity sarcoma trials. *Surgery* 91:17–23.

Tarpley, J. L., and M. J. Tarpley. 2002. Spirituality in surgical practice. *J Am Coll Surg* 194 (5): 642–47.

The SUPPORT Clinical Investigators. 1995. A controlled trial to improve care for seriously ill hospitalized patients. The study to understand prognoses and preferences for outcomes and risks of treatment (SUPPORT). *JAMA* 274 (20): 1591–98.

Whipple, A. O. 1942. Present day surgery of the pancreas. *N Eng J Med* 226:515.

Zimmerman, J. M. 1979. Experience with a hospice-care program for the terminally ill. *Annals of Surgery* 189 (6): 683–90.

Zimmerman, J. M. 1981. *Hospice-complete care of the terminally ill.* Baltimore: Urban and Schwarzenberg.

5 Sedation in Palliative Care and Its Impact on Nutrition

Kris C. P. Vissers, Jeroen G. J. Hasselaar, and Constans A. Verhagen

CONTENTS

5.1 INTRODUCTION

According to the definition of the World Health Organization, palliative care's objective is to improve the quality of life of patients suffering incurable diseases. The focus is on symptom control and, where possible, symptom prevention.

When symptoms such as pain, delirium, agitation, dyspnea, nausea/vomiting, or psychological distress prove to be refractory to other treatment options, sedation may be considered.

Questions regarding the utility of nutrition and hydration in sedated patients arise. It should be stressed that several patients in palliative care already need specific feeding arrangements, because the disease itself may be responsible for changes in digestion, absorption, and the possibility of food intake.

5.2 WHAT IS PALLIATIVE SEDATION?

The definition of palliative sedation is: "deliberately reducing consciousness so that the patient no longer experiences discomfort" (Levy and Cohen 2005). This describes the fact that patients are sedated to palliate refractory symptoms. Symptoms at the end-of-life are considered refractory when all conventional symptom treatment has failed to alleviate suffering within the available time frame and at an acceptable risk-benefit ratio (de Graeff and Dean 2007).

The following types of sedation can be identified: continuous deep sedation, proportional sedation, and intermittent sedation. Proportional sedation deliberately lowers the patient's consciousness to an extent that the refractory symptoms are no longer felt to be intolerable. If possible, the sedation will not be complete and communication may be preserved as long as experiencing discomfort is balanced against losing consciousness completely. Deep and continuous sedation (DCS) is the extreme form of palliative sedation used in those cases who continue to suffer during more superficial forms of palliative sedation. Intermittent sedation can be discontinued to permit reflection and discussion about the benefits and burdens of the sedation intervention by the healthcare team and the family and, if feasible, the patient. Theoretically, intermittent sedation may break an escalating cycle of refractory symptoms and permit the resumption of non-sedating palliation (Vissers, Hasselaar, and Verhagen 2007). Table 5.1 gives a summary of the characteristics of deep continuous and intermittent sedation.

Palliative sedation is an extraordinary sedation, because most physicians do not use this technique frequently. It is estimated that a physician performs this technique a mean of 0–5 times a year (Hasselaar et al. 2008). This results in a relatively low level of expertise, making the choice between the different types of palliative sedation difficult. The choice of the type of sedation will depend on the patient's general condition and life expectancy.

5.3 APPROPRIATE USE OF PALLIATIVE SEDATION

Once the diagnosis "incurable disease" is made, the patient and his relatives should be informed about the expected disease trajectory and the possible palliative care treatments that can and will be used to ensure optimal quality of life. As time and the disease progresses, the patient should also be informed about the scenarios for dying and potential associated complications. Within these specific scenarios, end-of-life decisions including the possibility of palliative sedation should be discussed. Patients and their relatives should receive information about the prognosis, the refractory nature of the key symptoms, and the risks and benefits of sedation. Before considering the use of palliative sedation, a non-resuscitation will must be documented from the conscious patient or proxy (Gonzalez Baron, Gomez Raposo, and Pinto Martin 2005; Levy and Cohen 2005; Plonk and Arnold 2005).

Prior to starting palliative sedation, the patient and proxies should have received extensive information regarding the different sedation options. Informed consent must be obtained from the patient or the patient's proxies and, if not already in place, an order to withhold cardiopulmonary resuscitation must be instituted before sedation is initiated.

According to national guidelines, palliative sedation is only indicated in the terminal phase of life, more specifically, in the last two weeks of life when intractable symptoms cause serious discomfort and no other treatment can provide relief of this discomfort within the available time frame (Morita et al. 2005; Verkerk et al. 2007). Predicting the exact moment of dying is not usually possible and patients and their relatives expect an intervention that alleviates symptoms. It is however critical to postpone the use of DCS until death is imminent to avoid serious problems and discomfort for the patient and his relatives.

Deep continuous palliative sedation has the objective to alleviate unbearable symptoms that are refractory and cannot be resolved in due time by less deep forms of sedation. Consultation should preferably be sought from palliative care experts who are skilled in identifying refractory symptoms and have experience in the whole spectrum of palliative sedation.

TABLE 5.1
Characteristics of Light Sedation, Intermittent Sedation, and Deep Continuous Sedation

Domain	Characteristics	Light Sedation	Intermittent	Deep Continuous
Medical	Imminent death	Often near future	Often near future	Prerequisite
	Refractory symptom(s)[a]	Often or difficult	Often or difficult	Prerequisite
	Titration of sedatives	Proportionally[b]	Proportionally	Until deep sleep
	Other medication (as indicated)	Full spectrum often orally	Full spectrum often orally	Limited for comfort only parenterally (S.C. or I.V.)
	Eating and/or drinking	Possible; often independently	Possible; often independently	Impossible
	Artificial feeding and/or hydration	If indicated	If indicated	Often counterproductive
Care	Monitoring symptom relief	Yes, input patient	Yes, input patient	Yes, observational
	Adequate feeding and/or hydration	Requires attention	Mainly intact	No issue (anymore)
	Special interventions (bladder catheter, bedsore prevention, mouth care, etc.)	Attention required	Seldom necessary	Always necessary
Social	Communication with patient	Slightly restricted	Normal at awakening	Impossible
	End-of-life rituals	Not yet necessarily	Not yet necessarily	Just before sedation
	Relatives are prepared for dying process	In principle but not inevitably imminent	In principle but not inevitably imminent	Yes
Ethical	Autonomy of patient	Still expressible	Still expressible	Must be cared for
	Life shortening	Not in effect or meant	Not in effect or meant	Not in effect or meant
	Less harmful/rigid alternatives are not available	Prerequisite	Prerequisite	Prerequisite
	Sedation is proportional to level of patient discomfort	Yes	Yes	Yes[c]
Legal	Objectives	No legal restrictions	No legal restrictions	No legal restrictions
	Regulations	According to medical guidelines and good clinical praxis	According to medical guidelines and good clinical praxis	According to medical guidelines and good clinical praxis
Other	Recommendation	Consultation if experience is limited	Consultation if experience is limited	Consultation if experience is limited

[a] No sedation for psycho-existential problems exclusively.

[b] Proportional sedation demands a careful titration of sedatives at the lowest dose possible aimed at symptom relief balanced with preservation of communication possibilities.

[c] Even deep and continuous sedation must be proportional. A less rigid sedation protocol is not effective or sound and ample reasoning suggests it is not effective.

TABLE 5.2
Criteria for Selecting Patients for Sedation

1. The illness is irreversible and death is expected imminently
2. The symptoms for which relief is sought are clearly defined and understood
3. These defined symptoms are unbearable for the patient and are truly refractory
4. Informed consent must be obtained from the patient or the patient's proxy
5. The patient and proxies have received extensive information relative to complete or deep sedation and the potential alternatives such as light sedative measures
6. Contraindications for sedation are absent
7. If not already in place, an order to withhold cardiopulmonary resuscitation must be instituted before sedation is initiated
8. Consultation should be sought from palliative care experts who are skilled in the use of sedation
9. Family members remain involved at the behest of the patient
10. The staff involved in the patient's care should be informed and engaged
11. Basic healthcare actions are maintained (such as prevention of bed sores, mouth care, continuation of essential drugs to prevent exaggeration of preventable symptoms under sedation, bladder catheter, and timely evacuation of stools)
12. Attention should be paid to personal care for the patient and proxies, with the availability of psychological support
13. Specifics of sedation medications and patient response will be documented in the medical record on a regular basis
14. After the patient has passed away, mourners and attending nurses must be offered an opportunity to discuss their feelings, remaining questions and experiences with the deceased

The medications used for the sedation must be documented in the medical record together with the patient's responses as observed by the treating physician, attending nurses, and next of kin. During palliative sedation, basic healthcare actions and care must be continued at a high level, such as prevention of bed sores, mouth care, and continuation of essential drugs to prevent exaggeration of preventable symptoms under sedation, bladder catheter, and timely evacuation of stools.

Special attention should be given to personal care for the patient and proxies. Lodging facilities should consist of a nice room, possibility for privacy for the family, and a place to rest. Finally, a dedicated team should be permanently available with attention to the multidimensional aspects of the palliative care trajectory. This team will be composed of a treating physician with special expertise in palliative care and palliative sedation, nurses trained in palliative care, psychologists, and consultants in spiritual care. Family members remain involved and attend the patient. The staff involved in the patient's care should be informed and engaged (Vissers et al. 2007).

The criteria for selecting patients for sedation are outlined in Table 5.2.

5.4 CURRENT PRACTICE IN PALLIATIVE SEDATION

A review of the role of sedation in palliative care (Hasselaar, Verhagen, and Vissers 2009) clearly showed the increasing interest in this technique since the turn of the century.

Three consecutive surveys conducted in the Flemish part of Belgium regarding the practices of end-of-life show that in 1998 deep sedation was not reported, whereas in 2001 and 2008 it was reported in respectively 8.2% and 14.5% of cases (Bilsen et al. 2009).

Surveys conducted in the Netherlands in 2003–2005 and 2007 provide information regarding the frequency of use and the practice of palliative sedation. It is important that, in 2005, the Royal Dutch Medical Association (RDMA) published a national guideline for palliative sedation

(RDMA 2007). In this guideline palliative sedation is considered a common medical practice as laid down in the Dutch Medical Treatment Act, making it mandatory for all physicians within the country.

These surveys also indicate that the implementation of national guidelines clearly changed the practice of palliative sedation. More physicians discussed sedation with patients some time in advance. Patient request for euthanasia before sedation occurred significantly less often in the second survey period (Hasselaar, Verhagen, Wolff et al. 2009).

5.5 GUIDELINES FOR PALLIATIVE SEDATION

There are very few guidelines on palliative sedation, mainly because of the absence of randomized controlled trials, which are impossible to perform in this frail population. Moreover, there is no reference treatment for the management of refractory symptoms at the end-of-life. Besides the already-mentioned guidelines issued by the RDMA, two other guidelines are worth mentioning (Morita et al. 2005; de Graeff and Dean 2007). These guidelines provide comparable recommendations regarding the different steps before, during, and after palliative sedation, considering the care for the patient, the family and relatives, and the caregivers. However, the subject of nutrition and hydration of sedated patients remains complicated and controversial.

The Dutch guidelines indicate that medically assisted nutrition in patients sedated for palliative symptom control is not an issue, because of the patient's condition and the commonly observed fact that terminally ill patients hardly have food intake prior to sedation. For hydration this guideline differentiates between patients who already refused fluid intake prior to sedation and those who still have sufficient oral or parenteral fluid intake. Depending on the competency of the patient, the issue of continuing or stopping will be discussed with the patient and/or the legal representatives. Food and fluid administration should only be considered when it does not harm the patient, does not cause unnecessary suffering, and does not represent a useless medical act (RDMA 2007).

The Japanese guidelines take a comparable but more moderate point of view, whereby artificial food and fluid administration must be made possible when the patient or the relatives request it. As in the Dutch guidelines, it is made clear that the patient and the proxies can only form an informed decision when all aspects of the sedation and consequences of nutrition and hydration are clearly and realistically explained (Morita et al. 2005).

5.6 NUTRITIONAL PATTERNS OF TERMINALLY ILL PATIENTS

Many terminally ill patients have a reduced oral intake that may be attributed to physical obstruction, anorexia/cachexia syndrome, generalized weakness, bowel obstruction, or loss of appetite (Good et al. 2008). The most important obstruction for nutritional intake is the fact that the patient usually becomes less conscious when death is imminent by a natural loss of physiological processes in the dying phase and therefore less able to take or receive nutrition orally.

Management of this condition may include medically assisted nutrition, which can be given via a tube inserted into any part of the gastrointestinal tract or intravenously. In a recent Cochrane review this technique was judged to involve ethical controversies (Good et al. 2008). First, there is no unanimity regarding the perception of medically assisted nutrition as a medical intervention or a basic provision of comfort. Secondly, the problem arises as to who should decide on artificial feeding and hydration in patients who are no longer competent to make their own decisions. The Cochrane review focused on the value of medically assisted nutrition in palliative care patients in general. The main findings are that there are no randomized or prospectively controlled trials on the subject and the prospective non-controlled trials are judged to be of low quality. Hence no recommendations regarding medically assisted nutrition can be made for palliative care patients according to the methods accepted by Cochrane reviews.

5.7 FEEDING AND HYDRATION IN TERMINALLY ILL PATIENTS

5.7.1 Beneficial Effects of Nutrition and Hydration

Hydration and feeding are considered essential for survival. Indeed, laymen consider nutrition and hydration a necessary part of basic human treatment of any patient at any stage of any disease. Nutrition and hydration are judged important to allow organs to function normally and to prevent hunger and thirst. Feeding and hydration are also considered as signs of love and caring. This explains the perception of people that withdrawing nutrition and, even more so, hydration will hasten death, which is considered controversial.

5.7.2 Detrimental Effects of Nutrition and Hydration

This elemental knowledge in medicine may not hold true for dying patients or for patients in an end stage of their disease. In terminally ill patients the objective of the treatment is inducing comfort and symptom control. Moreover, these patients often have renal and other organ failure. Excess liquid administration may cause fluid retention resulting in nausea, vomiting, aspiration, edema, and increased secretions. These conditions may in turn cause intolerable symptoms due to iatrogenic cardiac or lung failure.

There is no compelling evidence that withholding nutrition or hydration increases suffering in the dying patient. Table 5.3 summarizes the points to consider when making the decision on hydration.

5.7.3 Ethical Concerns Regarding Nutrition and Hydration

In the second edition of the IAHPC Manual of Palliative Care (Doyle and Woodruff 2009), the ethical dimension of hydration and nutrition is brought back to a medical question: "Will this particular intervention restore or enhance the quality of life of the particular patient?". If the answer is yes, and it can be justified on the best clinical grounds, then it is ethically right to do it. When, on the contrary, the answer is no, it should not be done.

There are other arguments to consider in the discussion of artificial hydration. Withholding fluids from a terminally ill patient may result in a dry mouth, but this can be well palliated topically by adjusted mouth care. Normally withholding hydration should result in thirst, but most dying patients do not complain of thirst.

A second concern in withholding fluids is the fact that dehydration may also provoke a diminished conscious state. Several reports and one randomized controlled trial showed no correlation between hydration and cognition in terminally ill patients (Dalal and Bruera 2004).

Dehydration may on the other hand be responsible for reduced urine output, which means less movement and less incontinence. Also, pulmonary secretions are diminished, thus reducing dyspnea

TABLE 5.3
Points to Consider when Making the Decision on Artificial Feeding and Hydration

Question
1. Is the patient capable of autonomous feeding/drinking?
2. Is the patient dehydrated?
3. Is the patient cachectic ?
4. Is the life expectancy longer than 2 weeks?
5. What are the symptoms caused or aggravated by dehydration?
6. Do the expected advantages of feeding outweigh the expected disadvantages?
7. Do the expected advantages of hydration outweigh the expected disadvantages?
8. Do the patient and family agree to artificial feeding/hydration?

TABLE 5.4
Possible Administration Routes of Nutrition and Fluids

Route	Nutrition	Fluid	Comments
Subcutaneous		√	24 hrs continuous infusion or intermittent administration
Intravenous	√	√	Peripheral or central line (may be present for other purposes)
Enteral	√	√	Nasogastric tube or gastrostomy
Proctoclysis		√	When other routes of hydration are not possible

and terminal congestion. The reduced gastrointestinal secretions will lessen nausea, vomiting, and diarrhea, and finally the risk of edema and effusions is reduced and existing ascites may be absorbed.

When the patient is not capable of independent oral intake, artificial feeding and hydration may be considered. The modalities for artificial feeding and hydration are outlined in Table 5.4. Artificial feeding and hydration by means of a drip may create the false hope of a reversible situation, and the drip forms a barrier between the patient and the relatives. Moreover, unnecessary feeding and hydration may induce vomiting and potentially aspiration, which could be harmful to the patient. Because the effects of artificial hydration in a terminal patient seem limited from a medical perspective, there is no reason for a general recommendation to continue or start artificial hydration during palliative sedation and the issue seems best decided on within the individual physician–patient relationship, as one guideline recommends (Morita et al. 2005).

The potential benefits and disadvantages of artificial feeding and hydration in terminally ill patients are summarized in Table 5.5.

5.8 NUTRITION IN SEDATED PATIENTS

There are no guidelines on nutrition in patients under palliative sedation. Therefore, the recommendations listed below are only expert opinion.

5.8.1 Important Points to Consider

A distinction should be made between deep continuous sedation and intermittent or light sedation. Only DCS will make autonomous feeding by the patient him of herself impossible and could, therefore, theoretically harm the patient.

5.8.2 Continuous Sedation

Patients eligible for deep continuous palliative sedation have a life expectancy that normally will not exceed 2 weeks. It has been estimated that 7 or 8 out of 10 patients that are indicated for continuous palliative sedation have already stopped oral intake before the start of sedation (Hasselaar, Verhagen, and Vissers 2009). Therefore most controversy surrounds patients with artificial hydration or with considerable oral intake at the time of starting continuous sedation. Many patients express, even early on in their disease, a disgust and aversion for food as it makes them nauseated, and induces vomiting and/or causes cramps and diarrhea. In these cases, no parenteral or

TABLE 5.5
Advantages and Disadvantages of Nutrition and Hydration According to Route

Advantages	Oral	Artificial
Medical		
Provides basic needs	yes	yes
Nutrition relieves hunger	yes	yes
Fluid relieves thirst		
Fluid prevents/alleviates symptoms such as: confusion, agitation, and neuromuscular irritability	yes	yes
Emotional		
Response to family's emotional concerns	yes	yes
Disadvantages		
Medical		
Fluid increases urine output, pulmonary secretions, risk of edema and ascites	yes	yes
Sedated patient does not present those symptoms	yes	yes
Emotional		
Instrumentation may give the impression of a curative intervention generates false hope for reversibility of the patient's situation	no	yes
Instrumentation creates barrier between patient and relatives	no	yes

intravenous feeding will be initiated either. Artificial feeding is expected to be a futile medical intervention in a dying patient and may even harm the patient with potential side effects.

In patients who already receive artificial oral or parenteral nutrition, the administration of food supplements will be halted for the same reasons as has been discussed for initiating artificial feeding above.

The controversy lies in the need for hydration (Dalal and Bruera 2004; Dalal, Del Fabbro, and Bruera 2009). In contrast to inadequate feeding for a restricted episode, withholding fluids from patients may be considered as an act that may shorten life, particularly when these patients have considerable oral intake at the start of continuous sedation. As long as the dying process induces the patient to stop the intake of fluids and death has been accepted, no ethical controversy will arise. But in cases where sedation prevents an adequate intake, uneasiness considering artificial hydration may arise. If death is expected within due time, artificial hydration may not change the outcome. Moreover, a nasal gastric drip or intravenous hydration may have numerous adverse effects including lung aspiration, worsening edema, increasing secretions and unnecessarily prolonging the naturally evolving dying process (Plonk and Arnold 2005). All these acts do have an important negative impact on the quality of life and the quality of dying. If death is not expected within a short time frame, sedation that interrupts adequate intake of fluids should not be undertaken as long as the patient himself is willing to continue intake.

On pure medical indications, it seems logical to stop food and fluid administration in patients whose death is imminent. When, however, death cannot be predicted to be imminent, intermittent sedation should be preferred.

5.8.3 Intermittent Sedation

For patients with refractory symptoms where intermittent sedation proves to be adequate, oral food and liquid intake will be possible and acceptable between periods of sleep. During intermittent sedation the patient has some respite and the general condition may improve to such a point that sedation is no longer needed or evolve to a natural dying phase. Intermittent sedation preserves the possibility of adequate food and fluid intake as far as the function of the body to digest and absorb has remained intact. This form of sedation does not influence the natural course and the patient himself will be able to express to what extent he may experience benefit and or harm from any intake. Nevertheless, during intermittent sedation, signs and symptoms of inadequate intake should be monitored carefully (Dalal et al. 2009). When feeding, the patient should be fully awake, reactive and able to swallow normally. Also, there should be adequate periods of awake time. This is especially true when signs of imminent dying are absent. On the contrary, as the condition of the patient deteriorates following the natural evolution of the underlying disease to a dying phase, feeding and fluid intake should not be forced, in order to prevent medically induced harm to the patient (Dalal and Bruera 2004).

5.8.4 Light Sedation

For those patients who have light or superficial sedation, oral feeding and drinking may be considered provided the patient is able to swallow normally and he remains in a phase in which feeding and drinking may be beneficial. All remarks under intermittent sedation hold true for this condition also. The main difference will be that the depth of superficial sedation may be changed according to the needs of the patient in order to sedate in proportion to the suffering experienced. Such a stepwise approach may evolve to a stage at which the patient is no longer able to maintain adequate food and fluid intake. Attending nurses and the responsible physicians should monitor intake cautiously.

5.9 ETHICAL CONSIDERATIONS OF NUTRITION

From an ethical point of view, the patient has the right to decide if fluid and food intake should be continued or stopped. The majority of patients under proportional, superficial, or intermittent sedation are capable of continuing or stopping drinking and eating according to their wishes and biological needs. In case of a need for artificial feeding and hydration, the decision to start or withhold such an intervention should be an act of shared decision making. Even potentially beneficial interventions should always be weighed against potential disadvantages. But as soon as a medical intervention has been judged advantageous, the patient or next of kin may insist on the proper execution of such treatment. The patient is always obliged to accept or refuse any intervention, even if a potential benefit can be expected. No patient has the right to force a medical intervention to be executed if the indication is missing. Of course any decision by the patient or next of kin can only be made based on accurate information provided by healthcare professionals. In cognitively impaired patients, who may no longer be able to express their own whishes, the next of kin have the obligation to reconstruct the most likely choice of their beloved one. In cases where the evidence for and against an intervention is less clear, or in cases where important patient values are at stake, shared decision making between professionals and the patient/family seems the best way to attain a good medical policy.

Any conscious and decisive patient has the right to exert his autonomous will to forego life-prolonging interventions.

When a patient, suffering incurable disease, has deliberately stopped eating and drinking in an attempt to hasten his death, the patient's decision should be respected. This may not limit access to palliative sedation, provided that there is a clear medical indication.

Ethical and moral problems arise in those situations where culture or religion dictate that life should be respected and maintained with medical interventions regardless of the terminal condition of the patient or his/her own wishes for withdrawal of medical treatment. Feeding and providing drinks is, in several cultures, synonymous with love and caring. The idea that a beloved terminally ill patient should also suffer hunger and thirst is unacceptable in those groups of people, even if it is not true from a medical perspective.

Cultural differences should of course be respected, though all efforts should be made to clearly explain the potential benefits and risks of medically assisted nutrition and hydration in continuously sedated patients. Moreover, a professional caregiver may never endanger the safety of his patient by applying a medically ineffective and even potentially harmful intervention based on cultural arguments only. However, worries should be addressed carefully, for example mouth care may be a very important treatment for both patient and relatives to clearly show that the patient is still a appreciated person during his final days or hours.

5.10 APPLICATIONS TO OTHER AREAS OF TERMINAL OR PALLIATIVE CARE

Palliative sedation is mainly an intervention aimed at controlling symptoms of the dying patient. In this stage of life considerations of maintaining organ functioning are no longer applicable. In earlier stages of palliative care the decisions will be made based on the patient's general condition, the life expectancy, and the patient's own will.

5.11 PRACTICAL METHODS AND TECHNIQUES

Intermittent and light sedation as a technique can be considered as a sedation in the operation room. The medications and the doses will be adapted according to the patient's needs. Care should be taken to switch essential oral medication to a parenteral route when the patient becomes unable to take them orally.

When the indication for deep continuous palliative sedation is clearly established and the patient and/or his proxies have provided informed consent, care should be taken to make sure that the patient and his family clearly understand that once the sedation is started there is no possibility for communication left. When necessary the essential medication should be administered parenterally, mainly by the subcutaneous route. Sedation can be achieved by increasing the dose of the sedatives already used by the patient. Theoretically sedation will be started with benzodiazepines. When this induces insufficient symptom control, additional hypnotics and antipsychotic drugs may be considered. For hospitalized or institutionalized patients where the treatment can be supervised by an anesthesiologist, the use of a narcoleptic drug as propofol can be indicated.

Increasing the dose of morphine to reduce the patient's consciousness is judged to be a medical error because the patient may become confused but not sedated. Moreover, increasing the dose of morphine may induce neurotoxicity, also indicated as "morphine-induced hyperalgesia," which is characterized by hyperalgesia, delirium, and myoclonus.

The nurses should follow a care program dedicated to patients under sedation. This includes observation of the primary symptoms that were the reason for applying sedation, and potential new problems. They should monitor the general sense of comfort and peace of the patient and next of kin. In patients with intermittent or superficial sedation they will monitor duration of sedation, depth of sedation, and the balance between preserving communication and palliation of existing complaints more intensively. Especially in these cases they should also monitor adequate intake and the level of consciousness during intake to prevent complications.

KEY POINTS

- There are three levels of palliative sedation that cover the whole spectrum of proportionally applied sedation in the palliative phase:
  - Intermittent sedation with restricted periods of induced sleep and consequently symptom control.
  - Light sedation whereby the degree of sedation is adapted to the patient's need, but communication and intake remain (partially) intact.
  - Deep continuous sedation.

- The role of nutrition and hydration depends on the patient's general condition, and ability and willingness to accept food and beverages.
- Deeply sedated patients cannot take oral food and drinks. In DCS in the palliative phase artificial feeding and hydration has no documented added medical value and it may even induce complications.
- For intermittent and lightly sedated patients, nutrition and hydration will be administered according to the patient's will.

SUMMARY POINT

- Palliative sedation consists of deliberately reducing the patient's level of consciousness to control symptoms in order to assure comfort. Palliative sedation in the strict sense of DCS is only indicated in patients whose death is imminent and who suffer symptoms that cannot be controlled otherwise.

REFERENCES

Bilsen, J., J. Cohen, K. Chambaere, G. Pousset, B. D. Onwuteaka-Philipsen, F. Mortier, and L. Deliens. 2009. Medical end-of-life practices under the euthanasia law in Belgium. *N Engl J Med* 361 (11): 1119–21.

Dalal, S., and E. Bruera. 2004. Dehydration in cancer patients: To treat or not to treat. *J Support Oncol* 2 (6): 467–79, 483.

Dalal, S., E. Del Fabbro, and E. Bruera. 2009. Is there a role for hydration at the end-of-life? *Curr Opin Support Palliat Care* 3 (1): 72–78.

de Graeff, A., and M. Dean. 2007. Palliative sedation therapy in the last weeks of life: A literature review and recommendations for standards. *J Palliat Med* 10 (1): 67–85.

Doyle, D., and R. Woodruff. 2009. *The IAHPC manual of palliative care*, 2nd Edition. IAHPC Press. Accessed March 2010.

Gonzalez Baron, M., C. Gomez Raposo, and A. Pinto Marin. 2005. Sedation in clinical oncology. *Clin Transl Oncol* 7 (7): 295–301.

Good, P., J. Cavenagh, M. Mather, and P. Ravenscroft. 2008. Medically assisted nutrition for palliative care in adult patients. *Cochrane Database Syst Rev* Oct 8 (4): CD006274.

Hasselaar, J. G., R. P. Reuzel, M. E. van den Muijsenbergh, R. T. Koopmans, C. J. Leget, B. J. Crul, and K. C. Vissers. 2008. Dealing with delicate issues in continuous deep sedation. Varying practices among Dutch medical specialists, general practitioners, and nursing home physicians. *Arch Intern Med* 168 (5): 537–43.

Hasselaar, J. G., S. C. Verhagen, and K. C. Vissers. 2009. When cancer symptoms cannot be controlled: The role of palliative sedation. *Curr Opin Support Palliat Care* 3 (1): 14–23.

Hasselaar, J. G., S. C. Verhagen, A. P. Wolff, Y. Engels, B. J. Crul, and K. C. Vissers. 2009. Changed patterns in Dutch palliative sedation practices after the introduction of a national guideline. *Arch Intern Med* 169 (5): 430–37.

Levy, M. H., and S. D. Cohen. 2005. Sedation for the relief of refractory symptoms in the imminently dying: A fine intentional line. *Semin Oncol* 32 (2): 237–46.

Morita, T., S. Bito, Y. Kurihara, and Y. Uchitomi. 2005. Development of a clinical guideline for palliative sedation therapy using the Delphi method. *J Palliat Med* 8 (4): 716–29.

Plonk, W. M., Jr., and R. M. Arnold. 2005. Terminal care: The last weeks of life. *J Palliat Med* 8 (5): 1042–54.

RDMA. 2007. Guideline Palliative Sedation. http://knmg.artsennet.nl/uri/?uri=AMGATE_6059_100_TICH_R193567276369746. Accessed March 2010.

Verkerk, M., E. van Wijlick, J. Legemaate, and A. de Graeff. 2007. A national guideline for palliative sedation in the Netherlands. *J Pain Symptom Manage* 34 (6): 666–70.

Vissers, K. C., J. Hasselaar, and S. A. Verhagen. 2007. Sedation in palliative care. *Curr Opin Anaesthesiol* 20 (2): 137–42.

6 Quality of Life and Aspects of Diet and Nutrition in Dying Children

Michelle Koh and Finella Craig

CONTENTS

6.1 INTRODUCTION

The Association for Children's Palliative Care (ACT, Table 6.1) defines palliative care for children with life-limiting conditions as "an active and total approach to care, from the point of diagnosis or recognition, embracing physical, emotional, social and spiritual elements through to death and beyond. It focuses on enhancement of QOL for the child/young person and support for the family" (ACT 2009).

Children with a diagnosis of a life-limiting or life-threatening condition (Table 6.2) should gain access to palliative care services at the time of diagnosis. When considering nutrition in paediatric palliative care, we have to address not only the issues during the end-of-life phase of the child's illness, but also in the early stages of their care, when they may have many months or years of life ahead.

TABLE 6.1
Key Facts About the Association of Children's Palliative Care (ACT)

- ACT was established in 1988
- One of ACT's co-founders, Sister Frances Dominica, founded the world's first hospice for children, Helen House, in Oxford, England
- ACT works across the United Kingdom to achieve the best possible quality of life and care for every child who has a life-limiting or life-threatening condition and their family

ACT has three strategic objectives

- Campaigning for improved provision of children's palliative care services
- Working with professionals to support the delivery of the best possible care
- Informing families and empowering them to have a voice in the development of the services and policies that affect them

Nutrition in children has an important role in a child's normal development and learning. In a child with life-limiting/life-threatening disease, it impacts his QOL, ability to recover from crises and overall prognosis. Samson-Fang et al. (2002) demonstrated that poor nutritional status in children with cerebral palsy was correlated with increased hospitalisations, doctor visits and decreased participation in usual activities.

An unsafe swallow, gastro-oesophageal reflux, food intolerance, abdominal pain and constipation are frequently encountered in children with developmental disabilities. Schwarz et al. (2001) showed that in these children, successful management of feeding problems results in significantly improved energy consumption and nutritional status, and decreased morbidity.

However, obesity can also be problem, for example in children with DMD and CP. This may be exacerbated in children requiring high-dose or long-term steroids as part of their treatment, such as oncology patients whose treatment may include steroid therapy, and boys with DMD, where the early introduction of steroids has an important role in preserving the child's mobility.

Feeding also affects the emotional and social bonds between a child and his parents. Feeding and nourishing one's child is a fundamental instinct for every parent. Problems and decisions surrounding feeding and nutrition can be emotive and potentially distressing for families.

6.2 NUTRITIONAL ASSESSMENT

Growth measurements and the use of growth percentile charts are fundamental to the examination of the paediatric patient. Mascarenhas, Zemel, and Stallings (1998) recommend that patients with chronic complex needs should have appropriate nutritional assessments including:

TABLE 6.2
Key Definitions in Children's Palliative Care

Life-Limiting Conditions

Conditions for which there is no reasonable hope of cure and from which children or young people will die. Some of these conditions cause progressive deterioration rendering the child increasingly dependent on parents and carers

Life-Threatening Conditions

Conditions for which curative treatment may be feasible but can fail, such as cancer. Children in long-term remission or following successful curative treatment are not included

Source: From Association for Children's Palliative Care (ACT). 2009. Children's palliative care definitions. http://www.act.org.uk.

- Medical and nutritional history including dietary intake
- Physical examination
- Anthropometrics (weight, length or stature, head circumference, mid-arm circumference, triceps skin fold thickness) and use of appropriate anthropometric charts
- Pubertal staging
- Skeletal maturity staging
- Biochemical tests of nutritional status: micronutrients, protein and fat profiles
- For patients at risk of fractures, bone density scans can be used to assess bone mineralisation and the risk of fracture

Working closely with the wider multidisciplinary team is essential for a comprehensive assessment. Speech and language therapists are expert in assessing the safety of a child's swallow and aspiration risk. They can recommend if the child will benefit from having the consistency of their food modified. They may also suggest whether further investigations such as video fluoroscopy will be helpful.

Dieticians will often take a detailed dietary history from families, including the child's past dietary preferences as well as their current intake. They also assess the child's energy requirements according to their age, size and diagnosis. Dieticians then work closely with families to recommend appropriate interventions (calorie supplements, feed, volume, regimen, etc.) and to monitor the effect of their recommendations.

Further investigations should be tailored to the specific feeding or dietary issues that are identified and will be considered in the corresponding sections.

6.3 FEEDING AND NUTRITIONAL DIFFICULTIES IN CHILDREN WITH LIFE-LIMITING/LIFE-THREATENING DISEASE

6.3.1 Mechanical Difficulties: Unsafe Swallow, Gastro-Oesophageal Reflux (GOR)

A significant proportion of children with life-limiting diagnoses have mechanical difficulties with feeding and GOR. For example, children with neurodevelopmental or metabolic disorders may have feeding difficulties from birth or early infancy. Other children with progressive disorders such as DMD may establish normal feeding before losing their ability to feed orally. As the child's oropharyngeal control diminishes, he is unable to suck, chew and swallow and to coordinate the sequence of actions. Ultimately, this not only leads to undernutrition but also poses a significant risk of the child aspirating food into his lungs (Morton, Wheatley, and Minford 1999).

Difficulties with feeding also prolong the time it takes to feed the child and feeding becomes a stressful and distressing experience instead of an enjoyable and nurturing time.

A large proportion of children with life-limiting conditions also have significant problems with GOR and its related complications. Sullivan (2008) demonstrated that children with neurodevelopmental disabilities commonly have foregut dysmotility causing dysphagia from oesophageal dysmotility, GOR and delayed gastric emptying.

Further investigations helpful in identifying the severity and complications include a pH or impedance study to identify degree of acid and non-acid reflux, and a chest x-ray if pulmonary aspiration is suspected. A CT scan may be appropriate if chronic aspiration is present and intensive management is being considered for the patient.

6.3.2 Gut Dysfunction (Dysmotility and Hypersensitivity)

It is increasingly recognised that children with severe neurological disorders may develop gut dysfunction as their neurological disease progresses. Their underlying diagnoses include progressive, neurodegenerative disorders as well as static neurological disorders. The gut dysfunction is characterised by dysmotility and hypersensitivity to milk feeds.

The underlying mechanisms and pathophysiology are not clearly known. Altaf and Sood (2008) summarised that the enteric nervous system modulates motility, secretions, microcirculation, and immune and inflammatory responses of the gastrointestinal tract. A primary defect in the enteric neurons or central modulation in children with developmental disabilities could adversely affect intestinal motility, neurogastric reflexes and brain perception of visceral hyperalgesia.

It is also postulated that antral dysmotility exacerbated after fundoplication and sympathetic overactivity may contribute to the gut dysfunction (Carachi, Currie, and Steven 2009). In addition, these children are often on proton pump inhibitors and H_2-receptor antagonists, resulting in gastric hypochlorhydria and small bowel bacterial overgrowth.

The prime symptoms of gut dysfunction in these children are abdominal pain when being fed and vomiting. If the child has a gastrostomy or nasogastric tube (NGT) left on free drainage, large volumes of aspirate (either bile-stained or non-bile-stained) reflux back.

Typically, these symptoms gradually resolve when the milk feeds are stopped and recur when the feeds are recommenced. Once the gut dysfunction is established, a notable feature is the degree of pain and distress even a small amount, either in volume or concentration, of milk feed can trigger.

Over time, the child not only fails to thrive, but also steadily loses weight and subcutaneous fat stores, eventually resulting in muscle wasting. The child inevitably develops pressure sores, and is at high risk of infection and respiratory failure.

Investigating these children is difficult as the gut dysfunction generally occurs at the end-stages of their underlying illness and they are unlikely to tolerate any invasive procedure such as an endoscopy or impedance study. The few children who have undergone an endoscopy and biopsy have shown an eosinophilic infiltration of their intestinal mucosa; however, the significance of this is unclear. In addition, as the investigations make little difference to their overall management, it is difficult to justify the burden of putting the child through the invasive procedures.

There has been no successful management strategy reported. The pain is refractory to opioid and neuropathic analgesia and only resolves when the child's feed is stopped. Promotility agents are used empirically to address the reflux and vomiting. The child eventually ends up in a cycle of having his feed stopped and substituted with an oral rehydration solution, such as Dioralyte, when the symptoms are too distressing, and then being re-started on milk feeds when he has had a few comfortable days. The distress induced by the feeds and the malabsorption mean that the child has inadequate caloric intake and drastic weight loss, and this ultimately contributes to his end-of-life event.

6.4 PHYSIOLOGICAL AND OTHER CONTRIBUTORY FACTORS

Anorexia and weight loss are common symptoms in the paediatric palliative care population.

In oncology children, poor appetite and cachexia are frequent at presentation, through their treatment and during disease progression. Their carbohydrate, protein and fat metabolism is altered via cytokine-mediated pathways. In addition to the catabolic effects of their disease, their therapy frequently induces mucositis, alters taste sensation and causes nausea, further depressing their appetite (Ward et al. 2009). Malnutrition is an adverse risk factor for compliance to the chemotherapy and radiotherapy treatment regimen, and for disease-free outcome (Gómez-Almaguer, Ruiz-Argüelles, and Ponce-de-León 1998; Sala, Pencharz, and Barr 2004).

It is also important to address any other symptoms such as pain, dry mouth and constipation that may contribute to the child's lack of appetite and inability to eat.

6.4.1 Psychological/Social Influences

Depression and mood disorders contribute to appetite changes, usually a depressed appetite. It is also well recognised that there is a two-way relationship between mood and nutritional intake, where one's food intake can also have an effect on how one feels.

It is also important to recognise that children and parents may be deeply anxious about weight gain, especially if steroids are part of their therapy or symptom management. Older children and adolescents worry about their body image, whilst rapid weight gain makes the physical care of an already dependent child more difficult.

The social and cultural background of the child also influences his nutritional state. A review by Darmon and Drewnowski (2008) demonstrated that whole grains, lean meats, fish, low-fat dairy products, and fresh vegetables and fruit are more likely to be consumed by groups with greater affluence. In contrast, the consumption of energy-dense, nutrient-poor diets are associated with less affluent families.

In the context of a life-limiting/life-threatening illness, this can have important implications for outcome and QOL. Nutrition-related disorders, such as iron deficiency anaemia or rickets, will compound the child's disability and affect his prognosis.

6.5 END-OF-LIFE CARE

It is well recognised that loss of appetite and loss of interest in food is common in children who are dying (Theunissen et al. 2007; Hechler et al. 2008). Fluid and caloric requirements decrease as their underlying illness causes a deterioration and activity levels decrease (Thompson, MacDonald, and Holden 2006).

Artificial hydration and feeds need to be given judiciously. If the child is already on artificial hydration, it is essential to reassess the child's likely fluid requirement and appropriately reduce the amount being given. If the child had previously been orally feeding, it is not usually beneficial to start artificial hydration. The child can be given frequent sips of fluid and allowed to eat as he wishes. Close attention should also be paid to mouth care and care of pressure areas.

At the end-of-life, artificial hydration could alleviate signs of dehydration, but worsen peripheral oedema, ascites, pleural effusions (Morita et al. 2005), respiratory distress and frequent urination (Thompson et al. 2006). The potential benefits of artificial hydration therapy need to be weighed against the distress of worsening fluid retention.

6.6 MANAGEMENT

The management of feeding problems and optimising a child's nutrition begins with an open discussion with the family and, if appropriate, the child. It is important to establish the family and child's priorities and for them to feel that their concerns are recognised.

An individualised rather than 'blanket policy' approach in addressing these issues is essential. Moreover, decision making about feeding is a dynamic process, with changing needs at different stages of illness.

This care and attention from an early stage helps the family build a relationship of trust and mutual respect with the professional team, making discussions and decision-making easier when the child is deteriorating and the difficult issues surrounding limiting or withholding feeds and fluids arise.

If at all possible and safe, oral feeding should be encouraged and preserved. The expertise of the SALT and dietician should be sought to determine if the child's food should be modified, such as having softened or pureed solids, or thickened fluids. The dietician may suggest fortifying the child's normal diet to make it more calorific (e.g., by the addition of cream, butter, oil, etc.) or additional supplementation (e.g., high-energy milkshakes, etc.). They are also best placed to advise when oral feeding alone is no longer adequate or safe and artificial feeding should be considered.

The impact of introducing artificial feeding should not be underestimated. Whilst for health professionals tube feeding is a common, everyday reality, it represents significant change in the child's physical care, the psychological impact on the child and family, and the social impact of planning life around a feeding regimen.

Artificial feeding is almost universally emotive for families. It often represents deterioration in the child's condition, a progression onto the 'next stage' of the disease. Parents may feel a sense of failure, as nourishing their child was primarily their responsibility, and guilt over depriving their child of the pleasure of orally feeding.

Petersen et al. (2006) examined the perceptions of gastrostomy tube feeding by caregivers of children with cerebral palsy. They found that most caregivers had an initial negative response when the gastrostomy was recommended. They generally perceived gastrostomy feeding as "unnatural". Parents persisted in orally feeding some children even though meals were an unpleasant experience (despite advice against oral feeding, in some cases). Although the children received a complete formula through the gastrostomy, some families gave other foods through the gastrostomy (juice, cereal, soup or table food). Understanding these attitudes can help clinicians to develop effective, family-centred, appropriate interventions for gastrostomy feeding in children with CP.

Resistance to tube feeding is also common from the children themselves. Younger children often resist NGT placements and older children are concerned about their body image—having a visible tube as well as potential weight gain. Home adaptations may be required to accommodate the increased care and the equipment that comes with artificial feeding, reinforcing the perception of disability that parents may resist.

Care planning for the child also becomes more difficult. The child's carers will need to be trained in giving the artificial feed and in managing any difficulties that may arise, such as the child 'vomiting up' their NGT. The various care settings include the child's school, respite care and extended family carers.

6.7 TUBE FEEDING

Several studies have supported the benefits of tube feeding. The indications for tube feeding are outlined in Table 6.3. Sullivan et al. (2005) reported that after the introduction of gastrostomy feeding in children with cerebral palsy, increase in weight and subcutaneous fat deposition were noted. Almost all parents reported a significant improvement in their child's health and a significant reduction in time spent feeding. In the study period, complications were rare, with no evidence of an increase in respiratory complications.

TABLE 6.3
Key Indications for Consideration of Tube Feeding

- Unsafe swallow and aspiration
- Inability to consume at least 60% of energy needs by mouth
- Total feeding time is greater than 4 hours a day. Oral feeding is unpleasant
- Weight loss or no weight gain for a period of 3 months (or sooner for younger children or infants)
- Weight-for-height less than second percentile for age and sex

Note: Thompson, MacDonald, and Holden (2006) recommend that tube feeding should be considered if one or more of the above are present.

6.7.1 Types of Feeding Tubes

6.7.1.1 Nasogastric Tubes

As the child's oral feeding begins to falter, the use of an NGT is usually the first intervention. For children who still retain some ability to orally feed, NGT feeding can be used as complementary or 'top-up' feeding in addition to their oral intake. In children whose swallow is deemed unsafe for any oral intake, oral-motor and taste stimulation should be encouraged and they should be included during mealtimes with the family.

There are two types of NGT commonly used. A long-term tube is made from silicone elastomer (known as 'silk tubes') and can be left in for 4–6 weeks. A short-term tube is made of polyvinyl chloride and needs to be changed every 5–7 days. Both tubes are easy to insert and can be changed by community nurses at the child's home or school.

6.7.1.2 Gastrostomy Tubes

For these reasons, when children require long-term tube feeding, a gastrostomy tube should be considered. These are now usually inserted by the percutaneous endoscopic route or, less commonly, by a formal surgical procedure. Both techniques can combine a gastrostomy tube insertion with a fundoplication should the child require this for management of GOR.

Once the gastrostomy tract is established, the gastrostomy tube can subsequently be changed for a skin-level gastrostomy device. These devices (commonly called gastrostomy 'buttons') sit flush with the skin and can be left in place for several months. They are easy to change and can be done in the outpatient setting or, if community nurses are trained, in the child's home.

Gastrostomy tubes can be used to administer medications but the feeds are special formulations, which are recommended and monitored by a dietician and prescribed by the child's GP.

6.7.1.3 Nasojejunal and Jejunostomy Tubes

Jejunal feeding is helpful with the management of GOR and the prevention of aspiration events. Jejunal tubes can be placed nasojejunally or as a jejunostomy. An NJT is difficult to accurately place and requires an x-ray to confirm its position. They are especially prone to displacement secondary to vomiting (as the main indication for their placement is GOR) and often require multiple, distressing reinsertions. If the child is able to tolerate an anaesthetic, the NJT should be regarded as a holding measure to protect the child from aspiration pneumonia, until a jejunostomy tube can be arranged.

A jejunostomy tube is inserted into the jejunum, either from the abdominal wall directly into the jejunum with a surgical procedure, or transgastrically via a previous gastrostomy.

A comparison of the different artificial feeding methods is outlined in Table 6.4 and Table 6.5.

6.7.1.4 Bolus and Continuous Tube Feeds

Tube feeding can be administered as multiple bolus feeds through the day, as a continuous feed or, most commonly, as a combination of both.

With bolus feeding, a relatively large volume of feed (typically 100–200 ml depending on the size of the child and what he will tolerate) is given over 15–30 minutes. Bolus feeding is a more physiological pattern of feeding, more convenient and allows the family more freedom in planning the feeds with their activities.

The disadvantages of bolus feeding are that the child is at higher risk of aspiration compared to continuous feeding and is more likely to have abdominal distension, nausea and diarrhoea.

For children unable to tolerate the larger bolus volumes, continuous feeding can be delivered via an infusion feed pump. It is generally given over an 8–10 hour period overnight in addition to 2–3 smaller bolus feeds or oral feeding during the daytime. Uninterrupted, continuous feeding over a 24-hour period is possible and considered for the child in whom any bolus feed induces GOR or pain. However, the child is attached to his feeding pump continuously and this may cause metabolic changes such as elevated insulin levels.

TABLE 6.4
Benefits and Complications of the Different Feeding Methods

Feeding method	Benefits	Complications
Nasogastric tube	Complements oral feeding in children with a faltering swallow or prolonged feeding time	Misplacement or migration of tube Exacerbation of GOR as the NGT keeps the gastro-oesophageal sphincter open Trauma during insertion of the NGT Local mucosal ulceration with long-term use Displacement of the NGT with vomiting and requiring repeated re-insertion Psychological impact of an NGT (child's refusing the tube insertion or body image issues)
Gastrostomy tube	In children requiring long-term tube feeding, a gastrostomy tube avoids regular NGT reinsertion A skin-level gastrostomy device is easily hidden under clothing and cosmetically more acceptable for the child	Infection or overgranulation of the gastrostomy stoma Leakage of the site Tube displacement Tube occlusion
Jejunostomy	Similar advantages to gastrostomy tubes As the feed is administered distal to the stomach, there is a reduced risk of GOR and pulmonary aspiration	Similar complications to gastrostomy tubes Jejunal feeds must be given as a continuous feed, not as a bolus feed As the feed is administered distally, there is an increased incidence of diarrhoea and feed intolerance
Total parenteral nutrition	Provides nutrition and calories to children who are unable to receive tube feeding or who are unable to absorb adequate nutrition enterally	Requires central venous access; line displacement or occlusion Line sepsis: in vulnerable, immunocompromised patients potentially fatal Cholestatic liver disease Metabolic disturbances Requires intensive support from a multidisciplinary nutrition team

6.8 TOTAL PARENTERAL NUTRITION

Total parenteral nutrition (TPN) in the context of a child's palliative care may be indicated as a short-term nutritional measure to support the child through times of crises or acute complications e.g., during postoperative recovery, chemotherapy-induced mucositis, etc. It is well recognised that in children with cancer, optimising nutrition reduces acute complications, treatment delays and drug dose alterations, and improves tumour response, time to first event (relapse or death) and survival (Bozzetti et al. 2009).

TPN may also be considered if the child has a malabsorption enteropathy or gut dysfunction. In this situation, TPN would be long-term management and would require homecare support. The decision to start TPN would need a multidisciplinary and ethical discussion. Gut dysfunction usually develops in the end stages of the child's illness and the ethics of commencing TPN in this setting need to be clearly discussed, taking into account the burdens of TPN versus benefits, and the family's priorities and ability to manage TPN at home.

TABLE 6.5
Symptom Management Guidelines

1. Gastro-oesophageal reflux	
The medical management of GOR includes:	i. Anti-secretory drugs (proton pump inhibitors and H_2-receptor antagonists) ii. Pro-motility agents (metoclopramide or domperidone) iii. Jejunal feeding
If symptoms persist, a surgical procedure can be considered:	iv. Nissen fundoplication: the fundus of the stomach is wrapped around the lower oesophagus, forming a valve at the junction of the oesophagus and stomach As the gastric fundus is used to fashion the anti-reflux valve, the stomach volume is reduced; the child may have some retching after the procedure. Small-volume, more frequent feeds are needed, and the retching usually, but not always, resolves after a few weeks or months. Some children may eventually vomit past the valve or the fundoplication wrap may become undone and need to be revised
2. Appropriate management of contributory symptoms:	
a. Pain	The management of gut-related pain is a stepwise approach of escalating analgesics: i. Simple analgesia (paracetamol) ii. Opiates (morphine) iii. Neuropathic agents as adjuncts (gabapentin or ketamine) iv. Non-steroidal anti-inflammatory drugs should be avoided as they have significant gastrointestinal side effects
b. Nausea	The following classes of antiemetics are appropriate for gut-related and vomiting-centre mediated nausea: i. Antihistamines (cyclizine) ii. Anticholinergics (transdermal hyoscine patch) iii. Phenothiazides (prochloperazine, levomepromazine)
c. Depression	The pharmacological management of depression and other psychological symptoms should be advised and reviewed regularly by a psychiatrist. Non-medical interventions, such as counselling, cognitive behavioural therapy or drama therapy, are also important to consider
3. Steroids as an appetite stimulant are rarely used in children as they have a high tendency to develop cushingoid, behavioural and psychological side effects	
4. Temporary cessation of feeding may have to be considered for children who have severe gut dysfunction. As previously described, these children have extremely distressing gastrointestinal symptoms, from which they may only obtain relief when their feed is stopped. A gradual reintroduction of feed and fluid can then be tried; feeds are upgraded and increased to an amount that the child is able to reasonably tolerate. The nutrition of these children is always balanced against the symptoms that their feed induces	

Note: This table lists the management approach for the specific symptoms that affect the feeding and nutrition in children with palliative care needs. Many of these management points can also apply to other areas of palliative care.

6.9 MULTIDISCIPLINARY TEAMWORK

A large number of professionals need to work together with the child and family to address the changing feeding and nutritional challenges for each child. This involves a SALT, dietician, GP, paediatrician, tertiary specialist and play therapist, and the palliative care, gastroenterology, surgical and psychology teams.

It is vital that these professionals are coordinated by the child's key worker. The community nurse usually fulfils this role and is the point of contact for the family and professionals, ensuring that communication is cascaded to everyone involved in the child's care. This is especially important, as the child is often cared for in multiple settings (e.g., home, school, hospital, respite care). It also facilitates an efficient response by professionals to changes in the child's condition.

ETHICAL ISSUES

The Royal College of Paediatrics and Child Health (RCPCH) has published an ethical framework to guide treatment decisions at the end-of-life (RCPCH 2004). It encourages parents and professionals to "enter a partnership of care, whose function is to serve the best interests of the child" and that "children should be informed and listened to so that they can participate as fully as possible in decision-making."

In the light of preceding court judgements, the RCPCH concludes "there is no obligation to give treatment which is futile and burdensome - indeed this could be regarded as an assault on the child" and that feeding and other medical treatment may be withdrawn if continuation is not in their best interests.

Another ethical dilemma we encounter is in managing gut dysfunction. Optimising the child's nutrition and weight gain has to be balanced with the day-to-day palliation of distressing symptoms, which often requires the reduction or cessation of feeds. In these situations, we encourage that decisions should be made in discussion with the wider multiprofessional team, the child and his parents, and regularly reviewed.

In conclusion, the family of Frances, a girl who died at age 13 of a neurodegenerative disorder, reflected: "Because a medical intervention is available, it does not always make it right and they need to consider the burden and benefit of any treatment they are recommending. That burden and benefit needs to take into account the whole family and extended carers" (*Archives of Disease in Childhood* 2005).

SUMMARY POINTS

- Poor nutrition in children with life-limiting and life-threatening illnesses has an adverse effect on their development, QOL and clinical outcome.
- The causes of poor nutrition in children with palliative care needs are often multifactorial and dynamic. They need to be reassessed regularly and interventions modified appropriately.
- Supplemental and tube feeding should be considered early and approached in a sensitive, family-centred manner.
- Assessing and supporting the child and family require an active, coordinated, multidisciplinary approach.
- The burden and benefits of each feeding and nutrition intervention need to be taken into account and decisions individualised for each child and family.

LIST OF ABBREVIATIONS

ACT Association for Children's Palliative Care
CP Cerebral Palsy
DMD Duchenne's Muscular Dystrophy
GOR Gastro-Oesophageal Reflux
GP General Practitioner
NGT Nasogastric Tube
NJT Nasojejunal Tube
QOL Quality of Life

SALT Speech and Language Therapy
TPN Total Parenteral Nutrition

REFERENCES

Altaf, M. A., and M. R. Sood. 2008. The nervous system and gastrointestinal function. *Developmental Disabilities Research Reviews* 14:87–95.

The mother and grandmother of Frances. 2005. Artificial feeding for a child with a degenerative disorder: A family's view. *Archives of Disease in Childhood* 90:979.

Association for Children's Palliative Care (ACT). 2009. Children's palliative care definitions. http://www.act.org.uk.

Bozzetti, F., J. Arends, K. Lundholm, A. Micklewright, G. Zurcher, M. Muscaritoli, and ESPEN. 2009. ESPEN guidelines on parenteral nutrition: Non-surgical oncology. *Clinical Nutrition (Edinburgh, Scotland)* 28:445–54.

Carachi, R., J. M. Currie, and M. Steven. 2009. New tools in the treatment of motility disorders in children. *Seminars in Pediatric Surgery* 18:274–77.

Darmon, N., and A. Drewnowski. 2008. Does social class predict diet quality? *The American Journal of Clinical Nutrition* 87:1107–17.

Gómez-Almaguer, D., G. J. Ruiz-Argüelles, and S. Ponce-de-León. 1998. Nutritional status and socio-economic conditions as prognostic factors in the outcome of therapy in childhood acute lymphoblastic leukemia. *International Journal of Cancer Supplement* 11:52–55.

Hechler, T., M. Blankenburg, S. J. Friedrichsdorf, D. Garske, B. Hübner, A. Menke, C. Wamsler, J. Wolfe, and B. Zernikow. 2008. Parents' perspective on symptoms, QOL, characteristics of death and end-of-life decisions for children dying from cancer. *Klinische Padiatrie* 220:166–74.

Mascarenhas, M. R., B. Zemel, and V. A. Stallings. 1998. Nutritional assessment in pediatrics. *Nutrition* 14:105–15.

Morita, T., I. Hyodo, T. Yoshimi, M. Ikenaga, Y. Tamura, A. Yoshizawa, A. Shimada et al. 2005. Association between hydration volume and symptoms in terminally ill cancer patients with abdominal malignancies. *Annals of Oncology* 16:640–47.

Morton, R. E., R. Wheatley, and J. Minford. 1999. Respiratory tract infections due to direct and reflux aspiration in children with severe neurodisability. *Developmental Medicine and Child Neurology* 41:329–34.

Petersen, M. C., S. Kedia, P. Davis, L. Newman, and C. Temple. 2006. Eating and feeding are not the same: Caregivers' perceptions of gastrostomy feeding for children with cerebral palsy. *Developmental Medicine and Child Neurology* 48 (9): 713–17.

Royal College of Paediatrics and Child Health (RCPCH). May 2004. Withholding or Withdrawing Life Sustaining Treatment in Children - A Framework for Practice. Second Edition. London: Royal College of Paediatrics and Child Health.

Sala, A., P. Pencharz, and R. D. Barr. 2004. Children, cancer, and nutrition—A dynamic triangle in review. *Cancer* 100 (4): 677–87.

Samson-Fang, L., E. Fung, V. A. Stallings, M. Conaway, G. Worley, P. Rosenbaum, R. Calvert et al. 2002. Relationship of nutritional status to health and societal participation in children with cerebral palsy. *The Journal of Pediatrics* 141:637–43.

Schwarz, S. M., J. Corredor, J. Fisher-Medina, J. Cohen, and S. Rabinowitz. 2001. Diagnosis and treatment of feeding disorders in children with developmental disabilities. *Pediatrics* 108:671–76.

Sullivan, P. B. 2008. Gastrointestinal disorders in children with neurodevelopmental disabilities. *Developmental Disabilities Research Reviews* 14:128–36.

Sullivan, P. B., E. Juszczak, A. M. Bachlet, B. Lambert, A. Vernon-Roberts, H. W. Grant, M. Eltumi, L. McLean, N. Alder, and A. G. Thomas. 2005. Gastrostomy tube feeding in children with cerebral palsy: A prospective, longitudinal study. *Developmental Disabilities Research Reviews* 47:77–85.

Theunissen, J. M., P. M. Hoogerbrugge, T. van Achterberg, J. B. Prins, M. J. Vernooij-Dassen, C. H. van den Ende. 2007. Symptoms in the palliative phase of children with cancer. *Pediatric Blood and Cancer* 49:160–65.

Thompson, A., A. MacDonald, and C. Holden. 2006. Feeding in palliative care. In *oxford textbook of palliative care for children*, ed. A. Goldman, R. Hain, and S. Liben, 374–86. Oxford: Oxford University Press.

Ward, E., M. Hopkins, L. Arbuckle, N. Williams, L. Forsythe, S. Bujkiewicz, B. Pizer, E. Estlin, and S. Picton. 2009. Nutritional problems in children treated for medulloblastoma: Implications for enteral nutrition support. *Pediatric Blood and Cancer* 53:570–75.

7 Nutrition and Quality of Life in Adults Receiving Palliative Care

Mick Fleming, Colin R. Martin, and Caroline J. Hollins Martin

CONTENTS

7.1 INTRODUCTION: THE IMPORTANCE OF NUTRITION DURING PALLIATIVE CARE

Palliative care refers to treatment and care delivered when the disease/illness is not responsive to curative treatment. The World Health Organization defines palliative care as 'an approach that improves the quality of life of patients and their families facing the problems associated with life threatening illness, through the prevention and relief of suffering by means of an early identification and impeccable assessment and treatment of pain and other problems, physical, psychosocial and spiritual' (WHO 2004). Palliative care and treatment strategies can also be used to manage the side effects of intrusive treatments within curative treatment. Often associated in the mind as being related to oncology and cancer, palliative care can be delivered to people experiencing any form of life-threatening illnesses such as chronic heart failure, respiratory disease, and neurological disorders such as motor neurone disease and multiple sclerosis. Palliative care can also be distinguished from end-of-life care. In the UK end-of-life care is written into clinical pathways concerned with the final days and hours of a person's life (DoH 2008; LCP 2008). The key aims of these care pathways are to improve quality of care of the dying in the last hours and days of life and to improve knowledge related to the process of dying.

Nutritional support is a recognised element of palliative care; it provides a useful strategy for the achievement of clinical outcomes and there are other comfort and ethical reasons for the justification of the use of nutrition during the provision of palliative care and end-of-life treatment. A range of diverse factors can impact on the nutritional status of palliative care patients (see Figure 7.1). Effects of the health condition such as dysphagia, metabolic responses to the health condition and treatment, and mood/thinking changes all contribute to a reduced ability for people who are receiving palliative

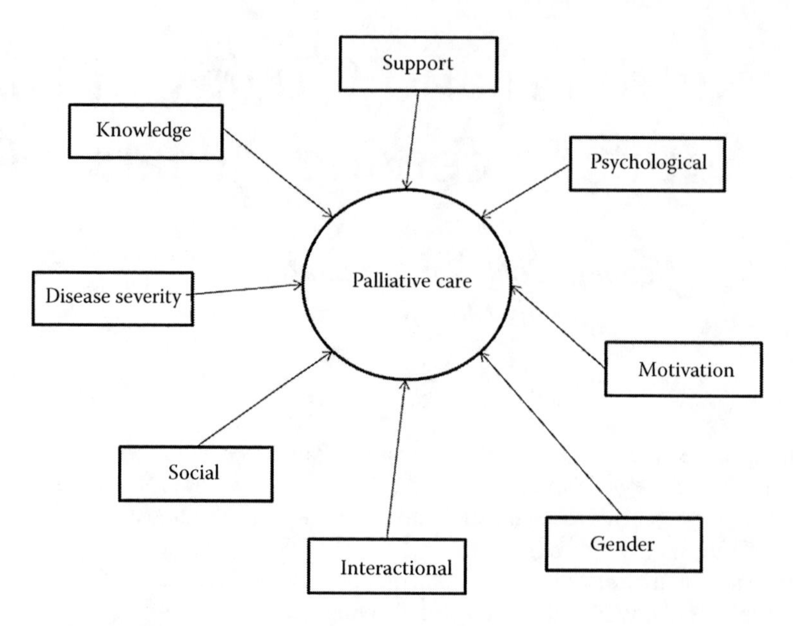

FIGURE 7.1 This figure illustrates examples of the diversity of factors that may impact on the nutritional status of palliative care patients.

care and treatment to maintain an adequate nutritional intake to satisfy their physical, psychological and social functioning needs (Hickson and Frost 2004; Sobotka et al. 2009). Inadequate hydration and malnutrition and the effects of this, such, as muscle wasting, vulnerability to infection, delirium and respiratory problems, are common potential risks for people receiving palliative care and treatment, particularly when people are near the end-of-life (Kutner 2005). The criteria for malnourishment and providing nutritional support are defined as:

- a body mass index (BMI) of less than 18.5 kg/m^2,
- unintentional weight loss greater than 10% in the last 3–6 months and
- a BMI of less than 20 kg/m^2 and unintentional weight loss greater than 5% in the last 3–6 months (NICE 2006).

The definition of the risk of malnutrition includes not eating or eating very little for the previous 5 days or longer and the bodies capacity for absorption and/or the need for increased nutritional need (NICE 2006).

Generic nutritional screening tools such as the Malnutrition Universal Screening Tool (Todorovic 2003) are commonly used in clinical practice. This specific screening tool has five steps that start with the measurement of BMI, unplanned weight loss, acute illness effects, risk for malnutrition and formulation of care plan.

Cachexia is a condition characterised by the signs of debilitation such as fatigue, muscle protein wasting, loss of weight, loss of body fat tissue, inflammation and loss of appetite (anorexia). The condition is seen as irreversible because of its association with progressive and terminal health conditions such as advanced cancer. Although a comorbid condition, it is a metabolic response to the health condition. Catabolic processes have been found in certain cancer conditions and the development of cachexia has been associated with the growth of tumours and the increasing competition for nutrients as the tumour develops (Argilés et al. 2005). Consequently, cachexia can occur even when the person has adequate nutritional intake. It has been found significantly in people who experience deteriorating health conditions such as cancer, neurological disorders, chronic cardiac failure and conditions relating to older age (Davidson et al. 2004; Kutner et al. 2005).

7.2 CATEGORIES OF NUTRITIONAL SUPPORT

Three categories of strategies for nutritional support can be found in the literature. A combination of these three nutritional strategies can also be used.

1. Support of natural nutritional intake: Wherever possible the health practitioners will seek to support and maintain natural routes of nutritional intake, especially in cases where use of the normal digestive system is not compromised. The aim of this type of intervention strategy is to ensure the correct amount and balance of the required nutrients are consumed, digested and metabolised. The most common strategy would be through the provision of oral supplements. A range of prescribed oral nutritional supplements (ONS) in the form of tablets, drinks and concentrated droplets can be administered in addition to a manageable diet. Mechanical aids for eating for people who can manage to chew, swallow and digest food have been recommended as an intervention strategy (NICE 2006).
2. Artificial methods of nutritional intake and hydration: There are two routes for the administration of artificial nutrition. Nutritional support using both routes is provided both in hospital and in the person's home:
   a. *Enteral route*. Considered a short-term nutritional intervention (4 weeks or less). This route is usually the first choice for nutritional support (Sobotka et al. 2009), essentially for people who do not have problems with the functioning of their gastrointestinal tract but are unable to swallow or feed orally. Nutrition is administered in two ways: into the stomach via a nasogastric tube or directly into the stomach via a percutaneous endoscopic gastromy, which is passed into the stomach through an incision into the abdominal wall.
   b. *Parenteral route*. Where the gastrointestinal tract is not functioning because of obstruction or the digestive system is not able to function or is preventing enteral feeding, nutrition is delivered into the body through a nonalimentary route via central or peripheral veins. Total nutrition that fully satisfies the energy requirements can be delivered through this parenteral route (TPN). Partial nutritional requirements can also be delivered by this route. The amount and type of nutritional mixture delivered is individualised and dependent on the nutritional needs of the person. A range of nutritional products such as amino acids, essential fatty acids, vitamins and other nutrients can be delivered. Peripheral veins are used where the need for the parenteral route is required for less than 14 days (NICE 2006). Where parenteral feeding is required for longer than 14 days a central vein is used to deliver the nutrients through a larger diameter intravenous catheter, which is placed directly into the superior vena cava or right atrium. Risk of infection and condition of the person are also considered when making clinical decisions about which parenteral route to use (Pittiruti et al. 2009). Hyperacidity, hyperglycaemia and refeeding syndrome can be consequences of the use of parenteral nutrition. Refeeding syndrome occurs within the first 3–4 days of reintroducing nutritional support and can be fatal. It is more likely to occur when high-calorie nutrition is rapidly reintroduced to malnourished people. The effects of the syndrome include low amounts of phosphate in the blood, electrolyte imbalances, the metabolism of fats, protein and glucose, thiamine deficiency and hypokalaemia (Mehanna et al. 2009). The effects are metabolic and can lead to cardiac, skeletal, respiratory and gastrointestinal disorders. The gradual reintroduction of nutritional support—50% of requirement over the first two days and then further gradual reintroduction up to optimal nutritional support with full biochemical monitoring—is recommended as a preventative measure (NICE 2006).
3. Dietary advice/counselling. Health practitioners can offer advice to both the person receiving palliative care and their carers/relatives. The aim of this strategy would be to

encourage positive eating habits such as the inclusion of high protein, carbohydrate and energy nutrition into diets. Often this strategy would not be used as a stand-alone intervention and would be delivered in conjunction with oral supplements (Baldwin and Weekes 2009). Clinical guidelines recommend that tailored information should be given alongside all forms of nutritional support about physical, psychological and social issues. In order to support the use of artificial feeding in people's homes and away from hospital, patients and their carers/relatives should be trained to manage, recognise the risks of and problem solve the process of artificial nutrition (NICE 2006).

7.3 ISSUES REGARDING NUTRITIONAL STATE, AND PALLIATIVE CARE AND TREATMENT

a. *Clinical rationale.* For many people receiving palliative care and treatment, suboptimal nourishment and malnutrition are comorbid complications of the health condition that they are experiencing. Nutritional support is often an indispensable part of their overall care and treatment (Sobotka et al. 2009). The aim of nutritional support may not be curative but it is nevertheless an integral strategy for maintaining quality of life for a period of time. The maintenance of a person's physical, psychological and social functioning requires adequate nutrition and hydration (Marin Caro, Laviano, and Pichard 2007). Clinical outcomes need to consider the specific nutritional needs of those receiving palliative care and treatment. Chronic obstruction caused by tumour growth prevents the digestion of adequate nutrition and starvation may be prevented by the administration of parenteral nutrition (Bozzetti et al. 2002). The disease process of pancreatic cancer is associated with pain, nausea, anorexia, early satiety and pancreatic insufficiency, and alteration in metabolic responses leads to weight loss, insufficient nutritional intake and cachexia (Davidson et al. 2004). There is a further acknowledgement within the literature that weight loss from cancer is different from simpler forms of starvation (Marin Caro et al. 2007). Details regarding the metabolic abnormalities and changes that lead to weight loss and cachexia are given. These metabolic changes render normal re-feeding ineffective in restoring nutritional status. Marin Caro et al. (2007) suggest cachexia accounts for 10–22% of all cancer deaths and summarises the range of clinical benefits of nutritional support for people with cancer as controlling cancer related symptoms, reducing postoperative complications and improving tolerance to treatment. These are sound justifications for the use of nutritional support and artificial feeding based on noncurative clinical outcomes, regardless of the ethical issues associated with comfort and quality of life.
b. *Ethical and cultural rationale.* Decisions about the use of nutritional support that does not have a curative/life-sustaining outcome are embedded within social, ethical and cultural belief systems about death for health practitioners, the person receiving palliative care and treatment, and relatives (Hughes and Neal 2000). However all three groups would aim to maintain comfort and quality of life. Hughes and Neal (2000) point out that the effects of malnutrition are uncomfortable and nutritional support can be justified on the grounds that it maintains the comfort and quality of life of the person. This is based on the assumption that nutritional support itself does not cause discomfort. Some artificial feeding can have uncomfortable side effects and fatal outcomes. Comfort care rather than life-sustaining treatments were seen as preferred by 70% of a sample within a total sample of 1266 aged 80 years or older who were admitted to intensive coronary care units in the United States (Somogyi-Zalud, Zhong, and Hamel 2002). The literature suggests the perceived importance of nutritional support, particularly artificial feeding and hydration, decreases as people reach the end-of-life. From a sample of 104, 97.1–99.0% of house officers believed that people who were seen as having the capacity to make the decision to end artificial feeding and

hydration should be able to refuse (Schildman et al. 2006). Tube feeding was considered as inappropriate for 20.5% of people experiencing dementia in the last 48 hours of life (Di Giullio et al. 2008). In comparison to other life-sustaining treatments, artificial nutrition is considered to be indispensable by health practitioners (Kaoruka et al. 2008). This view is shared by the general population and bereaved family members; 33%–50% believed that artificial hydration should be continued as the minimal standard until death. Ethical and cultural beliefs may well mediate these beliefs but 15%–31% also believed that artificial hydration relieved symptoms (Tatsuya et al. 2006). The withdrawal of artificial nutrition and hydration when they do not cause pain and discomfort has been questioned (Hildebrand 2000). The arguments within the literature are based on moral codes of ethics and do not explicitly consider quality of life issues. However some may point out that as nutrition and hydration are required to sustain life, withdrawal resulting in death extinguishes quality of life.

7.4 QUALITY OF LIFE

A number of factors have contributed to quality of life becoming a standard health outcome. Ideological shifts in health concepts such as the emergence of person-centred health provision have led to a focus on health and well-being rather than illness (Pais-Riberio 2004). Holism and consumerism place the person at the centre of health provision and from this there has been recognition of the multidimensional nature of the impact of illness on all parts of a person's life and functioning. Within palliative care treatment choices are of great importance to the person (Mystakidou et al. 2004). Health conditions affect psychological and social well-being as well as physical well-being. The individualised and personal nature of health and illness has also become more prevalent in modern health systems. Each person responds to a health condition in their own individual way. Two people at the same stage of the same illness will respond and react differently. Their behaviours in relation to their health condition will be determined by a number of nonphysical factors such as previous experiences, health attributions, emotional response and emotional environment. This is further indication of the multidimensional nature of the health concept. Definitions of health reflect this recognition and include physical, mental and social well-being within their scope (Marin Caro et al. 2007). Development in health technologies have led to populations living longer and it is the quality rather than quantity of that existence that is important to people. This is particularly apparent for those people that are living longer with ongoing and chronic health conditions. The debilitating nature of the health condition and the side effects of ongoing treatment will have an adverse impact on several domains of that person's life (Mystakidou et al. 2004).

Although developed for mental health services, Oliver, Huxley, and Bridges (1996) provide a taxonomy of the justification for the use of quality of life in (mental) health services: the importance of comfort not cure, complex health programmes require complex outcome measures, keeping the customer happy, re-emergence of the holistic perspective, quality of life is good politics (the emergence of the feel good factor), acceptable by patients and carers, common basis for multidisciplinary work, effective economic measurement, the achievability for studies of communities, the usefulness for evaluating community-delivered services, empirical measures are linked to theory and satisfaction with role performance is central to recovery.

7.5 DEFINITIONS OF QUALITY OF LIFE

Quality of life is a multidimensional but general concept that can be applied to a wide range of health conditions. It is distinct from the health condition itself (Oliver et al. 1996). Health-related quality of life is a multidimensional concept that focuses specifically on the impact of health, health treatments and illness on a person's physical, psychological and social functioning and well-being, and is an essential element of healthcare evaluation (Coons et al. 2000).

Common terms and themes such as multidimensional, well-being, satisfaction, expectations and functioning are prevalent in the quality of life literature. Definitions of quality of life and health-related quality of life do vary and this variation is determined by the philosophical and theoretical stance of the researcher. Subjective versus objective are the two dominant theoretical models of quality of life. The subjective model is individualised and places the person and their internal or perceived satisfaction with well-being and life at the heart of the investigation of quality of life. External factors such as culture, value system and the person's environment are seen as factors that influence the person's quality of life because it is these that determine their goals. Subjective measures of quality of life are concerned with the person's own view of their quality of life and are more likely to be self-report measures. The objective model does not see quality of life as being individually determined. There is an acceptance that quality of life is an external phenomena—observable, shared across communities/populations, measurable and associated with factors such as social contact, housing, role performance, functional ability and income (Oliver et al. 1996). There is an agreement that subjective and objective views of quality of life apply to two different dimensions of the concept of quality of life (Ruggeri et al. 2001).

7.6 ASSESSMENT OF QUALITY OF LIFE IN PEOPLE RECEIVING PALLIATIVE CARE

There is a consensus about the domains within quality of life measures. Mobility, self-care, usual activities, pain/discomfort and anxiety/depression are domains measured by the EQ-5D (see Figure 7.2) (EuroQol Group 1990). Physical functioning, role limitation due to physical problems, bodily pain, general health, vitality, social functioning, role limitation due to emotional problems and mental health are domains measured by the Medical Outcomes Short Form Health Survey 36 (SF-36) (see Figure 7.3) (Ware et al. 1993). This similarity between these two commonly used quality of life measures is reflected within other quality of life measures. Other commonly used health-related generic quality of life measures used in the literature include: the Nottingham Health profile, the Sickness Impact Profile, the Dartmouth Primary Care Co-operative Intervention Project Charts, the Quality of Well Being Scale and the Health Utilities Index (Coons et al. 2000). Within cancer treatment, tumour growth has been linked to functioning ability and studies compare measures of quality of life with measures of functioning ability such as the Karnofsky Performance Status Scale

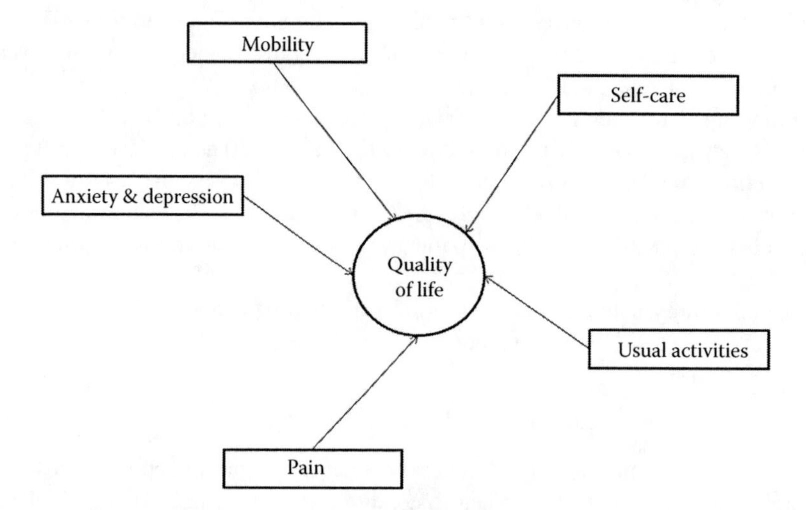

FIGURE 7.2 This figure illustrates the subscale domains of the EuroQol EQ-5D quality of life assessment tool. This is a quick, accurate and easy-to-administer quality of life assessment tool covering key dimensions which are of relevance to palliative care patients.

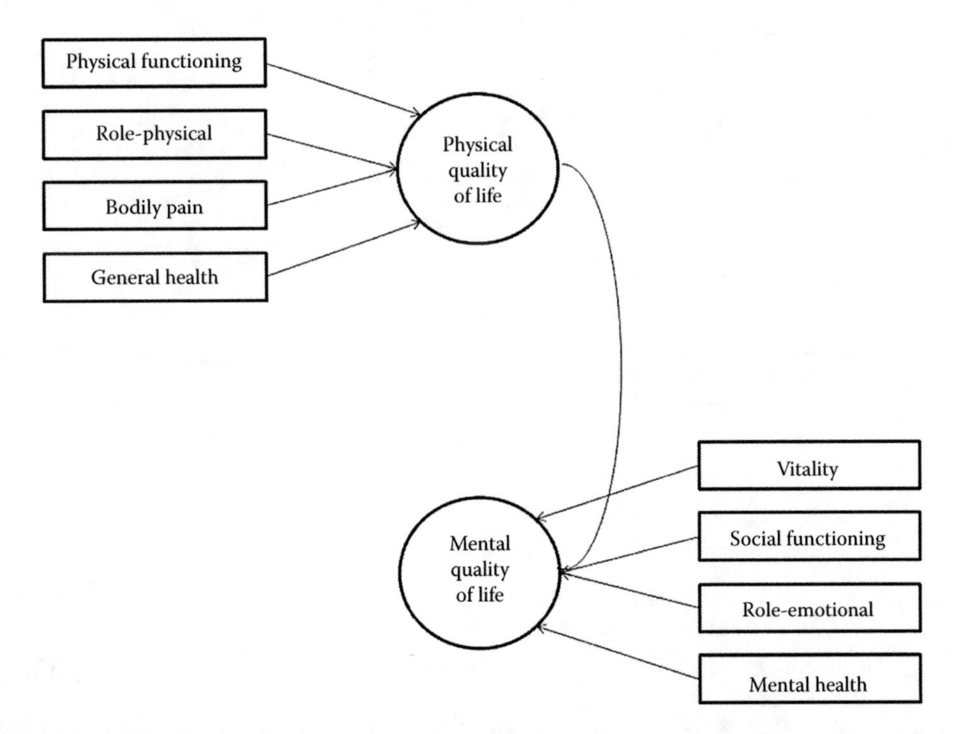

FIGURE 7.3 This figure illustrates the subscale and higher-order domains of the popular SF-36 quality of life assessment tool. This instrument allows the measurement of not only the eight subscale dimensions described, but also physical health and mental health component scores based on combinations of subscale results.

(Karnofsky and Burchenal 1949; Bozzetti et al. 2002). Specific palliative care quality of life measures incorporate physical functioning into the domains of the measure.

It has been argued that specific elements or domains relate to palliative and end-of-life care. Spirituality, existential issues (purpose and meaning of life), family members' perceptions of quality of care, symptom control and family support have been identified as specific to palliative and end-of-life care (Kaasa and Loge 2003). There are a number of factors that may impact on the accuracy of quality of life assessment in palliative care patients (see Figure 7.4). In their review of generic quality of life instruments, Coons et al. (2000) suggested choice of measure should be determined by the purpose of measurement, characteristics of client population and environment. Psychometric properties of quality of life instruments can influence the accuracy and sensitivity of quality if life assessments and issues relating to validity and reliability should be considered when selecting the most suitable quality of life measure (see Figure 7.5). The recommendation to clinicians and researchers working with people that are receiving palliative care is that whilst multidimensional measures should be used, these should have a limited number of items and should be based on the clinical outcomes and research question (Kaasa and Loge 2003).

Three specific quality of life measures for people receiving palliative care were found within the literature. The "Palliative Care Quality of Life Instrument" (Mystakidou et al. 2004) is a 28-item measure composed of 6 multi-item scales which are made up of 2 functional, 1 symptom, 1 choice of treatment and 1 psychological scale. There is a final single-item overall quality of life scale. The measure takes approximately 8 minutes to complete and when tested on people who have advanced stage cancer (test-retest reliability, $p < 0.05$ Spearman-rho; Cronbach's alpha coefficient >0.70), showed minimal reliability standards. Validity was also assessed using inter-item correlations, criterion validity and factor analysis. Fourteen of the 17 factors showed a correlation of >0.70

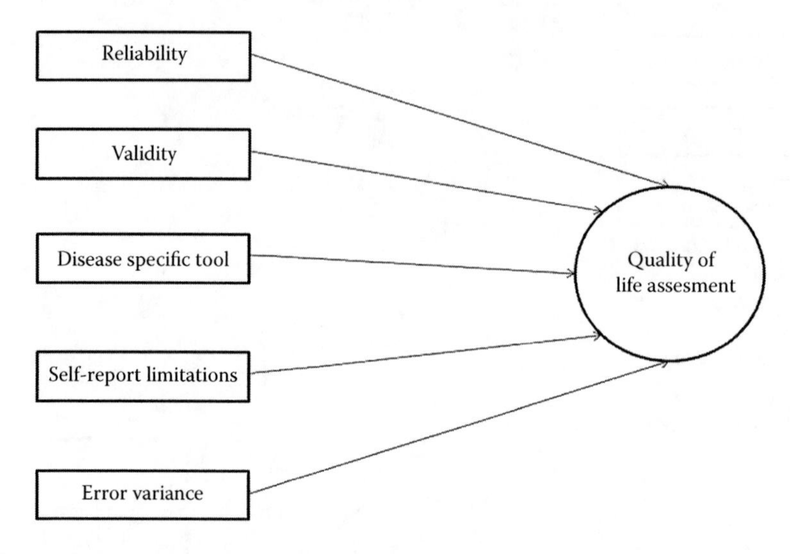

FIGURE 7.4 This figure illustrates examples of the multitude of factors that may impact on accuracy of quality of life assessment in palliative care patients.

or above. The authors concluded that the measure showed acceptable to very good reliability and validity (Mystakidou et al. 2004).

The Assessment of Quality of life at the End-of-life (AQEL) was developed for people who had cancer and were receiving palliative care. It is made up of 19 questions measuring physical, psychological, social, existential (ability to do what you want, meaningfulness, ability to feel joy), medical/care and global domains of quality of life (Axelsson and Sjoden 1998). Each of the 19 items is measured using a linear analogue scale from 0–10. It is considered to be a brief but comprehensive specific measure (Henoch, Axelsson, and Bergman 2010). Two studies were conducted with small samples (37 and 71). The existential domain was seen as strongly related to global quality of life and quality of life ratings became lower during the final 6 weeks of life (Axelsson and Sjoden 1998). Whilst the measure was described as valid and reliable, the domains within the measure were not supported by factor analysis, the social domain did not correlate well with similar domains from

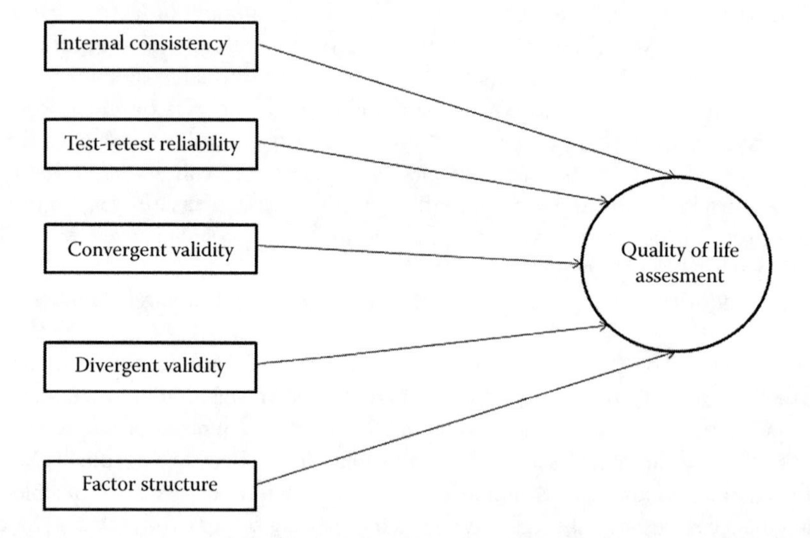

FIGURE 7.5 This figure illustrates examples of a variety of psychometric properties that are essential for the optimal accuracy and contextual sensitivity of a quality of life assessment tool for use in palliative care.

comparable measures and it was recommended that the measure should be viewed as 19 single items. A further recommendation was for further trails with larger sample sizes (Axelsson and Sjoden 1999; Henoch et al. 2010). A further validation study with a sample of 106 people found low internal consistency with the social domain within the 20-item version of the scale (dyspnoea item included for the study). The study confirmed that correlations with comparable measures were found for all the domains but that healthcare issues and physical and medical/healthcare worked best as individual items (Henoch et al. 2010).

The Spitzer Quality of Life Index (SQLI) is made up of 5 items scored on a 0–2 scale and was specifically designed for assessing clinical programmes within palliative care. The scale takes, on average, 1 minute to complete. Activity, daily living, health, support from family/friends and outlook make up the five items on the scale (Spitzer, Dobson, and Hall 1981). In subsequent studies the scale has demonstrated higher than acceptable levels of reliability and good content and convergent validity (Addington-Hall, MacDonald, and Anderson 1990).

The European Organisation for Research and Treatment of Cancer Quality of Life questionnaire has been used but this measure is not specifically designed for people receiving palliative care.

7.7 NUTRITION, NUTRITIONAL INTERVENTIONS, AND QOL

A search of the electronic databases using CINAHL, MEDline, PsycInfo and the British Nursing Index using the search terms nutrition AND palliative care AND quality of life was conducted. This search strategy identified 24 sources. A hand search found a further 3 sources relating to nutrition and quality of care. Only four of the sources accessed related directly to nutritional intake, palliative care and quality of life effects. The sources not directly relating to nutritional intake, palliative care and quality of life effects included people within samples that were diagnosed as having cancer, but it was not clearly identified if or how many of people within the sample were receiving or went on to receive palliative care. There also appears to be a crossover within the literature between palliative care and end-of-life care. The literature suggests that end-of-life care occurs anywhere between 2 months and 48 hours prior to death (DoH 2008) and end-of-life care may be part of palliative care. These two concepts are distinctly different and this is reflected in their definitions. These sources for the most part were not included within this section. Where they have been included the uncertainty about the numbers of the sample receiving palliative care will be indicated. The confounding effect of survival time on quality of life is potentially significant, as indicated in the two studies below, and so including studies where clients may be receiving curative treatment is likely to influence the conclusions drawn regarding the findings from studies measuring nutritional and quality of life outcomes.

There is an assumed link between weight loss, weight stability and quality of life; this association has been confirmed in recent studies. In samples where nutritional status and weight loss have been stabilised, resulting in an increase in length of time of survival, there has been consequent comparative increases in quality of life. Home parenteral nutrition was found to maintain the nutritional status of 69 people with advanced cancer. Survival ranged from 1 to 14 months and a third of people in the sample survived for more than 7 months (Bozzetti et al. 2002). Quality of life was measured using the Rotterdam Symptom Checklist Questionnaire at the start of the home parenteral nutrition intervention and then after the first month and then monthly. Fluctuations in scores showed a stabilisation of quality of life scores at the first month and continued until 2 months prior to death. Only those people that survived more than 3 months benefited from the stabilisation of nutritional status and quality of life (Bozetti et al. 2002). A similar association was found by Davidson et al. (2004). They divided a sample of 107 people with unresectable pancreatic cancer into two independent groups depending on the amount of weight loss after completing a nutritional intervention of oral supplements, food diaries and support for 8 weeks. Comparison from post hoc scores from the European Organisation for Research and Treatment of Cancer Quality of Life questionnaire between the two groups showed an association between weight stabilisation, longer survival and higher quality of life scores. Self-monitoring of nutritional intake for people with the digestive complications of pancreatic cancer was seen as being of limited value in this study.

The nutritional impact of dietary advice/counselling and dietary advice plus protein supplements was compared to as-usual nutritional intake in a group of people with colorectal cancer. The group of 111 were randomly assigned to one of the three groups and quality of life was measured using the European Organisation for Research and Treatment of Cancer Quality of Life questionnaire. Energy uptake and nutritional status improved in the first two groups and there was proportionate improvement in quality of life scores for the people in these two groups. Benefits to nutritional intake, energy levels and quality of life was maintained for a period of 3 months in the dietary advice/counselling group compared to the other two groups (Ravasco et al. 2005). This pattern of findings was only partially confirmed in a meta-analysis reviewing the results of five trials of dietary counselling with a pooled sample of 388 people (Halfdanarson et al. 2008). An overall statistically significant benefit on quality of life was not found in any of the five studies. Three studies showed benefits and two showed no benefit from dietary advice/counselling. The authors concluded that dietary intake did have positive clinical outcomes and is a justifiable intervention, but that the findings of the review could not confirm any significant relationship between dietary advice/counselling and improvements in quality of life.

Specific N-3 polyunsaturated fatty acids nutritional supplements have been found to stabilise weight and lead to improvements in quality of life (Marin Caro et al. 2007). These benefits have been found in people in cachectic states. Stabilisation and/or improvements in quality of life were proportionate to weight gain. The immunomodulating effects of these supplements were seen to produce benefits of improved immune function and mediate the metabolic effects and processes associated with tumour growth and development. These benefits required three weeks of oral supplementation at adequate levels to ensure sufficient concentrations were achieved (Marin Caro et al. 2007). Calorie intake, protein, calcium, iron, zinc, selenium, thiamine, riboflavin and niacin were all positively correlated with quality of life in 285 people with stomach cancer. The study also confirmed that better nutritional status was associated with improved quality of life (Tian and Chen 2005).

Enteral and parenteral nutrition was found to be beneficial in maintaining or improving nutritional status, increasing body composition and mass, and providing consequent improvements in quality of life (Bozzetti et al. 2002), particularly in people with advanced incurable cancer with associated malnutrition (Marin Caro et al. 2007). However, for those on home enteral nutrition, their quality of life has been found to be lower than the general population during treatment, especially for those who have cancer and are over the age of 45 years (Schneider et al. 2000). Survival time has been linked to the level of quality of life within people who receive palliative care. Many of these studies included above do not include assumed or real survival time as a potential influential variable in the assessment of quality of life. Similarly, the characteristics of people within the studies were heterogeneous in terms of cancer, goals of treatment received and tumour stage. The lack of homogeneity within the people and stage of cancer in these studies means that this review provides only limited and general clues as to the effects of nutritional status on quality of life and its relationship to people receiving palliative care.

7.8 APPLICATION TO OTHER AREAS OF HEALTH AND DISEASE

There are two key findings from the studies included within this chapter that are applicable to other areas of health and disease. Firstly, nutritional support stabilises and sometimes increases weight. This in turn provides people with the energy to help them to fulfil their physical, social and psychological functioning and goals, which have a proportionate positive effect on quality of life. These findings have a particular relevance in other conditions, not necessarily where palliative care is being delivered, but where there is a risk of undernourishment and/or gastric tract compromise such as recovery from complex surgery, injury, neurological conditions and cognitive functioning problems such as dementia. Secondly, quality of life is the only indicator that encompasses a range of physical, social and psychological domains. In modern twenty-first-century health care, where the emphasis is on person-centred and individualised health care, and in communities where people are living with long-term health conditions that would previously have resulted in death, quality of life provides health organisations with an ideally suited outcome measure for planning, targeting and evaluating health interventions.

Issues regarding quality of life for children and adolescents receiving palliative care have not been considered within this chapter. The issues regarding the complex effects of the disease process and treatment, nutritional support and the physical, psychological and social functioning needs of the child are similar to those of adults. There are added complexities such as parental support, the goals of treatment and parental decision making. These issues render the findings from studies included here only partially relevant.

DEFINITION OF KEY POINTS

- Body Mass Index – is a recognised measure of total body mass and body fat. The calculation involves dividing weight in kilograms by the square of height in metres. There is a criterion against which people can compare their final BMI to see if they are underweight, normal weight, overweight, obese or morbidly obese.
- Cachexia – refers to a condition of severe debilitation and loss of body mass. Characterised by significant weight loss, muscle atrophy and loss of energy, the process also includes a metabolic abnormality where the body breaks down its own tissues. The condition is often linked to metabolic processes arising from specific disease conditions such as "cancer cachexia".
- Digestive tract – referred to as the alimentary canal, it is the tract that passes from the mouth to the anus and traverses through the major organs that break down food into a form that can be absorbed as nutrients or expelled as waste products by the body.
- Enteral nutrition – is the process of providing shorter-term nutritional support for people who have a functioning gastric tract but are unable to swallow. Nutrition is delivered directly into the stomach through either a nasogastric tube or a tube that is inserted directly into the stomach via an incision in the abdominal wall.
- Nutrition – the provision of essential nutrients and chemicals usually in the form of food or food supplements in digestible form for use by the body for its effective functioning.
- Nutritional advice/counselling – any form of intervention that includes the provision of information directly to the person or carer with the purpose of altering/improving suitable nutritional intake.
- Parenteral nutrition – the process of providing longer-term nutritional support for people who do not have a functioning gastric tract and who require nutrition to be delivered through a nonalimentary route. Nutrition is delivered via central and/or peripheral veins depending on the length of time required to provide nutrition through this route.

SUMMARY POINTS

- Palliative care is concerned with treatments other than noncurative treatment. Treatments within the sphere of palliative care have the aims of optimising comfort, reducing the side effects of treatment and maintaining the quality of life of people. People experiencing chronic cardiac failure, renal disease, neurological conditions and cancer receive palliative care.
- End-of-life care refers to treatment that is provided during the last 2 months to hours of life and can be part of palliative care but is not the same as palliative care.

- The metabolic processes associated with specific disease process, and the direct physical effects of both the disease process and side effects of treatment can lead to malnutrition and other serious wasting conditions such as cachexia. These are common in people that receive palliative care.
- There is a sound clinical rationale for maintaining weight and nutritional intake. These are important elements of palliative care and can help to alleviate some of the metabolic and other physical effects of the disease process and treatment.
- Quality of life is a concept that, when applied to people receiving palliative care, covers all aspects of a person's physical, mental, spiritual and psychological functioning. It is a suitable measure for planning and evaluating outcomes for people receiving palliative care.
- A number of general and specific quality of life measures have been developed for measuring the quality of life of people receiving palliative care. The specific measures include spiritual, existential and family/friend support, three domains considered to be important and specific to palliative care.
- Weight stabilisation achieved through nutrition is key to maintaining physical, social and psychological well-being and these outcomes have a proportional effect on improvements in quality of life.
- Many studies include people with cancer and do not specifically include only those receiving palliative care, so the findings of these studies do not provide definitive ideas about how nutritional intervention influences the quality of life of people receiving palliative care. In the small number of studies including only people receiving palliative care, perceived or real length of survival influences quality of life outcomes. This is a key factor and its influence can only be understood from studies where people are receiving palliative care.

LIST OF ABBREVIATIONS

BMI	Body Mass Index
DoH	Department of Health
EN	Enteral Nutrition
HPN	Home Parenteral Nutrition
NICE	National Institute of Health and Clinical Excellence
ONS	Oral Nutritional Supplements
TPN	Total Parenteral Nutrition
WHO	World Health Organization

REFERENCES

Addington-Hall, J. M., L. D. MacDonald, and H. R. Anderson. 1990. Can the Spitzer Quality of Life Index help to reduce prognostic uncertainty in terminal care? *British Journal of Cancer* 62 (4): 695–99.

Argilés, J. M., S. Busquets, C. García-Martínez, and F. J. López-Soriano. 2005. Mediators involved in the cancer anorexia-cachexia syndrome: Past, present, and future. *Nutrition.* 29:977–85.

Axelsson, B., and P. O. Sjoden. 1998. Quality of life of cancer patients and their spouses in palliative home care. *Palliative Medicine* 12:29–39.

Axelsson, B., and P. O. Sjoden. 1999. Assessment of quality of life in palliative care-psychometric properties of a short questionnaire. *Acta Oncologica* 38 (2): 229–37.

Baldwin, C., and C. E. Weekes. 2009. Dietary advice for illness-related malnutrition in adults. *Cochrane Database of Systematic Reviews.* Issue 1, Art. No.: CD002009.

Bozzetti, F., L. Cozzaglio, E. Biganzoli, G. Chiavenna, M. De Cicco, D. Donati, G. Gilli, S. Percolla, and L. Pironi. 2002. Quality of life and length of survival in advanced cancer patients on home nutrition. *Clinical Nutrition* 21 (4): 281–88.

Coons, S. J., S. Rao, D. L. Keininger, and R. D. Hays. 2000. A comparative review of generic quality-of-life-instruments. *Pharmacoeconomics* 17 (1): 13–35.

Davidson, W., S. Ash, S. Capra, and J. Bauer. 2004. Weight stabilisation is associated with improved survival duration and quality of life in unresectable pancreatic cancer. *Clinical Nutrition* 23:239–47.

Di Giullio, P., F. Toscani, D. Villani, C. Brunelli, S. Gentile, and P. Spadin. 2008. Dying with advanced dementia in long-term care geriatric institutions a retrospective study. *Journal of Palliative Medicine* 11 (7): 1023–28.

DoH. 2008. *End-of-life Care Strategy – promoting high quality care for all adults at the end-of-life*. London: Department of Health.

EuroQoL Group. 1990. EuroQoL a new facility for the measurement of health related quality of life. *Health Policy* 16:199–208.

Halfdanarson, T. R., E. O. Thordardottir, C. P. West, and A. Jatoi. 2008. Does dietary counselling improve quality of life in c cancer patients? A systematic review and meta-analysis. *The Journal of Supportive Oncology* 6:234–37.

Henoch, I., B. Axelsson, and B. Bergman. 2010. The assessment of quality of life at the end-of-life (AQEL) questionnaire: A brief but comprehensive instrument for use in patients with cancer in palliative care. *Quality of Life Research* 19 (5): 739–50.

Hickson, M., and G. Frost. 2004. An investigation into the relationship between quality of life, nutritional status and physical function. *Clinical Nutrition* 23:213–21.

Hildebrand, A. J. (2000). Masking intentions: The masquerade of killing thoughts used to justify dehydrating and starving people in a "persistent vegetative state" and people with other profound neurological impairments. *Issues in Law & Medicine* 16 (2): 143–65.

Hughes, N., and R. D. Neal. 2000. Adults with terminal illness: A literature review of their needs and wishes for food. *Journal of Advanced Nursing* 32 (5): 1101–7.

Kaasa, S., and J. H. Loge. 2003. Quality of life in palliative care: Principles and practice. *Palliative Medicine* 17:11–20.

Kaoruka, A., M. Hiroaki, T. Miyako, and K. Ichiro. 2008. Japanese physicians' practice of withholding and withdrawing mechanical ventilation and artificial nutrition and hydration from older adults with very severe stroke. *Archives of Gerontology and Geriatrics* 46 (3): 263–72.

Karnofsky, D. A., and J. H. Burchenal. 1949. The clinical evaluation of chemotherapeutic agents in cancer. In *Evaluation of chemotherapeutic agents*, ed. C. M. MacLeod, pp. 191–205. New York: Columbia University Press.

Kutner, J. S. 2005. Terminal care: The last weeks of life. *Journal of Palliative Medicine* 8 (5): 1040–41.

LCP. 2008. The Liverpool Care pathway for the dying patient. www.mcpcil.org.uk.

Marin Caro, M. M., A. Laviano, and C. Pichard. 2007. Nutritional intervention and quality of life in adult oncology patients. *Clinical Nutrition* 26:289–301.

Mehanna, H., P. Nankivell, J. Moledina, and J. Travis. 2009. Refeeding syndrome-awareness, prevention and management. *Head & Neck Oncology* 1:4, 26 January 2009.

Mystakidou, K., E. Tsilika, V. Kouloulias, E. Parpa, E. Katsouda, J. Kourvaris, and L. Vlhas. 2004. The "Palliative Care Quality of Life Instrument (PLQI)" in terminal cancer patients. *Health and Quality of Life Outcome* 2:8, 12 February 2004.

NICE. 2006. Clinical Guideline 32. Nutrition support in adults: Oral nutrition support, enteral tube feeding and parenteral nutrition. www.nice.org.uk/CG032NICEguideline.

Oliver, J., P. Huxley, and K. Bridges, eds. 1996. *Quality of life and mental health services*. London: Routledge.

Pais-Riberio, J. L. 2004. Quality of life is a primary end-point in clinical settings. *Clinical Nutrition* 23:121–30.

Pittiruti, M., H. Hamilton, R. Biffi, J. MacFie, and M. Pertkiewicz. 2009. ESPEN guidelines on parenteral nutrition: Central venous catheters (access, care, diagnosis and therapy complications). *Clinical Nutrition* 28:365–77.

Ravasco, P., I. Montiero-Grillo, P. M. Vidal, and M. E. Camilo. 2005. Dietary counselling improves patient's outcomes: A prospective randomised, controlled trial in colorectal cancer patients undergoing radiotherapy. *Journal of Clinical Oncology* 23 (7): 1431–38.

Ruggeri, M., R. Warner, G. Bisoffi, and L. Fontecedro. 2001. Subjective and objective dimensions of quality of life in psychiatric patients: A factor analytic approach. The South-Verona Outcome Project 4. *British Journal of Psychiatry* 178:268–75.

Schildman, J., L. Doyal, A. Cushing, and J. Vollman. 2006. Decisions at the end-of-life: An empirical study on the involvement, legal understanding and ethical views of pre-registration house officers. *Journal of Medical Ethics* 32 (10): 567–70.

Schneider, S. M., I. Pouget, P. Staccini, P. Rampal, and X. Hebuterne. 2000. Quality of life in long-term home enteral nutrition patients. *Clinical Nutrition* 19 (1): 23–28.

Sobotka, L., S. M. Schneider, Y. N. Berner, T. Cederholm, Z. Krznaric, A. Shenkin, Z. Stanga, G. Toiga, M. Vandewoude, and D. Volkert. 2009. ESPEN guidelines on parenteral nutrition: Geriatrics. *Clinical Nutrition* 28 (4): 461–66.

Somogyi-Zalud, E., Z. Zhong, and M. B. Hamel. 2002. The use of life sustaining treatments in hospitalized persons aged 80 and older. *Journal of the American Geriatrics Society* 50 (5): 930–34.
Spitzer, W., A. Dobson, and J. Hall. 1981. Measuring the quality of life of cancer patients: A concise QL-Index for use by physicians. *Journal of Chronic Diseases* 34:585–97.
Tatsuya, M., M. Mitsunori, S. Makiko, H. Kei, A. Tomoko, I. Tatsuhiko, M. Tatsuhiro et al. 2006. Knowledge and beliefs about end-of-life care and the effects of specialized palliative care: A population based survey in Japan. *Journal of Pain and Symptom Management* 31 (4): 306–18.
Tian, J., and J. S. Chen. 2005. Nutritional status and quality of life of the gastric cancer patients in Changle county of China. *World Journal of Gastroenterology* 11 (11): 1582–86.
Todorovic, V. 2003. *The 'MUST' explanatory booklet: A guide to the Malnutrition Universal Screening Tool.* Redditch: BAPEN.
Ware, J. E., K. K. Snow, M. K. Kosinski, and B. Gandek. 1993. *The SF-36 Health Survey Manual and Interpretation Guide*. Boston, MA: The Health Institute, New England Medical Centre.
WHO. 2004. *Palliative care*: *The solid facts*. Geneva: World Health Organization.

8 Refractory Cancer Cachexia

D. Blum, R. Oberholzer, and F. Strasser

CONTENTS

8.1 INTRODUCTION

Involuntary weight loss is a common consequence of advanced cancer. Cachexia is a paraneoplastic syndrome and a major cause of involuntary weight loss. Cancer cachexia is defined by ongoing loss of skeletal muscle mass, a negative protein and energy balance, driven by reduced food intake and abnormal metabolism (Blum et al. 2010). In cancer cachexia not only weight declines, but also physical function. Cancer cachexia affects patients and their loved ones.

8.2 SIMPLE STARVATION

In clinical care of advanced cancer patients, oral nutritional intake is often impaired due to concurrent cancer-related or anti-cancer treatment-related complications (e.g., opioid-associated constipation, nausea, severe incident pain, shortness of breath, mucositis) or insufficient patient education on necessary diet in cachexia. This is labeled simple starvation (or secondary nutritional impact symptoms) and requires standardized assessment and management (Omlin and Strasser 2007).

8.3 PREVALENCE AND SIGNIFICANCE OF CANCER CACHEXIA

Cancer cachexia and its consequences are among the most common problems of advanced cancer patients (Strasser and Bruera 2002). Depending on the source, the prevalence of cancer cachexia in cancer patients ranges from 24%–80%. Survival is often limited to a few weeks to months. The difficulty in clinical practice is not only recognizing cancer cachexia and its underlying problems of nutritional intake, but managing cancer cachexia and its consequences like fatigue and decreased physical functioning. Accompanying symptoms like early satiety, nausea, and dysgeusia are major challenges for the treating healthcare professionals. The emotional and existential burden of the patients and their carers is often underestimated and can be overwhelming.

8.3.1 Phases

Different phases of cancer cachexia have been proposed recently (Fearon 2008; Argiles 2010). Early or pre-cachexia is defined as presenting early clinical and metabolic signs without the presence of significant involuntary weight loss. Cachexia syndrome is reached when weight loss reaches more than 5% or is ongoing. Patients with refractory cachexia have advanced muscle wasting with or without loss of fat. In terms of refractory cachexia, the prognosis of survival is too short to reverse depletion (Figure 8.1).

8.3.2 Current Management of Cachexia

Current management of cancer cachexia depends on the presence or absence of secondary nutritional impact symptoms and its phase. Pre-cachexia and cachexia demand standard cachexia management including pharmacological, nutritional, psychological, and physical interventions (Table 8.1).

8.3.3 Refractory Cachexia

The decline of physical function and the decrease of nutritional intake are part of the natural dying process. Therefore, it is paramount in clinical practice in palliative care to identify the point of no return in this decline. If this point of the disease has been diagnosed, cachexia is called refractory. There are completely different priorities in treatment of cachexia syndrome and refractory cachexia. The aim of this chapter is to help in the diagnosis of refractory cachexia.

8.3.4 Diagnosing Cachexia

Historically cancer cachexia was only described by weight loss. Cancer cachexia was then defined as weight loss (involuntary weight loss of 2% in 2 months or 5% in 6 months), anorexia (VAS 3/10), or impaired oral nutritional intake (<75% normal or <20 kcal/kg bodyweight).

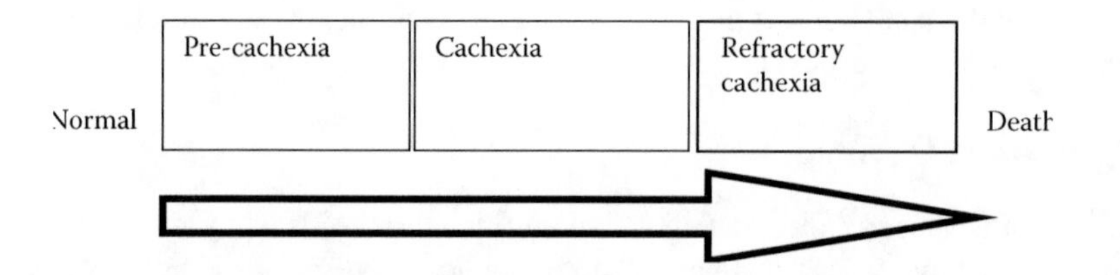

FIGURE 8.1 Cachexia trajectory. (Based on EPCRC work.)

TABLE 8.1
Interventions According to Cachexia Phase

Pre-cachexia	Cachexia	Refractory Cachexia
Monitor weight	Multimodal therapy	Symptom control
Prevention	Anticancer therapy	Symptom prevention
	Anticachexia therapy	Psychosocial/spiritual care
	Physical therapy	
	Psychosocial therapy	

Source: Based on EPCRC work.

International experts proposed, after a consensus meeting, a generic definition for cachexia/wasting disease associated with any form of chronic illnesses including cancer: weight loss with or without fat loss and, as additional criteria (three required for diagnosis): decreased muscle strength, reduced muscle mass, fatigue, anorexia, or biochemical alterations (anemia, inflammation, low albumin) (Evans et al. 2008).

The Patient-Generated Subjective Global Assessment (PG-SGA) is an assessment of nutritional risk in cancer patients which is widely used. Weight history generates a weight loss grade (0–5) and amount and type of food intake are also graded. The tool contains a functional status score and a list of 13 symptoms. A physical examination is part of the PG-SGA, and several factors potentially related to weight loss are assessed including comorbidities, age, cancer stage, the presence of fever, and use of corticosteroids.

In a Delphi consensus the European Palliative Care Research Collaborative (EPCRC) proposed a new definition of cancer cachexia based on the generic wasting disease definition for chronic illnesses and the PG-SGA (Table 8.2).

The EPCRC defines cancer cachexia as a multifactorial syndrome defined by an ongoing loss of skeletal muscle mass and a characteristic pathophysiology including a negative protein and energy balance, driven by a variable combination of reduced food intake and abnormal metabolism. Cancer cachexia cannot be fully reversed by conventional nutritional support and leads to progressive functional impairment (Figure 8.2).

The EPCRC proposes four domains to assess cancer cachexia. The domains are:

- stores
- intake
- potential
- performance

TABLE 8.2
Assessment Included in the PG-SGA

Weight loss
Condition
Metabolic stress
Physical examination
    Three categories: well nourished/at risk/malnourished

Source: From Bauer, J., S. Capra, and M. Ferguson, *Eur. J. Clin. Nutr.,* 56, 779, Aug. 2002.

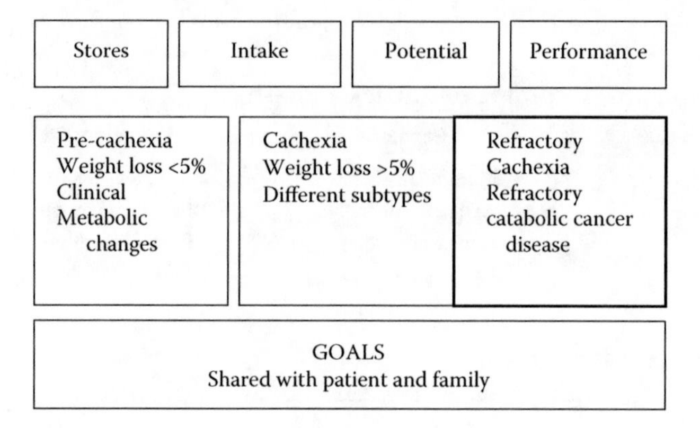

FIGURE 8.2 Diagnosing cancer cachexia. (Based on EPCRC work.)

The assessment of these four domains is designed for use as a screening tool to detect patients with cancer cachexia. It defines a set of key variables used to describe different phases of cancer cachexia, as a minimal data set and helps in terms of a clinical decision-guiding instrument to introduce/improve cancer cachexia treatment accordingly (Table 8.3).

8.3.5 Phases of Cachexia

Cachexia commonly worsens as cancer progresses. There is consensus that a staging of cachexia is necessary and three phases have been proposed:

- pre-cachexia
- cachexia
- refractory cachexia

Not all patients will go through all the proposed phases during their disease trajectory.

TABLE 8.3
Assessment According to Cachexia Domains

	Basic	Specialists
Storage		
Weight loss	PG-SGA Module weight loss	Weight loss history
Muscle mass	Change of mid-arm circumference	Native CT L4
Intake		
Eating-related symptoms	PG-SGA Presence of symptoms	Symptom quantitative scale
Nutritional intake	PG-SGA Module – Intake	1–2 day record (kcal, protein)
Secondary causes for decreased intake	PG-SGA Module – Presence NIS	Secondary-NIS quantitative scale
Potential		
Tumor catabolic activity	Presence of anticancer treatment	Tumor type, activity, response
Inflammation	Clinical signs	C-reactive protein
Performance		
Muscle strength	KPS	Chair raise time, get-up-and-go
Physical functioning	KPS	Subjective, mobility checklist
Psychosocial adaptation	Single item question	Cachexia-related suffering

Source: Based on EPCRC work.

Pre-cachexia, as a condition with no or very little weight loss (less than 5% of body weight loss in 6 months), is associated with anorexia, inflammation, and/or metabolic changes. These patients are at risk for progression to the cachexia syndrome. Therefore precachectic patients are the target group for cachexia prevention.

Patients with >5% weight loss in the last 6 months or with BMI <20 kg/m^2 and ongoing weight loss >2% are considered to be cachectic. Different phenotypes with different predominant features are under discussion and investigation. Furthermore, in obese patients, muscle loss can be masked by fat or fluid mass loss.

8.4 DIAGNOSING REFRACTORY CACHEXIA

Refractory cachexia is diagnosed clinically. Cachexia becomes refractory if the underlying disease is far advanced, rapidly progressive, and unresponsive to treatment, and the catabolism increased so that weight loss management is not possible or indicated. Refractory cachexia can often only be diagnosed after a defined treatment attempt.

Diagnosing refractory cachexia is close to diagnosing dying. However the symptoms associated with cachexia (i.e., anorexia, weight loss) are often used to diagnose approaching death even when cachexia is potentially still treatable.

In general the dying patient becomes bedbound, does not swallow food or drugs, and is comatose or semi-comatose. But all these symptoms are ambiguous and can occur in non-dying patients as well. Clinical prediction of survival (CPS) is subjective and dependent on assessment and experience. In clinical practice CPS is more likely to be overoptimistic than pessimistic. There are two validated prognostication tools: the Palliative Prognostic Score (PaP) includes CPS and a blood sample, whereas the Palliative Prognostic Index (PPI) contains only signs and symptoms (Table 8.4).

A combination of specific features within the four domains can diagnose refractory cachexia.

8.4.1 Stores

Weight loss is a key feature of cachexia. With weight loss above 5% the definition is reached as Tan et al. (2009) proved with new data that there is in fact a high correlation between weight loss and mortality. Due to an increase of adiposity in our population, weight loss can be substantial even when a normal BMI is still present. Weight loss measured by a scale is an easy to measure surrogate marker for the cachexia-defining muscle loss, because there is no clear consensus how to assess muscle loss in clinical practice. However a variety of methods are applicable: muscle loss can be assessed by clinical judgment, mid-arm circumference measurement, CT scan of the lumbar spine, MRI or DEXA, and bioimpedance analysis. If muscle loss exceeds 10% of muscle mass, the likelihood of refractory cachexia is strong.

TABLE 8.4
Items Included in the PaP Score

- Dyspnea
- Anorexia
- Karnofsky Performance Status
- Clinical prediction of survival
- Total white blood count
- Lymphocyte percentage

Source: From Glare, P., and K. Virik. *J. Pain Symptom Manage* 22, 891, Nov. 2001.

8.4.2 Intake

Social retreat and refusal of food are further common signs of approaching death. Living without food is possible up to 3 months and death occurs due to protein homeostasis. Anorexia per se does not define refractory cachexia, because it can often be surmounted by conscious control of eating.

Intake can be impaired by a variety of symptoms other than anorexia. Epidemiology studies support correlations between symptoms and weight loss (Walsh, Donnelly, and Rybicki 2000; Teunissen et al. 2007). Symptoms like mucositis and constipation occur frequently in advanced cancer (Strasser 2003). Other factors can impair the integrity from mouth to anus and act as secondary causes of impaired nutritional intake (S-NIS). Further, secondary causes of impaired nutritional intake involve shortness of breath, pain, fatigue, or depression and may also contribute to cachexia (Chiu et al. 2004).

The predominance of secondary nutrition intake symptoms is inversely related with refractory cachexia. Such S-NIS are treatable and potentially reversible. If there is severe structural or functional damage to the gastrointestinal tract, parenteral nutrition can be introduced if the treatment is monitored closely and a goal is defined.

8.4.3 Potential

The tumor per se is the main influence on survival, because high tumor activity and unresponsiveness to antitumor treatment are key features of a poor prognosis. Even though estimation of prognosis in a specific case is very difficult, stage and tumor types are predictive. Pragmatic tumor responsiveness tools are in the process of development.

C-reactive protein (CRP) as a marker for the inflammatory response in cancer has been proved to be prognostic for survival in studies in lung (Scott et al. 2002), pancreas, and gastric cancer. In the absence of infections, CRP can be a useful prognostication marker. Although a specific threshold for refractory cachexia is not defined, measurements above 150 mg/l are associated with high catabolic drive. Because of the potential influence of other underlying conditions (i.e., ongoing infection), it should never be used on its own. However, repetitive measurements can strengthen its prognostic value.

8.4.4 Performance

To estimate the impact of cachexia on patients' physical functioning, routine assessment of physical activity is recommended. The method of choice is patient-reported physical functioning (e.g., EORTC-QLQ-C30, patient-completed ECOG). Other methods may be physician-reported (e.g., Karnofsky Score) or objective methodologies (e.g., activity meter, checklists of specific activities). Low performance status is strongly associated with refractory cachexia, but possible reversible causes like delirium, depression, etc. must be excluded first.

For the assessment of psychosocial impact of cancer cachexia, a single screening question like: "How much do you feel distressed about your inability to eat?" is proposed. The Functional Assessment of Anorexia/Cachexia Therapy (FAACT) scale involves questions about psychosocial impact also (Ribaudo et al. 2001). Cachexia-related distress can arise as long as cachexia persists and resolve close to death due to other priorities. The assessment and treatment of cachexia-related suffering (CRS) are described in a separate chapter in this book.

8.5 TREATMENT

8.5.1 Palliative Cancer Care

For careful decision making in palliative care, the patient with cancer cachexia must be assessed. Decision making leads to the definition of a common intervention goal in general and it is paramount to ensure that the patient and the family understand and share these goals. Decision making is based on adequate communication.

Antineoplastic therapy can reduce the catabolic stimulus of the tumor and ameliorate cachexia (Giordano and Jatoi 2005). However, side effects from antineoplastic therapy can also aggravate symptoms. High catabolism can be reduced by antineoplastic therapies. Slow tumor progression due to tumor characteristics or chemotherapy with palliative intention does not necessarily lead to catabolism and can be overcome by nutritional interventions.

An attempt to increase nutritional intake is warranted if refractory cachexia is not proven. Secondary nutritional impact symptoms are actively searched and treated.

Conscious control of eating habits is the fundament of any nutritional intervention. Enriched nutrition like protein drinks is commonly used. Taste preferences may vary between patients and in a patient over time. If there is a severe structural barrier in the upper gastrointestinal tract, a percutaneous endoscopic gastrostomy tube (PEG tube) may be the device of choice in this situation. In severe structural or functional barriers in the intestines, as seen in chronic subileus due to peritoneal metastasis, parenteral nutrition may be preferable. Patients should be monitored for signs of refeeding syndrome. An evaluation after 10–14 days with measurement of pre-/albumin is indicated. If there is an increase in these parameters in the absence of complications, total parenteral nutrition (TPN) is continued and evaluated over time.

However, with such interventions, weight gain is not the target outcome, due to interference with fluid retention. Muscle mass, physical function, and well-being should improve if a attempt to improve nutritional intake is undertaken.

If anticancer treatment and nutritional interventions do not reach their predefined goals, refractory cachexia is evident. In refractory cachexia, therapeutic interventions have to focus on alleviating symptoms and avoiding complications and side effects.

8.5.2 Treatment of Refractory Cachexia

8.5.2.1 Nutritional Interventions

In refractory cachexia TPN should be stopped because the additional supply of calories in this situation is no longer efficient and causes only side effects. All efforts by the nutritionist to increase nutritional intake including behavioral interventions (conscious control of eating) should be reduced. Patients and their families are comprehensively informed that loss of appetite at this stage is often observed and attempts to force-feed the patient are futile. Possibilities of sharing other than sharing meals should be explained.

8.5.2.2 Pharmacological Interventions

In refractory cachexia it is important that pharmacological treatment does not replace other modes of care, i.e., psychological, social, or spiritual. A few drugs can play a role in alleviation of symptoms.

8.5.2.2.1 Corticosteroids

Corticosteroids improve appetite, oral food intake, and well-being in patients with advanced cancer. They are widely used to alleviate symptoms in refractory cachexia. Their exact mechanism of action is unclear, but their effects on mood are well known. An interaction with orexigenic hormones in the hypothalamus is discussed. Several studies have shown an improvement in appetite, food intake, and quality of life in advanced cancer patients taking corticosteroids. A meta-analysis summarizes six double-blind randomized controlled trials (Yavuzsen et al. 2005). Study duration ranges from 6 to 12 weeks and doses from 300 to 1200 mg methylprednisolone. However, in five of six studies benefits were dismissed over time (Popiela, Lucchi, and Giongo 1989).

Due to their broad effect, corticosteroids have a wide range of negative side effects like muscle myopathy, insulin resistance, and immune suppression. Adrenal insufficiency due to withdrawal can occur. Corticosteroids are recommended to alleviate symptoms in refractory cachexia for a short time.

8.5.2.2.2 Antidepressant 5-HT-antagonists

Antidepressants are widely used in advanced cancer. Appetite gain is a common side effect of antidepressants. A study with mirtazapine in patients with advanced cancer showed appetite stimulation (Riechelmann et al. 2007). The atypical neuroleptic drug olanzapin, used in anorexia nervosa, stimulated cachectic patients' appetite and raised ghrelin levels in a phase I study (Braiteh et al. 2008) (Table 8.5).

8.5.2.2.3 Progestins

Synthetic progestagenes have been used in the treatment of hormone-sensitive tumors. Due to their side effects, like appetite increase, they were investigated in cancer cachexia. Several prospective controlled randomized trials have been published and pooled in two systematic reviews (Maltoni, Nanni, and Scarpi 2001; Ruiz-Garcia, Juan, and Perez Hoyos 2002) and a Cochrane meta-analysis (Berenstein and Ortiz 2005). Several randomized controlled trials have shown that progestins improve appetite, caloric intake, and loss of fat tissue in patients with advanced cancer. However, improvement of physical function, fatigue, and lean body mass have not been demonstrated, but there is limited data for the use of progestins in refractory cachexia. Progestins are mainly recommended in cachexia when anorexia is the main cause for suffering after careful patient education. In refractory cachexia, progestins have limited benefit due to the relative overweight of other symptoms. Clinically relevant side effect such as thromboembolic events and edema, and the costs of the therapy have to be taken into account.

8.5.2.2.4 Cannabinoids

Throughout history mankind has used extracts from the plant *Cannabis sativa* as a recreational and therapeutical drug. Endocannabinoids are involved in the natural regulation of appetite.

The synthetic cannabinoid dronabinol (Delta-9THC) is approved as an antiemetic drug and as an appetite stimulant in HIV wasting. In cancer cachexia, after promising phase II trial results, two large placebo-controlled trials showed no clear improvement in appetite or quality of life (Strasser, Luftner, and Possinger 2006). Psychological symptoms like confusion and somnolence and physiological symptoms like tachycardia or hypotension occur in terms of adverse effects. In selected patients with predominantly chronic nausea or anxiety the use of cannabinoids can be an option.

TABLE 8.5
Key Facts of Depression and Antidepressants in Cachexia

Signs and symptoms

- Low mood, tearfulness, irritability, and distress
- Withdrawal, loss of interest or pleasure
- Physical symptoms or symptoms disproportionate to the degree of disease
- Feelings of hopelessness, helplessness, worthlessness, or guilt
- Suicidal behavior, requests for physician-assisted suicide/euthanasia, a wish to end it all, refusal of care

Therapy

- Tricyclic antidepressants (TCAs) or mirtazapine, or SSRIs
- Agitation and distress can be caused by delirium or adverse drug reaction and treated with benzodiazepines or neuroleptics
- Psychostimulants may help; stop if there is no benefit

Source: Based on EPCRC work.

8.5.2.2.5 Prokinetics

Long-acting prokinetics show an effect in patients suffering from chronic nausea, but they do not help in all patients. Still, based on good overall tolerability prokinetics can be used in refractory cachexia if nausea is a predominant symptom.

8.5.2.2.6 Other agents

Eicosapentaenoic acid (EPA) and cyclo-oxygenase inhibitors play a role in the treatment of cachexia but not in refractory cachexia. There is no data or experience for novel cachexia treatments like melatonin-receptor antagonists, and ghrelin and its analogues in refractory cachexia. Careful discussion is needed about which agents should be researched in this vulnerable patient population.

8.6 PSYCHOSOCIAL INTERVENTIONS AND EMOTIONAL SUPPORT

In refractory cachexia, patients and families should be carefully educated about the irreversible nature of their disease and be given time for acceptance. Meanwhile, patients and families are supported in finding ways other than sharing a meal in order to show their love and their care for each other.

8.7 APPLICATIONS TO OTHER AREAS OF TERMINAL OR PALLIATIVE CARE

Wasting disease was a major problem in HIV/AIDS patients in the first world and still is in the third world. Since the introduction of triple antiretroviral agents, loss of weight has become reversible in most AIDS patients. Patients who seemed to have refractory cachexia started to gain weight and physical function after having received antiretroviral therapy.

Translated into cancer research, this may indicate that along with successful anticancer therapy, cancer cachexia might be resolved. However there are anticancer therapies that can worsen cachexia per se or increase secondary nutritional impact symptoms and outweigh any benefit. There were anticachectic trials that were positive in AIDS and negative in cancer, challenging the straightforward comparability of these diseases.

Wasting and cachexia in other end-stage diseases like advanced COPD, cardiopathy or renal insufficiency have different dynamics than in advanced cancer patients. The point of no return where cachexia becomes refractory might be more difficult to define, because the decline might be slower or the phases of the disease more variable.

8.8 PRACTICAL METHODS AND TECHNIQUES

The first step is an active comprehensive multidimensional physical, psychological, social, and spiritual assessment of the patient and his family. This includes a good prognostication process with an estimation of survival and a discussion with the patient and his family.

Cachexia assessment covers the four domains:

Stores

A normal calibrated scale is sufficient to measure body weight. Patients should wear usual clothing without shoes. For repeated measurements the same scale should be used. Repeated measurements over time may increase accuracy. In patients with significant fluid retention, large tumor mass or obesity (BMI >30 kg/m^2), significant muscle wasting may occur in the absence of weight loss. In such patients a direct measure of muscularity is recommended.

Muscle loss can be measured by an L4/5 native CT scan or DEXA, but the same method should be applied each time.

Intake

Anorexia is usually measured on a VAS (0 no problem, 10 maximal problem). A score >3/10 or impaired oral nutritional intake (<75% than normal or <20 kcal/kg body weight) is part of the historic definition. Patients' estimation of overall food intake in relation to their normal intake may better reflect actual amount of food intake, although this can be affected by recollection bias.

The capacity to improve food intake by checking causes for simple starvation/secondary nutritional impact symptoms should be an integral part of the assessment.

There are several nutritional assessment tools in use. The patient-generated subjective global assessment (PG-SGA) is a frequently used validated method of nutritional assessment.

Full nutritional assessment in clinical practice is commonly done using a food diary analyzed by a nutritionist. Other methods such as a digital balance or photographs may also be used.

In refractory cachexia patients or proxies, estimation may be sufficient.

Potential

Patients suffering from certain cancer types are more prone to develop cancer cachexia, such as carcinomas from the gastrointestinal tract. Gastrointestinal and head and neck cancer are often associated with secondary nutritional impact symptoms due to disease or therapy. Different tumor dynamics or tumor burden (stable or progressive disease, stage, tumor kinetics, metastasis) have an impact on cachexia (Ravsasco et al. 2003). During progressive disease the tumor burden is a driver of increased metabolism and catabolism. A key component of cancer cachexia is this (hyper-) catabolic drive caused by systemic inflammation. CRP proved to be a robust marker to measure systemic inflammation. Sweating and night sweats or fever are a clinical sign.

Performance

A systematic review identified 135 different assessment tools (Helbostad et al. 2009). Simple and frequently used tools are the Karnofsky Performance Score (KPS) and ECOG, which are based on a physician's estimation. Patient-reported physical functioning is part of the EORTC-OLQ-C30.

Psychosocial impact should be assessed (e.g., items such as "how much do you feel distressed about your inability to eat?", "have you experienced feelings of pressure, guilt, or relational distress related to cachexia and weight loss?"). A single question asking about concerns regarding eating or the FAACT may be helpful for screening purposes. A validated tool, however, is lacking to date.

Refractory cachexia is suggested by significant weight loss, low intake, and low performance status, and proven by unresponsiveness to anti-cachexia treatment.

8.8.1 Interventions

In refractory cachexia therapeutic interventions focus on alleviating symptoms and avoiding complications. This often includes discontinuation of anticancer and nutritional treatment.

Steroids and antidepressants are commonly used drugs. Pharmacological treatment becomes less important. Psychosocial counseling at this stage becomes essential. Patients and their families are educated in possibilities of sharing other than taking meals together and supported in finding other ways to care.

KEY POINTS

- Cancer cachexia has a big impact on patients and families.
- Assessment of patients involves psychological, social, and spiritual issues.
- Monitor weight and muscle mass.
- Monitor and treat for secondary nutritional impact symptoms.
- Assess tumor dynamics and catabolism, and prognosticate carefully.

- Refractory cachexia is defined by unresponsiveness to anti-cachexia treatment.
- In refractory cachexia interventions alleviate symptoms and suffering.
- Complications are avoided by cessation of futile therapeutic attempts.
- Cachexia-related suffering is assessed and treated.

ETHICAL ISSUES

Diagnosing refractory cachexia is often a matter of debate. Cultural, religious, or legal issues arise. To admit that therapeutic attempts are no longer beneficial can be difficult for a treating team. Starting a therapeutic attempt is easier than stopping therapeutic attempts like chemotherapy or total parenteral nutrition because it can be overestimated as a symbol of hope, especially by relatives. Careful education about the nature of the disease and its trajectory prevents conflicts and reduces distress in teams or families.

SUMMARY POINTS

- Cachexia is a paraneoplastic syndrome and is a common cause of involuntary weight loss in advanced cancer.
- Associated symptoms like early satiety, nausea, and dysgeusia can impair nutritional intake. Other symptoms like pain or depression can impair nutritional intake. They are called secondary nutritional impact symptoms and require standardized assessment and management due to their reversibility.
- Manifest cachexia requires both standard management and pharmacological and nutritional interventions.
- Cachexia becomes refractory if the underlying disease is far advanced, rapidly progressive, and unresponsive to treatment, and catabolism so increased that weight loss management is not possible or indicated.
- Refractory cachexia can often only be diagnosed after a defined treatment attempt.
- The emotional and existential burden of the patients and their carers is often underestimated and can be overwhelming.
- In refractory cachexia therapeutic interventions focus on alleviating symptoms and avoiding complications. This often includes discontinuation of nutritional treatment attempts. Psychosocial counseling at this stage becomes essential.

ACKNOWLEDGMENTS

We thank Daniel Kauffmann, Librarian, and Nicole Schenk, Project Management, in the Cantonal Hospital St. Gallen, and all the collaborators participating in the EPCRC. We thank the international cancer cachexia experts, and last but not least we thank our patients.

LIST OF ABBREVIATIONS

BMI	Body mass index
COPD	Chronic obstructive pulmonary disease
CPS	Clinical prediction of survival
CRP	C-reactive protein
ECOG	Eastern Cooperative Oncology Group
EPCRC	European Palliative Care Research Collaborative
DEXA	Dual Energy X-ray Absorptiometry
FAACT	Functional Assessment of Anorexia/Cachexia Therapy

GI	Gastro intestinal
PaP Score	Palliative Prognostic Score
PG-SGA	Patient-Generated Subjective Global Assessment
PPI	Prognostic Index
S-NIS	Secondary nutritional intake symptoms
TPN	Total parenteral nutrition

REFERENCES

Argiles, J. M., S. D. Anker, W. J. Evans, J. E. Morley, K. C. Fearon, F. Strasser, M. Muscaritoli, and V. E. Baracos. May 2010. Consensus on cachexia definitions. *J Am Med Dir Assoc* 11 (4): 229–30.

Bauer, J., S. Capra, and M. Ferguson. Aug 2002. Use of the scored Patient-Generated Subjective Global Assessment (PG-SGA) as a nutrition assessment tool in patients with cancer. *Eur J Clin Nutr* 56 (8): 779–85.

Berenstein, E. G., and Z. Ortiz. 2005. Megestrol acetate for the treatment of anorexia-cachexia syndrome. *Cochrane Database Syst Rev* Apr 18:CD004310.

Blum, D., A. Omlin, K. Fearon, V. Baracos, L. Radbruch, S. Kaasa, and F. Strasser; European Palliative Care Research Collaborative (EPCRC). 2010. Evolving classification systems for cancer cachexia: Ready for clinical practice? *Support Care Cancer* 18:273–79.

Braiteh, F., S. Dalal, A. Khuwaja, H. David, E. Bruera, and R. Kurzrock. 2008. Phase I pilot study of the safety and tolerability of olanzapine (OZA) for the treatment of cachexia in patients with advanced cancer. *Journal of Clinical Oncology* 26 (May 20 suppl); abstr 20529.

Chiu, T. Y., W. Y. Hu, B. H. Lue, C. A. Yao, C. Y. Chen, and S. Wakai. 2004. Dyspnea and its correlates in Taiwanese patients with terminal cancer. *J Pain Symptom Management* 28:123–32.

Evans, W. J., J. E. Morley, J. Argilés, C. Bales, V. Baracos, D. Guttridge, A. Jatoi et al. 2008. Cachexia: A new definition. *Clinical Nutrition* 27:793–99.

Fearon, K. C. May 2008. Cancer cachexia: Developing multimodal therapy for a multidimensional problem. *Eur J Cancer* 44 (8): 1124–32. Epub Mar 28, 2008.

Giordano, K. F., and A. Jatoi. July 2005. The cancer anorexia/weight loss syndrome: Therapeutic challenges. *Curr Oncol Rep* 7 (4): 271–76.

Glare, P., and K. Virik. Nov 2001. Independent prospective validation of the PaP score in terminally ill patients referred to a hospital-based palliative medicine consultation service. *J Pain Symptom Manage* 22 (5): 891–98.

Helbostad, J. L., J. C. Hølen, M. S. Jordhøy, G. I. Ringdal, L. Oldervoll, and S. Kaasa; European Association for Palliative Care (EAPC) Research Network. 2009. A first step in the development of an international self-report instrument for physical functioning in palliative cancer care: A systematic literature review and an expert opinion evaluation study. *J Pain Symptom Management* 37:196–205.

Maltoni, M., O. Nanni, and E. Scarpi. 2001. High-dose progestins for the treatment of cancer anorexia-cachexia syndrome: A systematic review of randomised clinical trials. *Annals of Oncology* 12:289–300.

Omlin, A. G., and F. Strasser. 2007. Secondary causes of cancer-related anorexia: Recognition in daily practice by a novel checklist, a pilot study. *Journal of Clinical Oncology* 25:18S (supplementum; abstract 9058).

Popiela, T., R. Lucchi, and F. Giongo. 1989. Methylprednisolone as an appetite stimulant in patients with cancer. *Eur J Cancer Clin Oncol* 25:1823.

Ravasco, P., I. Monteiro-Grillo, P. M. Vidal, and M. E. Camilo. Dec 2003. Nutritional deterioration in cancer: The role of disease and diet. *Clin Oncol (R Coll Radiol)* 15 (8): 443–50.

Ribaudo, J. M., D. Cella, E. A. Hahn, S. R. Lloyd, N. S. Tchekmedyian, J. Von, and W. T. Leslie. 2001. Re-validation and shortening of the Functional Assessment of Anorexia/Cachexia Therapy (FAACT) questionnaire. *Quality of Life Research* 9:1137–46.

Riechelmann, R. P., I. Tannock, G. Rodin, and C. Zimmermann. 2007. Phase II trial of mirtazapine for cancer-related cachexia/anorexia. *Support Care Cancer* 15:775; abstract P197.

Ruiz-Garcia, V., O. Juan, and S. Perez Hoyos. 2002. Megestrol acetate: A systematic review usefulness about the weight gain in neoplastic patients with cancer. *Medicina Clinica (Barcelona)* 119:166–70.

Scott, H. R., D. C. McMillan, L. M. Forrest, D. J. Brown, C. S. McArdle, and R. Milroy. 2002. The systemic inflammatory response, weight loss, performance status and survival in patients with inoperable non-small cell lung cancer. *Br J Cancer* 87:264–67.

Strasser, F., J. Binswanger, T. Cerny, and A. Kesselring. 2007. Fighting a losing battle: Eating-related distress of men with advanced cancer and their female partners. A mixed-methods study. *Palliative Medicine* 21:129–36.

Strasser, F., and E. D. Bruera. 2002. Update on anorexia/cachexia. *Hematology/Oncology Clinics of North America* 16:589–617.

Strasser, F., D. Luftner, and K. Possinger. 2006. Comparison of orally administered cannabis extract and delta-9-tetrahydrocannabinol in treating patients with cancer-related anorexia-cachexia syndrome: A multicenter, phase III, randomized, double-blind, placebo-controlled clinical trial from the Cannabis-In-Cachexia-Study-Group. *J Clin Oncol* 24:3394–400.

Tan, B. H., L. A. Birdsell, L. Martin, V. E. Baracos, and K. C. Fearon. 15 Nov 2009. Sarcopenia in an overweight or obese patient is an adverse prognostic factor in pancreatic cancer. *Clin Cancer Res* 15 (22): 6973–79.

Teunissen, S. C., W. Wesker, C. Kruitwagen, H. C. de Haes, E. E. Voest, and A. de Graeff. 2007. Symptom prevalence in patients with incurable cancer: A systematic review. *J Pain Symptom Management* 34:94–104.

Walsh, D., S. Donnelly, and L. Rybicki. 2000.The symptoms of advanced cancer: Relationship to age, gender, and performance status in 1,000 patients. *Support Care Cancer* 8:175–79.

Yavuzsen, T., M. P. Davis, D. Walsh, S. LeGrand, and R. Lagman. 2005. Systematic review of the treatment of cancer-associated anorexia and weight loss. *J Clin Oncol* 23:8500–511.

Section II

Cultural Aspects

9 Nutrition and Hydration in Palliative Care: Japanese Perspectives

Tatsuya Morita

CONTENTS

9.1 INTRODUCTION

Recent literature has revealed marked differences in artificial hydration therapy for terminally ill cancer patients in Japan (Morita, Shima et al. 2002). This means that patients may undergo unnecessary suffering from over- or under-hydration. In addition to physical symptoms, artificial hydration and nutrition have a special meaning for patients and families as a metaphor for life. In Japan, recent efforts highlight the need to standize artificial hydration therapy, and the Japanese Society of Palliative Medicine developed a clinical guideline for artificial hydration therapy in terminally cancer patients. This chapter thus focuses on the current status of artificial hydration therapy in Japan, and describes: 1) the concept of a good death for Japanese, 2) the opinions of Japanese patients, families, and the general public on artificial hydration therapy, 3) the attitudes toward artificial hydration of physicians and nurses, and 4) the essence of the clinical guideline. We decided not to include research findings on the physical aspects of terminal dehydration because other chapters will deal with them.

9.2 CONCEPT OF A GOOD DEATH FOR JAPANESE

A good death is a core concept in understanding what we should do for each patient (Miyashita, Sanjo et al. 2007). A large-scale quantitative survey, followed by a qualitative study, was recently performed with the following primary aims: (1) to conceptualize dimensions of a good death in Japanese cancer care, (2) to clarify the relative importance of each component of a good death, and (3) to explore factors related to an individual's perception of the domains of a good death. In this study, the general population was sampled using a stratified random sampling method ($n = 2548$) and bereaved families from 12 certified palliative care units were surveyed ($n = 513$). We asked the subjects about the relative importance of 57 components of a good death. Explanatory factor analysis demonstrated 18 domains contributing to a good death. Ten domains were classified as "consistently important domains," including "physical and psychological comfort," "dying in a favorite place," "good relationship with medical staff," "maintaining hope and pleasure," "not being a burden to others," "good relationship with family," "physical and cognitive control," "environmental comfort," "being respected as an individual," and "life completion."

In the domains of a good death, some are strongly related to decision-making regarding artificial hydration (Table 9.1). First, many Japanese patients regard maintaining a good relationship with the family and medical staff as important. In some situations, patients do not always desire artificial hydration but families and/or medical staff want the patients to receive it. In this case, patients are likely to request artificial hydration to agree to the wishes of their families and even physicians. Second, the preference for a natural death and fighting against cancer are valued as important. While 66% of the respondents reported that "not being connected to medical instruments or tubes" is important for their good death, 78% maintained that "believing one has used all available treatments" is important. Whether or not a patient receives artificial hydration therapy may depend on his/her value of a natural death or fighting against cancer. Third, unawareness of death is a unique concept for Japanese. Over 80% of the respondents reported that they wish to continue "living as usual without

TABLE 9.1
Good Death Domains Related to Artificial Hydration Therapy in Japanese Population

Domain	Component	General Population, %	Bereaved Family, %
Good relationship with family	Believing that one's family will do well after one's death	92	91
	Family is prepared for one's death	92	91
Good relationship with medical staff	Trusting physician	96	98
Natural death	Dying a natural death	89	90
	Not being connected to medical instruments or tubes	66	68
Fighting against cancer	Believing that one has used all available treatments	78	79
	Fighting against disease until one's last moment	73	68
	Living as long as possible	42	39
Unawareness of death	Living as usual without thinking about death	85	88
	Dying without awareness of it	53	53
	Not being informed of bad news	44	42
Not being a burden to others	Not being a burden to family members	89	86
	Not making trouble for others	88	83

TABLE 9.2
Opinions about Artificial Hydration Therapy of the Japanese General Public

	Without Bereavement Experience (*n* = 949)	With Bereavement Experience				
		Noncancer, Institutions (*n* = 673)	Noncancer, Home (*n* = 264)	Cancer, Institutions (*n* = 525)	Cancer, Home (*n* = 86)	Cancer, PCUs (*n* = 548)
	% (n)	% (n)	% (n)	% (n)	% (n)	% (n)
Artificial hydration and nutrition should be continued as the minimum standard of care until death	38	40	41	42	33	50
Artificial hydration and nutrition relieve patient's symptoms	29	31	24	26	15	29

PCUs: Palliative care units.

thinking about death," and about 40% preferred "not being informed of bad news." Inadequate information on the benefits of artificial hydration therapy, preferred by patients themselves, could contribute to the increased use of artificial hydration in end-stage cancer. Finally, not being a burden to others is one important element. In Japanese clinical settings, family members usually assist in home parenteral nutrition and some patients feel that they are a heavy burden to their families.

In summary, the good death concept could explain how patients determine whether they do or do not receive artificial hydration therapy. The important domains include maintaining a good relationship with the family and medical staff, a natural death, fighting against cancer, unawareness of death, and not being a burden to others.

9.3 OPINIONS OF PATIENTS, FAMILIES, AND THE GENERAL PUBLIC

In the most recent and largest opinion-based survey, about 33–50% of the general public regarded artificial hydration therapy as the minimum standard of care and 30% believed that it relieved patients' symptoms (Table 9.2) (Morita, Miyashita et al. 2006). An education intervention trial indicated that a 1-hour education session lessened the belief that artificial hydration therapy is the minimum standard of care and that it promotes symptom relief (Table 9.3) (Miyashita et al. 2008). In this investigation, 1-hour educational lectures were held in Fukushima Prefecture, Japan. Meetings were held in a community center and the themes included the limitations of cancer treatment, life-prolonging treatment for end-of-life cancer patients, information about opioids, artificial hydration, and communication between patient and physicians. A pre-post survey was performed.

TABLE 9.3
Effects of 1-Hour Educational Intervention on Opinions about Artificial Hydration Therapy of the Japanese General Public

	Pre (%)	Post (%)	*p* Value
Artificial hydration and nutrition should be continued as the minimum standard of care until death	50	31	0.001
Artificial hydration and nutrition relieve symptoms	35	24	0.001

TABLE 9.4
Japanese Patients' and Families' Views on Artificial Hydration Therapy

	Patients (n = 62)	Family Members (n = 119)
Artificial hydration		
Prolongs a meaningless life	23%	24%
Worsens symptoms	55%	57%
Increases dependency	37%	26%
Withholding artificial hydration		
Cannot take sufficient nutrition	76%	85%
Leads to premature death	56%	84%
Worsens symptoms	23%	39%
Increases anxiety	21%	34%

Regarding the views of patients and families, a small investigation revealed the ambivalent nature of the problem. In this survey, 121 hospice inpatients with reduced oral intake and their families were interviewed to clarify concerns related to the reduced oral intake and artificial hydration therapy (Morita et al. 1999). About 80% of the patients and family members believed that withholding artificial hydration therapy means that patients "cannot take adequate nutrition," and about 60% of the patients and 80% of the family members believed that withholding artificial hydration therapy leads to premature death (Table 9.4). On the other hand, about 25% of the patients and family members believed that artificial hydration therapy "prolongs a meaningless life." Furthermore, about half of the patients and family members assumed that artificial hydration therapy would deteriorate physical symptoms, while about 30% reported that withholding it would deteriorate physical symptoms. In addition, 37% of the patients said that artificial hydration would increase dependency and 34% of the families reported that withholding artificial hydration would increase the anxiety levels of family members. Therefore, in short, some patients and families do wish for artificial hydration due to the expectation of an increased nutrient intake, alleviation of symptoms, and reduced anxiety (probably helplessness from "not doing anything valuable"), while some patients and families do not wish for it as it does not contribute to survival prolongation, they have no intent to prolong a "meaningless" life, it does not alleviate symptoms, and patients wish to avoid being a burden to others. The decision-making process is based on both medical facts and the values of each patient and family member.

9.4 ATTITUDES OF PHYSICIANS AND NURSES TOWARD ARTIFICIAL HYDRATION

Several nationwide surveys clarified physicians' and nurses' attitudes toward artificial hydration therapy. In the largest survey of physicians treating cancer patients (Morita, Shima et al. 2002), the authors surveyed a total of 584 physicians throughout the country to clarify physicians' attitudes toward terminal dehydration and identify the physician-related factors contributing to such attitudes. On hypothetically considering a gastric cancer patient with an estimated survival of 1 month and almost impossible oral intake due to intestinal obstruction, 50% chose intravenous hydration of 1000 ml/day, while 24% selected more than 1500 ml/day. For a lung cancer patient with cachexia, 58% chose 1000 ml/day, while 26% selected no hydration or 500 ml. Of notable findings, the physicians with more positive attitudes toward intravenous hydration were significantly less involved in end-of-life care, being more likely to regard the physiologic requirement of fluid and nutrition as important in initiating intravenous hydration, and more likely to believe that intravenous hydration is effective for symptom palliation and the minimum standard of care (Table 9.5). In this study, 40% of the physicians regarded intravenous hydration as the minimum standard of care and

TABLE 9.5
Determinants of Japanese Physicians' Decision to Perform Artificial Hydration Therapy

	Gastric Cancer (Intestinal Obstruction)			Lung Cancer (Cachexia)		
	Odds Ratio	95% CI	*p*	Odds Ratio	95% CI	*p*
Specialty (palliative medicine)	0.072	0.010–0.54	0.011	0.24	0.11–0.50	<0.01
Physician-perceived importance of "physiologic requirement"	1.89	1.34–2.66	<0.01	1.53	1.05–2.24	0.027
Belief that "intravenous hydration is effective for symptom palliation"	1.80	1.25–2.58	<0.01	2.23	1.51–3.28	<0.01
Belief that "intravenous hydration is the minimum standard of care"	1.37	1.07–1.76	0.012	2.16	1.63–2.87	<0.01

32% considered allowing a patient to die under dehydrated conditions as being ethically impermissible. These results corresponded to the findings of previous surveys whereby Japanese physicians were more likely to perform life-support therapy for terminal patients than Japanese-American doctors (Asai, Fukuhara, and Lo 1995) and 24% of Japanese oncologists regarded the withdrawal of life-supporting treatment as never being ethically justified (Asai et al. 1998). This attitude may be related to demands from patients and families themselves, as described above, and some physicians perform artificial hydration for terminal patients without a clear medical aim as a "symbol of caregiving." The survey concluded that, to provide "standardized" treatment for terminally ill cancer patients with a seriously reduced oral intake, the priority in hydration research should be to clarify the appropriate physiologic requirements of fluid and nutrition in dying patients, the effects of intravenous hydration on patient symptoms, and the reasons why physicians consider intravenous hydration therapy to be the minimum standard of care. The survey resulted in a subsequent series of observational studies to explore the effects of intravenous hydration on patient symptoms (Morita, Hyodo et al. 2006; Morita et al. 2005; Morita, Tei et al. 2002; Morita et al. 2001; Morita, Tei, and Inoue 2003; Morita et al. 1998; Morita et al. 2004). In one multicenter prospective study involving 226 consecutive terminally ill patients with abdominal malignancies, 1000 ml/day or more hydration was significantly associated with the deterioration of observer-rated edema, ascites, and pleural effusion, while there were no significant associations between the hydration volume and level of bronchial secretion, hyperactive delirium, communication capacity, agitation, myoclonus, or bedsores (Morita et al. 2005). These findings indicate that artificial hydration therapy could worsen peripheral edema, ascites, and pleural effusions, and that the potential benefits of artificial hydration therapy should be balanced with the risk of worsening fluid retention symptoms.

On the other hand, nurses have a somewhat different view from physicians (Miyashita et al. 2007a, b). Nurses generally perceive that artificial hydration therapy is not beneficial for terminally ill cancer patients, that artificial hydration is not always the minimum standard of care, and that maintaining hydration is a burden to patients (Table 9.6) (Miyashita et al. 2007a). In addition, in about 40% of cases in general hospitals, compared with 80% in certified palliative care units, nurses observed that patients and medical professionals adequately discuss the issue of artificial hydration, or physicians respect patients' and families' desires regarding artificial hydration (Table 9.7) (Miyashita et al. 2007b).

In summary, Japanese physicians' attitude toward artificial hydration is determined by (1) how physicians decide on the appropriate physiologic requirements of fluid and nutrition in dying patients, (2) how physicians evaluate the effects of intravenous hydration on patient symptoms, and (3) whether physicians regard artificial hydration therapy as the minimum standard of care. About 40% of Japanese physicians regard artificial hydration therapy as the minimum standard of care, while 20% of nurses have this opinion.

TABLE 9.6
Comparisons of Japanese Physicians' and Nurses' Views on Artificial Hydration Therapy

	Physicians (n = 584)	Nurses (n = 3328)	p
Artificial hydration alleviates the sensation of thirst	43%	20%	<0.0001
Artificial hydration alleviates fatigue	34%	19%	<0.0001
Withholding artificial hydration leads to loss of patients' trust	23%	19%	0.034
Withholding artificial hydration leads to loss of family's trust	26%	21%	0.010
Withholding artificial hydration shortens patient survival	29%	23%	0.002
Artificial hydration is a component of minimum standard of care	40%	22%	<0.0001
Maintaining a venous route is a burden to the patient	65%	71%	0.003

9.5 ESSENCE OF THE CLINICAL GUIDELINE

To minimize the actual treatment discrepancy and contribute to patient well-being by clarifying the optimal practice from empirical evidence and expert experience available, the Japanese Society of Palliative Medicine recently published a clinical guideline for artificial hydration therapy for terminally ill cancer patients using evidence-based and formal consensus-building methods (Morita et al. 2007).

The guideline is increasingly being accepted in Japan, and educational efforts are now ongoing. A preliminary nurse education program including a 5-hour interactive workshop based on the clinical guideline of the Japanese Society of Palliative Medicine improved nurses' knowledge, confidence, and self-reported practice, and was generally perceived as useful by nurses (Table 9.8) (Yamagishi, Tanaka, and Morita 2009). After the workshop, more than 80% of the nurses reported that they would more or much more frequently perform 6 of 8 recommended practices. This guideline includes general recommendations, specific recommendations (31 recommendations concerning medical aspects, 9 recommendations regarding nursing, and 7 recommendations concerning ethics), background descriptions, case examples, communication examples, a complete reference list, and structured abstracts of all relevant original articles. This chapter summarizes the essence of the clinical guideline.

TABLE 9.7
Japanese Nurses' Views on the Adequacy of Discussions Regarding Artificial Hydration for Terminally Ill Cancer Patients

	Oncology Nurse (n = 2735)	Palliative Care Unit Nurses (n = 593)	p Value
Patients and medical practitioners discuss the issue of artificial hydration adequately	39%	78%	<0.001
Medical practitioners discuss the issue of artificial hydration adequately	49%	79%	<0.001
Physicians respect the patient's/family's wishes regarding artificial hydration	42%	84%	<0.001

TABLE 9.8
Changes in Japanese Nurses' Practice Regarding Artificial Hydration Therapy

	More Frequently Performs	Unchanged
I will try to explore what worries the patients may have about not being able to eat	89%	3.9%
I will try to understand the patients' wishes and values concerning fluid infusion therapy	91%	3.9%
I will try to explore what worries the patients' families may have about the patients not being able to eat	91%	3.9%
I will observe the oral state and provide mouth care for thirst	93%	1.3%
I will ask the patients themselves about pain or how comfortable they are	89%	3.9%
I will modify infusion according to each patient's lifestyle (intermittent infusion, etc.)	82%	12%
I will advise physicians to perform subcutaneous administration if the peripheral IV route cannot be established	53%	29%
I will advise physicians to perform drug therapy that increases oral intake other than fluid infusion	68%	22%
I will advise physicians to reduce the volume of fluid infusion if ascites or pleural effusion is increased	67%	24%

9.5.1 Aims, Target Population, and Quality of Life

The primary aim of the guideline is thus to help clinicians make a clinical decision regarding artificial hydration therapy to ensure a better quality of care for terminally ill cancer patients.

The target population comprises adult cancer patients with incurable cancer, except for those with a primary head and neck, esophageal, and liver origin, without adequate oral intake refractory to appropriate palliative treatments who are likely to die within one to two months. The guideline defined "terminally ill cancer patients" as cancer patients with an estimated survival of 1–2 months or less, and recommended the clinical estimation of patient prognoses to be assessed by a multidisciplinary team on the basis of validated methods (e.g., the Palliative Prognostic Score or Palliative Prognostic Index). The targeted users are healthcare professionals who treat the target population described above.

The objective of this guideline is to improve the quality of life (QOL), dying, and death. The guideline assumes that the determinants of the QOL, dying, and death vary among individuals, and so a focus on individuality is essential to define what is important for each patient. Palliation of physical distress, peace of mind, having a good family relationship, not being a burden to others, completion of life, fighting against cancer, maintaining hope, and not being aware of death are good death elements that could be related to the decision-making process regarding artificial hydration therapy for Japanese.

9.5.2 Conceptual Framework

Figure 9.1 shows the conceptual framework used in this guideline. The guideline strongly recommends that clinicians respect patient and family values, individualize the treatment suitable for each patient, assess the situation comprehensively from a medical, practical, psychosocial, ethical, and legal point of view, and reevaluate the treatment efficacy periodically. On the basis of this conceptual framework, clinicians should first clarify that the general treatment goal is consistent

Clarify that the general treatment goal is consistent with patient and family values

↓

Comprehensive assessment
- Potential effects of artificial hydration therapy on patients' physical symptoms, survival, daily activities, and psycho-existential well-being
- Ethical and legal issues

↓

Decide on the treatment plan after discussions with patients and families

↓

Periodically reevaluate the treatment efficacy, and adjust the treatment suitable for each patient

FIGURE 9.1 Conceptual framework of the guideline of the Japanese Society of Palliative Medicine.

with patient and family values. Second, clinicians should comprehensively assess the situation, especially the potential effects of artificial hydration therapy on patients' physical symptoms, survival, daily activities, psychoexistential well-being, and ethical and legal issues. Third, clinicians should decide on a treatment plan after discussions with patients and families. Finally, and most importantly, clinicians should periodically reevaluate the treatment efficacy at planned intervals, and adjust the treatment suitable for each patient.

9.5.3 Development Process

The Hydration Guideline Task Force developed this guideline, following the Japanese national recommendation to develop a clinical guideline. The Task Force consisted of 32 experts: 6 palliative care physicians, 6 surgeons, 4 anesthesiologists, 3 medical oncologists, 2 home-care physicians, 5 nurses, a social worker, 2 bioethicists, a lawyer, and 2 epidemiologists. The Japanese Society of Palliative Medicine approved each member as possessing sufficient clinical and professional competency to complete this task. Employing a systematic literature review and the Delphi technique, the Task Force decided on recommendations using an original recommendation table for this project to effectively define each recommendation (Table 9.9).

TABLE 9.9
Recommendation Tables

A. Sufficient research evidence (level I or consistent findings from level II evidence) and sufficient clinical agreement. We strongly recommend the intervention, when the treatment is consistent with patient preference and the treatment effect is monitored

B. Fair research evidence (single or inconsistent findings from level II or level III–V evidence) and sufficient clinical agreement. We recommend the intervention, when the treatment is consistent with patient preference and the treatment effect is monitored

C. No research evidence available but fair clinical agreement. We can recommend the intervention, if the treatment is consistent with patient preference and the treatment effect is monitored

D. No research evidence to support the intervention available and inadequate clinical agreement. We recommend the indication of the intervention only in the specific situation that the patient desires the treatment after being fully informed and the treatment effect is closely monitored

E. Sufficient or fair research evidence (level I–V) and sufficient clinical agreement about the ineffectiveness or harmfulness of the treatment. We recommend not performing the intervention

9.5.4 Specific Recommendations

Among 31 recommendations regarding medical aspects, 9 recommendations for nursing, and 7 recommendations concerning ethics as specific recommendations, 5 recommendations on the general QOL, ascites, thirst, delirium, and bronchial secretion are described as examples.

9.5.4.1 General QOL

9.4.4.1.1 Rationale

In patients with a poor performance status, a preliminary randomized controlled trial demonstrated no significant improvement in patient-reported general well-being of 1000 ml/day compared with 100 ml/day hydration, and this finding is consistent with several observational studies.

On the other hand, some audit trials demonstrated that artificial hydration therapy could contribute to maintaining the QOL of patients with a better performance status. The backgrounds of patients who received marked benefits from this intervention include a better performance status, bowel obstruction, and estimated survival of several months or longer.

Available empirical evidence thus suggests that (1) artificial hydration therapy is ineffective in improving the overall QOL of cancer patients close to death and (2) artificial hydration therapy can be effective in improving the overall QOL of cancer patients with a better performance status, bowel obstruction, and estimated survival of several months.

9.4.4.1.2 Recommendations

R010: To improve the general QOL of terminally ill cancer patients who are expected to live for 1–2 months, are incapable of oral fluid intake due to intestinal obstruction, but show a performance status of 2 or better:

- Simple hydration at 1000–1500 ml/day (400–600 kcal/day, nitrogen (N) 0 g/day). [C]
- Hyperalimentation at 1500 ml/day (1000 kcal/day, N 5 g/day). [C]
- Simple hydration at 2000 ml/day (800 kcal/day, N 0 g/day). [D]
- Hyperalimentation at 2000 ml/day (1600 kcal/day, N 10 g/day). [D]

R011: To improve the general QOL of terminally ill cancer patients who are expected to live for 1–2 weeks, are incapable of oral fluid intake due to intestinal obstruction, and show a performance status of 3 or worse:

- Simple hydration at 1000–1500 ml/day (400–600 kcal/day, N 0 g/day). [D]
- Hyperalimentation at 1000–2000 ml/day (800–1600 kcal/day, N 5–10 g/day). [E]

R012: To improve the general QOL of terminally ill cancer patients who are expected to live for 1–2 weeks, are incapable of oral fluid intake due to progressive cachexia, and show a performance status of 3 or worse:

- Simple hydration at 1000–1500 ml/day (400–600 kcal/day, N 0 g/day). [E]
- Hyperalimentation at 1000–2000 ml/day (800–1600 kcal/day, N 5–10 g/day). [E]

9.5.4.2 Ascites

9.5.4.2.1 Rationale

We are aware of no intervention trials with the primary end-point of ascites. One large multicenter prospective observational study suggested that patients receiving 1000 ml/day or more hydration during the last 3 weeks experienced significantly more severe ascites than those receiving none or less than 1000 ml/day. This is consistent with another multicenter retrospective observational study, a nationwide opinion survey, and other small-scale observational studies.

Available empirical evidence thus suggests that (1) less than 1000 ml/day hydration is unlikely to worsen ascites, (2) 1500–2000 ml/day hydration can worsen ascites, and (3) volume reduction can alleviate ascites.

9.5.4.2.2 Recommendations

R020: To minimize ascites-related distress in terminally ill cancer patients who are expected to live for 1–2 months, are capable of oral fluid intake of 500 ml/day or more, and have symptomatic ascites:

- No artificial hydration therapy. [B]
- Artificial hydration therapy is limited to 500–1000 ml/day or less, if performed. [C]

R021: To minimize ascites-related distress in terminally ill cancer patients who are expected to live for 1–2 months, are incapable of oral fluid intake, and have symptomatic ascites:

- Artificial hydration therapy is limited to the volume of vomiting + 500–1000 ml/day or less, if performed. [C]

R022: To minimize ascites-related distress in terminally ill cancer patients who are expected to live for 1–2 months, are incapable of oral fluid intake, are receiving artificial hydration therapy at 2000 ml/day, and show the exacerbation of ascites:

- Artificial hydration therapy is limited to 1000 ml/day or less. [C]

9.5.4.3 Thirst

9.5.4.3.1 Rationale

One small randomized controlled trial demonstrated no significant benefits of an additional 1000 ml/day hydration compared with nursing care in terminally ill cancer patients with a median survival of 4 days, and this result is consistent with a well-conducted audit study which showed that nursing care without artificial hydration alleviated the sensation of thirst in most terminally ill patients. A large observational study demonstrated that patients receiving hydration of 1000 ml/day or more during the last 3 weeks showed significantly less objective findings of dehydration than those receiving none or less than 1000 ml/day, but the absolute difference was small and both groups demonstrated the consistent deterioration of objective dehydration. Several small observational studies revealed that the sensation of thirst was not linearly associated with the levels of blood urea nitrogen, sodium, protein, and the hematocrit, but could be significantly associated with hyperosmolarity, a decreased intravenous volume (measured by atrial natriuretic peptides), stomatitis, oral breathing, and anticholinergic medication.

Available empirical evidence thus suggests that (1) the sensation of thirst in terminally ill cancer patients is a multietiologic symptom, and hyperosmolarity and a decreased intravenous volume may contribute to symptom development, (2) artificial hydration can alleviate objective findings of dehydration to some extent, but a subjective sensation of thirst can be sufficiently alleviated by employing nursing measures without artificial hydration therapy. In patients with a better performance status and correctable dehydration, artificial hydration therapy appears effective in alleviating thirst, despite a lack of clinical observations on this selected study population.

9.5.4.3.2 Recommendations

R040: To alleviate thirst in terminally ill cancer patients who are expected to live for 1–2 months, are incapable of oral fluid intake due to intestinal obstruction, and have no fluid retention symptoms:

- Artificial hydration therapy at 1000–1500 ml/day. [C]

R041: To alleviate thirst in terminally ill cancer patients who are expected to live for 1–2 weeks or less, are capable of oral fluid intake, and have no fluid retention symptoms:

- Artificial hydration therapy at 500–1000 ml/day. [D]
- No artificial hydration therapy (nursing oral care only). [B]

R042: To alleviate thirst in terminally ill cancer patients who are expected to live for 1–2 weeks or less, are barely capable of oral fluid intake due to intestinal obstruction (peritonitis carcinomatosa), and have fluid retention symptoms:

- Artificial hydration therapy at 500–1000 ml/day. [D]
- Artificial hydration therapy increased from 1000 to 2000 ml/day. [E]
- No artificial hydration therapy (nursing-based oral care only). [B]

9.5.4.4 Delirium

9.5.4.4.1 Rationale

For patients with opioid-induced delirium, no controlled trials have accurately examined the effects of hydration therapy. Some observational studies suggested that dehydration was significantly associated with the reversibility of delirium, although the association seemed dependent on opioid use.

On the other hand, in patients close to death, a small randomized controlled trial demonstrated no significant benefits of 1000 ml/day hydration on improving the cognitive function of terminally ill cancer patients with a median survival of 4 days. A multicenter observational study failed to demonstrate beneficial effects of hydration to prevent agitated delirium and a Japanese historical control study also failed to demonstrate a decrease in the occurrence of agitated delirium using aggressive hydration and opioid rotation, contrary to a previous report from another group. These findings are consistent with several observations and case series suggesting that artificial hydration did not appear beneficial for improving the cognitive function in terminally ill cancer patients very close to death on a large scale.

Available empirical evidence thus suggests that (1) artificial hydration therapy can be useful in selected patients in combination with opioid rotation with opioid-induced delirium through the rapid clearance of toxic metabolites and (2) artificial hydration therapy has no benefits in improving delirium for most patients with organ failure.

9.5.4.4.2 Recommendations

R070: To alleviate delirium due to dehydration and morphine in terminally ill cancer patients, when other symptoms have been sufficiently palliated:

- Artificial hydration therapy (and opioid rotation, e.g., fentanyl). [B]

R071: To alleviate delirium due to no identifiable cause other than dehydration in terminally ill cancer patients, when other symptoms have been sufficiently palliated:

- Artificial hydration therapy at 1000 ml/day. [B]

R072: To alleviate delirium due to hypoxemia in terminally ill cancer patients with multiple lung metastases who are expected to live for 1–2 weeks, and have symptomatic pleural effusion and/or edema:

- Artificial hydration therapy at 1000 ml/day. [E]

R073: To alleviate delirium due to hepatic encephalopathy in terminally ill cancer patients with multiple liver metastases who are expected to live for 1–2 weeks, and have symptomatic ascites and/or edema:

- Artificial hydration therapy at 1000 ml/day. [E]

9.5.4.5 Bronchial Secretion

9.5.4.5.1 Rationale

We have encountered no intervention trials with a primary end-point of bronchial secretion. One large multicenter prospective observational study revealed no significant difference in the prevalence of bronchial secretion between patients receiving 1000 ml/day or more hydration during the last 3 weeks and those receiving no or less than 1000 ml/day. In that study, however, all patients had abdominal malignancy and the median hydration volume was relatively small (700 ml/day). Terminally ill cancer patients receiving a median of 1500 ml/day hydration experienced significantly more pronounced bronchial secretion than those receiving a median of 250 ml/day. This is consistent with an opinion-based survey and case report, suggesting that increased levels of hydration therapy could elevate the risk of developing bronchial secretion.

Available empirical evidence thus suggests that (1) a relatively large volume of hydration (e.g., 1500 ml/day or more) can worsen bronchial secretion and (2) in patients receiving a relatively small volume of hydration (e.g., <500–1000 ml/day), the hydration volume is minimally associated with the development of bronchial secretion.

9.5.4.5.2 Recommendations

R060: To alleviate bronchial secretion-related distress in terminally ill cancer patients who are expected to live for a few days:

- Artificial hydration therapy is reduced to 500 ml/day or less or discontinued. [B]

9.5.4.5.3 Application to other areas of palliative care

Artificial hydration therapy is closely associated with the palliative control of various symptoms, especially ascites, dyspnea, delirium, and bronchial secretion. Clinicians should maximize symptom control using an active combination of pharmacological, nonpharmacological, medical, and nonmedical strategies. In addition, a patient's decision regarding whether or not to receive artificial hydration reflects their values, or the concept of a good death, and, thus, could be related other medical decisions.

9.6 GUIDELINES

The guideline of the Japanese Society of Palliative Medicine summarizes the general recommendations (Table 9.10) (Morita et al. 2007). The author believes that this guideline is useful irrespective of cultural differences.

KEY FACTS REGARDING ARTIFICIAL HYDRATION FOR TERMINALLY ILL CANCER PATIENTS

- Artificial hydration is not only a medical, but also a psychological, social, and spiritual issue. Clinicians should make a decision from the viewpoint of a good death for each patient.
- An evidence-based guideline can be a useful resource to make clinical decisions.
- Periodic reevaluation is an important strategy to improve outcomes.

ETHICAL ISSUES

In the guideline, four specific recommendations are described as ethical recommendations (Asai et al. 1998). Of them, short descriptions of three recommendations are given as examples (Table 9.11).

TABLE 9.10
General Recommendations

[Respect for patient and family values, wishes, and individuality]
1. The aims of artificial hydration therapy should be consistent with the overall treatment goal on the basis of each patient and family value. Improvement of the laboratory findings and nutritional status alone is not a primary end-point for artificial hydration therapy
2. Patient and family wishes should be respected in the treatment decision
3. Artificial hydration therapy should be individualized for each patient and family situation. The routine use or non-use of artificial hydration therapy is not supported
[Evaluation]
4. The indication of artificial hydration therapy should be based on comprehensive assessment of the patient's overall quality of life, satisfaction, physical symptoms, survival, psychoexistential well-being, daily activities, and ethical and legal issues
5. Dehydration and/or water depletion in the terminal stage does not always cause discomfort to patients. Improvements in objective findings, such as laboratory findings, urine volume, and central venous pressure, are not primary end-points in artificial hydration therapy
6. The periodic reevaluation and timely adjustment of treatment regimens are essential to maximize the treatment benefit of artificial hydration therapy
[Maximization of the balance between benefits and burdens]
7. Artificial hydration therapy should maximize the balance between the benefits and burdens of artificial hydration therapy
[Importance of nursing and psychosocial care]
8. For terminally ill cancer patients suffering from a decreased oral intake, not only artificial hydration therapy, but pharmacological treatment to improve appetite, nursing care, psychosocial interventions, and support in the decision-making and daily activity are of great importance
[Summary of medical recommendations]
9. For terminally ill cancer patients with decreased oral intake due to a progressive malignancy-related etiology other than bowel obstruction and/or poor performance status, artificial hydration therapy alone is unlikely to improve the overall quality of life
10. For terminally ill cancer patients with a better performance status and decreased oral intake due to bowel obstruction, artificial hydration therapy can improve the overall quality of life
11. Artificial hydration therapy can worsen distress related to ascites, pleural effusion, and peripheral edema in terminally ill cancer patients
12. Artificial hydration therapy is unlikely to alleviate the sensation of thirst in terminally ill cancer patients. Intensive nursing care is of the utmost importance to alleviate the sensation of thirst
13. In some terminally ill cancer patients, artificial hydration therapy can contribute to improve the quality of life through alleviating opioid-induced delirium and acute dehydration/water depletion
14. Subcutaneous hydration is appropriate for terminally ill cancer patients in whom an intravenous line is difficult to place and/or is distressing

SUMMARY POINTS

- The good death concept could explain how patients determine whether they do or do not receive artificial hydration therapy. The important domains include maintaining a good relationship with the family and medical staff, a natural death, fighting against cancer, unawareness of death, and not being a burden to others.
- Many Japanese prefer artificial hydration therapy not only for medical, but also psychological, social, and spiritual reasons.

TABLE 9.11
Summary of Recommendations Regarding the Ethical Aspects of Artificial Hydration Therapy Listed in the Guideline of the Japanese Society of Palliative Medicine

1. When a patient's wish is consistent with what is in their best interests as assumed by medical professionals
   If a competent patient given sufficient information explicitly desires not to receive artificial hydration, physicians should not perform it on the basis of the patient's autonomy and assumed best interests
   If a competent patient desires not to receive artificial hydration but has insufficient information, physicians should first provide sufficient information and, meanwhile, can choose not to perform hydration
2. When a patient's wish is inconsistent with the best interests assumed by medical professionals
   If a competent patient given sufficient information explicitly desires to receive artificial hydration, physicians should first sufficiently reassess whether the patient's wish is explicit on being given sufficient information and whether medical professionals understand the individual values of each patient. After sufficient discussion with patients and medical professionals, the decision not to perform artificial hydration therapy is acceptable
   If a competent patient does not want to receive artificial hydration but has insufficient information, physicians should first provide sufficient information and, meanwhile, can choose whether or not to perform hydration according to the patient's condition
3. When a patient's wish is consistent with the best interests assumed by medical professionals, but is inconsistent with those of family members
   Physicians should: 1) first, sufficiently reassess whether the patient's and family's wishes are explicit given sufficient information, and whether medical professionals understand the individual values of each patient, and 2) coordinate a full discussion between patients and families to resolve any discrepancies. If a patient's wish is unchanged after sufficient discussion with him/her, the family, and medical professionals, the decision not to perform artificial hydration therapy is acceptable

- To minimize the actual treatment discrepancy and contribute to patient well-being, a clinical guideline is available from the Japanese Society of Palliative Medicine and increasingly being accepted in Japan.

NOTE

The clinical guideline (in Japanese) is available from the Web page of the Japanese Society of Palliative Medicine (http://www.jspm.ne.jp/).

REFERENCES

Asai, A., S. Fukuhara, and B. Lo. 1995. Attitudes of Japanese and Japanese American physicians towards life-sustaining treatment. *Lancet* 346:356–59.

Asai, A., Y. Miura, N. Tanabe, M. Kurihara, and S. Fukuhara. 1998. Advance directives and other medical decisions concerning the end-of-life in cancer patients in Japan. *Eur J Cancer* 34:1582–86.

Miyashita, M., T. Morita, Y. Shima, R. Kimura, M. Takahashi, and I. Adachi. 2007a. Physician and nurse attitudes toward artificial hydration for terminally ill cancer patients in Japan: Results of 2 nationwide surveys. *Am J Hosp Palliat Care* 24:383–89.

Miyashita, M., T. Morita, Y. Shima, R. Kimura, M. Takahashi, and I. Adachi. 2007b. Nurse views of the adequacy of decision making and nurse distress regarding artificial hydration for terminally ill cancer patients: A nationwide survey. *Am J Hosp Palliat Care* 24:463–69.

Miyashita, M., M. Sanjo, T. Morita, K. Hirai, and Y. Uchitomi. 2007. Good death in cancer care: A nationwide quantitative study. *Ann Oncol* 18:1090–97.

Miyashita, M., K. Sato, T. Morita, and M. Suzuki. 2008. Effect of a population-based educational intervention focusing on end-of-life home care, life-prolonging treatment and knowledge about palliative care. *Palliat Med* 22:376–82.

Morita, T., S. Bito, H. Koyama, Y. Uchitomi, and I. Adachi. 2007. Development of a national clinical guideline for artificial hydration therapy for terminally ill patients with cancer. *J Palliat Med* 10:770–80.

Morita, T., I. Hyodo, T. Yoshimi, M. Ikenaga, Y. Tamura, A. Yoshizawa, A. Shimada et al. 2005. Association between hydration volume and symptoms in terminally ill cancer patients with abdominal malignancies. *Ann Oncol* 16:640–47.

Morita, T., I. Hyodo, T. Yoshimi, M. Ikenaga, Y. Tamura, A. Yoshizawa, A. Shimada et al. 2006. Artificial hydration therapy, laboratory findings, and fluid balance in terminally ill patients with abdominal malignancies. *J Pain Symptom Manage* 31:130–39.

Morita, T., M. Miyashita, M. Shibagaki, K. Hirai, T. Ashiya, T. Ishihara, T. Matsubara et al. 2006. Knowledge and beliefs about end-of-life care and the effects of specialized palliative care: A population-based survey in Japan. *J Pain Symptom Manage* 31:306–16.

Morita, T., Y. Shima, I. Adachi, and Japan Palliative Oncology Study (J-POS) Group. 2002. Attitudes toward terminal dehydration of Japanese physicians: A nationwide survey. *J Clin Oncol* 20:4699–704.

Morita, T., Y. Shima, M. Miyashita, R. Kimura, and I. Adachi. 2004. Physician- and nurse-reported effects of intravenous hydration therapy on symptoms of terminally ill patients with cancer. *J Palliat Med* 7:683–93.

Morita, T., Y. Tei, and S. Inoue. 2003. Agitated terminal delirium and association with partial opioid substitution and hydration. *J Palliat Med* 6:557–63.

Morita, T., J. Tsunoda, S. Inoue, S. Chihara, O. Ishimoto, S. Shimada, N. Hisaoka, and M. Ito. 1998. The effect of hydration on death rattle and sensation of thirst in terminally-ill cancer patients. *Terminal Care* 8:227–32.

Morita, T., J. Tsunoda, S. Inoue, and S. Chihara. 1999. Perceptions and decision-making on rehydration of terminally ill cancer patients and family members. *Am J Hosp Palliat Care* 16:509–16.

Morita, T., Y. Tei, J. Tsunoda, S. Inoue, and S. Chihara. 2001. Determinants of the sensation of thirst in terminally ill cancer patients. *Support Care Cancer* 9:177–86.

Morita, T., Y. Tei, S. Inoue, A. Suga, and S. Chihara. 2002. Fluid status of terminally ill cancer patients with intestinal obstruction: An exploratory observational study. *Support Care Cancer* 10:474–79.

Yamagishi, A., F. Tanaka, and T. Morita. 2009. Artificial hydration therapy for terminally ill cancer patients: A nurse-education intervention. *J Pain Symptom Manage* 38:358–64.

10 Nutritional Support in Palliative Care: Chinese Perspectives

Meng-Yun Hsieh, Kuo-Chin Huang, Tai-Yuan Chiu, and Ching-Yu Chen

CONTENTS

10.1 INTRODUCTION

An ancient Chinese saying notes: "Kings place the people first, and the people place food first." Another adage follows the same theme: "Eating is as important as the emperor." Thus it is evident that Chinese society place much significance on food and food culture. The culmination of five thousand years of recorded history and the long-held traditional family-based ideology remain deeply ingrained in the people's hearts. Taiwanese people are adherent to these traditions, following the Confucian philosophy, and thus are good representatives of the core beliefs of traditional Chinese culture.

For many years, cancer has remained at the top of the list of the ten leading causes of death in Taiwan. Palliative care in Taiwan has developed rapidly following the approval of related legislation in the year 2000. Currently, with the exception of a few cases of amyotrophic lateral sclerosis, most are terminal cancer patients. The number of terminal cancer patients receiving palliative care has grown from 5.7% in 1997 (Lo 1997) to more than 30% of the total in 2008 (DOH 2009). Currently there are 41 hospice wards and 65 medical institutions providing combined care and house calls. While these statistics are much improved, more continued effort is needed.

Palliative care involves consideration of many bio-psycho-social-spiritual aspects, including different cultural backgrounds and socioeconomic factors. Ethnic minority populations now comprise over 25% of the US population, yet they represent less than 17% of patients enrolled in hospice (Crawley et al. 2000). In coming years, as more patients require palliative care, approaches with culture perspectives in mind will be much needed. For example, Chinese people expressed different concerns regarding the telling of bad news (Bowman and Singer 2001; Tse, Chong, and Fok 2003), the limitation of treatment, and the role of family in medical encounters (Muller and Desmond 1992). It is therefore crucial to take different ethnicity into consideration in palliative care.

Hospice and palliative care of terminal cancer patients has been the focus of much concerted deliberation. Individualized terminal care and cachexia in the dying have long been unavoidable dilemmas. Difficulty in eating or drinking often leads to anxiety in the patient's loved ones, who worry that the patient will starve to death and therefore become a "starving soul" after death. They also tend to pay attention to all the possible nutrients in the terminal stage. This attention to food is carried on after death, as people worship their ancestors by preparing feasts on the offering table. Thus the "Filial Piety" that all Chinese people follow and the family-centered culture are frequently interpreted as mandating the giving of more food, resulting in decisions often based on the family's philosophy, but not the patient's best interest (Kagawa-Singer and Blackhall 2001). It is similar in other Asian cultures (Blackhall 1999). Herein, the topic of nutritional and fluid administration in Chinese terminal patients is discussed. The following discussion mainly refers to terminal cancer patients as they make up the majority.

10.2 PREVALENCE OF ANOREXIA, CACHEXIA AND MALNUTRITION IN TERMINAL CANCER PATIENTS

According to estimations by the Taiwan Bureau of Health Promotion, the total cancer incidence in 2006 was 73,293 persons. The most common cancers were breast cancer, colorectal cancer, liver and biliary tract cancers in females, and liver and biliary tract cancers, colorectal cancer, and lung cancer in males. The Department of Health in Taiwan reported a total number of 38,913 cancer mortalities in 2008, averaging one cancer death every thirteen and a half minutes. According to the 2005 annual report of the World Health Organization, the number of cancer deaths in China was 1,890,200 persons, with over 1 million of these comprised of people under the age of 70 years old.

Terminal cancer patients often display multiple complicated symptoms and signs. Up to 80% of pain can now be sufficiently controlled (WHO 1995). However, other common symptoms such as lethargy and anorexia are often still recalcitrant to treatment. This, in turn, adds to the fear and anxiety for both the patient and family members, believing that the patient would therefore suffer from insufficient nutrition to combat disease. It is often then a difficult dilemma for health professionals regarding the administration of nutrition and fluid. A study conducted by the palliative care ward in National Taiwan University Hospital (NTUH) found that this moral dilemma was encountered in up to 25% of all patients (Figure 10.1) (Chiu et al. 2000). In Taiwan, the Natural Death Act was legislated in 2000 (the first country to do so in Asia) and the topic of artificial nutrition and hydration (ANH) is still one of the most conflicted of ethical dilemmas faced in palliative practice (Chiu et al. 2009).

Studies from the palliative ward at NTUH revealed that factors related to nutrition-related anorexia or decreased appetite comprise the largest proportion of the most common symptoms that terminal cancer patients experienced, including weakness (82.3%), anorexia (81%), weight loss (64.7%), pain (81%), and dysphagia (53.4%) (Table 10.1) (Chiu et al. 2000; Tsai et al. 2006).

10.3 CURRENT STATUS OF NUTRITIONAL SUPPORT IN PALLIATIVE CARE

Necessary aspects of nutritional support in palliative care should include statement and understanding of nutritional goal, formal nutritional consultations, consideration of pharmacological treatment, and educated choice between enteral and parenteral nutrition. Terminal cancer patients are a heterogeneous group, requiring individualized treatment; it is therefore important to design nutritional treatments tailored to each individual. In the early stage of disease or in those in whom starvation plays the primary role in weight loss (instead of the complex neuroendocrine mechanism), aggressive nutritional support may be considered. These may include, for example, (1) malignant bowel

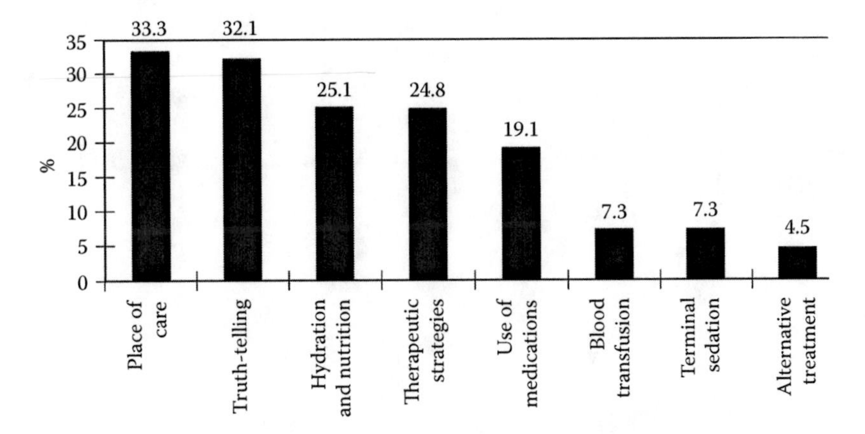

FIGURE 10.1 Types and frequency of ethical dilemmas during hospitalizations as assessed by health care workers. This figure depicts common ethical dilemmas encountered in palliative care. Of these, hydration and nutrition issues accounted for 25.1%; when combined, this represents the third most common ethical dilemma. (From Chiu, T. Y. et al., *J. Med. Ethics* 26, 353, 2000.)

obstruction caused by slow-growing tumors; (2) severe dysphagia due to radiation therapy in head and neck cancer patients; (3) anorexia due to psychological or economic factors; (4) postoperative anorexia and/or anorexia after aggressive chemotherapy (Doyle et al. 2005). Clinically, it is of great importance to recognize these patients and to estimate their predicted survival. Total parenteral nutrition should be reserved for patients whose predicted survival is longer than 2–3 months (Bozzetti et al. 2009). A detailed and multidisciplinary approach can help us to arrange for appropriately tailored treatments for each patient.

In the National Taiwan University Hospital palliative care ward, for example, the mean survival for terminal patients has been approximately 2–3 weeks. Referrals from other specialties were usually at a relatively late stage. Of these, 38.7% were unable to eat or drink at the time of admission, for which the most commonly attributed reason, in the opinion of the medical staff, was gastrointestinal tract disturbances. The inability to eat or drink reached 60.1% at 2 days before death, with cancer cachexia due to underlying pathology being the main cause (Table 10.2). For those who could still drink and eat at 2 days before death, nearly all of them needed help from their caregivers to facilitate food intake (Chiu et al. 2002). The percentage of patients receiving ANH started with 57% on admission, followed by a decrease to 46.9% 1 week after admission and then an increase again to 53.1% in the final 48 hours before death, which is still lower than the percentage on admission (Table 10.3).

At primary assessment of the patient, medical professionals first comprehensively evaluate the patient's predicted survival time and general nutritional status. Usually patients are encouraged to take more nutritional foods and to enjoy their delicious tastes. However, when patient survival is expected to be very limited, emphasis should be placed on the global improvement of quality of life (QOL), namely by carefully reassessing for incorrect or inappropriate types of foods, inappropriate time for food supply, oral hygiene or stomatitis, physiological causes, and any socioeconomic or emotional factors. Many patients who previously were unable to partake in oral intake may gradually increase nutrition by mouth. Through multidisciplinary care and increased family-patient interaction, a higher-quality, patient-centered management of the patient's medical care can be established. To provide holistic care, associated team members should consist of psychologists, chaplains (such as Buddhist monks/nuns), social workers, and volunteers, in addition to doctors and nurses.

Meanwhile, although hydration through a subcutaneous route is an option for terminal patients, it is still rarely used in Taiwan. Further exploration will be needed to understand its role in the Chinese culture (Chiu et al. 2002).

TABLE 10.1
Prevalence of Symptoms at the Time of Admission (By Primary Site of Cancer)

Primary Site	Symptoms (%)										No.
	Weakness	Pain	Anorexia	Weight Loss	Dysphagia	Dyspnea	Restlessness	Confusion	N/V	Insomnia	
Lung	80.0	78.0	76.0	69.4	48.0	60.0	52.0	58.0	42.0	48.0	50
Colon and rectum	62.5	79.4	91.7	60.9	62.5	45.8	58.3	25.0	55.0	45.8	25
Liver	83.3	70.8	85.3	58.3	41.7	58.3	37.5	52.0	62.5	45.8	25
Stomach	86.4	90.9	91.0	71.0	59.1	54.5	54.5	45.5	59.1	59.1	22
Head and neck	75.0	87.5	56.2	67.5	68.7	37.5	37.5	43.7	25.0	25.0	16
Cervix	90.0	60.0	90.0	70.0	50.0	80.0	30.0	50.0	40.0	50.0	10
Breast	70.0	70.0	90.0	70.0	70.0	60.0	70.0	80.0	50.0	50.0	10
Pancreas	80.0	100.0	90.0	80.0	60.0	60.0	60.0	40.0	60.0	40.0	10
Others	81.2	78.1	79.7	62.5	56.2	48.4	51.6	50.0	48.4	42.2	64
Total	82.3	81.0	81.0	64.7	54.7	53.4	50.0	48.7	48.3	44.8	232
p-value	0.662	0.478	0.125	0.861	0.644	0.483	0.511	0.168	0.414	0.751	

Source: With kind permission from Springer Science+Business Media: *Support Care Cancer*, Prevalence and severity of symptoms in terminal cancer patients: a study in Taiwan, 8, 2000, 311, Chiu, T. Y. et al., Table 1.

Note: This table shows common symptoms and their prevalence in a palliative care unit. Prevalence of anorexia, weight loss, and dysphagia related to malnutrition were 81.0%, 64.7%, and 54.7% respectively.

Chi-square test, *d.f.* = –8 (N/V, nausea and vomiting).

TABLE 10.2
Frequency and Causes of Inability to Eat or Drink in Terminal Cancer

	Admission		One Week after Admission		Two Days before Death	
Unable to Eat or Drink Orally?	**No**	**%**	**No**	**%**	**No**	**%**
Unable to	133	38.7	95	39.1*	164	60.1**
Able to	211	61.3	148	60.9	109	39.9
Total patients	344	100.0	243	100.0	273	100.0
Main Causes of Inability to Eat and Drink by Mouth (Multiple Choices)						
Consciousness disturbance	45	33.8	32	33.7	56	34.1
Head/neck tumor	34	25.6	26	27.4	27	16.5
Esophageal obstruction	15	11.3	13	13.7	11	6.7
GI disturbances	78	58.6	53	55.8	69	42.1
Systemic disorders including fatigue or anorexia	57	42.9	37	38.9	71	43.3
Emotional factors	11	8.3	8	8.4	9	5.5
Total impaired patients	133		95		164	

Source: With kind permission from Springer Science+Business Media: *Support Care Cancer*, Nutrition and hydration for terminal cancer patients in Taiwan, 10, 2002, 630, Chiu, T. Y. et al., Table 2.

Note: This table demonstrates the frequency of inability to eat or drink in terminal patient at different times (at admission, one week after admission, and two days before death) as well as its main causes. As disease progresses to terminal status, the frequency of inability to eat or drink increases; GI disturbances and impaired consciousness accounted for the main causes of this inability.

*$p < 0.01$: the ability decreased compared to the same patients ($n = 243$) at the time of admission.

**$p < 0.001$: the ability decreased compared to the same patients ($n = 273$) at the time of admission.

10.4 APPLICATIONS OF COMPLEMENTARY AND ALTERNATIVE MEDICINE IN PALLIATIVE CARE

In recent decades, Traditional Chinese Medicine (TCM) has become more popular, even though Western medicine is still regarded as the mainstay of modern medicine. The biggest difference between TCM and Western medicine rests in TCM's recognition of the human being functioning as a body-mind network rather than as separate distinct organ systems (Sagar and Wong 2008). Through the biological response modification, improvement of psycho-neuro-immunological function, improvement of symptom control and psychospiritual well-being, TCM has been shown to play a significant supportive role in patients being treated with conventional Western medicine. The different "Qi" deficiency and dysfunction could be relieved by TCM, which includes treatments with herbs, acupuncture, and "Qi-Gong." Theoretically, the different "Qi" disturbances should be treated with differing herbs and methods (Wong, Sagar, and Sagar 2001). There is evidence that fatigue, depression, pain, nausea and vomiting, myelosuppression, and poor appetite experienced by cancer patients could improve with TCM (Xu et al. 2007; Wong et al. 2001), but the target group of most studies were mostly those still receiving antitumor treatment regimens. Moreover, the idiosyncratic reactions and pharmacologic toxicities of herbs still also need to be addressed.

Most Chinese families place a certain value upon TCM, incorporating a variety of herbal remedies in their everyday diet. The homology between food and medicine is a common ideology in Chinese people. As the ancient medical texts of the "Yellow Emperor's Inner Canon" aptly illustrates: "food into the empty stomach is food; food into a patient is medicine." The concept of TCM places much significance on the balance between the two opposing forces of nature, "Yin" and "Yang," harmony between different "Qi"s, and emphasis on general well-being. Two sayings are

TABLE 10.3
Use of Artificial Nutrition and Hydration (ANH) in Terminal Cancer Patients

	Admission		One Week after Admission		Two Days before Death	
	No	%	No	%	No	%
Using ANH?						
Using	196	57.0	114	46.9*	145	53.1
Not using	148	43.0	129	53.1	128	46.9
Total	344	100.0	243	100.0	273	100.0
Types of ANH (Multiple Choices)						
Tube feeding	44	12.8	31	12.8	35	12.8
Parenteral						
1. Hydration and electrolyte	153	44.5	90	37.0**	118	43.2
2. Glucose	127	36.9	77	31.7	106	38.8
3. Other nutrients (albumin, amino acids, intrafat,.. etc)	66	19.2	37	15.2	50	18.3
Mean amount (ml) of I.V. fluid	862 ± 618		714 ± 528*		637 ± 420***	
Total	344		243		273	

Source: With kind permission from Springer Science+Business Media: *Support Care Cancer*, Nutrition and hydration for terminal cancer patients in Taiwan, 10, 2002, 630, Chiu, T. Y. et al., Table 3.

Note: This table represents the frequency of ANH use in terminal patients. One week after admission to palliative care unit, use of ANH significantly decreased. However, it increased again 2 days before death. As the disease progressed, mean amount of ANH amount decreased simultaneously.

*$p < 0.001$: decreased compared with the condition of the same patients ($n = 243$) at the time of admission.

**$p < 0.05$: decreased compared to the condition of the same patients ($n = 243$) at the time of admission.

***$p < 0.001$: decreased compared to the condition of the same patients ($n = 273$) at the time of admission.

central to these beliefs: "the basis of a healthy life and living is reliant upon food" and "food borrows from the strength of medicine, and medicine assists with the effects of food." In a broader sense, all the grains, fruits, vegetables, and/or meat we eat are simultaneously food and medicine, and "medicinal cooking" is the culinary combination of certain herbs and foods with known medicinal properties then cooked with an integration of traditional Chinese and modern methods with the aim of producing a healthy dish that simultaneously possesses vivid color, alluring scents, and enticing tastes. Because of this, many Chinese people hold the belief that proper diets can provide not only ample nutrition but also restore vitality.

Previous studies have shown that cancer patients in Taiwan have the highest rates of using complementary and alternative medicine (CAM) when compared to other countries (Ernst and Cassileth 1998). Patients frequently ask the question "if a certain kind of food can cure the cancer." Indeed, any Taiwanese health care practitioner, not only those in palliative care wards, may encounter these questions in daily practice. Common supplements such as "Antrodia cinnamomea," "Ganoderma," and "Cordyceps" are frequently asked about and are also commonly discussed amongst patients. Yet most of the CAM still lack substantiated evidence, while only a few have some animal studies or preliminary results. However, the philosophy of TCM encourages psychosocial support with compassion and healing intent, which is also the most central tenet of palliative care. A herbal diet carefully prepared with healthy food and herbs can be a symbol of love and benevolent intentions from the family and healthcare team. One study in a palliative care ward showed that these types of herbal diets were effective in reducing pain in cancer patients, thereby simultaneously improving the patients' QoL (Wu et al. 2008). In the NTUH palliative care ward, given that Western medicine was still the mainstream therapy, TCM was treated with an open attitude, seen as having a complementary and compassionate role.

Family members are allowed to take herbs or other treatment modalities to the patient after discussing the pros and cons thoroughly with their physicians. Moreover, volunteer members of the healthcare team regularly prepare herbal diets once a week for all patients, distributing food to patients at bedsides. These combined efforts can be good demonstrations of the spirit of holistic care.

10.5 MEANING OF NUTRITIONAL SUPPORT IN END-OF-LIFE CARE: PRACTICAL GUIDELINES

At different stages of disease progression, nutritional support takes on different meanings. Many studies emphasize that the goal of nutritional planning must be set in advance. In the early stages of disease, the treatment goal is geared toward curative care. Thus an important goal of nutritional support at this stage is to provide adequate physical strength to accommodate the needs of therapy. In many clinical guidelines for nutritional and fluid supplement for cancer patients, it has been suggested that routine screening of nutritional deficiencies should be performed at the time of tumor diagnosis in order to begin aggressive nutritional supplementation at the earliest possible time so as to facilitate subsequent treatment. When the disease progresses to the untreatable later stages, functional recovery should be the primary goal of nutritional supplementation. This, along with total psychosocial and somatic care of the patient, may help in symptom control. As the patient becomes weaker physically and begins to face impending death, the most important aspect of nutritional support becomes the improvement of QoL. Nevertheless, late referral, reluctance to discuss impending death, as well as social norms in Taiwan of withholding emotion with total acceptance all made a practical guideline difficult to generate. Also, in patients just transferred to the palliative ward, many were usually prescribed parenteral nutrition by their medical team if they experienced anorexia and decreased oral intake even in the face of limited survival. Thus, the cultural background and other unique needs of each patient cannot be overstated. With these types of concerns in mind, careful assessment of the nutritional needs with tailored nutritional supplementation and

TABLE 10.4
Nutritional Approaches at Different Stages of Diseases

Disease Status	Nutritional Assessment	Intervention	Goal
Early (disease directed)	1. Subjective global assessment of nutrition (SGA) 2. Mini nutritional assessment (MNA) 3. Thickness of skin fold 4. Weight and diet history 5. GI symptoms 6. Serum albumin level	1. Dietary advice 2. Enteral nutrition if indicated 3. Parenteral nutrition if indicated 4. Gastrostomy or surgical bypass if indicated	Cure the disease
Advanced (problem directed)	1. Assess the general well being 2. GI symptoms 3. Oral hygiene	1. Dietary advice 2. Symptomatic treatment 3. Medroxyprogesterone acetate and corticosteroids (appetite stimulant)	Function restoration
Terminal (goal directed)	1. Assess the general well being	1. Diet as tolerated 2. Comfort care 3. Family accompaniment and spiritual care	Quality of life

Note: This table outlines some considerations for choosing nutritional approaches, as there are differing goals for different disease stages.

treatment can then be truly in the patients' best interests. The nutritional approach at different disease stages is depicted in Table 10.4.

10.6 ETHICAL DILEMMA ISSUES OF NUTRITION AND FLUID SUPPORT IN TERMINAL CANCER PATIENTS

The continual primary theme or value in social structure among Chinese cultures throughout history has been the centrality of the family (Tong and Spicer 1994). From this arise the ideas of "Filial Piety," "honor the family," and "conformance to norms." As the family structure is traditionally hierarchical and patriarchal, older children have precedence over younger children, and male children over their female counterparts. Thus the eldest adult male customarily assumes the role of primary decision-maker. This central tenet of "family-first" is frequently deeply held and can influence the decision process throughout the entire clinical course, with the final decision often inclined toward the family's best interest but perhaps not the patient's (Charles and Chung 2002). Furthermore, one study suggests that Chinese people, compared to other cultural groups, are more likely to favor active life-sustaining medical interventions, with only a few requesting or even considering euthanasia (Hui et al. 1997).

ANH has been frequently regarded as an active life-sustaining treatment for patient and family. A study done by a palliative care ward in Taiwan found that in the majority of patients (80.6%), receiving ANH was considered an appropriate decision by the medical staff at admission. However, in some circumstances, the decision to implement ANH was only acceptable from a moral perspective. This issue can then result in conflict between the patient, family, and medical professionals. Some families insisted in using ANH against the advice of the medical professionals. This reason for the family to do so is that provision of food or drink is seen as the basic act of caring, and feeding carries a powerful symbolic and social significance, especially in Asia (McInerney 1992). Cessation of ANH is often believed to be against "Filial Piety" and thought to possibly shorten overall survival. In reality, a study in Taiwan found that ANH does not, in fact, significantly influence survival (Chiu et al. 2002).

Adequate communication is of paramount importance when dealing with such dilemmas. Conflicts related to the use of ANH were reported in about 25% of patients in 1998 (Chiu, Hu, and Chen 2000), with a decrease to less than 10% by 2001 (Chiu et al. 2002). Furthermore, since the majority of Taiwanese are Buddhists, it is usually believed that a "good death" can only be achieved in a Buddhist way. From the Buddhist point of view, death is but a process between different states of reincarnation (Zheng 1994). One may relay to the family members the Buddhist idea that excessive nutrition or hydration may not be conducive or appropriate for enlightenment and inspiration, both of which are helpful in achieving a better afterlife. Acknowledgement of this often relieves the family members' anxiety to a certain extent. It is also suggested for family members to attend to the patient by physically engaging the patient with body language such as touches and kisses, talking to the patients, and praying or chanting certain Buddhist phrases with them. In some cases, these actions could substitute the use of ANH and other life-sustaining treatment, which would otherwise have been regarded as the best possible care in the minds of family members. Other Chinese cultural considerations and beliefs regarding death are described in Table 10.5. If a strong conflict still exists, a therapeutic trial of ANH for a duration of several days may be reasonable; if the preset goals are not met after the trial, ANH can then be discontinued.

Based on previous studies, terminal cancer patients often have insufficient knowledge regarding ANH. Up to 62.9% of patients wish to have ANH, while only 24.4% of the patients have the correct knowledge and attitude regarding its use (Table 10.6); many patients still believe that ANH can be used to prevent dehydration and starvation. Previous experiences with use of nasogastric tubes, intravenous fluids, attitudes of healthcare professionals, and subjective social norms and stigmata

TABLE 10.5
Significant Influences on Views Regarding Death in Chinese Culture

Philosophy	Central Tenet	
Confucianism	Willing to die to preserve virtue. Barrier: You cannot know death if you don't know life.	One should not be afraid of death. If a nonvirtuous act is needed to preserve life, one would rather die. Discussion about death is socially unwise and unnecessary.
Buddhism	Belief in a new life after death. Barrier: Karma	Death is part of the process of the wheel of rebirth. Death is a way to Nirvana. The suffering in life is due to one's behavior, either in a previous life or this life.
Taoism	Life and death unified. Barrier: Superstition and spirit worship.	Life and death are natural processes. One becomes part of nature upon death, and one needs not grieve when facing death. The worship of spirits might save one in many ways.

Note: Several common philosophies integrated in daily life of Chinese people including Buddhism, Confucianism, and Taoism; This table depicts the differing attitudes toward death from these viewpoints.

TABLE 10.6
Knowledge of Artificial Nutrition and Hydration (n = 197)

Variables	Correct Response n (%)	Wrong Response n (%)	Not Clear n (%)
Peripheral intravenous route can only provide hydration	96 (48.7)	14 (7.1)	87 (44.2)
E xcessive ANH may increase the proliferation of cancer cells	63 (32.0)	29 (14.7)	105 (53.3)
ANH symbolizes the care of families	52 (26.4)	120 (60.9)	5 (12.7)
ANH is helpful to all patients at any stage of disease	49 (24.9)	117 (59.4)	31 (15.7)
ANH can prolong life for all patients	34 (17.2)	130 (66.0)	33 (16.8)
ANH can increase physical strength for all patients	32 (16.3)	136 (69.0)	29 (14.7)
ANH can prevent all patients from starving to death	11 (5.6)	175 (88.8)	11 (5.6)

Source: With kind permission from Springer Science+Business Media: *J Pain Symptom Manage*. Terminal cancer patients' wishes and influencing factors toward the provision of artificial nutrition and hydration in Taiwan,. 27, 2004, 206, Chiu, T. Y. et al., Table 2.

Note: Patient knowledge regarding ANH in terminal cancer patients is often insufficient or incorrect. Common incorrect views or inadequacies Chinese patients generally had about ANH are presented in this table.

TABLE 10.7
Key Features of Herbal Medicine

1. Herbal medicine is one of the common practices in Traditional Chinese Medicine (TCM). From a Chinese perspective, Western medicine is still the mainstream of treatment while TCM remains an important and common complementary method.
2. Herbal medicine aims to balance the disharmony between different "Qi"s in the human body.
3. Herbal remedies are not considered by the Food and Drug Administration (FDA) as drugs, but rather as dietary supplements.
4. Most Chinese families use a variety of herbal remedies in their everyday diet.
5. The effect of Chinese herbal medicine and palliative care nutritional support is scarce; future research should be focused on the quality of life (QOL) improvement.

Note: This table shows several important features of herbal medicine.

were the most significant variables relative to the perception of patients toward ANH (Chiu et al. 2004). Therefore, further continuing education with sufficient discussion and explanation remains essential.

10.7 CONCLUSION

From a Chinese cultural perspective, the importance of food intake cannot be overemphasized. Anorexia and cachexia of terminal cancer patients can be sources of distress for both patients and their families and also inevitable dilemmas for the healthcare team. TCMs and other herbal remedies are also frequently employed as augmentative treatments by concerned family members. For the terminal cancer patient, the most important task may be fastidious care with the purpose of QOL improvement (Table 10.7). Buddhist beliefs, widely held by Chinese cultures, also provide a supportive role. By encouraging continual communication between the healthcare team and patient's family members, it may be possible to achieve the ultimate goal of "peace for both the living and the dead."

SUMMARY POINTS

- Food represents much more than a source of energy; it also embodies family, love, and caring in Chinese culture, thus much distress in terminal patients can be attributed to or related to anorexia and cachexia.
- Traditional Chinese medicine and herbal remedies are frequently used as augmentative treatments in Chinese culture.
- The most important goal is still the improvement of quality of life.
- Buddhist beliefs can provide a supportive role in nutritional support in palliative care.

ACKNOWLEDGMENT

The authors would like to thank Dr. Po-Yu Shih for his editorial assistance.

LIST OF ABBREVIATIONS

ANH Artificial Nutrition and Hydration
TCM Traditional Chinese Medicine
QOL Quality of Life

REFERENCES

Blackhall, L. J., G. Frank, S. T. Murphy, V. Michel, J. M. Palmer, and S. P. Azen. 1999. Ethnicitiy and attitudes towards life sustanining technology. *Social Science Medicine* 48:1779–89.

Bowman, K. W., and P. A. Singer. 2001. Chinese senior's perspectives on end-of-life decisions. *Social Science Medicine* 53:455–64.

Bozzetti, F., J. Arends, K. Lundholm, A. Micklewright, G. Zurcher, and M. Muscaritoli. 2009. ESPEN Guidelines on Parenteral Nutrition: Non-surgical oncology. *Clinical Nutrition* 28:445–54.

Charles, K., and B. J. Chung. 2002. Culture and the End-of-Life: Chinese. *Journal of Hospice and Palliative Nursing* 4:173–78.

Chiu, T. Y., W. Y. Hu, S. Y. Cheng, and C. Y. Chen. 2000. Ethical dilemma in palliative care: A study in Taiwan. *Journal of Medical Ethics* 26:353–57.

Chiu, T. Y., W. Y. Hu, and C. Y. Chen. 2000. Prevalence and severity of symptoms in terminal cancer patients: A study in Taiwan. *Support Care Cancer* 8:311–13.

Chiu, T. Y., W. Y. Hu, R. B. Chuang, and C. Y. Chen. 2002. Nutrition and hydration for terminal cancer patients in Taiwan. *Support Care Cancer* 10:630–36.

Chiu, T. Y., W. Y. Hu, R. B. Chuang, Y. R. Cheng, C. Y. Chen, and S. Wakai. 2004. Terminal cancer patients' wishes and influencing factors toward the provision of artificial nutrition and hydration in Taiwan. *Journal of Pain and Symptom Management* 27:206–14.

Chiu, T. Y., W. Y. Hu, H. L. Huang, C. A. Yao, and C. Y. Chen. 2009. Prevailing ethical dilemmas in terminal care for patients with cancer in Taiwan. *Journal of Clinical Oncology* 27:3964–68.

Crawley, L., R. Payne, J. Bolden, T. Payne, P. Washington, and S. Williams. 2000. Palliative and end-of-life care in the African American community. *Journal of the American Medical Association* 284:2518–21.

Department of Health. 2009. *Medium-range policy plan from 2010–2013*. Taiwan: Department of Health.

Doyle, D., G. Hanks, N. I. Cherny, and K. Calman. 2005. *Oxford Textbook of Palliative Medicine*. 3rd ed., 520–46. USA: Oxford University Press.

Ernst, E., and B. R. Cassileth. 1998. The prevalence of complementary/alternative medicine in cancer: A systematic review. *Cancer* 83:777–82.

Hui, E., S. C. Ho, J. Tsang, S. H. Lee, and J. Woo. 1997. Attitudes toward life-sustaining treatment of older persons in Hong Kong. *Journal of the American Geriatrics Society* 45:1232–36.

Kagawa-Singer, M., and L. J. Blackhall. 2001. Negotiating cross-cultural issues at the end-of-life. *Journal of the American Medical Association* 286:2993–3001.

Lo, C. C. 1997. *The cost-and-effect analysis of hospice care*. Department of Health commissioned project, Taiwan.

McInerney, F. 1992. Provision of food and fluids in terminal care: A sociological analysis. *Social Science Medicine* 34:1271–76.

Muller, J. H., and B. Desmond. 1992. Ethical dilemmas in a cross-cultural context – A Chinese example, In Cross-cultural Medicine – A Decade Later. *Western Journal of Medicine* 157:323–27.

Sagar, S. M., and R. K. Wong. 2008. Chinese medicine and biomodulation in cancer patients – Part one. *Current Oncology* 15:42–48.

Tong, K. L., and B. J. Spicer. 1994. The Chinese palliative patient and family in North America: A cultural perspective. *Journal of Palliative Care* 10:26–28.

Tsai, J. S., C. H. Wu, T. Y. Chiu, W. Y. Hu, and C. Y. Chen. 2006. Symptom patterns of advanced cancer patients in a palliative care unit. *Palliative Medicine* 20:617–22.

Tse, C. Y., A. Chong, and S. Y. Fok. 2003. Breaking bad news: A Chinese perspective. *Palliative Medicine* 17:339–43.

Wong, R., C. M. Sagar, and S. M. Sagar. 2001. Integration of Chinese medicine into supportive cancer care: A modern role for an ancient tradition. *Cancer Treatment Reviews* 27:235–46.

World Health Organization. 1995. *Cancer pain relief and palliative care*. Geneva: World Health Organization.

Wu, T. H., T. Y. Chiu, J. S. Tsai, C. Y. Chen, L. C. Chen, and L. L. Yang. 2008. Effectiveness of Taiwanese traditional herbal diet for pain management in terminal cancer patients. *Asia Pacific Journal of Clinical Nutrition* 17:17–22.

Xu, L., L. X. Lao, A. Ge, S. Yu, J. Li, and P. J. Mansky. 2007. Chinese herbal medicine for cancer pain. *Integrative Cancer Therapies* 6:208–34.

Zheng, Xiaojiang, 1994. Philosophy of death in the Chinese (in Chinese). Taipei: Dong Da.

11 An Overview of the Indian Perspective on Palliative Care with Particular Reference to Nutrition and Diet

Nanda Kishore Maroju, Vikram Kate, and N. Ananthakrishnan

CONTENTS

11.1 INTRODUCTION

Provision of care as a palliative measure implies catering not only to the physical requirements of patients but also their spiritual, religious and personal beliefs. This definition seeks to affirm life and regard dying as a normal process while offering a support system to the patient and the patient's family to allow the patient to live as actively as possible until death (World Health Organization 2010).

Feeding the terminally ill has strong emotional elements for patients, relatives and doctors. For patients it is symbolic of their ability to survive their illness or gain more time. For their families it is the most basic act of caring and for doctors it is about providing succour and improving the quality of life (Jackson 2000). While the emotional elements of nutrition are very important, it is also important to realise that in the early stages of disease, the requirements of these patients are no less than a patient of any other reversible illness and a proper assessment and support has definite impact on their quality of life.

In putting together an Indian perspective on diet and nutrition in palliative care, it is essential to consider whether an Indian perspective is different from the global view and standards of care as established in the West. The obvious differences are mainly owing to the lack of emphasis on palliative medicine in the Indian healthcare system since it did not constitute one of the components of the primary healthcare system adopted by the state. Apart from this, the vast difference in availability of resources in terms of infrastructure and finance and also in human resources contributed to the lagging behind of palliative care in the Indian context.

11.2 RELEVANCE OF PALLIATIVE CARE IN INDIA

India is among the most populous nations of the world, accounting for close to one fifth of the world's population. The World Health Organization estimates an annual incidence of 1 million new cancer patients in India. About three quarters of these patients present at an advanced stage of malignancy where cure is almost impossible. That would tentatively put a figure of 750,000 new patients requiring palliative care yearly. The Government of India spends a mere 1.15% of its GDP on health, only a fraction of which is spent on cancer care (Chidambaram 2008). Ninety percent of resources allocated for cancer are spent on curative services. Of the noncancer patients requiring palliative care, such as HIV/AIDS patients, end-stage renal disease patients and patients with chronic medical diseases, only 10% receive reasonable care.

Palliative care is an emerging area of interest on India's healthcare map. There has been some improvement over the years, with an increase in the number of centres providing palliative care and guidance to people. There is improved awareness among the medical fraternity as well as laypeople regarding palliative care (Koshy 2009). However, against the backdrop of the sheer number of patients requiring palliative care, there are huge gaps in services, which need to be filled.

11.3 DIFFICULTY OF PALLIATIVE CARE IN INDIA

11.3.1 Resource Deficit

The most important obstacle in improving the reach and quality of palliative care in India is the mismatch between the demand and resources available. Of the 5% of GDP spent on healthcare, close to 4% is through private providers (WHO Statistical Information System 2010). This care is essentially profit oriented, cure centric and inaccessible to the poor of the country. A very large segment of the population is dependent on government-provided services, which are simply insufficient.

11.3.2 Government Policy

The only policy framed by the government for palliative care is as a component of the National Cancer Control Program. As a result, palliative care is invariably linked to advanced cancers alone. HIV/AIDS has received considerable attention but the stress here too is on awareness, prevention and antiretroviral therapy (Rajagopal and Venkateswaran 2003).

11.3.3 Attitudes of the Medical Fraternity

There is no dearth of advanced medical technology or know-how in the country and several centres have technology and expertise that match some of the best in the world. Most hospitals aspire towards a technology-intensive healthcare model. In several instances, rather than focusing on a symptom-based approach to these patients, doctors often prescribe anticancer medications or treatments which are costly, painful and ineffective. Ironically, while most chemotherapeutic drugs used in the West are easily available in the Indian market, it is near impossible to procure morphine owing to a very strict drug control policy (Mazza and Lipman 2003).

11.3.4 Lack of Open Communication

More than half of patients in India seeking cancer treatment are unaware of their diagnosis or treatment (Chandra et al. 1998). A major reason for this is explained by the phenomenon of collusion. In healthcare, collusion implies any information being withheld or not shared among individuals involved (Chaturvedi, Loiselle, and Chandra 2009). The family is a close-knit unit and can provide sustained and committed support. At the same time it can hamper effective open communication between the patient, physician and relatives, making it difficult and time consuming. In centres that are busy, communication is therefore half-hearted or absent (Rajagopal and Venkateswaran 2003).

11.3.5 Attitudes Towards Hospices

The hospices movement never really took off in India, in contrast to the developed countries where most of the care for dying is provided in hospices. Most patients who are terminally ill die either at their homes or in hospitals. The main reason for this is the perception of hospices as places where people without families die. Looking after the old and infirm is the norm in Indian families and the inability to do so is counted as failure on the part of the family.

11.4 FACTORS CONDUCIVE TO A GOOD PALLIATIVE CARE MODEL IN THE COUNTRY

11.4.1 Family

Families live as close-knit units in India and extended family members provide assistance where required. This could be a very useful asset as there is a universal trend towards shifting end-of-life care from hospital settings where healthcare professionals are in charge to the home-care setting where the family members are in charge of the care (Yates 1999).

11.4.2 Support Structures

Families can provide effective care only when backed by strong and sustained support from a palliative care unit. In the absence of such support, there may be a negative impact on the patients as well as their families. The experiment in the Indian state of Kerala called the Neighbourhood Network in Palliative Care (NNPC) is an initiative of the Pain and Palliative Care Society. This experiment involves a symbiosis between the existing government facilities, nongovernmental organisations, volunteers and patients' families (Figure 11.1). The huge success of this programme has set this as the benchmark of care in developing countries with limited resources.

11.4.3 Cancer Epidemiology

Among Indians residing all over the world, the lowest overall cancer incidence is among those residing in India. This is attributed to lifestyle and environmental factors. There are unique aspects of diet with a relative preponderance of vegetarianism and a high consumption of spices like turmeric which have anticarcinogenic properties (Rastogi et al. 2008).

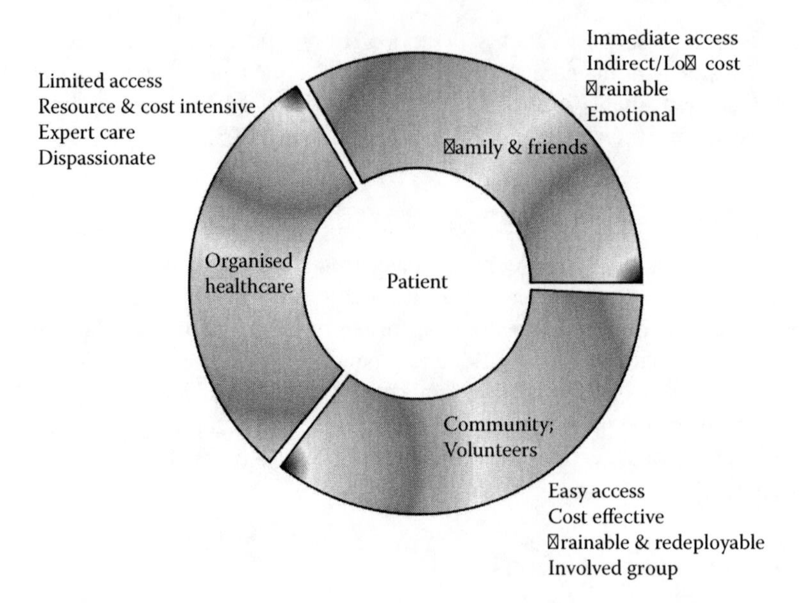

FIGURE 11.1 Integrated unit of care for palliation. This figure demonstrates the different providers of palliative care with the advantages and drawbacks of each group of providers. Complete and effective care is achieved by proportional inputs from the different groups. This proportional input depends on cultural, social and economic factors.

11.4.4 Complementary and Alternate Forms of Medicine

Alternative Indian systems of medicine like Ayurveda and Siddha have popular appeal and are also supported by government initiatives. Some principles of these forms of medicine are deeply ingrained in the culture of most Indians and are reflected in good food and lifestyle choices. Another area with positive impact is the practice of yoga. While there is no definite evidence regarding these forms of medicine or lifestyle on cancers or progressive diseases, their value in enriching the quality of life, physically and spiritually, is well established (Table 11.1).

11.5 OVERVIEW OF DIETARY AND NUTRITIONAL PRACTICES IN INDIA

India is a large country with varied geography, culture and food practices. While it is impossible to portray a uniform picture of India's dietary practices, the general trends in consumption and the components of a daily diet can be studied. Recent years have seen an improvement in caloric intake typified by an increase in consumption of cereals, and protein and fats, mainly as milk, milk products and designated flesh foods (meat).

TABLE 11.1
Key Features of Ayurvedic Medicine

1. Ayurveda literally means the "science of life" and is an ancient system of medicine which originated in India
2. It is a comprehensive system of medicine and attempts to maintain or restore health by achieving harmony between the individual and his environment
3. Ayurvedic medicine includes natural therapies including herbal medications, yoga, breathing exercises, massage and meditation
4. "Shaman" refers to a step in Ayurvedic disease management specifically related to palliation where the focus is more on the spiritual aspects of healing

A good description of the Indian diet was provided by Shetty in 2002. An average Indian consumes a diet to provide 2321 kcal/day, 70 g of protein and 31.3 g of fat. Cereals form a large component of the habitual Indian diet. Rice and wheat and their derivatives are the most common cereals consumed. A typical Indian diet consists of 488.1 g of cereals per consumption unit (CU) per day. In terms of weight, milk and milk products come second at 125.9 g/CU/day. Pulses and legumes are a very important source of vegetable proteins in the Indian diet. Animal fat accounts for only 27.5% of total fat consumed. Meat is restricted or avoided in several communities for religious reasons (Shetty 2002).

11.6 NUTRITIONAL ISSUES IN PALLIATIVE CARE

The goals of nutritional support as a part of palliative care change with progression of the disease. In the initial stages of the disease, food contributes to maintaining quality of life, and helps to provide for body's defences and healing, as well as meeting the metabolic requirements. As the disease progresses food has more of a social function than a nutritional one. Caregivers need to be aware of these changes and set realistic nutritional targets (Watson, Lucas, and Hoy 2005).

It is important to realise that as far as nutrition in palliative care is concerned, the final determinant is not how much nutrition the patient is receiving, but how he is receiving it. A small amount of food taken by mouth may meet a fraction of the patient's nutritional needs but counts far larger than a well-calculated parenteral drip.

In forming an approach to designing a nutritional programme for patients, we classify the patients based on their needs and abilities as follows (Figure 11.2).

a. Patients who are eating well
b. Patients who do not want to eat (due to cancer-associated anorexia)
c. Patients who cannot eat. This group can be further classified as:
   i. Troubled by nausea, vomiting and constipation.
   ii. Obstructed due to oropharyngeal, laryngeal, oesophageal, gastric growth (common in India).
   iii. Have disease- or treatment-related complications: intestinal obstruction, enterocutaneous fistulae (common in India).

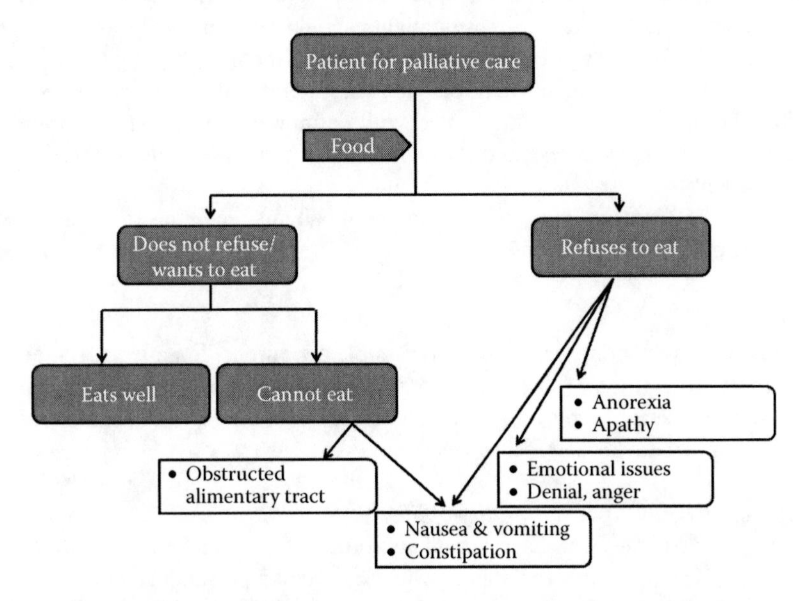

FIGURE 11.2 Classification of patients based on their needs and abilities. This figure shows the response of different groups of patients to food. This pathway can help providers choose the appropriate line of care.

Patients in the first two groups are usually at either end of the spectrum of patients requiring palliative care and can be managed without specialised care. Specialised care is required for patients who desire to eat but are unable to for various reasons.

A. Patients who are eating well
These patients are reasonably healthy and are receptive to the idea of making a comprehensive plan for their care. The main issues in the management of these patients are as follows:

1. Nutritional assessment to account for daily requirements and additional provision to cater for the illness and the treatment.
2. Nutritional supplements like mineral and vitamin supplements.
3. A plan for home management.
4. Preparing the patient and the family for the natural course of the disease.

B. Patients who do not want to eat
This group of patients need a much more supportive assessment of their condition. A failure to provide food to a patient is often perceived as a failure to provide care. Secondly, good intake provides some hope of improvement for the caregivers and patients. Reduced intake is seen as a sign of deterioration. These problems are especially common where open communication between patients, doctors and relatives is not encouraged.

The first step in the management of these patients is to have an open dialogue with the patient and the relatives. This may pave the way for more realistic targets to be set for these patients.

Anorexia as a component of advanced cancer has to be accepted and commonsense strategies to address this have to be evolved. Some common techniques to encourage intake in patients with anorexia are:

1. Smaller meals may appear more feasible to an anorexic, disinterested patient.
2. Limited exercise may stimulate appetite.
3. Patient's wishes with regard to the kind of food he wants to consume should be respected.

As the disease progresses the patient may be less responsive to feeding efforts. Evidence suggests that the best course of management in these patients should be to avoid invasive modes of nutritional support (Watson, Lucas, and Hoy 2005). Nevertheless there is a strong tendency to resort to tube feeding or to intravenous support in these patients. Enteral and parenteral routes of nutritional supplementation are invasive and are associated with definite complications. Restraining agitated patients to enable intravenous access and its maintenance may contribute to the suffering of the family and the patient.

The reasons tube feeding continues to be prevalent in patients receiving end-of-life care are multiple. Some of the arguments are given below:

1. *For prolonging life*
This is true in patients with nonprogressive or reversible conditions. In patients who are terminally ill with advanced cancer, there is no evidence for prolongation of life with tube feeds (Ackerman 2006). There is also evidence supporting an increased incidence of aspiration pneumonia in patients on tube feeds (Campbell-Taylor and Fisher 1987).

2. *Patients who are fed have a better quality of life*
This may be true for patients who have an appetite and yet are unable to eat due to causes like obstruction to the alimentary tract. In patients who are cachectic, no change in the quality of life is seen. On the other hand the tube may be an irritant and make life miserable for the patient. The tube may also prevent the patient from enjoying any food by mouth, however small the quantity may be.

The use of intravenous fluids for hydration in the palliative setting is still a common occurrence in most parts of the country. Many hospitals create a semblance of care by connecting an intravenous drip to the patient. This in most instances satisfies the relatives that "something is being done." However intravenous hydration has its own complications, does not benefit the patient and may well increase the patient's discomfort and pain.

Though communication is the key in avoiding these unnecessary steps, in common practice it may appear impossible for patients and their relatives to accept the inevitable. This is more so in the Indian setup where patients are usually unaware of their prognosis until the very end. The psychosocial conditions near the end-of-life are very complex and require a high level of experience on the part of the physician to address the fears and concerns of the caregivers.

C. Patients who cannot eat

This group of patients benefit from interventions of some kind. Among these patients, a large number are troubled by symptoms of nausea, vomiting, sore mouth and constipation. These complaints need to be addressed sympathetically. While complete relief is difficult, an attempt must be made to alleviate these symptoms.

Nausea and vomiting can be managed by taking small portions of food and eating it slowly. Some patients seem to tolerate cold foods better. 5-HT3 antagonists are reliable drugs to manage chemotherapy-associated vomiting and generic ondansetron tablets are effective.

There are a number of Ayurvedic preparations that are considered alternatives to allopathic drugs in the management of nausea, vomiting and constipation. A controlled clinical trial using a combination of an Ayurvedic (herbal) preparation (Misrakasneham) with a conventional laxative tablet (Sofsena) found this to be an acceptable alternative in morphine-induced constipation (Ramesh et al. 1998). Fresh ginger is one among several preparations with multiple beneficial properties used in controlling symptoms of nausea and vomiting (Ali et al. 2008).

Patients with an obstructed alimentary tract are the ones where a considered decision needs to be made in order to provide nutritional support. Cancers of the oral cavity, pharynx, larynx and oesophagus are extremely common in India. The majority of these cancers are advanced and are considered for palliative radiotherapy (Babu 2001).

Patients with oral cavity cancers present with large ulceroproliferative growths and intractable pain. Patients with large lesions involving the floor of the mouth and tongue have difficulty in swallowing. Those with malignant ulcers of the cheek may either have drooling of saliva and food, or discharge through an orocutaneous fistula. A considered assessment of patients must be taken to quantify the amount of oral intake. Where oral intake is severely impaired, a nasogastric tube may be placed for providing nutritional support during the period of treatment. Patients usually tolerate oral diet on completion of radiotherapy.

In patients with obstructing lesions of the larynx and pharynx, the options are limited to feeding by a nasogastric tube, a gastrostomy or a jejunostomy, at least until palliative radiotherapy facilitates oral feeding. A 16 or 18 Fr nasogastric tube can be inserted if there is a patent upper alimentary lumen. On successful insertion, the position of the tip of the tube in the stomach must be confirmed by a radiograph before the initiation of feeds. Most patients with appetite and thirst accept the tube easily despite the initial discomfort. Tube blockage is prevented by giving blenderised and strained feeds. The advantage over feeding gastrostomy or feeding jejunostomy is that an operative procedure can be avoided. Complications are tube blockage requiring change of tube, oesophageal ulceration and pain, nasal discomfort, sinusitis and aspiration pneumonia.

Feeding gastrostomy needs to be placed operatively as the proximal obstruction precludes placement of the tube endoscopically. A pharyngeal growth may render intubation difficult and hence a gastrostomy is placed operatively under local anaesthesia and sedation. The procedure is technically simple and inexpensive. The wide-bore Malecots catheter, which is used as the feeding tube, will accept incompletely blenderised food and makes feeding an uncomplicated process. The number of times that a feed has to be administered is also reduced as a relatively larger volume can be given at a time. However very large volumes carry the risk of regurgitation or reflux and should be avoided. A slipped gastrostomy tube can be easily replaced as a reliable epithelised gastrocutaneous track is formed.

Feeding jejunostomy is superior to a feeding gastrostomy in having a lower incidence of oesophageal regurgitation after feeds. Another indication for a feeding jejunostomy is delayed gastric emptying or an obstructing pyloric growth. The procedure is technically more difficult as compared to gastrostomy. Jejunostomy feeds need to be blenderised completely and administered slowly as a drip over 12–18 hours. A slipped jejunostomy tube can only be replaced operatively. The literature does not provide any guidance in choosing one procedure over the other and the choice of a jejunostomy or a gastrostomy depends on an individual assessment of each case. In our experience, when not contraindicated, patients find a gastrostomy easier to manage than a jejunostomy and it meets the nutritional demands of the patient (Figure 11.3).

Patients with obstructing lesions of the oesophagus have a number of procedures for palliation. The oesophagus has a relatively narrow lumen and the tumour usually obstructs the lumen relatively early in the course of the disease. These patients retain true hunger and thirst but are unable to take anything by mouth. An ideal palliative procedure should open up the lumen of the oesophagus rapidly and reliably to allow oral intake and swallowing of saliva.

Endoscopic placement of self-expanding metallic stents with or without dilation of the lumen achieves an immediate and lasting improvement in dysphagia. A study done at our centre recorded dysphagia scores and quality of life scores before and after the procedure and found a significant improvement on all counts. There was no procedure-related mortality and morbidity was acceptable (Maroju et al. 2006) (Figure 11.4).

Radiotherapy, either external beam alone or combined with intraluminal brachytherapy, is another option which is performed regularly in patients with advanced inoperable carcinoma oesophagus. However, this mode of palliation requires the patient to undergo therapy over 30–35 days and may require intermittent endoscopic dilatation. A study performed at our centre found good relief of symptoms with radiotherapy (Vivekanandam et al. 2001).

Endoscopic laser therapy using neodymium: yttrium-aluminium-garnet (Nd:YAG) laser photocoagulation of tumour tissue is yet another technique available to relieve distressing dysphagia. A large study from Chennai, India, found that, on average, 2.7 sessions of laser photocoagulation were required to relieve dysphagia in these patients (Rau, Harikrishnan, and Krishna 1994).

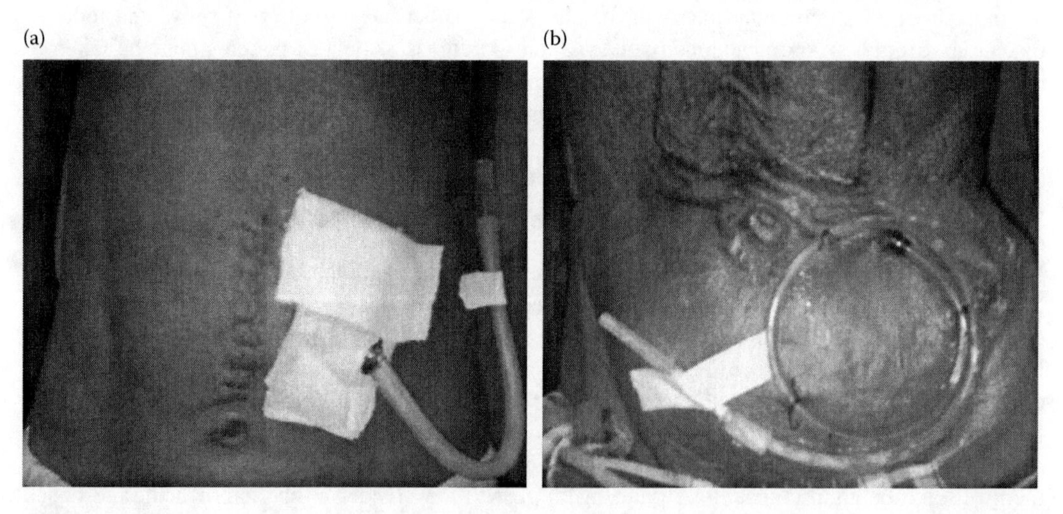

FIGURE 11.3 Enteral access for nutritional support. Enteral access can be achieved by (a) feeding gastrostomy or (b) feeding jejunostomy. Malecot's catheter for gastrostomy and nasogastric tube for jejunostomy are inexpensive options of achieving enteral nutrition in patients with oesophageal carcinoma. The difference in the calibre of the two tubes can be appreciated in this photograph. (Courtesy of Dr Vishnu Kumar.)

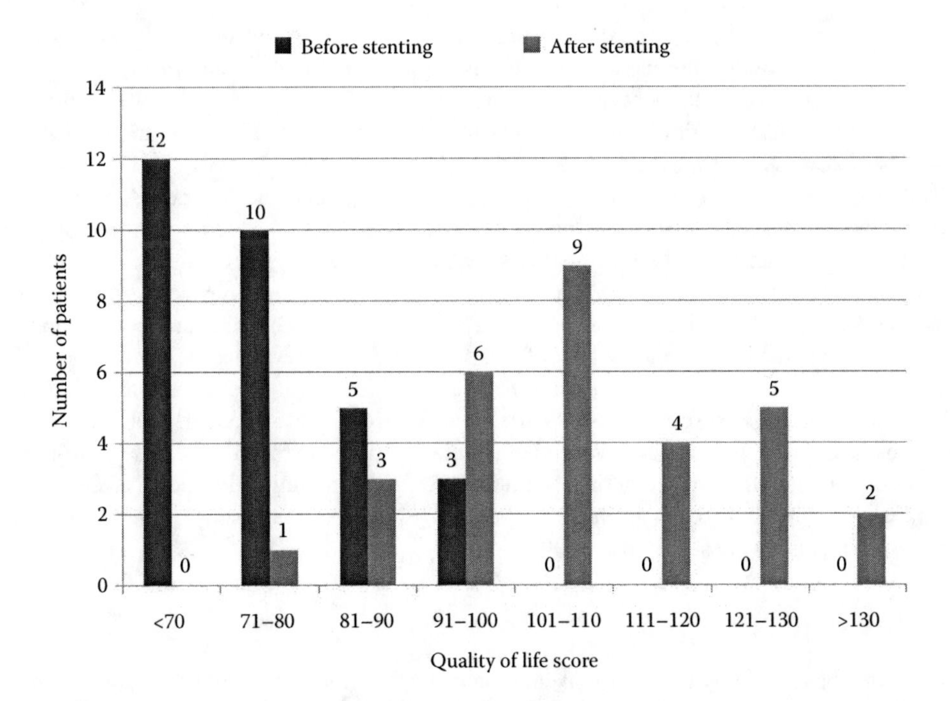

FIGURE 11.4 Quality of life after placement of self-expanding metallic stent in patients with oesophageal carcinoma. The quality of life was assessed by a self-prepared questionnaire and higher scores indicate a better quality of life. The figure shows a marked improvement in quality of life after placement of the stent. (Modified European Organisation for Research and Treatment of Cancer, QLQ C30.)

Another inexpensive alternative attempted by our centre is endoscopic injection of ethanol into the tumour. The drawback with this technique is the shorter period of relief from dysphagia.

Patients with carcinoma cervix treated by primary radiotherapy sometimes present with intestinal obstruction. These patients are very difficult to manage and the mortality as well as morbidity is very high. The decision to opt for surgery is difficult and is guided either by the presence of persistent abdominal pain, peritonism or by the failure of conservative management. Patients need to be counselled as the likelihood of ending up with an ileostomy is very high and the postoperative course is often stormy, with a high incidence of anastomotic dehiscence, wound infection and electrolyte disturbances.

ETHICAL ISSUES

Informed consent is the cornerstone of all medical treatments. It requires the capacity to retain and weigh up information as well as the ability to communicate a decision. In patients with severe neurological impairment like stroke disease or dementia these requirements are often not met. Depending on local law, a legal guardian or the treating physician might have to make a decision for the patient based on the patient's best interest. In palliative care situations it can be especially difficult to ascertain what constitutes this best interest.

Secondly, the amount of information required for the consent to be informed may worsen the already anxious or depressed patient's mood. It therefore requires careful consideration how much and which information is provided to the patient to not increase anxiety levels and mood problems. Furthermore the patient might be under considerable stress and pressure to make a number of decisions on medical care whilst also preparing a last will.

Ethical issues might also arise surrounding the availability of palliative care treatments. The best treatment might not be locally available or might not be funded.

Stents have superior results in the short term compared to radiotherapy (oesophageal obstruction) and surgery (gastric outlet obstruction), while long-term results favour radiotherapy and surgery respectively. To advise on treatment the physician needs to judge life expectancy well. This can be extremely difficult. Judging fitness for and risks of surgery is rather subjective and ethical issues around this often arise in clinical practice.

Whether to advise prophylactic treatment to prevent dysphagia (radiotherapy for oesophageal cancer for example) or an expectant strategy also needs ethical considerations. A prophylactic approach might take up valuable high-quality time in a relatively asymptomatic patient, while an expectant approach only takes up time when a problem has occurred. Prophylactic treatment might also have negative psychological effects (increased feeling of being ill) while an expectant approach might lead to the patient experiencing a lot of symptoms before undergoing the intervention.

Difficult ethical issues often arise regarding the question whether to start enteral feeding in patients with advanced or severe disease. While the evidence suggests that early tube feeding after severe strokes and tube feeding in advanced dementia should be avoided, relatives might push for such an intervention in the belief that the patient is suffering from hunger. Physicians face an ethical dilemma while trying not to upset relatives when conveying the treatment plan and acting in the patient's best interest at the same time.

SUMMARY POINTS

- Feeding the terminally ill has strong emotional elements for patients, relatives and doctors.
- Regional economic, social and cultural factors render the availability and provision of palliative care in India different from the Western models of care.
- The unique family structure in India, availability of support structures and acceptance of alternate forms of medicine are conducive to the development of a good palliative care model in the country.
- The main components of an Indian diet are cereals, pulses, fresh vegetables, fruits and milk.
- Patients can be classified as those who do not want to eat, those who cannot eat and those patients who consume a normal diet.
- Patients who do not want to eat due to cancer-related anorexia need a supportive approach with modifications in variety, quantity and texture of food.
- Patients who cannot eat due to mechanical reasons may benefit from interventional procedures like feeding tube insertion, oesophageal stenting, laser luminisation and radiotherapy.
- Overall, invasive procedures in the terminally ill should be avoided as they increase patient suffering without much nutritional benefit.

LIST OF ABBREVIATIONS

GDP Gross Domestic Product
NNPC Neighbourhood Network in Palliative Care
WHO World Health Organization

REFERENCES

Ackerman, R. J. 2006. Withholding and withdrawing potentially life-sustaining treatment. In *Principles and practice of palliative care and supportive oncology*, eds. A. M. Berger, J. L. Schister, and J. H. von Roenn, 697–706. Philadelphia: Lippincott, Williams, and Wilkins, Philadelphia.

Ali, B. H., G. Blunden, M. O. Tanira, and A. Nemmar, 2008. Some phytochemical, pharmacological and toxicological properties of ginger (Zingiber officinale Roscoe): A review of recent research. *Food Chem Toxicol* 46:409–20.

Babu, K. G. 2001. Oral cancers in India. *Semin Oncol* 28:169–73.

Chidambaram, P. "Budget 2008-09." *Government of India: Union budget & economic survey*. National Informatics Centre, Web. 16 Jan 2010. http://indiabudget.nic.in/ub2008-09/bs/speecha.htm.

Campbell-Taylor, I., and R. H. Fisher. 1987. The clinical case against tube feeding in palliative care of the elderly. *J Am Geriatr Soc* 35:1100–4.

Chandra, P. S., S. K. Chaturvedi, A. Kumar, S. Kumar, D. K. Subbakrishna, S. M. Channabasavanna, and N. Anantha. 1998. Awareness of diagnosis and psychiatric morbidity among cancer patients: a study from South India. *J Psychosom Res* 45:257–61.

Chaturvedi, S. K., C. G. Loiselle, and P. S. Chandra. 2009. Communication with relatives and collusion in palliative care: A cross-cultural perspective. *Indian J Palliat Care* 15:2–9.

Jackson, K. C., II. 2000. Nutrition and hydration problems in palliative care patients. *J Pharm Care Pain Symptom Control* 8:183–97.

Koshy, C. 2009. The palliative care movement in India: Another freedom struggle or a silent revolution? *Indian J Palliat Care* 15:10–13.

Maroju, N. K., P. Anbalagan, V. Kate, and N. Ananthakrishnan. 2006. Improvement in dysphagia and quality of life with self-expanding metallic stents in malignant esophageal strictures. *Indian J Gastroenterol* 25:62–65.

Mazza, D., and A. C. Lipman. 2003. Commentary: Palliative care in India, more than a matter of resources. In *Pain and palliative care in the developing world and marginalized populations: A global challenge*, eds. M. R. Rajagopal, D. Mazza, and A. C. Lipman, 129. New York: Haworth Medical Press.

Rajagopal, M. R., and C. Venkateswaran. 2003. Palliative care in India, more than a matter of resources. In *Pain and palliative care in the developing world and marginalized populations: A global challenge*, eds. M. R. Rajagopal, D. Mazza, and A. C. Lipman, 121–128. New York: Haworth medical Press.

Ramesh, P. R., K. S. Kumar, M. R. Rajagopal, P. Balachandran, and P. K. Warrier. 1998. Managing morphine-induced constipation: A controlled comparison of an Ayurvedic formulation and senna. *J Pain Symptom Manage* 16:240–44.

Rastogi, T., S. Devesa, P. Mangtani, A. Mathew, N. Cooper, R. Kao, and R. Sinha. 2008. Cancer incidence rates among South Asians in four geographic regions: India, Singapore, UK and US. *Int J Epidemiol* 37:147–60.

Rau, B. K., K. M. Harikrishnan, and S. Krishna. 1994. Oesophageal carcinoma: Laser palliation in 231 cases. *Ann Acad Med Singapore* 23:32–34.

Shetty, P. S. 2002. Nutrition transition in India. *Public Health Nutrition* 5:175–82.

Vivekanandam, S., K. S. Reddy, K. Velavan, V. Balasundaram, S. Rangarao, K. S. V. K. Subbarao, and M. Nachiappan. 2001. External beam radiotherapy and intraluminal brachytherapy in advanced inoperable esophageal cancer: JIPMER experience. *Am J Clin Oncol* 24:128–30.

"WHO definition of palliative care." *World Health Organization*. WHO, Web. 16 Jan 2010. http://www.who.int/cancer/palliative/definition/en/.

"WHOSIS WHO statistical Information system." *World Health Organization*. WHO, Web. 16 Jan 2010. http://apps.who.int/whosis/data/search.jsp.

Watson, M., C. Lucas, and A. Hoy. 2005. *Oxford handbook of palliative care*. New York: Oxford University Press.

Yates, P. 1999. Family coping: Issues and challenges for cancer nursing. *Cancer Nursing* 22:63–71.

12 Cultural Aspects of Forgoing Tube Feeding in American and Hong Kong Chinese Patients at the End-of-Life

Helen Yue-lai Chan and Samantha Mei-che Pang

CONTENTS

12.1 INTRODUCTION

In an era of burgeoning medical technology, medicine has been developed extensively to intervene in all life processes so as to challenge the notion that humans are mere mortals. Problems related to eating, such as dysphagia, anorexia and cachexia, would not be life threatening as they could be dealt with by simply inserting a tube for feeding. Tube feeding emerged for the sake of providing nutrition and hydration support as a measure for acute conditions. In some situations, however, it is used for the remaining days when the person loses swallowing ability. This is not limited to patients with terminal illness, but also includes those in a persistent vegetative state (PVS) or when the disability rendered by their disease is irreversible, such as advanced dementia and severe stroke, and there is little or no reasonable hope of recovery. To them, withholding or withdrawing tube feeding would result in death within a predictable time frame, while its administration can support their life for months or years.

This chapter compares the cultural differences in tube-feeding decisions between Caucasian American and Hong Kong Chinese communities. Culture here can be understood as having two layers: ethnic cultural differences and medical cultural differences in care (Pang et al. 2007). The comparison is achieved by first examining the discourse on the legalization of forgoing tube feeding in the two communities, and then uncovering the implicit meaning of tube feeding and eating in the two cultures.

12.2 A TALE OF TWO COMMUNITIES

Of the various treatments to sustain life, tube feeding has been at the heart of debates throughout the decades, particularly in situations when death is not yet imminent. From the legal point of view, it has been agreed in both the American and Hong Kong communities that, first, a patient who is mentally competent can refuse treatment after having been properly informed of the treatment's nature and its benefits, risks, possible alternatives and consequences. Second, there is no moral difference between withholding and withdrawing life-sustaining treatment. The ethical issue that remains unresolved is whether tube feeding in some situations should be considered as medically futile. On one hand, it can successfully deliver sufficient nutrition and hydration to support the patient's life. On the other, it fails to improve the underlying incapacitating condition. This different line of thinking leads to divergent conclusions in which tube feeding is either regarded as an extraordinary medical treatment which could be forgone or as basic sustenance care which should always been in place. The plights of patients in several precedents in the United States have exemplified the dilemma.

Dating back to 1976, the case of Karen Ann Quinlan was the first landmark case related to treatment-limiting decisions in the community. Karen, despite having survived cardiopulmonary arrest, had suffered from irreversible brain damage. After several months of trial, her parents acknowledged that her condition could not be improved by the ventilator and so requested its removal. The New Jersey Supreme Court, taking the right to privacy into consideration, recognized the individual's right to refuse life-sustaining medical interventions. The mechanical ventilator was eventually withdrawn, but she was able to breathe on her own and lived for nine more years with the support of tube feeding. Her parents later explained that since there seems a moral distinction between the mechanical ventilator and the feeding tube, they did not request the removal of the feeding tube (Quinlan and Quinlan 1977). Another young lady, Nancy Cruzan, was also on a feeding tube after going into a PVS in a road accident in 1983. Her family requested that it be removed, as they believed it was not in Nancy's best interest. With the establishment of clear and convincing evidence that she would not want her life to be sustained through artificial means, the feeding tube was regarded as a life-sustaining treatment and therefore removed. Subsequently, the federal Patient Self-Determination Act was passed by the U.S. Congress in 1990 to encourage the preparation of advance directives by informing the patients of their rights to prospective autonomy regarding future treatment decisions. Its establishment, however, has not put the debate to an end.

The tragic case of Terri Schiavo sparked heated debate over tube feeding again. She was in a prolonged coma after being found collapsed at home in 1990. Due to a disagreement between her husband and parents on the diagnosis and Terri's wish for the use of life support measures, the legal battle lasted for years and the feeding tube was repeatedly inserted and removed according to court decisions over the period. Publicity surrounding the case later even induced the President, the Pope and advocacy groups to express their political and religious views of tube feeding. The competing views and uncertainties regarding prognostication and clinical outcomes in this case highlight the complexity inherent in tube-feeding decisions.

The issue did not raise similar concerns in the Hong Kong community. Given that the medical technology in Hong Kong and the United States is of a similar level of advancement and the development of health care is comparable, local awareness concerning treatment-limiting decisions lags far behind that in the United States (see Table 12.1). Over the years, the most prominent case in the community was that of Ah-Bun, who appealed to the Chief Executive in 2004 to request euthanasia after having been quadriplegic for 17 years as a result of an accident. Instead of setting the scene for an open debate on life-sustaining treatment decision in local society, most attention was drawn to providing psychosocial support for him (Pang 2006).

There has never been any case before the Hong Kong court to challenge the treatment-limiting decision on forgoing tube feeding. Whilst specific legislation on advance directives has not yet been established to give it statutory recognition, an advance refusal of treatment would still be honoured provided

TABLE 12.1
Timeline of Events Related to Treatment-limiting Decisions in the United States and Hong Kong

← Karen Quinlan's case → (1976–1985)

Natural Death Act passed (since 1976)

← Nancy Cruzan's case → (1983–1990)

Enactment of the Patient Self Determination Act (PSDA) in the United States (since 1990)

← Terri Schiavo's case → (1990–2005)

Ah Bun's case (2004)

Consultation on advance directives by the LRC of Hong Kong (2004)

Report on advance directives by the LRC of Hong Kong (2006)

Consultation on advance directives by the FHB, Hong Kong (2009)

Note: LRC, Law Reform Commission; FHB, Food and Health Bureau.

that it met the criteria for validity under the principles of common law. To confirm the practice of forgoing life-sustaining treatment as ethically and legally acceptable in clinically appropriate situations, a set of guidelines was formulated to provide guidance for health professionals (Hospital Authority 2002). The concept of advance directives was first introduced to the community in 2004 when the Law Reform Commission (LRC) conducted a consultation on the matter (Law Reform Commission of Hong Kong 2004). Although media attention was attracted, it lasted only a short period of time, with limited public discussion. Most of the relevant dialogue was limited to the professional field (Pang et al. 2006). It is therefore not surprising that the Commission later, in 2006, reported that the concept is new to the community, where most people have little knowledge in this respect, so it would be premature to formulate a statutory framework for it at the moment (Law Reform Commission of Hong Kong 2006). The Commission also proposed a model form of advance directive in the report, to enable individuals who wish to prepare an advance directive to enhance the validity of their advance refusal.

The model form was an important initiative but both healthcare and legal professionals were reluctant to implement it. The definition of life-sustaining treatment in the form was in an all-embracing format that included all kinds of treatments that "have the potential to postpone the patient's death," so simply choosing the option of "do not consent to receive any life-sustaining treatment" meant to decline all of them, including artificial nutrition and hydration (ANH). This was challenged, as different treatments involve a range of benefits, risks and burdens that might be acceptable or unacceptable to the individual (E.C. Hui, personal communication, October 24, 2006).

Upon receiving diverse opinions, the Food and Health Bureau also issued a consultation paper on Introduction of the Concept of Advance Directives in Hong Kong in 2009 in response to the recommendations of the LRC (Food and Health Bureau 2009). A major change to the model form is noted. In particular, the decision about ANH has been separated from the long list of life-sustaining treatments as an independent option, underscoring the fact that it might be a point of contention. As can be seen in some of the aforementioned American cases, tube feeding is the only intervention used to sustain a person's life. Forgoing it would definitely end the person's life, but this poses an ethical challenge if withholding food and fluids is justifiable when death is not yet imminent. The meaning of providing food and fluids in the Chinese culture also plays an important role in the decision, which will be further elaborated later in this chapter.

12.3 TO DEBATE OR NOT TO DEBATE

We cannot say that awareness relating to treatment-limiting decision making is not improving in the Hong Kong community, but clearly the majority of the general public has not participated actively in the relevant discussion. One possible explanation rests in the disparity of enthusiasm on open debate and inquiry between the two cultures, which can be illustrated by two stories from the philosophy classics of East and West.

In Plato's work *Euthyphro*, Euthyphro accused his father of murder. His arguments were repeatedly challenged by Socrates through a dialectic method of inquiry (Plato 1997). A similar incident was discussed in *Mencius*, when a student asked Mencius how Shun, who was an emperor renowned for his filial piety, would react if his father was accused of murder (Mencius 2003). Mencius said that although Shun would arrest his father accordingly, he would then cast aside the empire and secretly carry his father on his back to the edge of the sea and live happily with him there. Regardless of the distinct actions of the two sons, the stories show that the approaches to a solution in the two cultures are dissimilar. The inquiry and debate between Socrates and Euthyphro enables critical examination of the issues and claims raised in the incident and challenges the implicit beliefs and values. This eventually results in maturation in the reasoning. Shun, however, realizes his obligations to his father intuitively without needing to clarify his act with rational justification. This provides a coherent explanation for the lack of an open debate or court case related to treatment-limiting decisions in the local community. Likewise, healthcare decisions are often understood as family matters that should be dealt with internally rather than as a public affair to be widely debated in general

(Fan 1997). Perhaps exposing disputes between family members to the public may suggest a lack of harmony in the family and result in the entire family losing face.

12.4 TUBE-FEEDING DECISION IN THE CULTURAL CONTEXT

The above section reveals that the Chinese are less likely to openly discuss treatment decisions than Americans, though this does not necessarily mean that it is not of concern to them or that there is not any conflict in the family or the community. In contrast to placing emphasis on the principle of autonomy like Americans, in Hong Kong the medical decision is usually based on the best interests of the patient and the treatment utility is often open to interpretation. When there is difficulty in defining whether tube feeding is a basic care that health professionals are obliged to provide or an extraordinary measure, how tube feeding and eating are understood in the culture would therefore influence the treatment decision. This will be elaborated in the following paragraphs.

The dying trajectory of persons with advanced dementia is less definite than that of patients with terminal cancer, thus questions concerning tube feeding are often raised. Certain points along the illness trajectory of dementia are critical for decisions on the provision of tube feeding (Figure 12.1), which may be complicated given the progressive cognitive and functional deterioration. Comparing tube-feeding decisions between the two cultures can therefore reveal the differences in their underpinning values and beliefs. Given this backdrop, a dementia unit in Boston (Boston Care Unit, BCU) and a long-term care unit in Hong Kong (Hong Kong Care Unit, HKCU) were purposely recruited for examination. Both units are committed to providing quality care and have credible reputations (Pang et al. 2007).

Two major differences in medical practices were observed in the two units. First, the BCU strongly upheld hospice philosophy with its core values of compassion, comfort and dignity. Based on a consensus that letting the disease take its natural course and providing comfort care only is in the patient's best interests, forgoing tube feeding is an institutional practice. The HKCU follows the model of conventional medicine, a culture in which life preservation is the predominant embedded value. Tube feeding is commonly instituted to residents who fail to obtain a sufficient dietary intake or are at risk of aspiration during oral feeding. Second, the BCU has a standard procedure of advance proxy care planning, which allows a surrogate to make treatment decisions on behalf of the mentally incompetent person. The HKCU also values the involvement of patients' families in treatment decisions, though their right to a proxy treatment decision is not granted legally.

12.5 TUBE FEEDING AS AN OPTION OR A SOLUTION

Treatment decisions in the BCU are made on two grounds: advance decisions based on personal wishes and advance proxy decisions focusing on comfort care. The first pattern, which represents an enactment of the principle of respect for autonomy, honours the treatment decisions indicated in advance directives. Of the ten participants included in the ethnographic study, five had made advance directives before they became mentally incapacitated.

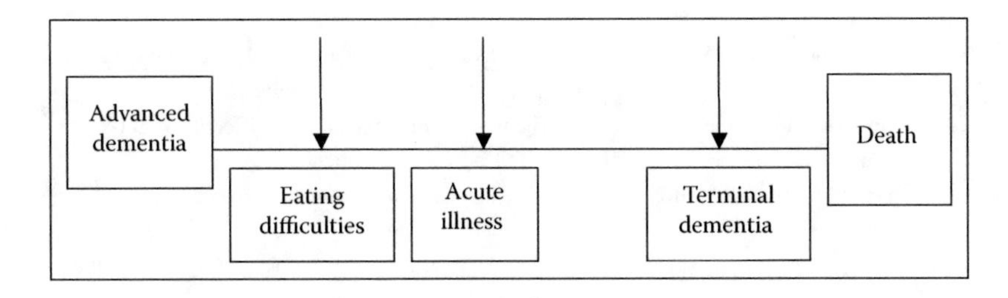

FIGURE 12.1 Critical decision points on tube feeding.

The second pattern is based on a consensual agreement between the family members and healthcare professionals on the patient's best interests. When the families come to the point of considering placing their sick family member in a facility for end-of-life care, their primary concern is usually that they have chosen the right place for their loved ones for optimal care at the close of their life. Since the BCU has an institutional policy of no tube feeding, this was also a critical decision point, compelling family members to examine the meaning of tube feeding as a form of life-sustaining treatment. Among families who had decided to place their loved ones in the BCU, there was a consensus that tube feeding for the sake of prolonging life was not in the best interests of the person. Generally, they did not support tube feeding for three reasons. First, the tube placement would cause discomfort, while insufficient intake and the subsequent weight loss might not. Second, they perceived the declining swallowing ability as a natural progression of the disease. The patient's deterioration was often rationalized, as "it is the disease that is taking him away." Third, they were convinced that the healthcare team would offer better care alternatives for their loved ones.

An analysis of the interviews with the healthcare team in the HKCU, however, reveals arguments in support of tube feeding. First, in contrast to the predominant belief among the BCU informants, a consensual view in the HKCU held that tube feeding was to provide nutrition essential for basic sustenance; it became a medical treatment only when the tube was used to administer medicine. Second, given the different levels of sophistication in terms of medical technology, the reasons for withholding cardiopulmonary resuscitation should not apply to the decision on tube feeding. Third, preserving life is the primary obligation of the health professionals as implied by the principle of "do no harm." The swallowing problem is considered as a medical problem emerging from the disease and as such requires medical intervention. Fourth, in weighing the risk of aspiration between tube feeding and hand feeding, health professionals favour the former as they believe that they would be better protected from legal liability should the patients suffer aspiration. Fifth, the burdens of tube feeding on patients cannot outweigh its benefits in reversing malnutrition and dehydration to prevent other complications such as susceptibility to infection. Above all, they could not bear the thought of completely forgoing tube feeding. Comparisons between the two cultures are listed in Table 12.2.

12.6 EATING CAN NEVER BE REPLACED

As noted in the book *Food in Chinese Culture: Anthropological and Historical Perspectives* (Chang 1977), Chinese culture is renowned for being food-oriented; there is an old saying that "To the people, food is all-important." Liu (2004) further contends that eating is not just meant to meet physiological

TABLE 12.2
Comparison of Values and Beliefs Underpinning Tube-feeding Decisions in the Two Cultures

BCU	HKCU
The declining swallowing ability is a natural progression of the disease	The declining swallowing ability is a degenerative life process
Compassion, comfort and dignity as care goals	Life preservation is the primary obligation of health professionals
Tube feeding is a medical intervention	Tube feeding became a medical treatment only when it was used to administer medications
The healthcare team would be able to offer better care alternatives	The nature of tube feeding is different from other life-sustaining treatments
Tube placement would cause discomfort	Tube feeding is a basic sustenance care that reverses malnutrition and dehydration.
	The risk of aspiration is higher in oral feeding than tube feeding

needs; being able to eat a good amount is a blessing. Among the 20 prospective case studies recruited in the HKCU, feeding tubes were instituted to 18 patients on admission, though none of their family members took it to be a permanent means of delivering food. Fourteen families therefore requested that oral feeding be resumed after the patients' condition stabilized (Pang et al. 2004).

Unlike in American society, where people are used to greeting their loved ones through kisses and hugs or with terms of endearment, such as "sweetheart" or "honey," Chinese people are more reserved in expressing their affection to their loved ones. "Doing something special for a person" is their common way of showing care and concern for their loved ones. Among such special gestures, preparing the person's favourite food carries the symbolic meaning of "pointing to the heart (dian xin)."

This notion has deep roots in the Chinese culture, as revealed in several traditional stories in *The Twenty-four Paragons of Filial Devotion* (Wang 1992). For example, Jiang Shi's wife travelled long distances every day to bring back water from a river for her mother-in-law because she did not like the flavour of the well-water. In another story, Tanzi's parents had eye diseases that the physicians said could only be cured by drinking deer's milk. Tanzi pretended to be a deer and came to the does to nurse milk. He continued to get the milk for his parents in this way for weeks and they eventually began to recover their sight. Yu, another devoted son, even fed his sick father with his own flesh as a kind of medicine, while lady Tan fed her mother-in-law with her breast milk because she was too senile and could not chew food on her own. Likewise, the act of feeding is a way to show support and fulfil the filial obligations (Wu and Barker 2008). In the study, although less dramatic than the above stories, some family members found themselves engaged with the patients in a meaningful way through hand feeding, as characterized in the following two cases (Pang et al. 2007).

> An 85-year-old woman admitted to the HKCU with tube feeding one year ago. The patient tried every means to pull out the tube. Her children did not feel comfortable putting her in restraints. They finally decided to work closely with the healthcare team to hand feed the patient. They found that a syringe was the best utensil for feeding the patient.

> Another female patient's only daughter had dedicated her life to taking care of her mother. She had attempted to hand feed her mother when she was first put on the tube. She dared not feed her mother openly because the nurses had warned her that aspiration would endanger her mother's life.

Their sentiments were closely connected to the patient's ability to resume oral feeding and they perceived the use of tube feeding as their failure to care, as characterized in the following two cases.

> A 69-year-old woman started tube feeding after an episode of stroke. She wore a sad expression and frowned most of the time. Her husband requested that the healthcare team try hand feeding, but the speech therapist indicated that the patient had lost the capability to swallow. In the interview, the husband repeatedly uttered, "What else can I do?"

> A 90-year-old man started tube feeding one year ago while receiving mechanical ventilation for treatment of a chest infection. The patient frequently stated that he was hungry because he had not eaten any food. In the interview, his daughter expressed regret over having consented to the invasive treatment that had rendered her father unable to eat by mouth.

Through examining the meaning of eating and providing food in the Chinese culture, one can understand that the act of feeding, which is meaningful to both the patient and family members, can hardly be replaced by tube feeding.

12.7 DIFFERENT CULTURES, SAME CONCERN

On comparing the two cultures, one may tend to contrast them down to details in order to point out the differences. In the study, however, similarities noted in the tube-feeding decisions in the two cultures are more revealing. Regardless of the differences in the ethnic and medical cultures, the patients in the two places are being afflicted by diseases that intrude upon their existence. In the words of Pellegrino and Thomasma (1981), all patients are facing *the fact of illness* that wounds their humanity and deprives them of some of the freedoms most fundamental to being human. Family members who witness the process often feel obliged to promote the comfort of their vulnerable sick relative. It is already clear that comfort care is the focus in the BCU. In the HKCU, apart from expressing their love and care through hand feeding, another reason for family members to request forgoing tube feeding was also because they hoped the care for their loved ones would be for their comfort, as exemplified in the following case.

> An 89-year-old man broke both hips. Once hospitalized, he was put on tube feeding and provided with a conservative treatment for his fractured hips. He strongly rejected the feeding tube and made every attempt to pull it out. His arms were restrained but he tried every position in bed to release himself from the constraints. While frequent reinsertion of the feeding tube traumatized his naso-oesophageal passage, his mobility was reduced due to restlessness in bed. His son questioned whether it would be better to forgo tube feeding.

The son of this old man considered tube feeding as invasive and possibly causing discomfort to his father; he eventually decided to forgo it. His wish was "to feed his father with his favourite food as long as his father could eat." However, in some situations, also out of a wish to maintain the loved one's comfort, ANH may be administered. The old lady who was hand-fed by syringe as mentioned earlier experienced a remarkable health decline six months after the practice because of aspiration pneumonia. In such acute conditions, standard methods, including intravenous infusion, antibiotics, oxygen therapy and nasogastric tube, were instituted. The patient died six days later.

Reinstating the ANH for the patient in the last phase of life is indeed in line with the notion of "doing something for the person." Its purpose is to relieve the patient from the possible sense of hunger and thirst, since totally withholding food and fluids and letting the patient starve and dehydrate to death seems more torturous and inhumane. In the Chinese tradition, dying with a "full stomach" is an element of a good death. Hence, criminals sentenced to death are also given a last supper before their execution so that they will not become "hungry ghosts." Maintaining the best possible appearance at the moment of death also helps to preserve the patient's dignity.

Although there is evidence to support the notion that death resulting from dehydration is usually painless and peaceful, it is distressing for family members to witness the patient's prolonged dying process and unsightly appearance. There were also family members in the BCU who could not tolerate the sight of the patient's downward deterioration and thus refrained from visiting the patient. Perhaps the tubes at that moment are given for the "comfort" of the family members as well as the patient. This explains why all patients in the HKCU died with either tube feeding or both tube feeding and intravenous or subcutaneous hydration for artificial fluid support, as illustrated in Figure 12.2.

12.8 APPLICATIONS TO OTHER AREAS OF TERMINAL OR PALLIATIVE CARE

It is not the intention of this chapter to compare, in evaluative terms, the cultures and their impacts. The discussion above helps to delineate the cultural issues in treatment decisions which may also be applicable to other areas of terminal or palliative care. First, the discrepancy in the enthusiasm for discussing treatment decisions in the two communities is highly likely related to the differences in culture of open dialectics and interrogations. It is not surprising that Chinese people would consider treatment decisions, not only those limited to tube feeding, as a family issue rather than a public affair for discussion and debate. Such decisions are commonly made collectively but within the caring entity, with the patient's best interests and advice from health professionals being taken into consideration. Second, tube-feeding decisions in both communities are grounded on the wish

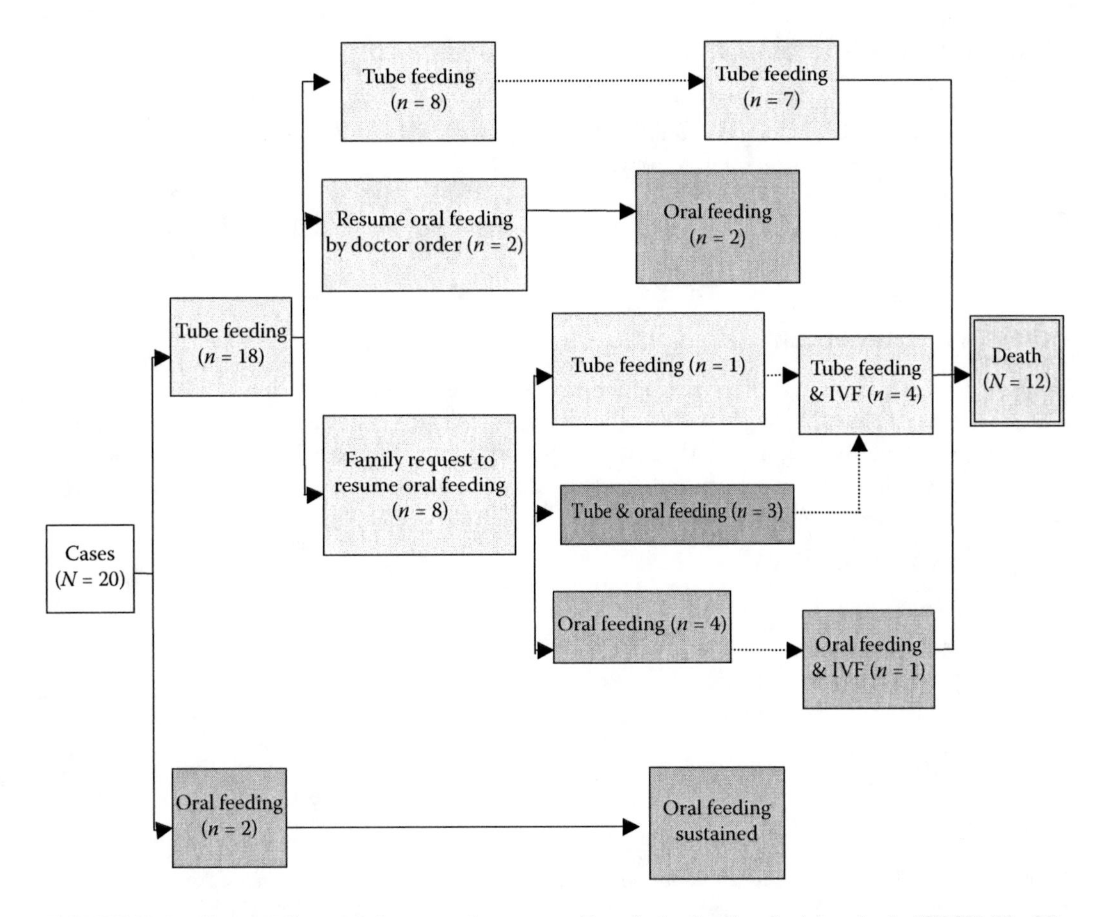

FIGURE 12.2 Consort diagram of prospective case studies of tube feeding decisions in the HKCU ($N = 20$).

to promote comfort for the sick. Since the understanding of comfort is subject to interpretation, the decision may vary across different contexts.

12.9 FEATURES OF TUBE-FEEDING DECISIONS IN CHINESE CULTURE

Chinese people are more reserved in their expression of emotions. Preparing the favourite foods of their loved ones carries a symbolic meaning of expressing care, love and dedication. Due to the underpinning meaning, family members often try all possible ways to encourage oral feeding. However, this does not necessarily mean that tube feeding would be denied in the culture. It is considered as the last resort when oral feeding fails, so that they can still "try to do something" for their loved ones.

ETHICAL ISSUES

Apparently there is still no consensus on the nature of tube feeding for patients with grave prognosis in the two communities. The utility of tube feeding in these patients also remains in doubt. Though it helps in the delivery of nutrients and fluid to the sick, its administration is only for prolonging their dying process, and sometimes the burdens it brings may outweigh its benefits. Should tube feeding be considered as basic sustenance care or extraordinary medical treatment? From the perspective of family members, witnessing the sick relative on long-term tube-feeding support with little or no hope of recovery and leaving the sick relative to starve and dehydrate to death seem equally torturous. Whatever the decision, emotional distress may ensue.

SUMMARY OF KEY POINTS

- A decrease in swallowing ability is perceived as a disease complication requiring intervention in the Hong Kong community, whereas it is considered as a natural process in the illness trajectory in American society.
- Treatment decisions are rarely discussed or debated openly in Chinese culture.
- Preparing food is a usual way for Chinese to express their love and support for their loved ones.

ACKNOWLEDGMENTS

The qualitative data and part of the discussion in this chapter are primarily drawn from the second author's article (Pang et al. 2007) as the basis for further analysis. The authors would like to thank all the patients' family members and healthcare providers again for sharing their views and concerns regarding tube feeding.

LIST OF ABBREVIATIONS

ANH	Artificial nutrition and hydration
BCU	Boston Care Unit
HKCU	Hong Kong Care Unit
LRC	Law Reform Commission
PVS	Persistent vegetative state

REFERENCES

Chang, K. C. 1977. *Food in Chinese culture: anthropological and historical perspectives.* New Haven: Yale University Press.

Fan, R. 1997. Self-determination vs. family-determination: two incommensurable principles of autonomy. *Bioethics* 11:309–22.

Food and Health Bureau. 2009. *Consultation Paper on Introduction of the Concept of Advance Directives in Hong Kong.* Hong Kong SAR Government.

Hospital Authority. 2002. *Guidelines on life sustaining treatment in the terminally ill.* Hong Kong: Hospital Authority Head Office.

Law Reform Commission of Hong Kong. 2004. *Consultation paper on substitute decision-making and advance directives in relation to medical treatment.* Hong Kong SAR Government.

Law Reform Commission of Hong Kong. 2006. *Report on substitute decision-making and advance directives in relation to medical treatment.* Hong Kong SAR Government.

Liu, J. 2004. *Chinese foods* (Trans: Wang, W. W.). Hong Kong: Chinese Intercontinental Press.

Pang, M. C. S., P. M. B. Chung, Y. M. I. Chung, W. K. A. Leung, P. White, T. Y. Chui, and K. S. Chan. 2004. The decision making of hand/tube feeding for patients with advanced dementia and its impact on their quality of life. *Modern Nursing Education & Research* 1(3): 138–43. [in Chinese]

Pang, S. M. C. 2006. Editorial comment. *Nursing Ethics* 13:103–4.

Pang, M. C., K. S. Wong, L. K. Dai, and K. L. Chan. 2006. An analysis of lay and professional views on advance directives and life-sustaining treatment preferences at the end-of-life. *Chinese Medical Ethics* 19:11–15. [in Chinese]

Pang, M. C. S., L. Volicer, P. M. B. Chung, Y. M. L. Chung, W. K. A. Leung, and P. White. 2007. Comparing the ethical challenges of forgoing tube feeding in American and Hong Kong patients with advanced dementia. *Journal of Nutrition, Health and Aging* 11:495–501.

Plato. 1997. *Defence of Socrates; Euthyphro; Crito* (Trans: Gallop, D.). New York: Oxford University Press.

Mencius. 2003. *Mencius* (rev. ed.) (Trans: Lau, D. C.). Hong Kong: Chinese University Press.

Pellegrino, E. D., and D. C. Thomasma. 1981. *A philosophical basis of medical practice.* New York: Oxford University Press.

Quinlan, J., and J. Quinlan. 1977. *Karen Ann: The Quinlans tell their story.* New York: Doubleday and Company.

Wang, Z. ed. 1992. Er shi si xiao (*The Twenty-four Paragons of Filial Devotion*). Hong Kong: Xing Hui Tu Shu. [in Chinese]

Wu, S., and J. C. Barker. 2008. Hot tea and juk: The institutional meaning of food for Chinese elders in an American nursing home. *Journal of Gerontological Nursing* 34:46–54.

Section III

General Aspects

13 Stents in the Gastrointestinal Tract in Palliative Care

Iruru Maetani

CONTENTS

13.1 INTRODUCTION

Even now, many gastrointestinal (GI) malignancies are significantly advanced and incurable at presentation. Unresectable malignancies frequently lead to luminal obstruction and reobstruction after surgical resection caused by local recurrence or lymph node metastasis may occur.

The consequences of GI obstruction can be serious, including intolerance of oral intake and deterioration of quality of life. Stents now play a significant role in relieving obstructive symptoms in these patients. Regarding the esophagus, plastic prostheses have been used for a long time, but were associated with frequent serious complications. Introduced in the early 1990s, self-expandable metallic stents (SEMS) (Table 13.1) are more flexible and provide a significant decrease in the incidence of stent-related complications, as well as use in other organs such as the duodenum and colorectum. Although conventional treatment for obstruction of the GI tract has been palliative surgery, such as gastroenterostomy or colostomy, the fact that unresectable GI obstruction is often

TABLE 13.1
Key Features of Self-Expandable Metallic Stents (SEMS)

1. SEMS are cylinder-shaped devices made with metal alloy wires and are used to treat obstructions in many organs
2. The shapes and sizes vary depending on the manufacturer
3. The diameter of SEMS is chosen according to the organ of placement
4. The radial force and degree of foreshortening differ between stent types
5. Before deployment, SEMS is mounted in a thinner catheter
6. After deployment, the stent is gradually expanded by the radial force of the SEMS
7. Metal mesh wires are deeply embedded in the wall, which helps to prevent migration
8. Interstices of metal mesh allow tissue to pass into the stent lumen, sometimes causing stent blockage. Coated stent may prevent this phenomenon

Note: This table lists the key facts of self-expandable metallic stents, including basic structure, and behavior of SEMS.

a preterminal event may make less invasive stent placement preferable. Therefore, the use of SEMS for GI obstruction is now significantly increasing.

13.2 ESOPHAGUS

13.2.1 Malignant Esophageal Stricture

The main etiology of esophageal obstruction is esophageal cancer, but some cases are caused by cancer extension or metastasis from other malignancies. The rising incidence of esophageal cancer over the past two decades has coincided with a change in histologic type and primary tumor location, owing to the increasing incidence of adenocarcinoma of the esophagus in the United States and Western Europe.

Such obstructions often cause dysphagia. For the approximately 50%–60% of esophageal cancer patients who cannot undergo resection at diagnosis due to distant metastases, extensive invasion or a poor health condition, most of whom have short life expectancy, the primary goal of palliative care is rapid relief of dysphagia. Although a variety of palliative treatments for relieving malignant dysphagia are available, including stents, brachytherapy, chemotherapy, and ablative procedures, the use of stents has increased markedly.

13.2.2 Stent Placement

Thanks to its straight anatomy, efforts to place a stent in the esophagus have a long history. Semi-rigid plastic prostheses like the Celestine tube were commonly used in the 1970s and 1980s, but were associated with a higher rate of complications, particularly perforation, a life-threatening event. Advancements in stent technology then led to the development of SEMS for the esophagus, with the first experience reported in 1990 (Domschke et al. 1990). Composed of metallic wires, SEMS have the strong advantage of greater flexibility. Before deployment, they are mounted in a thinner delivery system. With these characteristics, esophageal stenting has become easier, safer, and less invasive. In prospective comparison studies, SEMS have shown fewer complications than plastic stents and significantly greater safety (Knyrim et al. 1993), and now account for most endoprostheses used for esophageal obstruction (Figure 13.1). Recently, self-expandable plastic stents (SEPS) have also become commercially available.

The first generation of uncovered stents had the drawback of allowing reobstruction as a result of tissue growth through the wire mesh of the stent, leading to recurrent dysphagia in 20%–30% of cases. These have been mostly replaced with covered SEMS, which are not subject to this problem, but lack integration into the esophageal mucosa and are more likely to migrate than uncovered stents. In a comparative study, albeit a retrospective analysis, tumor ingrowth was more frequent in the uncovered group whereas stent migration was more frequent in the covered group (Saranovic et al. 2005).

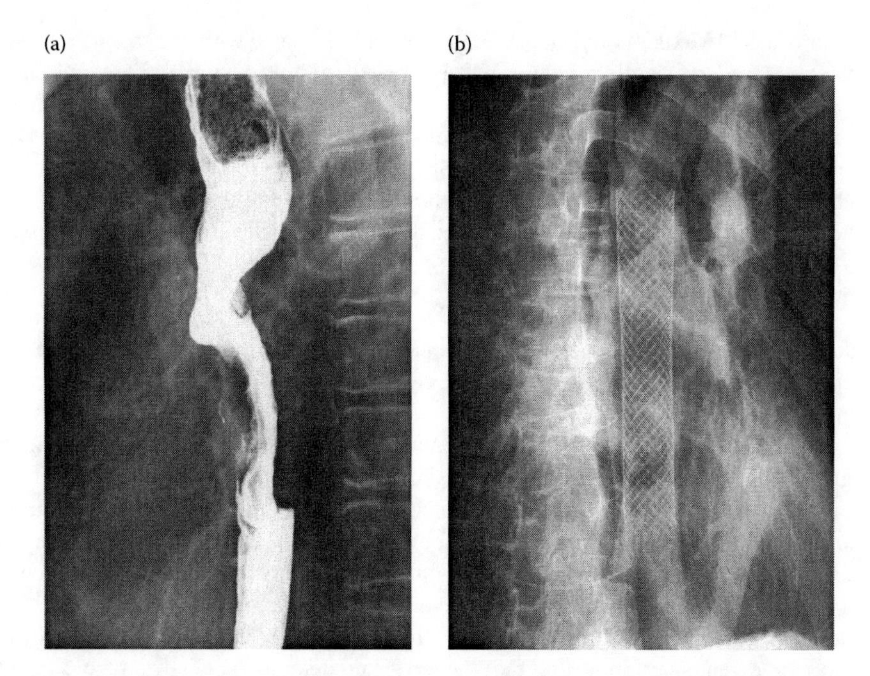

FIGURE 13.1 Stent placement for esophageal cancer. (a) Contrast study showing stricture of the mid part of the esophagus. (b) A metallic stent was placed and deployed at the optimal position.

In addition, covered SEMS are generally used as an effective treatment in sealing esophagorespiratory fistula (ERF) caused by cancer development, although they were reported to have a high rate of reopening (Shin et al. 2004).

13.2.3 Practical Methods and Techniques

The procedure can be performed under conscious sedation. The SEMS is usually placed under a combination of endoscopic and fluoroscopic control, but can be placed under fluoroscopy alone. Fluoroscopic visualization of the stricture is facilitated by endoscopic clips, contrast injection in the submucosal layer, and external skin markers. A guidewire is then passed through the endoscope across the stricture. When too narrow or tight to allow passage by the delivery catheter, predilation with a balloon dilator may be required. A stiff guidewire may also be helpful. The stent is gradually deployed with position adjustment under fluoroscopic control. Finally, the endoscope is then reinserted to confirm correct stent positioning.

13.2.4 Efficacy and Complications

The technical success rate of stent placement in the esophagus is approximately 100% and an improvement in dysphagia score is obtained in 83%–100% of patients (Morgan and Adam 2001). In terms of ERF, successful closure with covered SEMS is achieved in 67%–100% of patients (Morgan and Adam 2001). Although studies assessing quality of life (QOL) after palliative stenting using EORTC questionnaires have reported conflicting results, a recent study with a disease-specific instrument (EORTC QLQ-OES 18 symptom score) reported that palliative stenting provided significant improvement in all QOL scales (Madhusudhan et al. 2009).

Perforation, bleeding, aspiration, and severe pain occur in about 20%–30% of patients as a procedure-related complication (Siersema, Marcon, and Vakil 2003). Delayed complications following stent placement occur in 35%–45% of patients and include bleeding, fistula formation, gastroesophageal (GE) reflux, stent migration, food bolus obstruction, and tumor overgrowth at either end of the stent

(Siersema, Marcon, and Vakil 2003). Tumor overgrowth can be treated with placement of an additional stent or ablative procedures, while migration can be treated with retrieving a migrated stent with an endoscope and placing a second stent. Complete migration of a stent out of the stomach may lead to bowel obstruction or perforation. Although prior chemoradiotherapy is generally considered to increase life-threatening complications after placement of SEMS, a recent analysis with 200 patients suggests that prior chemoradiotherapy did not affect either the incidence of life-threatening complications and survival after stenting (Homs et al. 2004), indicating the need for further evaluation of this issue.

13.2.5 Cervical Esophagus and GE Junction

Two specific methodological conditions require consideration. With regard to proximal esophageal cancer, stent placement for esophageal stricture close to the upper esophageal sphincter (UES) was previously difficult using SEMS. Recently, however, successful outcomes have been reported: one large study indicated that despite major complications in 21%, stent placement in patients with malignant stricture close to the UES is feasible and well tolerated, and although eight (8%) patients complained of globus sensation, no patient required stent removal (Verschuur, Kuipers, and Siersema 2007). The other is stenting across the GE junction, usually performed for esophageal adenocarcinoma or gastric cardia cancer. The main problems here are possible migration and GE reflux. Placement of an uncovered stent may prevent stent migration, while antireflux stents may prevent reflux in patients in whom the stent crosses the GE junction. However, their efficacy remains controversial: one recent study indicated that they offer no demonstrable advantage over the combination of a standard open stent and proton pump inhibitor medication (Sabharwal et al. 2008).

13.3 STOMACH AND DUODENUM

13.3.1 Gastric Outlet Obstruction

Gastric outlet obstruction (GOO) is common in patients with unresectable malignancies such as gastric, pancreatic, or periampullary cancers. GOO usually causes a variety of obstructive symptoms, including nausea, vomiting, or bloating, and usually leads to poor or no oral intake in affected patients. In those with severe GOO through which gastric juice cannot pass, dehydration and electrolyte dehydration is often present. Since most of these patients have limited life expectancy, the primary goal of palliative care is rapid relief of obstructive symptoms and resumption of oral intake.

Although conventional therapy in patients with unresectable malignant GOO has been palliative surgery such as gastrojejunostomy, this surgery carries significant risks of morbidity and mortality (Weaver et al. 1987), and frequently causes delayed gastric emptying (Doberneck and Berndt 1987). Most patients unsuitable for surgical palliation do not ingest food orally and often require placement of a decompression tube (i.e., nasogastric or gastrostomy tube). Further, chemotherapy and radiotherapy are often ineffective. Against this background, stent placement has recently emerged as a new alternative to surgical palliation.

13.3.2 Stent Placement

For anatomical reasons—long access route, sharp angulation, and loop formation of the delivery system in the stomach—stent placement for GOO is technically difficult. Initial reports were for patients with post-operative anatomy (e.g., after Whipple's operation) (Kozarek, Ball, and Patterson 1992). We first reported duodenal stenting in a patient with normal anatomy using a peroral placement technique in 1994 (Maetani et al. 1994).

The initial lack of dedicated systems meant that in the early period the over-the-wire (OTW) method using esophageal stent was mostly used (Maetani et al. 2002) (Figure 13.2). However, the placement technique was markedly complicated and difficult. First-generation dedicated enteral stents became available in the late 1990s (Soetikno et al. 1998). This type of stent is mounted in a

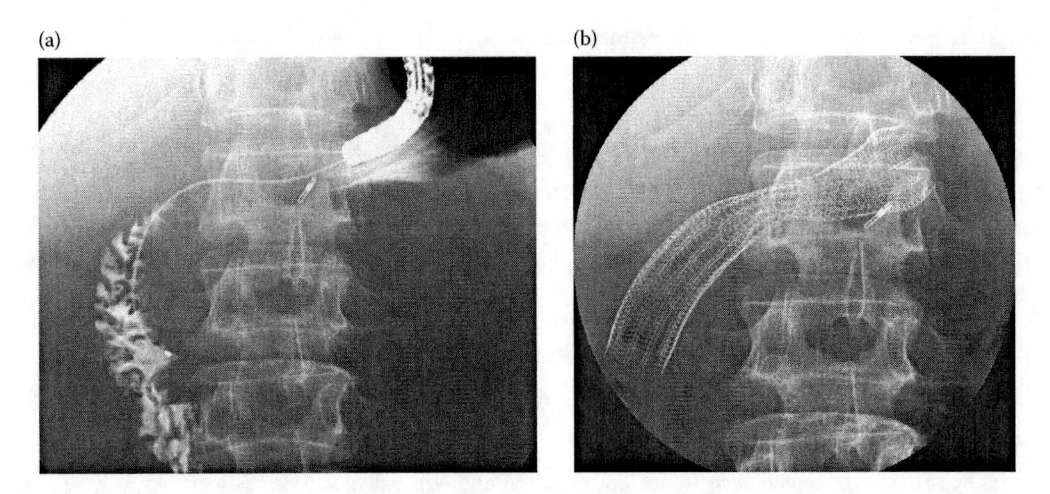

FIGURE 13.2 Stent placement in patients with recurrent gastric cancer. (a) Contrast study through the endoscope showing stenosis at gastroduodenostomy due to recurrent gastric cancer. (Arrow: clip for a marker of the oral end of the stenosis.) (b) Plain x-ray photo showing a successfully placed stent.

slim delivery system, which can be inserted through the endoscope. The through-the-scope (TTS) method makes it much easier to place SEMS in the pyloro-duodenal region.

Most patients with pancreatobiliary cancers have both biliary as well as gastroduodenal obstruction. Duodenal obstruction occurs most frequently following biliary stricture. In some patients, stenosis of the CBD and duodenum occurs simultaneously. Because placement of a duodenal stent hampers access to the ampulla for biliary stenting, the biliary stent should be placed first, when possible, followed by the duodenal stent (Figure 13.3). When the duodenal stent is placed prior to

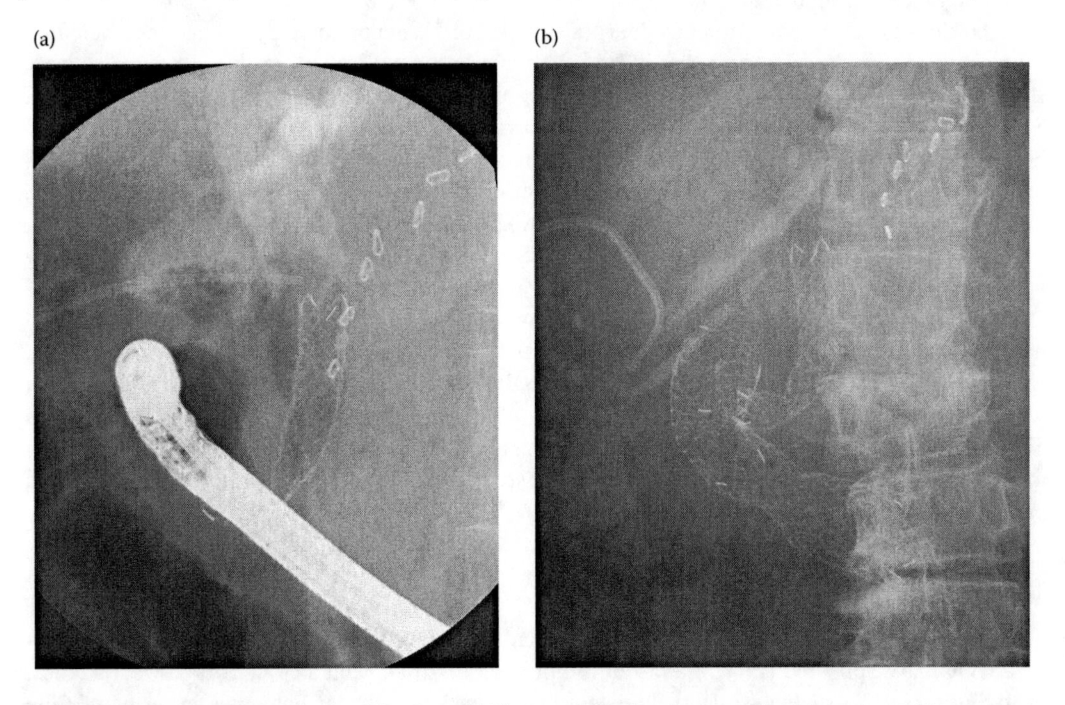

FIGURE 13.3 Placement of a combination of biliary and duodenal stents. For this patient with pancreatic cancer, biliary and duodenal stricture (pars III) occurred simultaneously. (a) Biliary SEMS was first placed endoscopically, followed by placement of the duodenal stent. (b) Plain x-ray photo the day after stenting showing both stents placed in the T configuration.

the biliary stent or the duodenoscope cannot pass through a severe duodenal stricture, percutaneous biliary drainage may be required.

13.3.3 Practical Methods and Techniques

Of the two procedures mentioned (OTW and TTS), the TTS procedure is generally used because of its significant ease of use. However, the diameter of the delivery catheter is 10–10.5 Fr, requiring a therapeutic endoscope with a large working channel. A guidewire is passed across the stricture under endoscopic and fluoroscopic control. Once a guidewire is successfully passed through the stricture, the delivery system is advanced along it, positioned in the stricture, and deployed by pulling back the outer sheath. Finally, contrast is injected to confirm correct positioning of the SEMS and the endoscope is removed.

13.3.4 Efficacy and Complications

A review of 1046 published cases reported technical and clinical success rates were 96% and 89%, respectively (Jeurnink et al. 2007). Reasons for clinical failure were the presence of duplicated distal stenosis, dissemination, and deteriorated peristalsis due to neural invasion.

The most frequently used system to score oral intake is the Gastric Outlet Obstruction Scoring System (GOOSS), with 0 = no oral intake, 1 = liquid only, 2 = soft solids, and 3 = low-residue or full diet (Adler and Baron 2002). A systematic review suggested that the GOOSS score is significantly improved following stent placement (Jeurnink et al. 2007), but a more recent study using radionuclide scanning indicated that gastric emptying function remains delayed after stenting in many patients (Maetani et al. 2008).

The only study to objectively evaluate QOL score before and after stenting, using the EORTC QLQ-C30 and QLQ-STO22 instruments, found that placement was associated with acceptable QOL outcomes (Schmidt et al. 2009).

According to a systematic review (Jeurnink et al. 2007), major early complications, including migration and stent dysfunction, occur in 7%, and major late complications in 18%. These are mostly stent migration and obstruction caused by tumor in- or over-growth, hyperplasia or food impaction. Stent obstruction occurs more frequently than stent migration. Tumor-related stent obstructions can be managed by placement of a second stent or ablative procedures (Maetani et al. 2002), while placement of an additional stent may be chosen for stent migration. Minor complications, such as pain, nausea, or vomiting, are not frequent (9%) (Jeurnink et al. 2007), while life-threatening complications like perforation and bleeding are rare. SEMS with significant flexibility and blunt ends may be helpful in preventing ulcer formation and perforation (Maetani, Isayama, and Mizumoto 2007).

Covered stents may prevent tumor ingrowth and mucosal hyperplasia, but are more likely to migrate than uncovered stents without integration into the gastroduodenal mucosa. In addition, when a covered SEMS is placed covering the ampulla, subsequent endoscopic biliary intervention will become impossible. A recent study (Maetani et al. 2009) comparing covered and uncovered SEMS for GOO indicated no advantage to coating, and the covered group required reintervention more frequently despite similar outcomes. Further study to determine the significance of coating in patients with GOO is warranted.

13.3.5 Stent Placement versus Gastrojejunostomy

To date, only two randomized comparisons of stent placement and gastrojejunostomy in patients with GOO have appeared (Fiori, Lamazza, Volpino et al. 2004; Mehta et al. 2006). Most studies, including these two studies, suggest that stent placement offers better outcomes in terms of time to resumption of oral intake and hospital stay. According to a systematic review, however, stenting has a higher clinical success rate and fewer minor complications, but a higher rate of recurrence of obstructive symptoms, suggesting that stenting may be more favorable in patients with a relatively short life expectancy, while gastrojejunostomy is preferable in those with a more prolonged prognosis (Jeurnink et al. 2007). Presently, however, because malignant GOO is usually a preterminal event with very limited life expectancy, stent placement appears a more reasonable palliative procedure for most such patients. Further randomized comparison is warranted.

13.4 COLORECTUM

13.4.1 Colorectal Obstruction

Acute colorectal obstruction usually requires decompressive procedures and may be life threatening if untreated. It is most frequently caused by colorectal cancer and rarely by extrinsic invasive tumors due to pelvic malignancies (i.e., bladder cancer, ovarian cancer, etc.). There are two main indications for stenting using SEMS in the colorectum: palliative treatment in patients with unresectable colorectal obstructions and presurgical decompression for potentially curable patients. Presurgical application of SEMS is described in a subsequent section of this chapter; the present section focuses on the former indication only.

13.4.2 Stent Placement

The first application of a SEMS for the colorectum was reported in 1991 (Dohmoto 1991). Since no dedicated stent system was available at that time, placement in the long and tortuous colon was difficult, and was significantly complicated by the need for various modifications and an overtube (Maetani et al. 2004). With the development of dedicated TTS stents, technical and clinical success rates with proximal colonic stenting are now comparable to those with distal colonic stenting (Repici et al. 2007).

13.4.3 Practical Methods and Techniques

The TTS procedure is more commonly selected, particularly in patients with proximal colonic obstruction. Radiologic placement without endoscopic support is used in some cases of left-sided colonic obstruction. TTS placement of colorectal stents is similar to that for GOO, with two points of difference. First, passing the guidewire across the stricture is more challenging: because angulation of the stricture is sometimes acute and the colonic wall is thin, the guidewire should be gently manipulated to avoid perforation. Second, predilation with a balloon catheter presents a risk of perforation and is therefore dangerous. Subsequent procedures, however, including delivery and deployment of SEMS, are the same as for GOO stenting (Figure 13.4). If successful, bowel obstructions are dramatically and instantaneously relieved.

13.4.4 Efficacy and Complications

In a systematic review of 96 previously published series involving 1198 cases (palliation, 791 patients), technical and clinical success rates in patients treated palliatively were 93% and 91%, respectively (Sebastian et al. 2004).

Among adverse findings, the perforation rate in this review was 3.8% (Sebastian et al. 2004), and showed a significant association with predilation (17.7%), indicating that balloon dilation should not be conducted prior to stent placement. Of a total of 45 perforations, 29 (64.4%) required emergency surgical intervention. Migration was the most frequent problem, occurring in 11.8% (Sebastian et al. 2004), two-thirds of which occurred within a week of stent placement. Risk factors for stent migration are widely considered to be the use of a covered stent, dilation prior to stent placement, use of laser treatment, and use of chemoradiotherapy. Migrated stents are usually excreted from the anus. The review indicated that the rate of reobstruction was 7.3% (Sebastian et al. 2004), caused by tumor ingrowth, tumor overgrowth, fecal impaction, migration, etc. The most frequent cause was tumor ingrowth, which is usually treated by placement of an additional stent.

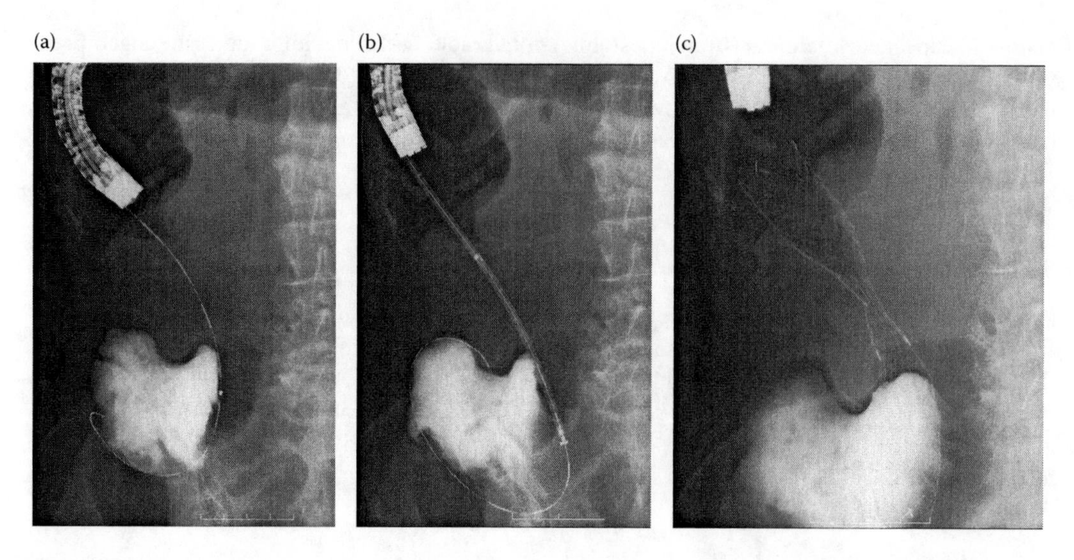

FIGURE 13.4 Colonic stenting. (a) Contrast study through the endoscope showing obstructive colon cancer in the ascending colon. A guidewire was successfully passed across the stricture. (b) The delivery catheter was introduced through the endoscope and passed across the stricture. (c) A SEMS was successfully placed and deployed.

Although one report found that covered SEMS were effective in preventing tumor ingrowth (Repici et al. 2000), the more frequent late migration in the covered group in a later study comparing outcomes with uncovered and covered SEMS indicates that there is no advantage to covered SEMS for palliative purposes (Lee et al. 2007).

Other complications, including pain, diarrhea, and minute bleeding, occur less frequently and are usually not serious. Although there is no consensus on whether stent placement in the lower rectum provides effective and comfortable palliation, one retrospective study indicated placement of SEMS in patients with malignant rectal obstruction within 5 cm of the anal verge may provide adequate palliation, albeit with some risk of pain. These patients should be counseled about pain, incontinence, and tenesmus before considering stent placement.

The cumulative mortality rate is less than 1%. The systematic review suggested that it was 0.58% and most cases were associated with perforation (Sebastian et al. 2004).

13.4.5 Stent Placement versus Surgical Alternatives

Two randomized studies have compared palliative stenting to colostomy (Fiori, Lamazza, De Cesare et al. 2004; Xinopoulos et al. 2004). Results showed that stent placement offered better outcomes, such as shorter hospital stay and shorter procedure time. Both studies were small, with a limited number of patients however, warranting a larger randomized study. A meta-analysis comparing colonic stenting with open surgery for malignant bowel obstruction indicated that colonic stenting offers rapid relief from symptoms with less chance of the need for stoma creation in the terminal phase of illness, but data on quality of life and economic evaluation were limited (Tilney et al. 2007). These two factors require further evaluation.

13.5 APPLICATION OF STENTING TO OTHER AREAS OF PALLIATIVE CARE

Esophageal SEMS are used for the treatment of benign esophageal strictures and esophageal perforations or leaks. Temporary placement of covered SEMS can be considered. Regarding the former, 12 studies have reported on 168 patients who underwent SEMS placement for benign esophageal strictures due to various etiologies, including achalasia, caustic stricture, and anastomotic stricture, among others (Siersema 2009). Regarding the use of SEMS for benign strictures, the main problem is the frequent occurrence of hyperplastic tissue ingrowth or overgrowth. Although SEPS was developed to overcome these problems, they were shown to have another drawback of frequent migration. Biodegradable stents are considered to represent a promising alternative to these existing stents (Stivaros et al. 2009), although performance will require full evaluation. The other purpose is sealing esophageal perforations or leaks. The main causes of esophageal perforation are iatrogenic injury, Boerhaave's syndrome, or foreign body ingestion. Although the use of hemoclips or glue is effective in small ruptures, stenting is usually required for larger ruptures.

Few reports have described stenting for benign GOO (Bae et al. 2004). Temporary placement of a SEMS or use of a biodegradable stent is potentially effective for refractory benign gastroduodenal strictures.

Colorectal stenting has a significant role in colorectal cancer, not only as palliation but also as a bridge to surgery. Presurgical placement of a SEMS is beneficial for colon decompression, allowing a one-stage scheduled operation after adequate bowel preparation. This approach is now widely accepted and is becoming common practice for acute bowel obstruction due to curative malignancy without distant metastasis or locally extensive invasion. In addition, some reports about stenting for benign colorectal obstruction due to various etiologies have appeared (Forshaw et al. 2006). In general, the stent is left in place for a long time or is used as a 'bridge to surgery.' Although offering effective decompression, it has the significant drawback of frequent complications, particularly in acute diverticular disease (Forshaw et al. 2006).

ETHICAL ISSUES

As noted above, stent placement is a safe and effective procedure in patients with incurable GI obstructions. However, patients may encounter complications, including migration and reobstruction in 10%–30%, although severe procedure-related complications are rare. In most patients with complications, reintervention may be required. In addition, 5%–15% of patients may not obtain symptom relief even after stenting. The provision of appropriate information before the procedure is therefore important, including potential complications, ineffectiveness, and the inability to remove a stent.

SUMMARY POINTS

- Currently, self-expandable metallic stents play an important role in the palliation of GI obstruction. The chief advantage of this treatment is less invasiveness compared to surgical alternatives and rapid relief of obstructive symptoms.
- The success rate of stenting is relatively high and serious procedure-related complications are rare. Ten to thirty percent of patients may encounter recurrent stent dysfunction due to stent migration, obstruction, etc. However, most stent dysfunctions are manageable by placement of a second stent.
- A larger randomized comparison with surgical alternatives is lacking and is warranted for further objective evaluation of this procedure.
- Even currently available stents should be revised to reduce the occurrence of complications and prolong stent patency.

LIST OF ABBREVIATIONS

ERF	Esophagorespiratory fistula
GE	Gastroesophageal
GI	Gastrointestinal
GOO	Gastric outlet obstruction
OTW	Over-the-wire

QOL	Quality of life
SEMS	Self-expandable metallic stent
SEPS	Self-expandable plastic stent
TTS	Through-the-scope
UES	Upper esophageal sphincter

REFERENCES

Adler, D. G., and T. H. Baron. 2002. Endoscopic palliation of malignant gastric outlet obstruction using self-expanding metal stents: Experience in 36 patients. *Am J Gastroenterol* 97:72–78.

Bae, J. I., J. H. Shin, H. Y. Song, and G. H. Lee. 2004. Treatment of a benign anastomotic duodenojejunal stricture with a polytetrafluoroethylene-covered retrievable expandable nitinol stent. *J Vasc Interv Radiol* 15:769–72.

Doberneck, R. C., and G. A. Berndt. 1987. Delayed gastric emptying after palliative gastrojejunostomy for carcinoma of the pancreas. *Arch Surg* 122:827–29.

Dohmoto, M. 1991. New method-endoscopic implantation of rectal stent in palliative treatment of malignant stenosis. *Endoscopia Digestiva* 3:1507–12.

Domschke, W., E. C. Foerster, W. Matek, and W. Rodl. 1990. Self-expanding mesh stent for esophageal cancer stenosis. *Endoscopy* 22:134–36.

Fiori, E., A. Lamazza, A. De Cesare, M. Bononi, P. Volpino, A. Schillaci, A. Cavallaro, and V. Cangemi. 2004. Palliative management of malignant rectosigmoidal obstruction. Colostomy vs. endoscopic stenting. A randomized prospective trial. *Anticancer Res* 24:265–68.

Fiori, E., A. Lamazza, P. Volpino, A. Burza, C. Paparelli, G. Cavallaro, A. Schillaci, and V. Cangemi. 2004. Palliative management of malignant antro-pyloric strictures. Gastroenterostomy vs. endoscopic stenting. A randomized prospective trial. *Anticancer Res* 24:269–71.

Forshaw, M. J., D. Sankararajah, M. Stewart, and M. C. Parker. 2006. Self-expanding metallic stents in the treatment of benign colorectal disease: Indications and outcomes. *Colorectal Dis* 8:102–11.

Homs, M. Y., B. E. Hansen, M. Van Blankenstein, J. Haringsma, E. J. Kuipers, and P. D. Siersema. 2004. Prior radiation and/or chemotherapy has no effect on the outcome of metal stent placement for oesophagogastric carcinoma. *Eur J Gastroenterol Hepatol* 16:163–70.

Jeurnink, S. M., C. H. Van Eijck, E. W. Steyerberg, E. J. Kuipers, and P. D. Siersema. 2007. Stent versus gastrojejunostomy for the palliation of gastric outlet obstruction: a systematic review. *BMC Gastroenterol* 7:18.

Knyrim, K., H. J. Wagner, N. Bethge, M. Keymling, and N. Vakil. 1993. A controlled trial of an expansile metal stent for palliation of esophageal obstruction due to inoperable cancer. *N Engl J Med* 329:1302–7.

Kozarek, R. A., T. J. Ball, and D. J. Patterson. 1992. Metallic self-expanding stent application in the upper gastrointestinal tract: Caveats and concerns. *Gastrointest Endosc* 38:1–6.

Lee, K. M., S. J. Shin, J. C. Hwang, J. Y. Cheong, B. M. Yoo, K. J. Lee, K. B. Hahm, J. H. Kim, and S. W. Cho. 2007. Comparison of uncovered stent with covered stent for treatment of malignant colorectal obstruction. *Gastrointest Endosc* 66:931–36.

Madhusudhan, C., S. S. Saluja, S. Pal, V. Ahuja, P. Saran, N. R. Dash, P. Sahni, and T. K. Chattopadhyay. 2009. Palliative stenting for relief of dysphagia in patients with inoperable esophageal cancer: Impact on quality of life. *Dis Esophagus* 22:331–36.

Maetani, I., H. Isayama, and Y. Mizumoto. 2007. Palliation in patients with malignant gastric outlet obstruction with a newly designed enteral stent: A multicenter study. *Gastrointest Endosc* 66:355–60.

Maetani, I., S. Ogawa, H. Hoshi, M. Sato, H. Yoshioka, Y. Igarashi, and Y. Sakai. 1994. Self-expanding metal stents for palliative treatment of malignant biliary and duodenal stenoses. *Endoscopy* 26:701–4.

Maetani, I., T. Tada, J. Shimura, T. Ukita, H. Inoue, Y. Igarashi, H. Hoshi, and Y. Sakai. 2002. Technical modifications and strategies for stenting gastric outlet strictures using esophageal endoprostheses. *Endoscopy* 34:402–6.

Maetani, I., T. Tada, T. Ukita, H. Inoue, M. Yoshida, Y. Saida, and Y. Sakai. 2004. Self-expandable metallic stent placement as palliative treatment of obstructed colorectal carcinoma. *J Gastroenterol* 39:334–38.

Maetani, I., T. Ukita, T. Tada, M. Ikeda, M. Seike, H. Terada, and E. Kohda. 2008. Gastric emptying in patients with palliative stenting for malignant gastric outlet obstruction. *Hepatogastroenterology* 55:298–302.

Maetani, I., T. Ukita, T. Tada, H. Shigoka, S. Omuta, and T. Endo. 2009. Metallic stents for gastric outlet obstruction: Reintervention rate is lower with uncovered versus covered stents, despite similar outcomes. *Gastrointest Endosc* 69:806–12.

Mehta, S., A. Hindmarsh, E. Cheong, J. Cockburn, J. Saada, R. Tighe, M. P. Lewis, and M. Rhodes. 2006. Prospective randomized trial of laparoscopic gastrojejunostomy versus duodenal stenting for malignant gastric outflow obstruction. *Surg Endosc* 20:239–42.

Morgan, R., and A. Adam. 2001. Use of metallic stents and balloons in the esophagus and gastrointestinal tract. *J Vasc Interv Radiol* 12:283–97.

Repici, A., D. G. Adler, C. M. Gibbs, A. Malesci, P. Preatoni, and T. H. Baron. 2007. Stenting of the proximal colon in patients with malignant large bowel obstruction: Techniques and outcomes. *Gastrointest Endosc* 66:940–44.

Repici, A., D. Reggio, C. De Angelis, C. Barletti, P. Marchesa, A. Musso, P. Carucci et al. 2000. Covered metal stents for management of inoperable malignant colorectal strictures. *Gastrointest Endosc* 52:735–40.

Sabharwal, T., M. S. Gulati, N. Fotiadis, R. Dourado, A. Botha, R. Mason, and A. Adam. 2008. Randomised comparison of the FerX Ella antireflux stent and the ultraflex stent: Proton pump inhibitor combination for prevention of post-stent reflux in patients with esophageal carcinoma involving the esophago-gastric junction. *J Gastroenterol Hepatol* 23:723–28.

Saranovic, D., A. Djuric-Stefanovic, A. Ivanovic, D. Masulovic, and P. Pesko. 2005. Fluoroscopically guided insertion of self-expandable metal esophageal stents for palliative treatment of patients with malignant stenosis of esophagus and cardia: Comparison of uncovered and covered stent types. *Dis Esophagus* 18:230–38.

Schmidt, C., H. Gerdes, W. Hawkins, E. Zucker, Q. Zhou, E. Riedel, D. Jaques, A. Markowitz, D. Coit, and M. Schattner. 2009. A prospective observational study examining quality of life in patients with malignant gastric outlet obstruction. *Am J Surg* 198:92–99.

Sebastian, S., S. Johnston, T. Geoghegan, W. Torreggiani, and M. Buckley. 2004. Pooled analysis of the efficacy and safety of self-expanding metal stenting in malignant colorectal obstruction. *Am J Gastroenterol* 99:2051–57.

Shin, J. H., H. Y. Song, G. Y. Ko, J. O. Lim, H. K. Yoon, and K. B. Sung. 2004. Esophagorespiratory fistula: Long-term results of palliative treatment with covered expandable metallic stents in 61 patients. *Radiology* 232:252–59.

Siersema, P. D. 2009. Stenting for benign esophageal strictures. *Endoscopy* 41:363–73.

Siersema, P. D., N. Marcon, and N. Vaki. 2003. Metal stents for tumors of the distal esophagus and gastric cardia. *Endoscopy* 35:79–85.

Soetikno, R. M., D. R. Lichtenstein, J. Vandervoort, R. C. Wong, A. D. Roston, A. Slivka, H. Montes, and D. L. Carr-Locke. 1998. Palliation of malignant gastric outlet obstruction using an endoscopically placed Wallstent. *Gastrointest Endosc* 47:267–70.

Stivaros, S. M., L. R. Williams, C. Senger, L. Wilbraham, and H. U. Laasch. 2010. Woven polydioxanone biodegradable stents: A new treatment option for benign and malignant oesophageal strictures. *Eur Radiol* 20:1069–72.

Tilney, H. S., R. E. Lovegrove, S. Purkayastha, P. S. Sains, G. K. Weston-Petrides, A. W. Darzi, P. P. Tekkis, and A. G. Heriot. 2007. Comparison of colonic stenting and open surgery for malignant large bowel obstruction. *Surg Endosc* 21:225–33.

Verschuur, E. M., E. J. Kuipers, and P. D. Siersema. 2007. Esophageal stents for malignant strictures close to the upper esophageal sphincter. *Gastrointest Endosc* 66:1082–90.

Weaver, D. W., R. G. Wiencek, D. L. Bouwman, and A. J. Walt. 1987. Gastrojejunostomy: Is it helpful for patients with pancreatic cancer? *Surgery* 102:608–13.

Xinopoulos, D., D. Dimitroulopoulos, T. Theodosopoulos, K. Tsamakidis, G. Bitsakou, G. Plataniotis, M. Gontikakis et al. 2004. Stenting or stoma creation for patients with inoperable malignant colonic obstructions? Results of a study and cost-effectiveness analysis. *Surg Endosc* 18:421–26.

14 Artificial Nutrition, Advance Directives, and End-of-Life in Nursing Homes

Cheryl Ann Monturo

CONTENTS

14.1 INTRODUCTION

More than 30% of people living in nursing homes in the United States die there or within a short time after transfer to an acute care facility, highlighting the need for an increased focus on delivery of palliative care services (Center for Disease Control and Prevention 2002). A significant part of this care requires consideration of the resident's preferences for life-sustaining treatment. One manner in which these preferences are communicated is through advance directives (ADs) executed by the residents. Although a variety of treatments may be addressed, artificial nutrition (AN) has attracted significant attention. In the recent case of Terri Schiavo, a young American nursing home resident in a persistent vegetative state receiving AN, commentary spread across the world, including a papal address. In light of society's continuing struggle with this life-sustaining treatment, this chapter addresses nursing home care, ADs, and AN for those at the end-of-life.

14.2 NURSING HOMES

14.2.1 Personnel to Meet the Demands

As individuals live longer with serious illness, many require skilled care that can be found in long-term care facilities also known as nursing homes or care homes (The Care Commission 2009). Increasingly, these facilities are becoming the place for many to die with an expectation that this number will rise significantly in coming years (Center for Disease Control and Prevention 2002). With these numbers comes an increased demand for staff to care for more residents. The Center for Medicare and Medicaid Services in the United States recently provided minimum guidelines on appropriate staffing for nursing homes, concluding that 90% of the homes were already deficient in meeting these standards (Abt Associates 2001). Poorer staffing translates into more residents per staff member, causing the potential for significant workplace stress and higher rates of staff turnover. This lack of stability further erodes the quality of care in general and palliative care in particular.

In some instances residents who are capable of eating may receive AN due to poor staffing. These residents require hand feeding and in the absence of family or volunteers to assist, may not receive adequate nutrition because of the time it takes to feed them. Although some may feel that AN is more expedient and will provide all the necessary nutrients, residents are deprived of the innate social nature of mealtime.

14.2.2 Palliative Care Services

More residents not only demand higher staffing ratios, but staff capable of providing overall as well as palliative care. Recent research documents the lack of appropriate palliative care services in nursing homes such as the inconsistency of care with patient preferences (Teno et al. 2004) and the lack of awareness that palliative care should be delivered to specific residents (The Care Commission 2009). Statistics are available on multiple aspects of palliative care, however for the purposes of this chapter, the focus will remain on life-sustaining treatments, specifically AN.

14.2.3 Palliative Care Education

The lack of palliative care in nursing homes may be attributed to inadequate attention by staff development departments within homes (International Council of Nurses 2002), as well as the absence of proper education within basic nursing curricula (McDonnell et al. 2009; The Care Commission 2009). Further, with higher staff turnover rates, the effectiveness of educational programs is limited, requiring educators to continually re-educate new groups of employees. Consideration of these educational needs is important to fostering appropriate educational programs in nursing homes (Table 14.1).

Although there is a significant body of literature on the palliative care educational needs of nursing home staff, there are few studies on the effect of systematic organized education in this area. In one study, the presence of a palliative care program in a group of nursing homes positively impacted the knowledge level and attitudes of staff (Stillman et al. 2005). It is clear that education is a positive force in improving palliative care, however historical events in the regulation of nursing homes may add to the difficulty in realizing appropriate palliative care.

14.2.4 Regulations

Nursing home regulations exist for the protection and welfare of residents. In Ireland, both publicly and privately owned nursing homes are subject to regulations (Health Information and Quality Authority 2008), recognizing the need for palliative care knowledge and basic skills (An Bord Altranais 2009). Scotland's Commission for the Regulation of Care recently reported mixed results on the provision of palliative care in care homes (The Care Commission 2009).

TABLE 14.1
Palliative Care Education in Nursing Homes

- Examine the underlying culture of the institution
  - Survey staff and administrators
  - Capture beliefs and values
  - Include a values clarification exercise
- Develop a plan for palliative care education
  - Use multiple strategies
  - Provide the basics first
  - Include plans for remediation
  - Provide support for staff to attend
  - Plan ahead for continuing education
- Include all parts of the organization in educational sessions
  - Administration, clinical, and support staff
  - "Buy in" is essential for success
- Develop an advance care planning protocol
  - Identify key staff who will approach residents and families
  - Identify a timeline for completion of the process from admission
  - Reinforce need for consistency of message to residents and families
- Develop a standard advance directive
  - Begin with a standardized document to avoid omissions
  - Allow for additions by residents and families
- Reinforce necessary documentation
  - Document advance care planning process
  - Document resident's preferences on an advance directive
  - Standardize the location for all documentation
- Reinforce the ongoing process
  - Preferences may change so continuous communication is key
  - Support of resident and family

Note: This table presents key steps in the process of initiating a palliative care education program in a nursing home. The process includes the mechanics as well as the need to incorporate psychosocial and cultural aspects of program development. In addition, ongoing support, evaluation, and readjustment of the program is necessary to maintain a healthy and viable palliative care education program.

Abuse and neglect in the mid-twentieth century U.S. nursing homes necessitated the institution of regulations to insure adequate nutrition and hydration. These regulations utilized resident weight as an indicator of nutritional adequacy unless further documentation identified a reason that this goal could not be achieved (Omnibus Budget Reconciliation Act 1987). A resident's refusal to eat or drink was not considered in applying this regulation, thereby increasing the possibility that AN would be instituted to maintain compliance. In addition to OBRA 1987, U.S. nursing homes receiving funds from Medicare (a federally funded program) or Medicaid (a state-funded program) must collect specific nutritionally related data on each resident as part of the Minimum Data Set (MDS) (Table 14.2).

Although weight may be one indicator of poor nutrition, it is one of many that must be assessed in the palliative care population. Difficulty in standardization of procedures and equipment lead to inaccuracies in reporting of actual weights. Disease processes and aging also affect the weight in terms of measuring lean body mass, fat, and extracellular fluid changes (Monturo and Strumpf 2007). Fear of litigation and/or loss of institutional accreditation may increase the use of AN without considering the residents' preferences and quality of life, or that weight loss is a common indicator of impending death (Center for Gerontology and Health Care Research Brown Medical School 2004).

TABLE 14.2
Minimum Data Set (MDS) Nutritional Parameters

- Oral problems
- Height and weight
- Weight change
- Altered taste
- Hunger
- Uneaten meals
- Food intake
- Use of nutrition support
- Use of mechanically altered food
- Use of therapeutic diets

Note: The MDS is a data repository for information collected on all residents in nursing homes receiving state or federal funding in the United States. This data is used to assess residents, but is also extensively used for research purposes as it is easily accessible through internet sites.

14.2.5 Cognitive Impairment

Dementia results in many neurodegenerative impairments, including eating difficulties in its final stages. Recent statistics show that 70% of those with dementia are expected to receive end-of-life care in nursing homes (Mitchell et al. 2005). Although the use of AN is not exclusive to those residents with dementia, reports show that it is highest in those with significant cognitive impairments (Mitchell et al. 2003). In addition to dementia, those with other forms of cognitive impairment, such as a individuals in a persistent vegetative state, a minimally conscious state, or a coma, are unable to eat normally and therefore AN may be provided.

14.3 ADVANCE DIRECTIVES

ADs are considered the written result of advance care planning and must not exist in isolation as simple documents (Figure 14.1, Table 14.3). ADs may be standardized to include certain language, such as those in individual U.S. states, or may be available to the general public. Routinely, ADs contain directions to allow or refuse specific medical treatments. In this manner they may also be called 'living wills.' Another form of AD is the power-of-attorney for healthcare decisions. This AD identifies an individual who will make decisions for the resident should they no longer be able to communicate their own wishes. These two types of ADs may also be combined into one document, such as Five Wishes offered by the organization *Aging with Dignity*. In some Asian cultures, ADs are viewed as a liberal model for decision-making and one that is not central to normal familiar relationships (Chan 2004). Although advance care planning and ADs exist in numerous forms in many countries, the United States continues to experience much difficulty with this issue, specifically as it relates to AN. For that reason, much of this section is dedicated to information derived from the United States.

14.3.1 Historical Evolution

In the latter part of the twentieth century, the literature focused on advance care planning and specifically ADs in the United States, originating from legal mandates and the right to die movement, unlike the previous focus on "do not resuscitate" orders and a less autonomous environment (Figure 14.2). The first right to die case was that of Karen Ann Quinlan, a young nursing home resident in a persistent vegetative state supported on a respirator. Although the case involved

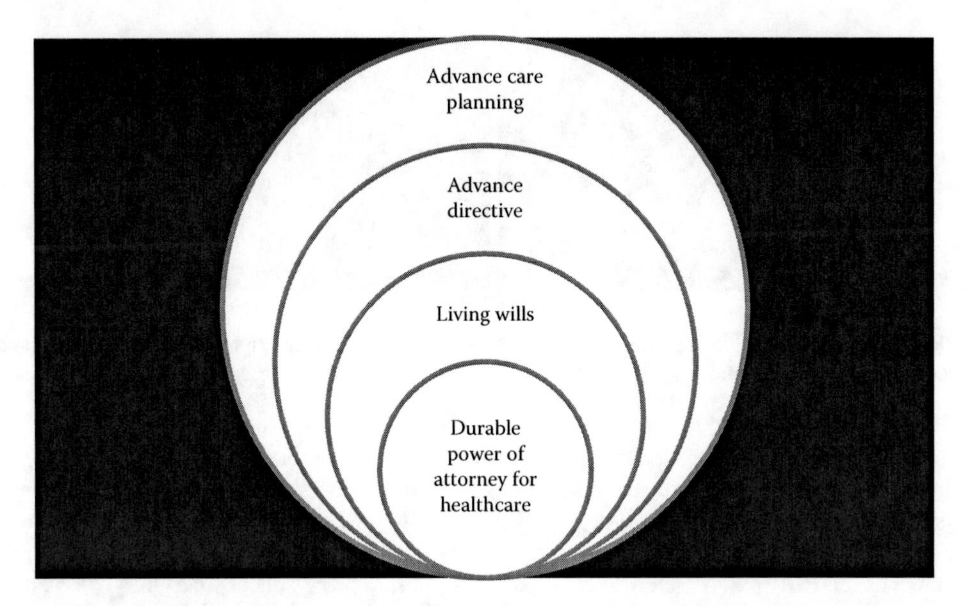

FIGURE 14.1 Advance directives. Advance care planning is the overarching and inclusive approach to advance directive development.

discontinuation of a respirator, removal of AN was also an option, but one which was not acceptable to her family at that time. Ms. Quinlan died 9 years later of pneumonia while still receiving AN.

Numerous cases arose after Ms. Quinlan, focused on withdrawal of treatment, sometimes including AN. At this time, some believed there was a difference between withdrawal of AN and withdrawal of antibiotics, respirators, or other medical treatments. Seven years after the Quinlan decision, medical and ethical experts found no difference between AN and other life-sustaining treatments (The President's Commission for the Study of Ethical Problems in Medicine and Biomedical and Behavioral Research 1983). Despite this ruling, societal struggles concerning this life-sustaining treatment continued in the United States. As a result of a newborn case, federal regulations known as the "Baby Doe Directives" were imposed preventing withdrawal or withholding of nutrition and fluids from a newborn based solely on a disability.

In 1990, as a result of the Nancy Cruzan case, the U.S. Supreme Court provided support for individual states' rights in upholding a requirement to provide clear and convincing evidence of an

TABLE 14.3
Key Features of an Advance Directive

- It is a document but should be supported by a plan of care
- An AD provides directions for care when an individual is unable to communicate
- ADs may be modified over time
- Actual templates or documents vary with country/state
- ADs may be developed using two basic forms: a living will and a durable power of attorney for healthcare
- ADs are considered legally valid in some areas
- ADs may also be seen as an "individual's voice"
- Enforceability of advance directives also varies with locale
- There is no expiration date on an advance directive
- ADs require preparation prior to execution of the document

Note: Advance directives vary according to locale, however they contain basic information necessary to communicate the preferences of residents no longer able to describe their wishes.

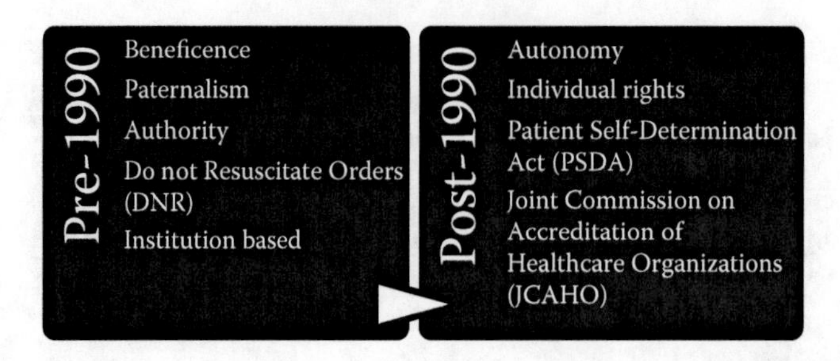

FIGURE 14.2 Historical evolution of advance directives. As a result of the right to die movement, a focus emerged on autonomy and individual rights after years of paternalism and authority-based decision-making. More formal advance directives arose from this evolution post-1990.

individual's wishes concerning treatment (Cruzan v. Director Missouri Health Department 1990). Similar to Ms. Quinlan, Ms. Cruzan was a young woman in a persistent vegetative state, however in this case the issue was withdrawal of AN. Eventually, Ms. Cruzan's AN was discontinued at the request of her family after they provided additional evidence of her wishes. At the same time, a U.S. act known as the Patient Self Determination Act was put into place concerning ADs. Upon admission to a nursing home, staff were required to ask residents if they possessed an AD and to provide information regarding the right to complete an AD (Omnibus Budget Reconciliation Act 1990).

Despite court rulings, ethics panel results, and federal acts, other cases continued to appear, evoking strong emotions. The case of Ms. Terri Schiavo, the most recent involving AN to reach national attention, continued the debate, although in this instance the issue was which surrogate had power over this decision—a spouse or a parent. In all these cases, individuals did not have previous documented treatment wishes, ADs, and therefore discussions led to surrogate decision-making, court-appointed guardians, and/or a best interest standards.

14.3.2 Usefulness of Advance Directives

The presence and successful use of ADs is variable (Center for Gerontology and Health Care Research Brown Medical School 2004; Monturo and Strumpf 2007; Teno et al. 1997). Some report that given the number of years that ADs have been available, there continues to be poor utilization and that this venture has essentially failed (Fagerlin and Schneider 2004). Others would argue that the combination of palliative care education, planning, and AD can work; however more focus must be placed on the plan and education than merely on a document (Monturo and Strumpf 2007; Stillman et al. 2005).

Limited data exists on the incidence or frequency with which preferences for AN appear in ADs. One study reported a high rate of AN preferences (94%) in ADs, although this was likely attributed to the existence of a previously conducted palliative care study in these nursing homes (Monturo and Strumpf 2007).

14.4 ARTIFICIAL NUTRITION

AN is known by many different names including enteral nutrition, parenteral nutrition, and tube feedings. Hydration is frequently included when discussing AN; however these two treatments are distinct. Although both are delivered as a fluid, hydration is simply intravenous fluids with minimal sodium or dextrose, depending on the formulation, whereas enteral (tube feeding) and parenteral nutrition contain micro- and macronutrients necessary to sustain life. AN originated as a means to nourish those unable to ingest food and fluids due to temporary or chronic illness. Although the success of AN is widespread in the literature, its overuse in palliative care and in severe cognitive impairments such as advanced progressive dementia or persistent vegetative states may create ethical dilemmas for residents, families, and healthcare providers (Monturo 2009).

14.4.1 Enteral Nutrition History

Enteral nutrition or "tube feeding" is more common in nursing homes and thus will be the focus of this discussion. This treatment dates to ancient times and throughout the centuries has taken on a variety of different forms (Randall 1990). Technological advances in surgical procedures led to the development of the percutaneous endoscopic gastrostomy (PEG) tube. Placement of this tube afforded patients a decreased risk of complications. The three-fold increase in placement of gastrostomy tubes in older adults over the past 20 years (DeFrances, Cullen, and Kozak 2007) may be due in part to the relative ease of PEG tube placement.

14.4.2 Enteral Nutrition Use

The use of AN in U.S. nursing homes is well documented and, as noted earlier, appears to be higher in those with advanced cognitive impairment (Mitchell et al. 2003); therefore the majority of literature on enteral nutrition in nursing homes focuses on those with dementia. There is little evidence that AN is prescribed for those with dementia in other parts of the world. The rate of AN in the United States may also vary by individual nursing home, state, community (rural vs. urban), and by nursing home culture (Gessert, Elliott, and Peden-McAlpine 2006; Mitchell et al. 2003; Palan Lopez et al. 2010; Teno et al. 2002). Despite the significant number of U.S. nursing home residents receiving AN, there is no evidence to support that this treatment is beneficial to those with dementia (Candy, Sampson, and Jones 2009). Unlike orally ingested food, delivery of enteral nutrition is not free from complications. These complications may be mechanical and therefore directly related to the tube, or physiological (Figure 14.3). As a result, efforts should be made to avoid AN in end-of-life care and instead consider viable alternatives.

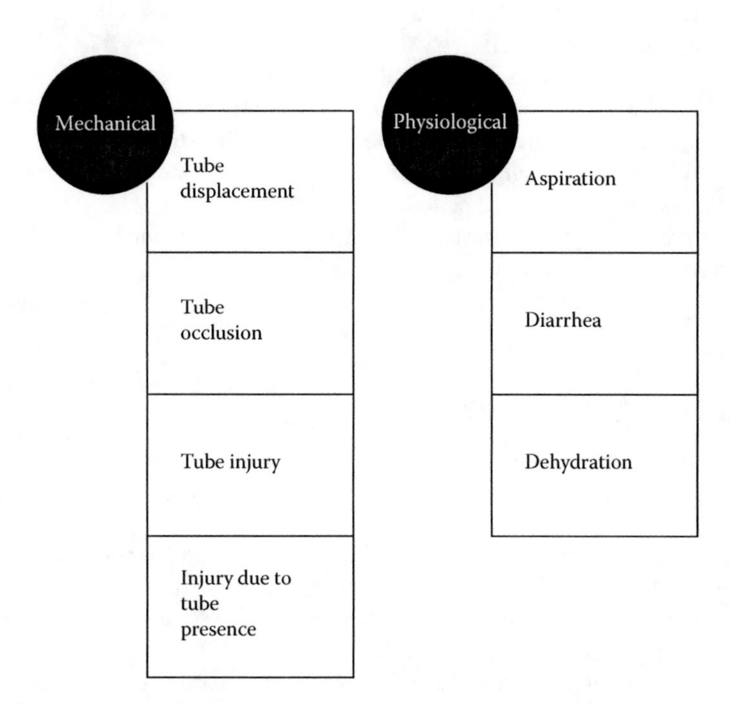

FIGURE 14.3 Enteral nutrition complications. Complications with enteral nutrition are divided into two categories: mechanical and physiological. Mechanical complications are associated with the actual device, the tube, whereas physiological complications encompass the body's reaction to enteral nutrition.

TABLE 14.4
Guidelines for Alternatives to Artificial Nutrition

Intact Swallowing Function	Swallowing Deficit
Adjust food consistency for ease of ingestion	Determine limitations for oral intake[a]
Determine likes/dislikes and tailor menu	Provide frequent mouth care
Encourage family/friends to bring appropriate foods	Provide frequent skin care
Arrange food attractively on small plates	Instill lubricant eye drops for dry eyes
Provide small frequent meals	Encourage family to assist with physical care
Medicate as necessary to control pain and/or nausea	Medicate as necessary to control pain and/or nausea
Be aware of resident's wishes	Encourage other nurturing activities in place of food (singing, massage, reading, music, photographs)
Goal is not nutritional repletion, but comfort or pleasure	Goal is comfort and helping to replace the "food connection" between resident and family

Note: For those individuals who choose not to accept artificial nutrition at the end-of-life, there are alternatives. This table offers suggestions for those with intact swallowing function as well as those with a swallowing deficit.

[a] For those with a swallowing deficit, families must consult with healthcare providers concerning the limitations for oral intake since the risk of aspiration must be discussed and a decision made to either accept or reject the idea of providing tastes or sips of food/fluids at the request of the resident at the end-of-life.

14.5 PRACTICAL GUIDELINES FOR ALTERNATIVES TO ARTIFICIAL NUTRITION

Without the potential for alternatives to AN, practitioners would be forced into a black and white decision to initiate, maintain, withhold, or withdraw AN in end-of-life situations. To avoid this dilemma and to assist the resident and family through the grieving process, guidelines have been developed to address both those residents with an intact gag/swallowing reflex and those with some level of swallowing deficit (Table 14.4).

These guidelines contain ways to provide oral nutrition or fluids for those with intact swallowing function, but more importantly provide other means to comfort residents without the need for food. Historically, eating and feeding are viewed as nurturing or caring functions. For many, food is an integral part of secular as well as religious holidays. Food is also central to gatherings for mourning or grieving a loss, assuring that all will be fed and nurtured.

In this respect practitioners must develop different methods to reconnect or maintain the connection between residents and families at end-of-life. These methods must be based on knowledge of the family and resident, information that may be discovered during the advance care planning process (Monturo 2010).

KEY FEATURES OF NURSING HOMES

- Regardless of country, nursing homes provide care for those unable to care for themselves.
- Some may provide only custodial care, while others may have subacute and rehabilitation units.
- Nursing homes are not limited to the care of older adults. Younger adults with life-limiting or severely debilitating and chronic conditions are also treated.
- Nursing homes are regulated so as to provide safe and effective care to all residents. These regulations differ based on country/state.
- Some nursing homes may be modeled on a hospital type ward with individual rooms off a corridor and no access to a kitchen.
- Other nursing homes offer a more home-like and inviting milieu such as the new Green Houses featuring central kitchens and great rooms with resident rooms off this space.

- The cost of nursing home care is variable across countries and may be the responsibility of the resident, the family, the insurance company, the health service, the state and federal governments, or a combination of these entities.

ETHICAL ISSUES

The use of AN in end-of-life care is not supported by research and it is not beneficial to those with dementia, according to recent results from the Cochrane Collaboration (Candy et al. 2009). Despite this, some nursing home residents with dementia or other terminal illnesses continue to receive AN. Perhaps the recent notoriety of the Terri Schiavo case and John Paul II's papal address on AN highlight an ethical dilemma: is artificial nutrition a medical treatment or basic life support? Notwithstanding the ethics panel's findings from more than 20 years ago, individuals continue to struggle with the notion of "not feeding" or starving a loved one. Starvation is a highly emotive word and one filled with individual images of pain and suffering. Similarly the emotions connected with the meaning of food are based on individual values and beliefs and comprise one's life story (Monturo 2009; Monturo 2010). Examination of the meaning of food and individual nursing home cultures may provide insight as to the necessary changes and ongoing intensive palliative care education required for compassionate and clinically appropriate end-of-life care for nursing home residents.

SUMMARY POINTS

- Nursing homes will increasingly provide a substantial portion of end-of-life care.
- The lack of appropriate palliative care education in nursing homes is well documented.
- Advance directives are one part of the advance care planning process.
- The right to die movement began the discussions of withdrawal and withholding of life-sustaining treatments such as artificial nutrition.
- Artificial nutrition is a viable option for treatment of temporary illnesses.
- Artificial nutrition is not beneficial in those with advanced dementia.
- Nursing home culture and geographic community may affect the rate of artificial nutrition delivered in that particular home.
- An ethical dilemma exists for some who believe that artificial nutrition is synonymous with food and that withdrawal or withholding this treatment is tantamount to starvation.
- Examination of the meaning of food for residents and families is necessary to plan appropriate end-of-life care.

ACKNOWLEDGMENTS

The author gratefully acknowledges the John A. Hartford Foundation Building Academic Geriatric Nursing Capacity (BAGNC) for their continuing financial support through a postdoctoral fellowship. Many thanks also go to Dr. Neville Strumpf at the Hartford Center for Geriatric Nursing Excellence and Center for Geriatric Nursing Science at the University of Pennsylvania School of Nursing, Dean Don Barr, Dr. Ann Stowe, and Dr. Charlotte Mackey from the West Chester University of Pennsylvania College of Health Sciences and the Department of Nursing for their continuing support.

LIST OF ABBREVIATIONS

AD	Advance directive
AN	Artificial nutrition
MDS	Minimum Data Set
OBRA	Omnibus Budget Reconciliation Act
PEG	Percutaneous endoscopic gastrostomy

REFERENCES

Abt Associates. 2001. Report to Congress: Appropriateness of minimum nurse staffing ratios in nursing homes. Phase II final report (Center for Medicare and Medicaid Services ed.), Baltimore, MD. http://www.allhealth.org/BriefingMaterials/Abt-NurseStaffingRatios(12-01)-999.pdf. Accessed 14 February 2010.

An Bord Altranais. 2009. Professional guidance for nurses working with older people (Altranais AB ed.), Dublin. http://www.nursingboard.ie/en/publications_current.aspx. Accessed 14 February 2010.

Candy, B., E. L. Sampson, and L. Jones. 2009. Enteral tube feeding in older people with advanced dementia: Findings from a Cochrane systematic review. *International Journal of Palliative Nursing* 15:396–404.

Center for Disease Control and Prevention. 2002. The national nursing home survey: 1990 summary. *Vital Health Statistics*. Series 13:No.152.

Center for Gerontology and Health Care Research Brown Medical School. 2004. Facts on dying: Policy relevant data on care at end-of-life. CHCR Brown University. http://www.chcr.brown.edu/dying/usastatistics.htm. Accessed 17 December 2004.

Chan, H. M. 2004. Sharing death and dying: Advance directives, autonomy and the family. *Bioethics* 18:87–103.

Cruzan v. Director, Missouri Department Health, 497 U. S. 261. (1990).

DeFrances, C. J., K. A. Cullen, and L. J. Kozak. 2007. National hospital discharge survey: 2005 annual summary with detailed diagnoses and procedure data. *Vital Health Statistics*. Series 13: No. 165.

Fagerlin, A., and C. E. Schneider. 2004. Enough: The failure of the living will. *Hasting Center Report* 34:30–42.

Gessert, C. E., B. A. Elliott, and C. Peden-McAlpine. 2006. Family decision-making for nursing home residents with dementia: Rural-urban differences. *Journal of Rural Health* 22:1–8.

Health Information and Quality Authority. 2008. National quality standards for residential care setting for older people in Ireland (HIQUA ed.), Dublin. www.hiqua.ie. Accessed 14 February 2010.

International Council of Nurses. 2002. Peaceful death: Recommended competencies and curricular guidelines for end-of-life care. http://www.aacn.nche.edu/publications/deathfin.htm. Accessed 14 February 2010.

McDonnell, M. M., E. McGuigan, J. McElhinney, M. McTeggart, and D. McClure. 2009. An analysis of the palliative care education needs of RGNs and HCAs in nursing homes in Ireland. *International Journal of Palliative Nursing* 15:446–55.

Mitchell, S. L., J. M. Teno, S. C. Miller, and V. Mor. 2005. A national study of the location of death for older persons with dementia. *Journal of the American Geriatrics Society* 53:299–305.

Mitchell, S. L., J. M. Teno, J. Roy, G. Kabumoto, and V. Mor. 2003. Clinical and organizational factors associated with feeding tube use among nursing home residents with advanced cognitive impairment. *Journal of the American Medical Association* 290:73–80.

Monturo, C. 2009. The artificial nutrition debate: Still an issue...after all these years. *Nutrition in Clinical Practice* 24:206–13.

Monturo, C. A. 2010. The meaning of food: A cultural model of community identity and social memory. Unpublished manuscript.

Monturo, C. A., and N. E. Strumpf. 2007. Advance directives at end-of-life: Nursing home resident preferences for artificial nutrition. *Journal of the American Medical Directors Association* 8:224–28.

Omnibus Budget Reconciliation Act. 1987. In *Medicare and Medicaid requirements for long-term care facilities*, 42, CFT Part 483.

Omnibus Budget Reconciliation Act. 1990. 42 U.S.C. (1395cc(a) (I)(Q), 1395 mm (c)(8), 1395cc(f), 1396a(a)(57), 1396a(a)(58), and 1396a(w) ed).

Palan Lopez, R., E. J. Amella, N. Strumpf, J. M. Teno, and S. L. Mitchell. 2010. The influence of nursing home culture on the use of feeding tubes. *Archives of Internal Medicine* 170:83–88.

Randall, H. T. 1990. The history of enteral nutrition. In *Clinical nutrition: Enteral and tube feeding*, 2nd ed. J. L. Rombeau, and M. T. Caldwell, 614. Philadelphia: Saunders.

Stillman, D., N. Strumpf, E. Capezuti, and H. Tuch. 2005. Staff perceptions concerning barriers and facilitators to end-of-life care in the nursing home. *Geriatric Nursing* 26:259–64.

Teno, J. M., K. J. Branco, V. Mor, C. D. Phillips, C. Hawes, J. Morris, and B. E. Fries. 1997. Changes in advance care planning in nursing homes before and after the patient Self-Determination Act: Report of a 10-state survey. *Journal of the American Geriatrics Society* 45:939–44.

Teno, J., B. R. Clarridge, V. Casey, L. C. Welch, T. Wetle, R. Shield, and V. Mor. 2004. Family perspectives on end-of-life care at the last place of care. *Journal of the American Medical Association* 291:88–93.

Teno, J. M., V. Mor, D. DeSilva, G. Kabumoto, J. Roy, and T. Wetle. 2002. Use of feeding tubes in nursing home residents with severe cognitive impairment. *Journal of the American Medical Association* 287:3211–12.

The Care Commission. 2009. Better care every step of the way. Scottish Commission for the Regulation of Care. http://www.carecommission.com/images/stories/documents/publications/reviewsofqualitycare/better_care_every_step_of_the_way_-_april_2009.pdf. Accessed 14 February 2010.

The President's Commission for the Study of Ethical Problems in Medicine and Biomedical and Behavioral Research. 1983. *Deciding to forego life-sustaining treatment*. Washington, D.C.: U.S. Government Printing Office.

15 Support for Hydration at End-of-Life

Robin L. Fainsinger

CONTENTS

15.1 INTRODUCTION

The controversial topic of dehydration and rehydration of palliative care patients is complicated and has many different aspects to consider. The divergence of opinion is well illustrated by the following quotes: "Research is limited but suggests that artificial hydration in imminently dying patients influences neither survival nor symptom control" (Soden et al. 2002) and "The best available evidence suggests that hydration of advanced cancer patients plays an important role in maintaining cognitive function and is therefore an important factor in the prevention and reversal of delirium in this population" (Lawlor 2002).

Differences in medical opinions are further complicated by other complex issues illustrated by the following: "terminal dehydration is a controversial topic, weighted heavily with historic symbolism and strong religious, societal and cultural conflicts" (Huffman and Dunn 2002). Consideration of a case example can be helpful in illustrating aspects of these issues: A 65-year-old man who has been active and in good health notes that he has lost 4–5 kg of weight over the previous few months. He is investigated and a liver biopsy confirms liver metastases from a probable pancreatic primary cancer. He develops nausea and vomiting and presents to the emergency room of the local hospital where he is found to have clinical evidence of dehydration. He is given intravenous fluids for rehydration and subsequently improves, and is discharged home. As the patient develops increasing abdominal pain over the next few weeks he requires increasing morphine doses to keep him comfortable. He expresses a desire to remain at home. He and his wife discuss goals of care and advanced directives with their family physician and indicate that their worldview is that everything possible should be done to maintain life. As the patient develops episodic nausea and vomiting he is changed to subcutaneous morphine which is increased up to 120 mg subcutaneously per day. As the patient's oral intake is suboptimal, the palliative homecare nurse and family physician suggest the option of parenteral hydration with hypodermoclysis. This is subsequently started to ensure

TABLE 15.1
Issues for Healthcare Professionals to Consider

1. Various expressions of opinion
2. Information on pathophysiology and biochemical changes
3. Conflicting research outcomes
4. Conflicting family and cultural expectations
5. Variability in consensus statements
6. Unique circumstances of each patient and family

that the patient receives at least one liter of fluid overnight. At this point their two children return home to provide extra support for their mother in caring for their father. The daughter works as a hospice nurse and does not believe in the value of parenteral hydration. The son is a nephrologist who argues that hydration is essential for normal renal function to avoid the accumulation of morphine metabolites and the associated risk of side effects. The parents are aware of their children's different opinions, but continue to rely on their relationship with their family physician and homecare nurse, and their advice and direction as to appropriate management.

This case example demonstrates some of the complex issues that are considered when debating this controversial topic. Regardless of the setting and circumstances, the common ground in the discussion is the desire to keep patients as comfortable as possible and avoid futile management and procedures. Differences of opinion start to emerge when considering what may be futile in the provision of hydration at the end-of-life. Healthcare professionals trying to make these decisions with patients and families need to consider a variety of expressions of opinion, information on pathophysiology and biochemical changes, a variety of research outcomes, family and cultural expectations, and variability in consensus statements. The unique trajectory and circumstances of each patient and family has to be considered as we attempt to make an individual decision on whether or not to use parenteral hydration (Table 15.1).

15.2 BACKGROUND TO THE HYDRATION CONTROVERSY

It is important to understand at the outset that encouraging palliative care patients to maintain a reasonable oral intake to prevent fluid deficit is not a point of controversy. The opposing viewpoints in literature reports revolve around the use of supplemental parenteral hydration, and include clinical and ethical viewpoints (Craig 1994; Fainsinger and Bruera 1994). The traditional arguments for and against the use of parenteral hydration are summarized in Table 15.2.

The standard medical approach to fluid deficits is to initiate or maintain parenteral hydration. As a result we can expect that in most countries patients dying in hospitals will have an intravenous line, with the exception of patients with a sudden deterioration or unexpected death. This has been demonstrated by a study where 73 of 106 cancer patients dying in a Canadian acute care hospital had intravenous fluids administered (Burge, King, and Wilson 1990). A more recent report suggests that artificial hydration may no longer be considered routine hospital practice for palliative care patients. In this retrospective study (Soden et al. 2002) in an English hospital 65% of patients were hydrated during the last week of life and only 46% were actually being given hydration when they died.

In our setting in Edmonton, Canada, we sought to understand the routine practice of physicians involved in end-of-life care regarding the application of parenteral hydration for patients in a palliative care unit and an acute care hospital while being followed or not being followed by the palliative care program at the acute care site (Lanuke, Fainsinger, and deMoissac 2004). There were 50 consecutive patients for each of the three cohorts included in this retrospective chart review. The majority of patients received hydration with a range of 66–98% of patients receiving parenteral hydration during the last week of life. However the volume of hydration was significantly lower and the use of hypodermoclysis was significantly higher in the palliative care unit site.

TABLE 15.2
Arguments for and Against the Use of Parenteral Hydration

No parenteral hydration

- Comatose patients do not experience symptom distress
- Parenteral fluids prolong dying
- Incontinence and need for catheters will be reduced
- As a result of decreased gastrointestinal fluid there will be less nausea and vomiting
- Problems with cough and pulmonary edema will be limited by decreased respiratory secretions
- Decreased problems with edema and ascites
- Dehydration may be a natural anesthetic in decreasing patient awareness and suffering
- Parenteral hydration may limit patient mobility and be uncomfortable

Use parenteral hydration

- Terminally ill patients are more comfortable with parenteral hydration
- Parenteral hydration does not prolong life
- Restlessness, confusion, and neuromuscular irritability can be increased by fluid deficit
- Parenteral hydration should be an option for terminally ill patients complaining of thirst
- This is a minimum standard of care
- This is a reasonable quality of life measure
- Withholding treatment to other compromised patient groups may begin with withholding parenteral hydration for palliative care patients

It would seem reasonable to argue that a policy of maintaining intravenous hydration with volumes in excess of three liters per day in advanced palliative care populations is likely to cause significant problems. In this circumstance we can anticipate complications such as increased respiratory and gastrointestinal symptoms. Conversely, a review of reports arguing against hydration at the end-of-life suggests that healthcare professionals looking after palliative care populations may be reacting to overuse of intravenous fluids with the conclusion that the complete opposite approach of no parenteral hydration is preferable. This belief has been reinforced by many anecdotal literature reports suggesting that palliative care patients appear to die comfortably without parenteral hydration. However review of the literature does indicate that these reports are primarily based on unsubstantiated data.

The argument has been made that there are other issues to consider (Fainsinger and Bruera 1994):

1. Confusion and restlessness in the general population is well recognized as a consequence of fluid deficit. Similar problems of agitated delirium have frequently been reported in palliative care populations.
2. Pre-renal failure is known to be caused by decreased intravascular volume and glomerular filtration rate as a consequence of fluid deficit. We know that opioid metabolites accumulate in patients with renal failure, resulting in confusion, myoclonus, and seizures.

The problem of agitated delirium and terminal restlessness is frequently reported and discussed in palliative care literature. The focus of management of these problems is frequently on the need for pharmacological management, including sedation, and often omits consideration of the role of parenteral hydration. We have noted that the severity of agitated delirium requiring sedation decreased to as low as 3% in our palliative care unit. We hypothesized that this was a result of changing our practice to include more frequent use of parenteral hydration with hypodermoclysis, opioid sequential trials when toxicity is noted, and less sedating treatments for agitated delirium. Our experience is worth comparing with a retrospective chart review of patients dying at St. Luke's Hospital in Cape Town, South Africa, where 29% of patients required sedation for agitated delirium. In this setting no patients were treated with parenteral hydration and patients requiring sedation were given significantly higher doses of opioids (Fainsinger et al. 1998). Subsequent reports from our integrated regional palliative care service in Edmonton has suggested that agitated delirium appears to be a less prevalent problem in our different settings where parenteral hydration is common practice, compared with requirements for sedation as reported at other international locations (Lanuke et al. 2004; Fainsinger, deMoissac et al. 2000; Fainsinger, Waller et al. 2000).

Our group has continued to argue that dehydration could be a reversible component of agitated delirium, which may be missed if we focus exclusively on sedative pharmacological solutions to this common and distressing symptom (Fainsinger and Bruera 1997). We do not consider that it is logical for a patient to receive medications for agitated delirium, myoclonus, and seizures if these problems could be prevented or improved for some patients by a more liberal use of parenteral hydration.

15.3 CLARIFYING TERMINOLOGY

Reviews on this topic have taken issue with the inaccurate use and description of dehydration (Lawlor 2002). Fluid deficit should be understood as water loss with or without electrolytes that includes subtypes of volume depletion and dehydration. Dehydration is total body water deficit that is mainly intracellular and is associated with hypernatremia. Volume depletion is a deficit in the intravascular fluid volume and may be isotonic, hyponatremic, or hypernatremic (Figure 15.1).

A number of factors need to be considered using history, physical examination, and laboratory findings to assess for the risk or presence of fluid deficit. The fluid deficit symptoms to consider include behavior and cognitive changes, fatigue, thirst, nausea, and dry mouth. Dry mouth, decreased skin turgor, postural hypotension, tachycardia, decreased jugular venous pressure, sunken eyes, and decreased sweating are considered classical signs of fluid deficit. Nevertheless these problems have to be interpreted with caution as they may be associated with other causes such as aging, cachexia, advanced cancer, and side effects seen with frequently used medications. In some situations laboratory tests can provide further helpful information. Elevated levels of urea, creatinine, plasma proteins, hematocrit, and sodium are often seen in volume-depleted patients.

15.4 HYDRATION RESEARCH

There are three dimensions that need to be considered when reviewing the research on the use of hydration for palliative care patients (Table 15.3).

The acknowledgement of fluid deficit as a cause of renal failure is not considered controversial. Parenteral hydration is accepted as standard management in many settings, however the impact of fluid deficit and rehydration on renal function and electrolyte balance in palliative care patients,

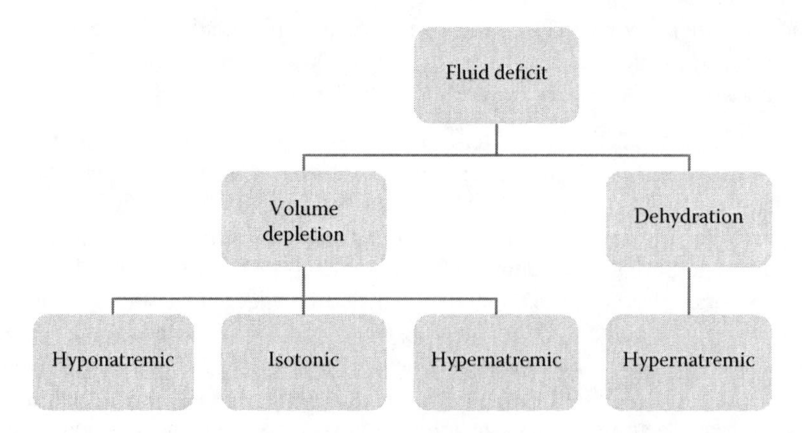

FIGURE 15.1 Fluid deficit subgroups.

TABLE 15.3
Dimensions of Palliative Care Hydration Research

1. Association between biochemical findings and hydration status
2. Association between biochemical findings and clinical symptoms
3. Association between hydration status and clinical symptoms

particularly in the last few days of life, is uncertain. There is some evidence that parenteral hydration does have an impact in decreasing abnormal biochemistry, particularly renal function, in the last week of life (Fainsinger 1999; Morita et al. 1998).

While much of the early literature on determining the association between hydration status and clinical symptoms in early literature is based on anecdotal opposing viewpoints in case reports, there have been a number of subsequent reports attempting to look at this issue more carefully. Burge (1993) studied the quantitative assessment of the dehydration experience in advanced cancer patients and concluded that parenteral hydration on the basis of fluid intake and laboratory measures was not helpful if the aim was to reduce thirst. McCann, Hall, and Groth-Juncker (1994) investigated symptom prevalence and management of hunger and thirst in palliative care patients not receiving parenteral hydration and concluded that the symptoms of hunger, thirst, and dry mouth were well managed with oral hydration and mouth care.

Ellershaw, Sutcliffe, and Saunders (1995) considered the association of symptoms and dehydration in 82 patients where parenteral hydration was not provided. There was no significant association between the level of hydration and the outcome measures of respiratory tract secretions, thirst, and dry mouth. However the association of renal failure and possible consequences of agitated delirium was not assessed.

Our group assessed the impact of our change of practice with regard to parenteral hydration and cognitive impairment in a retrospective chart review of 117 and 162 patients admitted to our palliative care unit in 1988–1989 and 1991–1992. We concluded that our results suggested that routine cognitive assessment, opioid rotation, and hydration could reduce the frequency of agitated delirium in our population. Although we believe that parenteral hydration had a significant impact, it was not possible to determine relative contributions of our change in practice (Bruera et al. 1995).

Lawlor et al. (2000) reported a prospective delirium study of 113 patients with advanced cancer. Reversibility was associated with psychoactive medications and dehydration. This study concluded that although delirium is multifactorial, the use of hypodermoclysis for parenteral hydration may be a potentially useful reversible measure.

Bruera et al. (2005) published the first randomized, controlled, double-blind study of parenteral hydration in terminally ill cancer patients. This was a multicenter study where patients with clinical and biochemical evidence of dehydration, and history of an oral intake of less than one liter of fluid per day were randomly assigned to receive 1000 ml (treatment group) or 100 ml (placebo group) of normal saline over four hours for two days. The outcome measures were patient- and investigator-rated symptoms of fatigue, sedation, myoclonus, hallucinations, and a global sense of well-being. A significant improvement in sedation and myoclonus scores were noted in the hydration treatment group.

There have been three reviews on this topic (Burge 1996; Viola, Wells, and Peterson 1997; Good et al. 2009) that have all concluded that it is impossible to draw firm conclusions regarding clinical care based on the research evidence.

15.5 SOCIAL, CULTURAL, AND ETHICAL ISSUES

Family and patient attitudes, level of comfort with end-of-life issues, education, healthcare professionals' biases, and level of education all have an influence on decisions with regard to parenteral hydration.

It is unfortunate that artificial nutrition and hydration are often considered as the same issue in ethical and clinical discussion papers. This can be confusing, as the arguments and rationale for providing nutritional calories via artificial means as opposed to hydration alone deserve to be considered independently.

Morita et al. (1999) considered patient and family perceptions regarding rehydration to identify factors contributing to decision making. Patient performance status, fluid retention symptoms, denial, physician recommendations, and beliefs with regard to hydration effect on patient distress, and family anxiety regarding withholding rehydration were all significantly associated with the decision-making process. The most important factors determining rehydration were the patient's performance status, fluid retention symptoms, denial, and care receiver's beliefs regarding the effects of rehydration on symptom distress.

Issues of importance to family caregivers regarding parenteral hydration use in advanced cancer patients were considered in a Canadian study (Parkash and Burge 1997). Symptom distress issues, ethical and emotional considerations, information between healthcare professionals and families, and culture were all important factors influencing the caregivers. The perceived benefit of parenteral hydration was central to the ethical, emotional, and cultural considerations involved in the decisions of caregivers.

An article (Bodell and Weng 2000) on the values of the Jewish faith regarding terminal dehydration provides a good illustration of some of the problems in applying cultural and ethnic research and opinion. This report generated responses varying from descriptions of this as an "excellent article" (Schur 2000) to "extremely offensive in its references to Jewish people" (Rothstein 2000).

A core ethical principle of healthcare decision making is the importance of patient autonomy. Using this principle it has been proposed that voluntary cessation of drinking and the refusal of parenteral hydration is a legal right that could provide an alternative to physician-assisted suicide. Miller and Meier (1998) have suggested that using this option along with standard palliative care treatment "offers patient's a way to escape agonizing, incurable condition that they consider to be worse than death, without requiring transformation of the law and medical ethics." Quill et al. (1998) argued that voluntary cessation of drinking "may be acceptable to a patient and physician and do not require fundamental changes in the law."

Craig (2008) has argued passionately that a blanket policy of no hydration, as endorsed in a national guideline in the United Kingdom, is ethically indefensible. The primary concern is that the value of hydration is underestimated and could increase deaths associated with palliative sedation. Craig (2004) has devoted a book to this issue, in which she states "My personal role in the hydration debate has been to highlight the ethical, legal and medical dangers of a regime of sedation without hydration in the dying and draw attention to the plight of dissenting relatives."

15.6 OPTIONS FOR ALTERNATIVE HYDRATION

There is no controversy that the most convenient route for correction of fluid deficits would be improving or increasing oral intake. Where this is not possible or inadequate, there are some circumstances where the benefits of parenteral hydration need to be considered. We need to understand that we are not necessarily all seeing patients in the same trajectory of illness. Clinical circumstances change over time, and a physically independent and cognitively normal patient at an early stage of a palliative care illness will be viewed differently from the same patient a number of months later who has become physically dependent and cognitively impaired.

If a decision is made to use parenteral hydration (Table 15.4), we need to consider the type of fluid, volume, and options for route of administration. In acute care institutions the traditional route of choice has been intravenous hydration. However there are many disadvantages such as difficulty finding venous access, pain, infection, mobility limitations, and need to replace displaced lines, particularly with less cooperative or agitated patients.

TABLE 15.4
Alternatives to Oral Hydration

1. Intravenous fluids
2. Nasogastric tubes or percutaneous gastrostomy
3. Hypodermoclysis
4. Rectal hydration

15.6.1 Nasogastric Tubes and Gastrostomy

Nasogastric tubes are often uncomfortable for patients and prolonged use, particularly in palliative care populations, should be avoided as far as possible. Head and neck or esophageal cancer patients with increasing dysphagia may benefit from nutrition as well as hydration given via a percutaneous gastrostomy. The goals of care with regard to parenteral nutrition need to be reviewed as patients deteriorate. We need to recognize that it can be difficult to discontinue management and the ease of access with percutaneous gastrostomy can result in ongoing nutrition and hydration in some circumstances where this might otherwise not have been started.

15.6.2 Hypodermoclysis

The use and safety of hypodermoclysis has been well documented and reported, and there have been studies in palliative care populations demonstrating ease of administration with minimal side effects. The application of hypodermoclysis is simple and is associated with minimal discomfort. A subcutaneous needle is inserted and attached to a fluid line, which can be run using gravity or an infusion pump. Minimal training for insertion and surveillance is required, and families can be trained to use this option very easily at home. There is evidence that hypodermoclysis is being increasingly used in acute care settings (Lanuke et al. 2004). The standard recommendation is to use solutions with electrolytes, as nonelectrolyte solutions may draw fluid into the interstitial space. Rates of infusion are usually limited to a maximum of 100 to 120 ml per hour. However in some situations patients can tolerate boluses of up to 500 ml per hour for a maximum of two to three hours per day. These bolus administrations should be administered over one hour at a time every eight to twelve hours.

The use of hypodermoclysis has been aided by adding hyaluronidase to promote absorption. The doses used have ranged from 150 to 750 units per liter. However, anecdotal reports suggesting good absorption without hyaluronidase resulted in evidence demonstrating that patients can receive hypodermoclysis without hyaluronidase (Centeno and Bruera 1999). It is now standard practice in our setting to give patients hypodermoclysis without the addition of hyaluronidase, with the most common range between 40 and 80 ml per hour. However, recombinant human hyaluronidase is now being used in clinical studies and may have a future role in improving the absorption of subcutaneously administered fluids (Pirrello, Ting Chen, and Thomas 2007).

15.6.3 Rectal Hydration

Intravenous hydration can be uncomfortable, expensive, and difficult to maintain in settings such as the home, while even hypodermoclysis can be too expensive or complicated in some situations. The potential advantage of fluid administered rectally, particularly in resource-limited developing countries, prompted reports of rectal hydration use in terminally ill patients (Bruera, Pruvost, and Schoeller 1998). Rectal hydration was noted to be well tolerated with minimal side effects in the majority of patients. The mean daily volume, hourly rate, and duration of therapy was reported as 1035 ± 150 ml per day, 224 ± 58 ml per hour, and 14 ± 8 days, respectively. Rectal hydration appears to be a safe, effective, and low-cost technique for rehydration that may have an application in limited, poorly resourced terminally ill palliative care populations.

KEY POINTS

- Fluid deficit, dehydration, and rehydration of palliative care patients is complicated and has been a controversial issue in end-of-life care.
- It is important to understand the definitions and use of terminology for fluid deficit, dehydration, and volume depletion.
- Artificial nutrition and hydration are not the same issue and should be considered independently in ethical and clinical discussion.
- Individual patients' and families' social, religious, and cultural background can have a major influence in determining clinical management.
- Hypodermoclysis is a safe and convenient alternative when oral hydration is inadequate.
- There is an extensive and growing literature on this topic that includes much opinion and some research and is unlikely to provide any black and white answers for the foreseeable future.

SUMMARY POINTS

- There is consensus that fluid deficit is a cause of renal failure, and that hypodermoclysis is a safe and effective way of providing parenteral hydration.
- There is some evidence that parenteral hydration in palliative populations may result in better biochemical parameters at the end-of-life.
- There is a body of evidence to suggest that if palliative care patients are not provided with parenteral hydration, medications such as opioids should be gradually decreased to avoid accumulation and problematic and unnecessary side effects.
- The major clinical issue in this controversy is the consideration of whether parenteral hydration will cause benefit or harm to palliative care patients unable to sustain an adequate oral intake.
- We need to consider the individual circumstances, anticipated prognosis, and trajectory of the patient's illness in evaluating the potential benefits of parenteral hydration in end-of-life care (Dalal, Del Fabbro, and Bruera 2009).

REFERENCES

Bodell, J., and M. A. Weng. 2000. The Jewish patient in terminal dehydration: A hospice ethical dilemma. *Am J of Hospice and Palliative Care* 17 (3): 185–88.

Bruera, E., J. J. Franco, M. Maltoni, S. Watanabe, and M. Suarez-Almazor. 1995. Changing pattern of agitated impaired mental status in patients with advanced cancer: Association with cognitive monitoring, hydration, and opioid rotation. *J Pain & Sympt Manage* 10:287–91.

Bruera, E., M. Pruvost, and T. Schoeller. 1998. Proctoclysis for hydration of terminally ill cancer patients. *J Pain Sympt Manage* 15:216–19.

Bruera, E., R. Sala, M. A. Rico, J. Moyano, C. Centeno, J. Willey, and J. L. Palmer. 2005. Effects of parenteral hydration in terminally ill cancer patients: A preliminary study. *J of Clin Oncology* 23 (10): 2366–71.

Burge, F. I., D. B. King, and D. Wilson. 1990. Intravenous fluids and the hospitalized dying: A medical last rite? *Cam Fam Physician* 86:883–86.

Burge, F. I. 1993. Dehydration symptoms of palliative care cancer patients. *J Pain & Symptom Manage* 8:454–64.

Burge, F. I. 1996. Dehydration and provision of fluids in palliative care. What is the evidence? *Can Fam Physician* 42:2383–88.

Centeno, C., and E. Bruera. 1999. Subcutaneous hydration with no hyaluronidase in patients with advanced cancer. *J Pain & Sympt Manage* 17 (5): 305–6.

Craig, G. M. 1994. On withholding nutrition and hydration in the terminally ill: Has palliative medicine gone too far? *J of Medical Ethics* 20:139–43.

Craig, G. 2004. Challenging Medical Ethics 1: No water – No life: Hydration in the dying. Fairway Folio (Christian Publishing Services), Cheshire, UK.

Craig, G. 2008. Palliative care in overdrive: Patients in danger. *Am J of Hospice and Palliative Care* 25 (2): 155–60.

Dalal, S., E. Del Fabbro, and E. Bruera. 2009. Is there a role for hydration at the end-of-life? *Curr Opin Support Palliat Care* 3:72–78.

Ellershaw, J. E., J. M. Sutcliffe, and C. M. Saunders. 1995. Dehydration and the dying patient. *J Pain Sympt & Manage* 10:192–97.

Fainsinger, R. L., and E. Bruera. 1994. The management of dehydration in terminally ill patients. *J of Palliative Care* 10:55–59.

Fainsinger, R. L., and E. Bruera. 1997. When to treat dehydration in a terminally ill patient? *Supportive Care Cancer* 5:205–11.

Fainsinger, R. L., W. Landman, M. Hoskings, and E. Bruera. 1998. Sedation for uncontrolled symptoms in a South African hospice. *J of Pain & Sympt Manage* 16 (3): 145–52.

Fainsinger, R. L. 1999. Biochemical dehydration in terminally ill cancer patients. *J of Palliative Care* 15 (2): 59–61.

Fainsinger, R. L., D. deMoissac, I. Mancini, and D. Oneschuk. 2000. Sedation for delirium and other symptoms in terminally ill patients in Edmonton. *J of Palliative Care* 16 (2): 5–10.

Fainsinger, R. L., A. Waller, M. Bercovici, K. Bengtson, W. Landman, M. Hosking, J. M. Nunez-Olarte, and D. deMoissac. 2000. A multi-centre international study of sedation for uncontrolled symptoms in terminally ill patients. *Palliative Medicine* 14:257–65.

Good, P., J. Cavenagh, M. Mather, P. Ravenscroft. 2009. Medically assisted hydration for adult palliative care patients (Review). The Cochrane Collaboration. Published in The Cochrane Library, Issue 4.

Huffman, J. L., and G. P. Dunn. 2002. The paradox of hydration in advanced terminal illness. *J Am Col Surg* 194 (6): 835–39.

Lanuke, K., R. L. Fainsinger, and D. deMoissac. 2004. Hydration management at the end-of-life. *J of Palliative Medicine* 7 (2): 257–63.

Lawlor, P. 2002. Delirium and dehydration: Some fluid for thought? *Support Care Cancer* 10:445–54.

Lawlor, P. G., B. Gagnon, I. L. Mancini, J. L. Pereira, J. Hanson, M. E. Suarez-Almazor, and E. D. Bruera. 2000. Occurrence, causes, and outcome of delirium in patients with advanced cancer. *Arch Int Med* 160:786–94.

McCann, R. M., W. J. Hall, and A. Groth-Juncker. 1994. Comfort care for the terminally ill patients. The appropriate use nutrition and hydration. *JAMA* 272:1263–66.

Miller, F. G., and D. E. Meier. 1998. Voluntary death: A comparison of terminal dehydration and physician-assisted suicide. *Ann Intern Med* 128:559–62.

Morita, T., T. Ichiki, J. Tsunoda, S. Inoue, and S. Chihara. 1998. Biochemical dehydration and fluid retention symptoms in terminally ill cancer patients whose death is impending. *J of Palliative Care* 14 (4): 60–62.

Morita T, J. Tsunoda, S. Inoue, and S. Chihara. 1999. Perceptions and decision-making on rehydration of terminally ill cancer patients and family members. *Am J of Hospice and Palliative Care* 16 (3): 509–16.

Parkash, R., and F. Burge. 1997. The family's perspective on issues of hydration in terminal care. *J of Palliative Care* 13 (4): 23–27.

Pirrello, R. D., C. Ting Chen, and S. H. Thomas. 2007. Initial experiences with subcutaneous recombinant human hyaluronidase. *J Palliat Med* 10 (4): 861–64.

Quill, T. E., D. E. Meier, S. D. Block, and J. A. Billings. 1998. The debate over physician-assisted suicide: Empirical data and conversant views. *Ann Intern Med* 128:552–58.

Rothstein, J. M. 2000. Out of context? *Am J of Hospice and Palliative Care* 17 (5): 297.

Schur, T. G. 2000. Life and afterlife in Jewish tradition. *Am J of Hospice and Palliative Care* 17 (5): 296–97.

Soden, K, A. Hoy, W. Hoy, and S. Clelland. 2002. Artificial hydration during the last week of life in patients dying in district general hospital. *Palliative Medicine* 16 (6): 542–43.

Viola, R., A. G. A. Wells, and J. Peterson. 1997. The effects of fluid status and fluid therapy on the dying: A systematic review. *J of Palliative Care* 13 (4): 41–52.

16 Palliative Treatment of Dysphagia

Christian Selinger

CONTENTS

16.1 INTRODUCTION

The term 'dysphagia' means difficulties in swallowing. In a clinical context 'dysphagia' is however used to describe a variety of problems that can be encountered while trying to get food and fluid into and through the upper part of the digestive system. Dysphagia can occur because of obstruction in the mouth or head and neck area, through disturbances in the neuromuscular process that moves fluid or food from the pharynx to the stomach, and obstruction of the oesophagus. Gastric outlet obstructions causing regurgitation of stomach content will also be discussed, as they are often encountered and the same principles of care apply.

16.2 PATHOPHYSIOLOGY AND ANATOMY OF DYSPHAGIA

16.2.1 Neuromuscular Dysphagia

To propel food or fluid from the mouth to the stomach, a series of complex neurological and muscular actions is required: Voluntary muscles of the pharynx move the food or fluid into the proximal oesophagus, from where it is moved further by involuntary smooth muscle action to the stomach.

The neurological ability to swallow can be impaired by a variety of conditions encountered in the terminal or palliative care setting. Central or peripheral nervous system illnesses like cerebrovascular disease, intracranial haemorrhages, dementia, primary and secondary cerebral tumours, Parkinson's disease, and motor-neuron disease can cause neurological dysphagia at oropharynx level. Diseases affecting voluntary muscles directly (myotonic dystrophy for example) can also cause dysphagia. The voluntary swallowing should be assessed clinically by a speech and language therapist and if needed by video-fluoroscopy. Patients might still be able to move the food or fluid to the oesophagus but they could be at high risk of aspirating the content into the trachea and lungs, which can lead to aspiration pneumonia. Increasing the viscosity of the food and fluid can increase the safety of swallowing in cases of mild to moderate neuromuscular dysphagia. Should these measures not lead to a safe swallow, the appropriateness of establishing an alternative enteral feeding route (nasogastric tube (NG), percutaneous endoscopic gastrostomy (PEG), percutaneous endoscopic jejunostomy (PEJ), radiologically introduced gastrostomy (RIG)) needs to be discussed. In some circumstances it might be appropriate to accept a risk of aspiration rather than intervene to establish an alternative feeding route.

A range of diseases can impair the smooth muscle actions of the oesophagus though they are infrequently seen in palliative care. In severe cases of systemic sclerosis, for example, an alternative enteral feeding route (NG, PEG, PEJ, RIG) can be used (Figure 16.1).

16.2.2 Dysphagia by Oral, Head and Neck Cancers

Tumours of the mouth, pharynx and larynx can cause direct obstruction, prohibiting effective swallowing. Furthermore, surgery or radiotherapy can lead to dysphagia. In most cases alternative enteral feeding needs to be established via PEG, PEJ, RIG or surgically placed jejunostomy (SPJ).

16.2.2.1 Oesophageal and High Gastric Obstruction

Oesophageal and high gastric tumours can cause direct obstruction of the upper gastrointestinal (GI) tract. However other intrathoracic tumours (e.g., lung cancers or lymphadenopathy) can also cause dysphagia by external compression. Palliative efforts will often aim to reopen the lumen of the oesophagus, which can be achieved by radiotherapy or placing a stent over the tumour. Alternatively, a different enteral feeding route can be established.

16.2.2.2 Gastric Outlet Obstruction

Obstruction at low gastric or pyloric level is caused by gastric ulceration or malignancy, while duodenal-level obstructions are often caused by pancreatic neoplasms or primary duodenal tumours. Treatment options include reopening of the narrowed segment by stent placement, surgical gastrojejunostomy or formation of an SPJ.

16.3 APPLICATIONS TO OTHER AREAS OF TERMINAL OR PALLIATIVE CARE

While maintenance of nutrition is the main aim of dysphagia treatment in a palliative care setting, other aspects also need consideration. If lesions in the upper GI tract cause full or near full obstruction of the lumen, the patient is at high risk of aspiration of saliva and, in some cases, gastric juices. Treatments that reopen the lumen will allow nutrition but also improve the chest of the patient and greatly reduce the risk of severe aspiration pneumonia. Quality of life (QOL) should also improve.

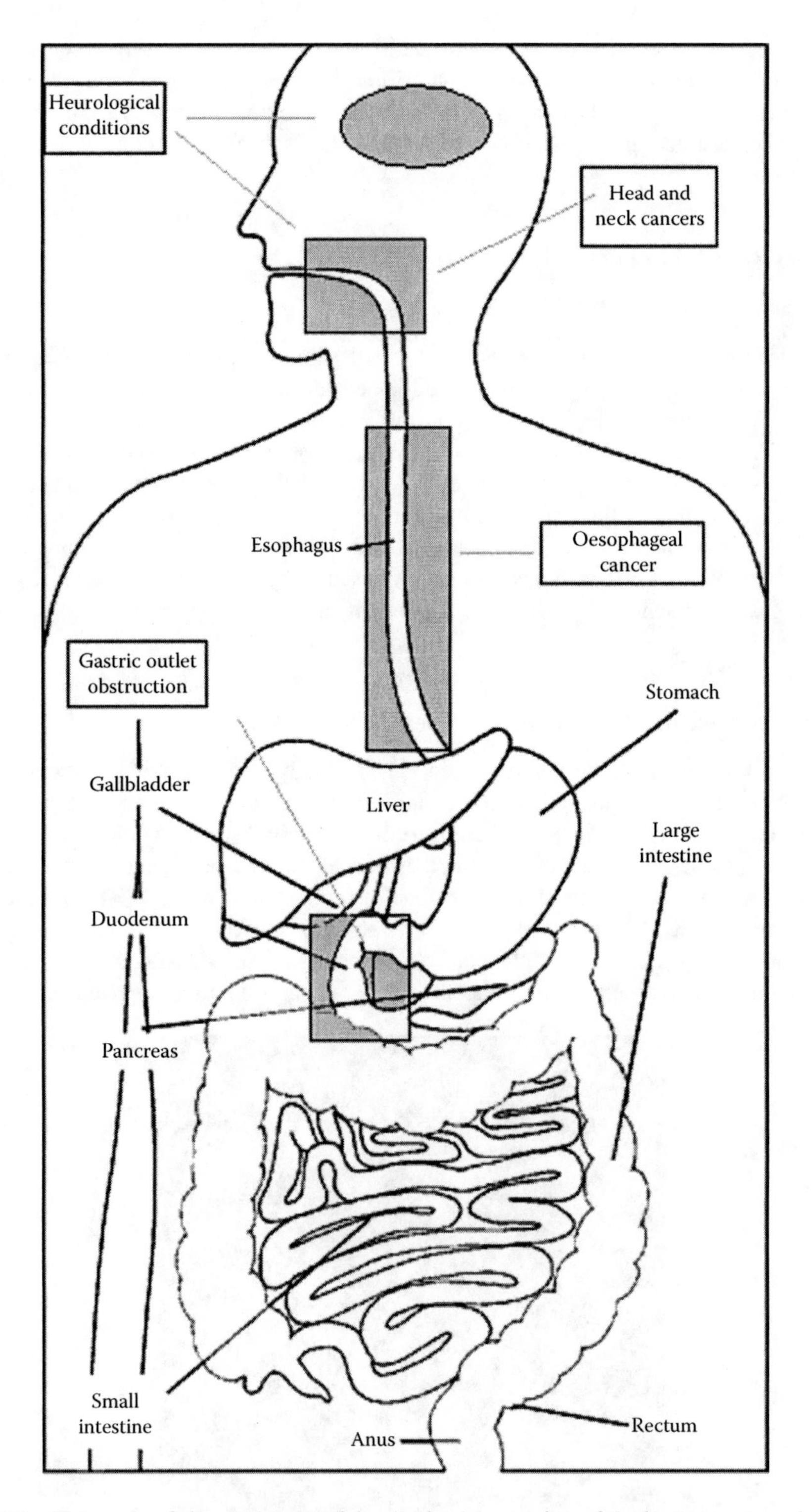

FIGURE 16.1 Pictogram of sites and types of dysphagia. An overview of the human anatomy highlighting areas where dysphagia can arise from.

The patient does not need to spit out saliva, which may not be seen as socially acceptable in public spaces. The ability to enjoy at least some oral nutrition should also positively influence QOL.

Furthermore the ability to take enteral medication can be extremely useful. It avoids the need for an injection when fast-acting pain relief is required and allows the use of medications only available for enteral use.

16.4 PRACTICAL PROCEDURES AND TECHNIQUES

16.4.1 Nasogastric Tube (NG) Insertion

Nasogastric feeding tubes are fine-bore plastic tubes designed to produce a safe feeding route for the short to medium term. They can be placed at the bedside and patients rarely experience any discomfort during placement. Little training is required, making them widely available inside hospitals and hospices. The correct placement of the tube should be established via aspiration and pH-testing of gastric fluid (pH < 5.5) or demonstration of the tube tip below the diaphragm on chest x-rays if pH-testing fails (National Collaborating Centre for Acute Care 2006). NG tubes fall out relatively frequently but can be better secured with a nasal bridle. Occasionally discomfort is caused by irritation to the throat. However in cases of neuromuscular dysphagia a risk of regurgitation and aspiration of gastric content into the lungs remains. Any obstructive upper GI tract pathology is not amenable to NG feeding.

16.4.2 Endoscopically Placed Feeding Tubes

Feeding tube placement via a flexible endoscope is normally performed in dedicated endoscopy units. In most cases conscious sedation and antibiotic prophylaxis is used. The endoscope is passed into the stomach, via transillumination to the abdominal wall, a suitable site is identified and using an aseptic technique local anaesthetic is placed. A large-bore cannula is placed through the abdominal wall into the stomach and a thread is fed into the stomach. This thread is pulled to the mouth and the feeding tube is connected to it. By removing the thread back through the abdominal wall, tube placement is achieved. These tubes can be used long term (Figures 16.2 and 16.3). The main risks involved in PEG placements are wound infections, perforation and leakage

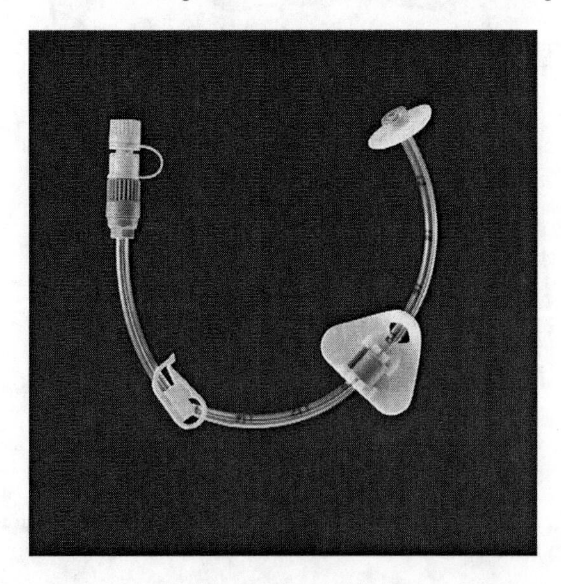

FIGURE 16.2 PEG set. Standard set used for PEG placement. (Reproduced with kind permission from Fresenius Kabi.)

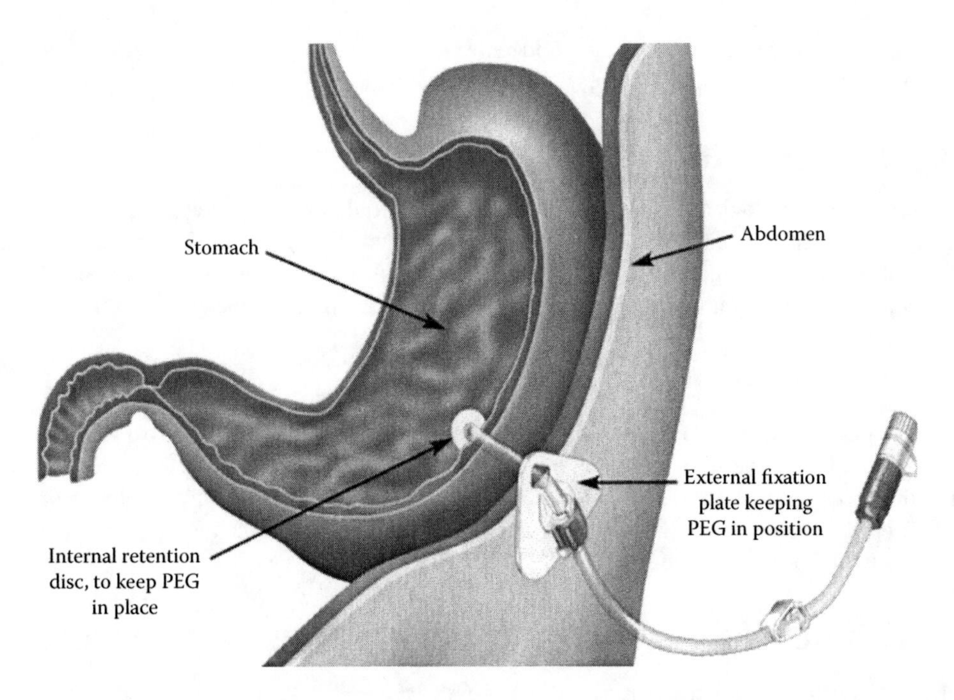

FIGURE 16.3 PEG set and placed in situ. A cut view demonstrating a PEG tube positioned in the stomach. (Reproduced with kind permission from Fresenius Kabi.)

into the peritoneal cavity, and bleeding. Complications occur in up to 15.4% of patients (Wollman et al. 1995). Large hiatus hernias, surgical scars in the upper abdomen and previous gastric surgery are relative contraindications. In some cases an endoscopic placement of a jejunostomy can be feasible.

16.4.3 Radiologically Induced Gastrostomy

Radiological placement requires local anaesthesia but rarely conscious sedation. There is a reduced risk of cardiovascular or respiratory compromise compared to endoscopic placement. An NG tube will be used to inflate the stomach to allow radiological detection. Ultrasound can be used to avoid accidental hepatic punctures. The stomach will then be punctured through the abdominal wall and dilators will be used to open up the puncture site. A tube will then be placed through the stomach wall. Risks involved are the same as for PEG placement, but the complication rate seems lower (Wollman et al. 1995).

16.4.4 Stents

Stents can be placed under radiological or combined endoscopic and radiological guidance. The procedure requires conscious sedation as pain is frequently experienced during placement. Self-expanding metal stents (SEMS) consist of a tightly knit metal mesh that is rolled onto an introducer measuring 5–7 mm in diameter. Placement of the closed stent over the tumour will be guided by x-ray and/or endoscopy. The stent will be released, opening up to its full diameter of 16–23 mm, reopening the lumen at the obstruction site and allowing passage of food again. A risk of stent obstruction by food bolus remains and patients should chew carefully and sometimes stick to a mash-consistency diet. Larger stent diameters seem to reduce the risk of food bolus obstruction (Verschuur et al. 2007). Short-term risks include perforation, heavy bleeding and significant pain, while stent migration and obstruction by tumour overgrowth are longer-term risks (Selinger et al.

2008). Patients experiencing significant acid reflux after oesophageal stent placement should be treated with oral proton pump inhibitors.

16.4.5 Surgically Placed Feeding Tubes

If endoscopic or radiological placement of a feeding tube fails or is impossible due to changes in anatomy, a surgically placed feeding jejunostomy can be used. Though it is a short procedure, placement usually requires a general anaesthetic and can be performed with a mini-laparotomy or using laparoscopy. Wound infection, perforation and leakage into the peritoneal cavity are the main risks.

16.4.6 Surgical Bypass Procedures

In cases of gastric outlet obstruction, a surgical bypass can establish an alternative route allowing food to proceed from the stomach to the proximal intestine. Under general anaesthetic a proximal small bowel loop will be anastomosed to the stomach. This is a relatively invasive procedure and therefore has a considerable risk (mainly of the anaesthetic, failure of the anastomosis and wound infections) in palliative care patients.

16.5 EVIDENCE FOR DYSPHAGIA TREATMENT ACCORDING TO INDICATION

16.5.1 Neurological and Muscular Disorders

16.5.1.1 Stroke Disease

Strokes caused by either infarction or haemorrhage of the brain can affect swallowing severely. Neurological improvement can often be seen in the first few weeks after a stroke. Alternative feeding routes like NG, PEG or RIG are commonly used to allow nutrition. In a large multicentre randomised controlled clinical trial (RCT), Dennis, Lewis, and Warlow (2005) compared early tube feeding with avoidance of tube feeding for seven days after an acute stroke. A nonsignificant reduction of death was found in the early feeding group. This reduction however came at the expense of an excess of survivors with poor neurological outcome who would have otherwise died. Based on these findings, early tube feeding cannot be recommended. The trial also addressed the issue of NG versus PEG tube insertion in stroke disease. PEG feeding showed no benefit over NG feeding and a small nonsignificant increase in death rate was found in the PEG group (Dennis et al. 2005). This finding is in contrast to a Cochrane meta-analysis (Bath, Bath-Hextal, and Smithard 1999) that found nonsignificant improvements in mortality and nutritional status in PEG patients compared to NG patients. No clear guidance can be derived from the current evidence. PEG tubes however offer the advantage of a more secure placement and do not cause irritation to the patient's throat (Table 16.1).

TABLE 16.1
Treatment Options by Cause of Dysphagia

Type of Dysphagia	NG Tube	PEG/RIG Tube	Surgical Jejunostomy	Stent	Surgical Bypass	Radiotherapy
Neuromuscular problems	+	++	(+)	–	–	–
Head and neck cancers	++	+	(+)	–	–	–
Oesophageal cancer	(+)	(+)	(+)	++	–	++
Gastric outlet obstruction	–	–	(+)	++	++	–

Note: An overview of treatments and their feasibility in respect to cause of dysphagia. –, not feasible; (+), feasible but rarely advised; +, feasible; ++, preferred.

16.5.1.2 Motor-Neuron Disease

When motor neuron disease affects the bulbar region, dysphagia develops. This is of great concern as dehydration and malnutrition will further weaken muscles and thereby hasten the development of respiratory insufficiency and death (Langmore, Kasarskis, and Manca 2006). Poor appetite and the inability to self-feed may also contribute to weight loss. Whether PEG feeding leads to better nutrition, improved quality of life and longer survival has not been tested in an RCT. Of seven case-control studies addressing the effect of PEG feeding on survival, four found no difference, while three reported a longer survival. The two studies with a stronger, prospective design found a survival benefit (Mazzini et al. 1995; Chio et al. 2002). Only three of the seven studies report on nutritional status, but all show positive effects. QOL aspects have not been well studied so far. Based on the current level of evidence, PEG feeding should be advised in cases of motor neurone disease.

16.5.1.3 Dementia

Loss of interest in food and dysphagia occur late in the course of dementia. While over a third of U.S–based nursing home residents with dementia were tube fed, this practice is not currently used in other parts of the world (Sampson, Candy, and Jones 2009). No RCT has been conducted to assess whether PEG feeding in advanced dementia influences survival, nutritional status or QOL. Based on six case control studies, a Cochrane review (Sampson et al. 2009) concluded that there is "insufficient evidence for the effectiveness of enteral feeding for older people with advanced dementia on survival, quality of life, nutrition and pressure ulcers, function and behavioural or psychiatric symptoms of dementia."

16.5.2 Other Neuromuscular Diseases

Dysphagia caused by other neuromuscular disorders has not been subject to systematic studies. A case series on PEG placement for neurological indications has included patients suffering from brain tumours, Parkinson's disease and multiple sclerosis (Zalar et al. 2004). Nutritional improvement was seen in all cases, but this heterogenous cohort study without controls does not allow generalisation of this finding. Clinicians should make individual assessments of possible risks and benefits before initiating PEG feeding in such patients.

16.6 HEAD AND NECK TUMOURS

Mucositis and dysphagia caused by treatment for head and neck cancers often necessitate temporary or permanent tube feeding (Mekhail et al. 2001). While patients seem to prefer PEG over NG tubes, a retrospective series found that PEG tubes were associated with more dysphagia at 3 and 6 months and with a greater need for pharyngoesophageal dilatation of strictures (Mekhail et al. 2001). PEG tubes were required for significantly longer periods than NG tubes. There is a need to confirm these findings in a prospective setting, but a recent trial was terminated prematurely due to patients' reluctance to be randomised (Corry et al. 2008). Metastatic seeding to the PEG site is a major concern in head and neck cancers, which has been reported in up to 0.98% of cases (Ruz et al. 2005). This is generally attributed to the pull technique used in PEG placement, when the tube is pulled through the upper GI tract containing the tumour. The push technique used during RIG placement should avoid this risk, but a case of tumour spread to the RIG site has also been reported (Hawken et al. 2005). Complication rates following RIG placement are higher than those seen after PEG placement (Grant et al. 2009). Given the problems associated with PEG use in head and neck cancers, the views of the patient are vital when deciding on the choice of tube feeding method.

16.6.1 Oesophageal and High Gastric Obstruction

In cases of malignant oesophageal and high gastric obstruction, treatment can either be focussed on re-establishing the natural upper GI tract or on establishing an alternative feeding route (PEG

TABLE 16.2
Stent versus Radiotherapy for Oesophageal Cancer

	Advantages	Disadvantages
Stent	Quicker improvement of dysphagia Widely available	High rate of late complications Dysphagia improvement not as well sustained
Radiotherapy	Better long-term results Less complications	Slower onset of improvement Need for tertiary referral and travel

or RIG). Generally the former is preferred as this allows the pleasure of eating and eliminates the inability to swallow saliva. The lumen can be reopened by reducing the tumour bulk (radiotherapy or endoscopic ablative therapy) or by placement of an SEMS. Advances in SEMS have led to a decrease in the use of endoscopic treatment modalities (laser therapy, bipolar cautery, argon plasma coagulation, injection of caustics) (Kozarek 2003). Most patients will be offered palliation either by SEMS or radiotherapy. External palliative radiotherapy is given in one session (Homs, Steyerberg et al. 2004). Endoluminal radiotherapy often requires three sessions (Bergquist et al. 2005). SEMS insertion can be achieved with a 48-hour hospital stay in 50% of cases and produces an improvement in dysphagia in 94% of patients (Selinger et al. 2008).

Two RCTs have shown that SEMS lead to a quicker and better improvement in dysphagia at 1 month when compared to radiotherapy (Homs, Steyerberg et al. 2004; Bergquist et al. 2005). Improvement of dysphagia was however better sustained at 3 months in the external radiotherapy group (Homs et al. 2004). External and endoluminal brachytherapy were both associated with better overall quality of life when compared to SEMS (Homs, Essink-Bot et al. 2004; Bergquist et al. 2005). Stent insertion is often associated with periprocedural chest pain (over 10%). Serious acute complications occur in around 5%; longer-term issues including stent migration, food bolus obstruction and tumour overgrowth affect 25% of SEMS patients (Selinger et al. 2008). The main side effects of external radiotherapy are short-lived dysphagia and odynophagia, nausea, a dry mouth and mild skin burns.

A cost-effectiveness study based on the findings of the endoluminal brachytherapy versus SEMS trial found that due to the higher initial costs of the three sessions of therapy total healthcare-related costs were twice as high as in the SEMS group (Wenger et al. 2005). Cost-effectiveness modelling using U.S–(Medicare)-based health care costs suggest that external radiotherapy might be more cost effective than SEMS (Da Silveira and Artifon 2008). The findings of these studies cannot be generalised as healthcare-related costs and availability of treatments will differ from country to country. In the United Kingdom SEMS is available in most District General Hospitals while radiotherapy requires referral to a tertiary centre, leading to a delay in treatment and need for travel. Treatment options should therefore be discussed with the patient and the patient's preference, local availability of treatment, prognosis, side effects and likelihood of cost effectiveness should be taken into consideration. While patients with a shorter life expectancy will benefit most from SEMS insertion, radiotherapy should be considered in individuals with a life expectancy of 3 months or longer (Table 16.2).

16.6.2 Gastric Outlet Obstruction

Gastric outlet obstruction (GOO) is most commonly caused by neoplastic processes in the head of pancreas. Lower gastric and pyloric obstruction due to benign or malignant ulceration and tumour growth as well as hepatobiliary tumours can also cause GOO, which leads to the accumulation of gastric content and subsequent vomiting. A surgical jejunostomy feeding tube placed distal to the lesion guarantees adequate nutrition. Gastric fluid will however continue to cause nausea and vomiting. It is therefore preferable to either re-establish the natural orifice or to construct an alternative

TABLE 16.3
Stent versus Gastrojejunostomy for Gastric Outlet Obstruction

	Advantages	Disadvantages
Stent	Quicker improvement of symptoms Relatively minor procedure Short hospital stay	High rate of late complications Improvement not as well sustained
Gastrojejunostomy	Better long-term results Less complications in later phase	Delayed gastric emptying Longer hospital stay Requires fitness for surgery and anaesthesia

route of gastric emptying via a surgical bypass (in most cases a gastrojejunostomy (GJJ) connecting proximal small bowel to the stomach).

Pancreatic tumours are common and 15%–20% of patients will experience GOO due to locally advanced tumours (Jeurnink et al. 2007). It is rather controversial whether a prophylactic GJJ is advisable. Hueser et al. (2009) found in their meta-analysis of two RCTs and one prospective non-randomised study that prophylactic GJJ at the time of biliary bypass formation leads to significantly lower occurrences of GOO than an expectant strategy (19% versus 1.6%, $p < 0.001$). Morbidity and mortality for the combined procedure including a GJJ were similar to those of a biliary bypass only operation. However, given the advances in endoscopic management of biliary obstruction, this seems to be a comparison with a nonstandard treatment: A Cochrane review (Moss, Morris, and MacMathuna 2006) concluded that SEMS insertion should be used as the standard treatment approach for malignant distal biliary tree obstruction. Morbidity and mortality of a GJJ compare unfavourably to endoscopic biliary SEMS insertion. Given that at least 80% of patients with a pancreatic neoplasm will not experience GOO, major "prophylactic palliative" surgery on the gastric outflow tract should probably not be recommended over a watch-and-wait strategy.

When GOO occurs, treatment choices include SEMS and surgery (Tables 16.3 and 16.4). SEMS insertion is a relatively minor procedure with a high initial success rate, but around 25% experience late complications like stent occlusion, GI bleeding and intestinal perforation (Kim et al. 2009). Open or laparoscopic GJJ has a lower risk of late complication and recurrence of obstructive symptoms but is associated with delayed gastric emptying (lasting 8 days or longer) in the initial postoperative phase (Jeurnink et al. 2007). Two randomised studies comparing GJJ and SEMS included only a total of 45 patients and do not allow firm conclusions to be drawn. A systematic review largely based on noncomparative studies included 1216 patients and found clinical success rates of 89% for SEMS and 72% for GJJ ($p = 0.1$) (Jeurnink et al. 2007). Major early and late complications occurred with equal frequency for both interventions, but GJJ required longer hospital stays (13 versus 7 days). Survival was much longer in the GJJ group. This is likely due to selection bias as the majority of patients in this review were from non-randomised studies. QOL aspects and cost effectiveness have not been studied well. Patients with shorter life expectancy are likely to benefit more from SEMS, while GJJ offers preferable longer-term results.

TABLE 16.4
Key Features of Gastric Outlet Obstruction (GOO)

GOO is caused by obstruction of the outflow tract of the stomach
Common underlying conditions are cancers of the stomach, duodenum and the pancreas and occasionally benign ulceration of the stomach
GOO leads to accumulation of fluid in the stomach and subsequent vomiting
Subsequently dehydration and malnutrition develops

Initial SEMS success rates do not differ for pancreatic or gastric malignancies but stent collapse occurs significantly more often with gastric carcinomas, while other serious complications (GI bleeding, perforation) are more commonly seen in pancreatic carcinoma patients (Kim et al. 2009). Adjuvant chemotherapy may improve the long-term results of SEMS.

ETHICAL ISSUES

Informed consent is the cornerstone of all medical treatments. It requires the capacity to retain and weigh up information as well as the ability to communicate a decision. In patients with severe neurological impairment like stroke disease or dementia these requirements are often not met. Depending on local law, a legal guardian might consent for the patient or the treating physician might have to make a decision for the patient based on what is in the patient's best interest. Especially in palliative care situations it can very difficult to ascertain what constitutes this best interest.

In order to make consent informed, a patient needs to be given enough information to understand the procedure, its risks and possible outcomes. Anxiety and low mood occur commonly in palliative patients. Therefore, how much and which information is provided to the patient to not increase anxiety levels and mood problems requires careful consideration. Furthermore the patient might be under considerable stress and pressure to make a number of decisions on medical care whilst also preparing a last will.

Ethical issues might also arise regarding the availability of palliative care treatments. The best treatment might not be locally available or might not be funded.

Stents provide fast and effective relief from dysphagia caused by upper GI tract obstruction and have superior results in the short term compared to radiotherapy (oesophageal) and surgery (GOO). Results at three months however favour radiotherapy and surgery. To advise on treatment the physician needs to be able to judge life expectancy well. This can be extremely difficult. Judging fitness for and risks of surgery is rather subjective and ethical issues regarding this often arise in clinical practice.

Whether to advise prophylactic treatment to prevent dysphagia (radiotherapy for oesophageal cancer for example) or an expectant strategy also needs ethical consideration. A prophylactic approach might take up valuable high-quality time in a relatively asymptomatic patient, while an expectant approach only takes up time when a problem has occurred. Prophylactic treatment might also have negative psychological effects (increased feeling of being ill) while an expectant approach might lead to the patient experiencing a lot of symptoms before undergoing the intervention.

Difficult ethical issues often arise regarding the question of whether to start enteral feeding in patients with advanced or severe disease. While the evidence suggests that early tube feeding after severe strokes and tube feeding in advanced dementia should be avoided, relatives might push for such an intervention in the belief that the patient is suffering from hunger. Physicians face an ethical dilemma when trying not to upset relatives when conveying the treatment plan and acting in the patient's best interest at the same time.

SUMMARY POINTS

- Dysphagia in the palliative care setting can arise from neuromuscular problems or obstruction of the upper GI tract.
- Treatment options include the creation of alternative feeding routes (NG, PEG and RIG), therapy to reopen the natural lumen of the GI tract (stents, endoluminal therapy and radiotherapy) and creation of alternative drainage of the stomach with surgery.
- The choice of treatment depends on the patient's overall state of health, fitness to undergo interventions and personal choice.
- PEG, NG and RIG provide a safe feeding route, but the appropriateness of the intervention depends on the underlying condition.

- Stents are a very effective way of treating obstructive dysphagia and have favourable results at 1 month, but carry a high risk of long-term complications.
- Surgery or radiotherapy have better long-term results than stents, but are not as effective in the short term.

LIST OF ABBREVIATIONS

GI	Gastrointestinal
GJJ	Gastrojejunostomy
GOO	Gastric outlet obstruction
NG	Nasogastric tube
PEG	Percutaneous endoscopic gastrostomy
PEJ	Percutaneous endoscopic jejunostomy
RCT	Randomised controlled clinical trial
RIG	Radiologically introduced gastrostomy
SEMS	Self-expanding metal stent
SPJ	Surgically placed jejunostomy

REFERENCES

Bath, P. M. W., F. J. Bath-Hextal, and D. Smithard. 1999. Interventions for dysphagia in acute stroke. *Cochrane Database of Systematic Reviews*. Issue 4. Art. No.: CD000323.

Bergquist, H., U. Wenger, E. Johnsson, J. Nyman, H. Ejnell, E. Hammerlid, L. Lundell, and M. Ruth. 2005. Stent insertion or endoluminal brachytherapy as palliation of patients with advanced cancer of the esophagus and gastroesophageal junction. Results of a randomized, controlled clinical trial. *Disease of the Esophagus* 18:131–39.

Chio, A., G. Mora, M. Leone, L. Mazzini, and D. L. Cocito. 2002. Early symptom progression rate is related to ALS outcome: A prospective population based study. *Neurology* 59:99–103.

Corry, J., W. Poon, N. McPhee, A. D. Milner, D. Cruickshank, S. V. Porceddu, D. Rischin, and L. J. Peters. 2008. Randomized study of percutaneous gastrostomy versus nasogastirc tubes for enteral feeding in head and neck cancer patients treated with (chemo)radiation. *Journal of Medical Imaging Radiation Oncology* 52:503–10.

Da Silveira, E. B., and E. L. Artifon. 2008. Cost-effectiveness of palliation of unresectable esophageal cancer. *Digestive Disease and Science* 53:3103–11.

Dennis, M. S., S. C. Lewis, and C. Warlow. 2005. Effect of timing and method of enteral tube feeding for dysphagic stroke patients (FOOD): A multicentre randomised controlled trial. *The Lancet* 365:764–72.

Grant, D. G., P. T. Bradley, D. D. Pothier, D. Bailey, S. Caldera, D. L. Baldwin, and M. A. Birchall. 2009. Complications following gastrostomy tube insertion inpatients with head and neck cancer: A prospective multi-institution study, systematic review and meta-analysis. *Clinical Otolaryngology* 34:103–12.

Hawken, R. M., R. W. Williams, M. W. Bridger, C. B. Lyons, and S. A. Jackson. 2005. Puncture site metastasis in a radiologically inserted gastrostomy tube: Case report and literature review. *Cardiovascular Interventional Radiology* 28:377–80.

Homs, M. Y., E. W. Steyerberg, W. M. Eijkenboom, H. W. Tilanus, L. J. Stalpers, J. F. Bartelsman, J. J. van Lanschot et al. 2004. Single dose brachytherapy versus metal stent placement for the palliation of dysphagia from oesophageal cancer: Multicentre randomised trial. *The Lancet* 364:1497–504.

Homs, M. Y., M. L. Essink-Bot, G. J. Borsboom, E. W. Steyerberg, and P. D. Siersema. 2004. Quality of life after palliative treatment for oesophageal carcinoma – A prospective comparison between stent placement and single dose brachytherapy. *European Journal of Cancer* 40:1862–71.

Hueser, N., C. W. Michalski, T. Schuster, H. Friess, and J. Kleef. 2009. Systematic review and meta-analysis of prophylactic gastroenterostomy for unresectable pancreatic cancer. *British Journal of Surgery* 96:711–19.

Jeurnink, S. M., C. H. J. van Eijck, E. W. Steyerberg, E. J. Kuipers, and P. D. Siersema. 2007. Stent versus gastrojejunostomy for the palliation of gastric outlet obstruction: A systematic review. *BMC Gastroenterology* 7:18.

Kim, J. H., H. Y. Song, J. H. Shin, H. T. Hu, S. K. Lee, H-Y. Jung, and J. H. Yook. 2009. Metallic stent placement in the palliative treatment of malignant gastric outlet obstructions: Primary gastric carcinoma versus pancreatic carcinoma. *American Journal of Roentgenology* 193:241–47.

Kozarek, R. A. 2003. Endoscopic palliation of esophageal malignancy. *Endoscopy* 35:S9–13.

Langmore, S. E., E. J. Kasarskis, M. L. Manca, and R.K. Olney. 2006. Enteral tube feeding for amyotrophic lateral sclerosis/motorneuron disease. *Cochrane Database of Systematic Reviews.* Issue 4. Art. No.: CD004030.

Mazzini, L., T. Corra, M. Zaccala, G. Mora, M. Piano, and M. Galante. 1995. Percutaneous endoscopic gastrostomy and enteral nutrition in amyotrophic lateral sclerosis. *Journal of Neurology* 242:695–98.

Mekhail, T. M., D. J. Adelstein, L. A. Rybicki, M. A. Larto, J. P. Saxton, and P. Lavertu. 2001. Enteral nutrition during the treatment of head and neck carcinoma: Is a percutaneous endoscopic gastrostomy tube preferable to a nasogastric tube? *Cancer* 91:1785–90.

Moss, A. C., E. Morris, and P. MacMathuna. 2006. Palliative biliary stents for obstructing pancreatic carcinoma. *Cochrane Database of Systematic Reviews.* Issue 2. Art. No.: CD004200.

National Collaborating Centre for Acute Care. February 2006. *Nutrition support in adults: Oral nutrition support, enteral tube feeding and parenteral nutrition.* National Collaborating Centre for Acute Care, London. Available from www.rcseng.ac.uk.

Ruz, I., J. J. Mamel, P. G. Brady, and M. Cass-Garcia. 2005. Incidence of abdominal wall metastasis complicating PEG tube placement in untreated head and neck cancer. *Gastrointestinal Endoscopy* 62:708–11.

Sampson, E. L., B. Candy, and L. Jones. 2009. Enteral tube feeding for older people with advanced dementia. *Cochrane Database of Systematic Reviews.* Issue 2. Art. No.: CD007209.

Selinger, C. P., P. Ellul, P. A. Smith, and N. C. Cole. 2008. Oesophageal stent insertion for palliation of dysphagia in a UK District General Hospital: Experience from a case series of 137 patients. *QJM: An International Journal of Medicine* 101:545–48.

Verschuur, E. M., E. W. Steyerberg, E. J. Kuipers, and P. D. Siersema. 2007. Effect of stent size on complications and recurrent dysphagia in patients with esophageal or gastric cardia cancer. *Gastrointestinal Endoscopy* 65:592–601.

Wenger, U., E. Johnsson, H. Bergquist, J. Nyman, H. Ejnell, J. Lagergren, M. Ruth, and L. Lundell. 2005. Health economic evaluation of stent or endoluminal brachytherapy as a palliative strategy in patients with incurable cancer of the oesophagus or gastro-oesophageal junction: Results of a randomized trial. *European Journal of Gastroenterology Hepatology* 17:1369–77.

Wollman, B., H. B. D'Agostino, J. R. Walus-Wigle, D. W. Easter, and A. Beale. 1995. Radiologic, endoscopic, and surgical gastrostomy: An institutional evaluation and meta-analysis of the literature. *Radiology* 197:699–704.

Zalar, A. E., C. Guedon, E. L. Piskorz, A. Sanchez Basso, and P. Ducrotte. 2004. Percutaneous endoscopic gastrostomy in patients with neurological diseases. Results of a prospective multicenter and international study. *Acta Gastroenteroligica Latinoamericana* 34:127–32.

17 Fatigue in Hospice Cancer Patients: How Do Nutritional Factors Contribute?

Yeur-Hur Lai and Shiow-Ching Shun

CONTENTS

17.1 INTRODUCTION

Fatigue is one of the most common problems experienced by cancer patients (Table 17.1), and non-cancer patients with life-threatening diseases. The prevalence of fatigue has been reported as up to 99% of patients receiving active treatment (Radbruch et al. 2008) for patients with cancer. For those with terminal cancer, the range is from 52%–81% (Okuyama et al. 2008). In addition, in our previous hospice study on terminal cancer patients, they generally experienced moderate to severe levels of fatigue (Tsai et al. 2007). Fatigue has been found to be closely linked to decreasing performance (Okuyama et al. 2008; Tsai et al. 2007) and to quality of life.

17.2 DEFINITION OF CANCER-RELATED FATIGUE (CRF)

Fatigue is a complex, multifactorial phenomenon that has been recognized in multiple dimensions including temporal, physical/sensory, affective/emotional, cognitive/mental, and behavioral (Piper, Lindsey, and Dodd 1987). Patients use different words or phrases to describe their different domains of fatigue (Table 17.2). Due to its complexity, cancer-related fatigue (CRF) has various definitions. Fatigue has been defined as a "subjective feeling of tiredness, weakness or

TABLE 17.1
Key Facts of Cancer-Related Fatigue

1. Fatigue is the most common symptom among cancer patients during the cancer trajectory
2. Fatigue is a subjective feeling and self-reporting is the only method to measure patients' level of fatigue
3. Fatigue is viewed as having multiple dimensions including severity, physical, affective, cognitive, and behavioral
4. Healthy people could experience fatigue and the level of fatigue generally decreases after taking a rest or with good sleep for one night; however, cancer-related fatigue cannot be relieved with one night's good sleep
5. The mechanism of cancer-related fatigue has not been understood until now
6. Cancer-related fatigue can be caused by cancer itself and the side effects of cancer-related treatments
7. Assessing treatable contributing factors (such as nutrition assessment, pain, anemia, or activity level) and managing the problems can decrease the level of fatigue

lack of energy" (Radbruch et al. 2008, 15) and "an unusual and persistent sense of tiredness that can occur with cancer or cancer treatment, that may affect both physical and mental capacity, and that is unrelieved by rest" (National Comprehensive Cancer Network 2003). The National Comprehensive Cancer Network (NCCN) has also defined CRF as a "distressing, persistent, subjective sense of tiredness or exhaustion related to cancer or cancer treatment that is not proportional to recent activity and interferences with usual functioning" (National Comprehensive Cancer Network 2010, FT1).

TABLE 17.2
Dimensions of Fatigue and Words/Phrases Used to Describe Fatigue

Dimensions	Definition	Words or Phrases to Describe
Temporal	Related to the timing, onset, pattern, and duration of fatigue	Continuous, steady, generalized, affecting whole body, constant, periodic, description of daily pattern (worse in the morning, the afternoon, evening, no consistent daily pattern)
Physical/sensory	Related to the feelings of general and muscular weakness, exhaustion, and their severity and quality	Barely able to move, worn out, dragged out, sleepy, drowsy, exhausted, no energy, sluggish, low energy, wiped out, weak, weak legs (legs feel weak), general weakness, tired, muscle weakness, muscles ache, head feels heavy, arms feel weak, ache all over, body feels heavy all over, desire to close eyes, desire to lie down, breathless
Affective/emotional	The emotional response to fatigue or distress evoked by fatigue	Loss of ability, overcome, stuck, helpless, vulnerable, frustrated, listless, feel upset, feel nervous, feel sad, feel tense, distressed, feel depressed, unpleasant, loss of future
Cognitive/mental	Reflecting the impact of fatigue on concentration processes and including the meaning that patients attribute to fatigue	Hard to concentrate, difficulty thinking, have trouble in remembering things, confused, have trouble paying attention, make more mistakes than usual, forgetful, thoughts easily wander, impatient, conserving energy, planning every move
Behavioral	Reflecting the changes in physical performance, impact of fatigue symptoms on activities of daily living	Fatigue interferes with the following aspects: general activity, mood, walking ability, normal work, relations with other people, enjoyment of life, ability to concentrate, sleep habits

Source: Adapted from Shun, S.C., *Psychometric testing of three fatigue instruments with cancer outpatients in Taiwan*, College of Nursing, University of Utah, Salt Lake City, 2005.

Note: The table shows words/phrases that patients might use to describe their fatigue based on different domains. Healthcare providers should know about these words and it will help in identifying their problems in fatigue.

The criteria for a diagnosis of CRF, based on the International Classification of Diseases-10 (ICD-10), are "significant fatigue, diminished energy or increased need to rest, disproportionate to any recent change in activity level has been present everyday or nearly every day during the same 2-week period in the past month" (Cella et al. 2001). Five out of ten additional symptoms are required to make the diagnosis of CRF syndrome, including generalized weakness, diminished concentration or attention, decreased motivation or interest in engaging in usual activities, insomnia or hypersomnia, or marked emotional reactivity to feeling fatigued.

Finally, Yennurajalingam and Bruera (2007) also proposed the concept of "clinical fatigue" as being better for clinical assessment and management of fatigue. Clinical fatigue includes three components: "(1) generalized weakness, resulting in inability to initiate certain activities; (2) easy fatigability and reduced capacity to maintain performance; and (3) mental fatigue resulting in impaired concentration, loss of memory, and emotional liability" (Yennurajalingam and Bruera 2007, 297).

Taken together, although several definitions or terms pertaining to fatigue in cancer patients have been proposed, these definitions indicate that CRF is a subjective, generalized condition of weakness and a distressing experience that is not easily relieved by rest. It also suggests that CRF is a multifactorial phenomenon.

17.3 PATHOPHYSIOLOGY OF FATIGUE

The pathophysiology of fatigue is complex and not precisely understood. However, there are several assumptions or models (Table 17.3) that can be used to study the potential pathophysiological mechanisms or causes of fatigue (Ryan et al. 2007; Glaus 1998; Radbruch et al. 2008). The European Association for Palliative Care (EAPC) has approached fatigue by differentiating between primary and secondary fatigue (Radbruch et al. 2008). Primary fatigue is hypothesized to be associated with the "tumor itself." Primary fatigue is hypothesized to be caused either by "peripheral mechanisms, such as energy depletion" or by "central mechanisms such as dysregulation of the hypothalamic-pituitary-adrenal (HPA) axis or serotonin metabolism" (Radbruch et al. 2008). Taking together, the fatigue mechanism is thought to be linked to serotonin dysregulation and a proinflammatory

TABLE 17.3
Models for Potential Mechanisms or Causes of Fatigue

Assumptions or Models	Author (Year)	Hypothesis
Psychophysiological fatigue theory	Grabdjean (1961)	Cumulative effect of day-to-day causes of fatigue due to intensity and duration of physical and mental work, psychological causes, and illness, pain, and nutrition
Integrated fatigue model	Piper (1987)	Potential 14 patterns of causes for fatigue including changes in energy and energy substrate pattern, etc.
Central and peripheral mechanisms of fatigue	Gibson and Edwards (1989)	Impairment in central mechanisms (e.g., hypothalamus-anterior pituitary-adrenal cortex-axis dysfunction, serotonin dysregulation, cytokine dysregulation) or peripheral mechanisms (e.g., ATP dysregulation) may cause fatigue by affecting the metabolic effects and energy supply
Psychobiological-entropy model	Winningham and Barton-Burke (2000)	Energy consumption and producing process across the process of energy, organic functioning, and entropy. Factors to enhance energy will decrease fatigue and increase function

Note: This table summarizes the possible mechanisms for causing fatigue. Several pathophysiological mechanisms (e.g., hypothalamus-anterior pituitary-adrenal cortex–axis (HPA) dysfunction, serotonin dysregulation, cytokine dysregulation) have been reported but most of them were correlated to HPA dysfunction; therefore, those hypotheses are included in the central and peripheral mechanism. Data are summarized from Ryan (2007) and Glaus (1998).

cytokine dysregulation and disturbance in the HPA-axis dysfunction (Ryan et al. 2007). However, there are still no consistent findings to fully support this mechanism.

Secondary fatigue is associated with cancer-concurrent symptoms or treatment-related side effects (Radbruch et al. 2008) and is a multifactorial phenomenon. These may include anemia, cachexia, malnutrition, infection, fever, dehydration, dyspnea, pain, mucositis, side effects from sedative drugs or opioids, etc. Similarly, cancer care researchers have also proposed multidimensional models to explain CRF experiences. Piper's Integrated Fatigue Model (Piper et al. 1987) focuses on the factors causing CRF. Fatigue has also been viewed as a multifactorial model with the energy consumption and producing process based on Winningham's Psychobiological-Entropy Model of Functioning (Winningham and Barton-Burke 2000). In this model, fatigue is discussed from three points of views: energy, entropy, and organic functioning (Winningham and Barton-Burke 2000). Therefore, factors that enhance energy will decrease fatigue and increase function.

In sum, although the pathophysiology mechanism is not fully understood, the mechanisms and models explored above suggest a possible connection between proinflammatory cytokines and CRF. Furthermore, based on a mechanism proposed by EAPC (Radbruch et al. 2008), clinically, fatigue has been found to be related to cancer itself, its concurrent symptoms/distress and side effects. How these factors influence terminal cancer patients' nutrition and fatigue will be discussed in the following section.

17.4 MALNUTRITION AND CANCER-RELATED FATIGUE IN TERMINAL PATIENTS

Although the possible link between proinflammatory cytokines and fatigue has been hypothesized, a lack of sufficient information still inhibits the direct implication of cytokines in clinical practice (primary fatigue). Thus, we sought to identify those clinical factors that might be directly related to terminal patients' fatigue (secondary fatigue). Among these factors, malnutrition has been identified as closely linked to patients' lack of energy and fatigue (Neuenschwander and Bruera 1998). Due to the lack of sufficient evidence, this discussion will not include the particular kinds of foods or nutrients thought to decrease terminal patients' fatigue. For the purpose of this chapter, we will focus more on those important factors or causes related to nutrition/malnutrition and fatigue in terminal cancer patients.

17.4.1 MALNUTRITION, CACHEXIA, AND FATIGUE

Malnutrition is found to be a prevalent problem among cancer patients. Bozzetti's (2009) nutrition status survey of 1000 cancer outpatients found that a significant weight loss (≥10%) and a nutritional risk score of ≥3 were observed in 39.7% and 33.8% of patients, respectively. An Asian hospice study in terminal cancer patients' nutrition intake and hydration status (Chiu, Hu, and Chen 2000) showed that 38.7% of patients admitted to hospice were unable to take water or food orally. Even worse, 39.1% and 60.1% of these patients could not eat or drink orally one week after admission and 48 hours before death, respectively. Malnutrition in cancer patients can be caused by insufficient caloric intake, protein deficiency, fluid electrolyte imbalance (e.g., sodium, potassium, calcium, and magnesium), lack of ferritin, anemia, and insufficient vitamins (e.g., B1, B6, and B12) (National Comprehensive Cancer Network 2010; Radbruch et al. 2008). This results in further weight loss and decreased physical performance. Weight loss among terminal cancer patients is complex and multifactorial, is likely related to cachexia, and contributes to patients' fatigue (Yennurajalingam and Bruera 2007).

Cachexia is one of the most prevalent problems in terminal cancer patients. Although the mechanism of cancer-related cachexia is not well understood, it is hypothesized that endogenously produced cytokines are the major mediators (Jaskowiak and Alexander 1998). Cancer cachexia is characterized as having anorexia, and experiencing weight loss and abnormal changes in metabolism. The specific changes in carbohydrates, proteins, and lipids include the increase of endogenous glucose production, lactate recycling, hepatic gluconeogenesis, skeletal muscle catabolism, hepatic protein synthesis, and hepatic lipogenesis and lipolysis, as well as a decrease in glycogen stores, insulin sensitivity, skeletal muscle synthesis, lipoprotein lipase activity, and lipid stores (Jaskowiak and Alexander 1998). Abnormal protein metabolism, such as increased proteolysis in skeletal muscle, can further lead to loss of functional lean body mass, muscle wasting, tiredness, energy decrease, weakness, and then fatigue (Jaskowiak and Alexander 1998).

17.4.2 Malnutrition Related to Anorexia, Treatments, and Cancer

Anorexia/loss of appetite is frequently found in cancer patients undergoing anticancer treatments such as chemotherapy. Patients on chemotherapy might experience changes in taste, anorexia, and loss of appetite. For terminally ill cancer patients, anorexia could be caused by a lack of activity, decreasing bowel movements, and the effects related to the illness, and it could become even worse and a prologue to cachexia. Previous studies by the authors (Tsai et al. 2007) and by Okuyama et al. (2008) identified similar findings in that hospice cancer patients' fatigue was associated with decreasing appetite.

17.5 CANCER-RELATED SYMPTOMS DIRECTLY INFLUENCING FOOD INTAKE AND FATIGUE

17.5.1 Head and Neck Cancer-Related Problems

Patients with head and neck cancers have been reported as having a relatively high risk of malnutrition. The irradiation of head and neck areas might destroy the salivary gland, leading to dry mouth, which would influence food intake and therefore lead to malnutrition (Chasen and Bhargava 2009). In addition, head and neck cancer patients, particularly those with oral cavity cancers, may have more difficulties in taking food orally while undergoing a wide range of tumor resection and reconstruction. The dysfunction from the damage to food-taking organs, such as the tongue, buckle tissues, teeth, or nerves, might all lead to problems on various levels, including chewing and swallowing difficulties. Any of these problems could lead to oral intake difficulties and malnutrition.

17.5.2 Gastrointestinal System-Related Problems and Malnutrition

With gastrointestinal tract cancers, metastasis and treatments in this area of the body may prevent normal food intake or digestion. For example, patients with gastric cancer receiving stomach resection may decrease normal food intake or nutrient absorption. Patients with esophageal cancers may experience problems swallowing. For patients in a terminal condition, liver metastasis may cause ascites. Severe ascites with abdominal distension and edema may decrease appetite and general physical activities, and may further decrease bowel movement. This may lead to worsening conditions in appetite and food intake.

Constipation is also a frequent problem in terminally ill cancer patients. About 50% of terminal cancer patients have reported this problem (Sykes 1998). Constipation in terminal cancer patients can result from long-term bed rest (inactivity/immobilization), intestinal obstruction due to tumor in the bowel wall, or external compression. It may also stem from secondary effects of disease, such as inadequate food intake, low-fiber diet, dehydration, and other complications. It might be also related to certain medicines, such as the side effects of opioids. Constipation may lead to even worse food intake, and this can become a vicious cycle in which the patient receives decreasing nourishment/energy and becomes more fatigued.

Nausea and vomiting are also common problems in advanced cancer patients (Lagman et al. 2005). From 30–70% of terminal cancer patients are reported to have such problems (Lagman et al. 2005; Maree and Wright 2008). The causes of nausea and vomiting in terminally ill cancer patients are complex. These can be related to drugs (such as opioids), ascites, intestinal obstruction, constipation, liver metastasis, irritation of the GI tract, increasing intracranial pressure, movement-associated nausea, and severe mood disturbances such as anxiety (Mannix 1998).

Taken together, symptoms related to GI tract disturbance may interfere with normal food-intake processes and cause weight loss and malnutrition. In Bozzetti's study (2009), weight loss was greater in upper gastrointestinal cancers and in advanced stages of disease. Our previous study in hospice cancer patients' fatigue supported the inferences that patients' fatigue was related to both overall symptom severity as well as to some GI tract-related individual symptoms, such as nausea, vomiting, lack of appetite, and dry mouth (Tsai et al. 2007). These factors could be due in part to cancer cachexia and to a further decrease in patients' energy, causing them to develop more fatigue and weakness.

17.6 COMMON PHYSICAL SYMPTOMS RELATED TO FOOD INTAKE AND FATIGUE

Pain is one of the most distressful symptoms among terminal cancer patients. Moderate to severe cancer pain may interfere with patients' daily life, general activity, eating, sleeping, etc. (Lai et al. 2009). Such patients, therefore, have a greater possibility of developing malnutrition and severe fatigue.

Similarly, dyspnea and shortness of breath may expend patients' energy and decrease their physical performance. This may decrease food intake due to lack of motivation and energy. In Tsai et al. (2007) and Okuyama et al. (2008), it was found that dyspnea is the symptom most associated with terminal cancer patients' fatigue. Other symptoms commonly found in terminal cancer patients include anemia, fever or active infection, and sleep restriction (National Comprehensive Cancer Network 2010). These may be related to terminal cancer patients' fatigue. Anemia can result directly from disease or can be a long-term side effect of treatments, and it has been found to be closely related to patients' fatigue (Cella et al. 2004).

In conclusion, the general lack of energy, weakness, and multiple symptoms in terminal cancer patients may cause further bed rest, worsen the physical condition, and increase patients' fatigue. Symptoms related to the GI tract and the head and neck area may decrease food intake and decrease physical function, causing further weakness and fatigue. Other symptoms, such as anemia (Cella et al. 2004), dyspnea, pain, infection, and fever can worsen fatigue. These factors should all be carefully assessed and monitored for managing fatigue in terminal cancer patients.

17.7 PSYCHOLOGICAL DISTRESS, FATIGUE, AND MALNUTRITION

For most terminal cancer patients, the psychological-spiritual-related factors play important roles in cancer patients' fatigue experiences. Depression, a sense of hopelessness, and anxiety are common forms of psychological distress. For patients with depression or feelings of hopelessness, it is meaningless to eat. This inference has been preliminarily supported by our findings in a study of hospice cancer patients' fatigue (Tsai et al. 2007) and by a study in Japan (Okuyama et al. 2008). In Brown and Kroenke's review (2009) of cancer patients' fatigue across studies of 12,103 cancer patients, this fatigue was shown to be strongly related to patients' depression and anxiety. The more depression and psychological distress a patient had, the more fatigue could occur due to inactivity and lack of sufficient energy from lost appetite, etc., which could lead to malnutrition.

17.8 MANAGING CANCER-RELATED FATIGUE IN TERMINAL CANCER PATIENTS: INTEGRATING NUTRITION-RELATED FACTORS

The management of CRF, particularly in terminal cancer patients, is a challenging issue. As the terminal condition, and assessment and management of terminal cancer patients' fatigue are

TABLE 17.4
Clinical Assessment of Cancer-Related Fatigue

1. To take patient disease status and treatment history
2. To assess patient fatigue characteristics (such as intensity, pattern, duration, and interference in daily life caused by fatigue)
3. To assess current activity level and type of exercise patients can do
4. To assess patients' physical distress (such as pain, anemia, sleep disturbance, nausea, vomiting, etc.)
5. To assess patients' psychological/emotional distress (depression, anxiety, uncertainty, etc.)
6. To assess comorbidities (such as infection, cardiac dysfunction, pulmonary dysfunction, etc.)
7. To assess nutritional status and obstacles or problems related to food intake (such as weight loss, caloric intake, fluid electrolyte imbalance, cachexia anorexia, or dehydration)

complex and multidimensional, nutrition-related factors should be integrated into both assessment and management (National Comprehensive Cancer Network 2010; Radbruch et al. 2008). Furthermore, due to the subjective nature of CRF, the assessment and management of CRF should be individualized with multifactorial concerns (Berger 2003; National Comprehensive Cancer Network 2010; Radbruch et al. 2008). Therefore, based on the research of the EAPC (Radbruch et al. 2008) and the NCCN, clinical assessment of CRF in terminal cancer patients, as shown in Table 17.4, should include the following basic components: (1) patients' history—disease status and treatment; (2) fatigue characteristics (such as intensity, pattern, duration, and interference in daily life caused by fatigue); (3) current activity level and type of exercise they can do; (4) assessment of physical distress (such as pain, anemia, sleep disturbance, etc.); (5) assessment of patients' psychological/emotional distress (depression, anxiety, uncertainty, etc.); (6) assessment of comorbidities (such as infection, cardiac dysfunction, pulmonary dysfunction, etc.); and (7) basic nutritional status and obstacles or problems related to food intake (such as weight loss, caloric intake, fluid electrolyte imbalance, cachexia anorexia, or dehydration). These are summarized in Table 17.5.

For the management of fatigue in patients at the end-of-life stage, four major approaches are suggested by the NCCN (2010). These include (1) patient/family education and counseling, (2) general

TABLE 17.5
Practical Assessment of Nutritional Status

Basic Assessment

1. To collect patients' history, including disease status and treatment experiences
2. To collect body weight and height and change of body weight within one month
3. To record caloric intake daily and intake and output
4. To check fluid electrolytes (e.g., sodium, potassium, calcium, magnesium), ferritin, Hgb, and albumin
5. To assess any signs of dehydration
6. To assess the dietary preferences

Specific Assessment: Assess Problems Related to Food Intake

1. To assess oral health including teeth, swallowing function, and oral mucus
2. To assess physical distress especially for pain, nausea/vomiting, dry mouth, ascites, constipation, shortness of breath, etc
3. To assess psychological distress, such as depression, anxiety, sense of uncertainty, hopelessness, fear of death, etc

strategies for management of fatigue, (3) specific nonpharmacologic strategies, and (4) specific pharmacologic interventions. In patient/family education and counseling, information about known patterns of fatigue and assessing/managing families'/patients' expectations about fatigue are important. General strategies for management of fatigue should include such strategies as (1) energy conservation (such as setting priorities, resting and activity pacing, conserving energy for valued activities), and (2) applying distraction and relaxation. In specific nonpharmacologic strategies, "activity enhancement" and "applying psychological interventions" to "decrease emotional distress" are suggested. In activity enhancement, clinicians should focus on treating those physical problems or symptoms related to the terminal condition, to help patients gain more energy and to increase their daily activities. Nutrition consultation should be applied to help patients achieve better intake and keep a higher energy level.

Finally, using pharmacological strategies to decrease patients' physical symptoms, such as pain, sleep disturbance, mood distress, etc., can further comfort patients and decrease fatigue. Managing anemia would be another important strategy to decrease fatigue. Medication used to directly manage CRF still remains to be examined. However, corticosteroids have been reported to provide some help in decreasing fatigue in terminal cancer patients (Carroll et al. 2007). The most appropriate types and dosages of corticosteroids used for terminally ill cancer patients, however, have not yet been determined.

In conclusion, CRF is a complex and multifactorial phenomenon. Therefore, careful assessment and individualized management of CRF in terminally ill cancer patients are indicated. Malnutrition and cachexia are problems related to CRF. Therefore, problems or symptoms from disease, and side effects from treatments that are related to patients' nutrition intake and cachexia, should be carefully assessed and managed to decrease the fatigue problems in terminal cancer patients.

ETHICAL ISSUES

The primary ethical issues related to managing nutrition for CRF in terminal cancer are to minimize those factors interfering with patients' nutrition intake. The most important issue is to discuss nutrition issues with patients and family members and to find the best strategies to keep patients comfortable and to decrease severe fatigue (beneficence).

SUMMARY POINTS

- Cancer-related fatigue (CRF) is among the most prevalent problems experienced by terminally ill cancer patients. CRF should be carefully assessed and managed individually.
- Factors or problems related to malnutrition should be identified and managed to decrease CRF.
- Patients with cancers, metastasis, or symptoms in the GI tract or in the head and neck areas might have a higher risk of developing malnutrition compared to other types of cancers. These patients may need to be assessed, particularly for their nutrition status and fatigue due to malnutrition problems.
- Psychological distress, such as anxiety and depression, should be carefully assessed, for these problems may influence patients' willingness to eat and thus develop further malnutrition problems and related fatigue.
- Nutritional factors should be integrated into the multidimensional assessment and management of CRF in terminally ill cancer patients.

LIST OF ABBREVIATION

CRF Cancer-Related Fatigue

REFERENCES

Berger, A. 2003. Treating fatigue in cancer patients. *Oncologist* 8 (Suppl 1) : 10–14.

Bozzetti, F. 2009. Screening the nutritional status in oncology: A preliminary report on 1,000 outpatients. *Supportive Care in Cancer* 17:279–84.

Brown, L. F., and K. Kroenke. 2009. Cancer-related fatigue and its associations with depression and anxiety: A systematic review. *Psychosomatics* 50:440–47.

Carroll, J. K., S. Kohli, K. M. Mustian, J. A. Roscoe, and G. R. Morrow. 2007. Pharmacologic treatment of cancer-related fatigue. *Oncologist* 12 (Suppl 1): 43–51.

Cella, D., K. Davis, W. Breitbart, and G. Curt. 2001. Cancer-related fatigue: Prevalence of proposed diagnostic criteria in a United States sample of cancer survivors. *Journal of Clinical Oncology* 19:3385–91.

Cella, D., J. Kallich, A. Mcdermott, and X. Xu. 2004. The longitudinal relationship of hemoglobin, fatigue and quality of life in anemic cancer patients: Results from five randomized clinical trials. *Annals of Oncology* 15:979–86.

Chasen, M. R., and R. Bhargava. 2009. A descriptive review of the factors contributing to nutritional compromise in patients with head and neck cancer. *Supportive Care in Cancer* 17:1345–51.

Chiu, T. Y., W. Y. Hu, and C. Y. Chen. 2000. Prevalence and severity of symptoms in terminal cancer patients: A study in Taiwan. *Supportive Care in Cancer* 8:311–13.

Glaus, A. 1998. Fatigue in patients with cancer. Analysis and assessment. *Recent Results in Cancer Research* 145:I–XI, 1–172.

Jaskowiak, N. T., and H. R. Alexander. 1998. The pathophysiology of cancer cachexia. In *Oxford textbook of palliative medicine,* 2nd ed., eds. D. Doyle, G. Hanks, N. I. Cherny, and K. Calman, 534–47. Oxford: Oxford University Press.

Lagman, R. L., M. P. Davis, S. B. Legrand, and D.Walsh. 2005. Common symptoms in advanced cancer. *Surgical Clinics of North America* 85:237–55.

Lai, Y. H., S. L. Guo, F. J. Keefe, L. Y. Tsai, S. C. Shun, Y. C. Liao, I. F. Li, C. P. Liu, and Y. H. Lee. 2009. Multidimensional Pain Inventory-Screening Chinese version (MPI-sC): Psychometric testing in terminal cancer patients in Taiwan. *Supportive Care in Cancer* 17:1445–53.

Mannix, K. A. 1998. Gastrointestinal symptoms: Palliation of nausea and vomiting. In *Oxford textbook of palliative medicine,* eds. D. Doyle, G. W. C. Hanks, and N. Macdonald, 489–98. Oxford: Oxford University Press.

Maree, J. E., and S. C. Wright. 2008. Palliative care: A positive outcome for cancer patients? *Curationis* 31:43–49.

National Comprehensive Cancer Network. 2003. Cancer-Related Fatigue [Online]. http://www.nccn.org.

National Comprehensive Cancer Network. 2010. Cancer-Related Fatigue [Online]. http://oralcancerfoundation.org/treatment/pdf/fatigue-NCCN.pdf. Accessed 17 March 2010.

Neuenschwander, H., and E. Bruera. 1998. Asthenia. In *Oxford textbook of palliative medicine,* eds. D. Doyle, G. W. C. Hanks, and N. Macdonald, 573–82. Oxford: Oxford University Press.

Okuyama, T., T. Akechi, Y. Shima, Y. Sugahara, H. Okamura, T. Hosaka, T. A. Furukawa, and Y. Uchitomi. 2008. Factors correlated with fatigue in terminally ill cancer patients: A longitudinal study. *Journal of Pain and Symptom Management* 35:515–23.

Piper, B. F., A. M. Lindsey, and M. J. Dodd. 1987. Fatigue mechanism in caner patients: Developing nursing theory. *Oncology Nursing Forum* 14:17–23.

Radbruch, L., F. Strasser, F. Elsner, J. F. Goncalves, J. Loge, S. Kaasa, F. Nauck, and P. Stone. 2008. Fatigue in palliative care patients—an EAPC approach. *Palliative Medicine* 22:13–32.

Ryan, J. L., J. K. Carroll, E. P. Ryan, K. M. Mustian, K. Fiscella, and G. R. Morrow. 2007. Mechanisms of cancer-related fatigue. *Oncologist* 12 (Suppl 1): 22–34.

Shun, S. C. 2005. *Psychometric testing of three fatigue instruments with cancer outpatients in Taiwan.* Salt Lake City: College of Nursing, University of Utah.

Sykes, N. P. 1998. Constipation and diarrhea. In *Oxford textbook of palliative medicine,* eds. D. Doyle, G. Hanks, N. I. Cherny, and K. Calman, 513–25. Oxford: Oxford University Press.

Tsai, L. Y., I. F. Li, Y. H. Lai, C. P. Liu, T. Y. Chang, and C. T. Tu. 2007. Fatigue and its associated factors in hospice cancer patients in Taiwan. *Cancer Nursing* 30:24–30.

Winningham, M. L., and M. E. Barton-Burke. 2000. *Fatigue in cancer: A multidimensional approach.* Sudbury: Jones and Bartlett.

Yennurajalingam, S., and E. Bruera. 2007. Palliative management of fatigue at the close of life: It feels like my body is just worn out. *JAMA* 297:295–304.

18 Taste Alteration in Palliative Care

Takumi Kawaguchi, Yumiko Nagao, and Michio Sata

CONTENTS

18.1 INTRODUCTION

Sufficient food intake is indispensable for maintaining nutritional status as well as quality of life in patients with cancer (Kawaguchi et al. 2006). Food intake is affected by multiple factors including sensory properties. Texture, temperature, and appearance of food are properties that regulate food intake (Kawaguchi et al. 2006). In addition, taste is a notable factor in sensory-specific satiety, as shown in Figure 18.1 (Rolls, Hetherington, and Burley 1988).

In patients with cancer, taste alterations are frequently seen because of not only therapeutic intervention such as chemotherapy and radiotherapy, but also cancer itself (Ravasco 2005). Taste alteration causes a decrease in dietary food intake and subsequent malnutrition. Malnutrition is a primary morbidity and has an impact on quality of life in patients with cancer (Ottery 1994). Thus, the management of taste alterations is important in palliative care (Table 18.1).

18.2 TYPES OF TASTE ALTERATIONS

Two types of taste alterations are seen in patients with cancer. Hypogeusia and ageusia are changes in taste acuity. Dysgeusia and phantogeusia are changes in taste quality (Hong et al. 2009) (Table 18.2).

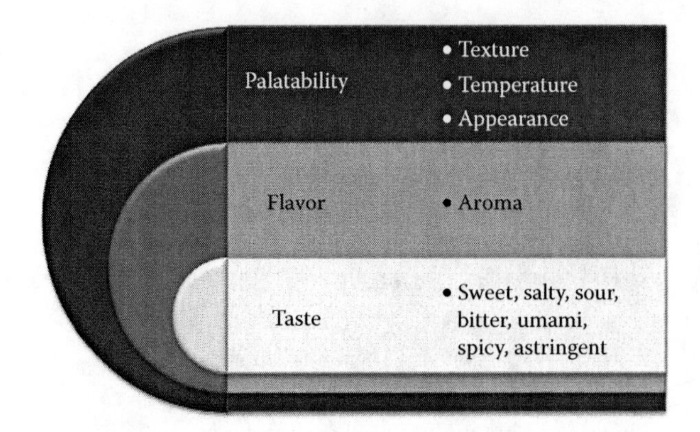

FIGURE 18.1 Factors associated with dietary food intake. This figure shows factors associated with dietary food intake. In addition to taste, flavor and palatability affect dietary food intake.

18.2.1 Assessments of Taste Alteration

Taste alteration is assessed by taste acuity and recognition and detection thresholds are determined for any of the five basic tastes: sweet, sour, salty, bitter, and umami (a Japanese word for delicious) (Wismer 2008). This examination can assess precise taste alteration; however it is not always available for patients in palliative care because of its complicated procedure.

Taste alteration can be assessed by questionnaires. Among a variety of patient-reported tools for taste alteration, the 14-questionnaire scored tool is evaluated in patients with advanced cancer (Hutton, Baracos, and Wismer 2007). The tool shows a significant correlation between the self-perceived chemosensory experience, energy intake, and quality of life (Hutton et al. 2007), suggesting a usefulness in palliative care.

18.2.2 Mechanisms of Taste Alteration

Taste alterations are induced by anticancer therapy and/or cancer itself (Ravasco 2005). Although the mechanisms of taste alteration are largely unknown, impairment of sensory receptor cells and zinc deficiency are well-known causative factors for taste alteration (Hong et al. 2009). Turnover rates of sensory receptor cells for taste are about 7–10 days. Since these high turnover cells are sensitive for radiation and chemotherapy (Hong et al. 2009), anticancer therapy may cause taste alteration. Zinc is a trace element that is involved in the sensitivity of taste (Henkin et al. 1976). Some anticancer agents bind with zinc and inhibit an activation of sensory receptor cells. In addition, a depletion of serum zinc is frequently seen in patients with hypermetabolism, malnutrition, and cachexia (Hong et al. 2009). Abnormalities in digestive

TABLE 18.1
Key Features of Taste

1. Taste is the sense that distinguishes the flavor or savor of dissolved substances by contact with the taste receptors on the tongue
2. Humans can detect seven taste qualities: sweet, sour, salty, bitter, umami, spicy, and astringent
3. Taste alterations are frequently seen in patients with cancer, because of not only therapeutic intervention, but also cancer itself
4. Taste alterations reduce interest in food, resulting in decreased dietary food intake and subsequent malnutrition
5. Malnutrition is a major morbidity and reduces quality of life in patients with cancer

TABLE 18. 2
Definitions of Taste Alterations

Abnormalities	Definition
Changes in taste acuity	
Hypogeusia	Decreased sensitivity to taste perception
Ageusia	Loss of taste perception
Changes in taste quality	
Dysgeusia	Distorted sensitivity to taste perception
Phantogeusa	Perception of metallic or salty taste

tract also affect taste sensitivity and other possible mechanisms of taste alteration are summarized in Table 18.3.

18.3 PRACTICAL METHODS AND TECHNIQUES

18.3.1 Modification of Food

18.3.1.1 Flavors

Since taste is modified by flavors, adding flavor to foods is a strategy to alleviate taste alteration (Schiffman 2007) (Figure 18.2). In patients with breast or lung cancer, aromatic flavors improved nutritional status and physical function compared to those in the control group (Schiffman 2007). In addition, flavoring is reported to enhance patient compliance and quality of life (Steinbach et al. 2009).

18.3.1.2 Palatability

Temperature of food is an important palatability regulating food intake (Smith, Smith, and Houpt 2010) (Figure 18.1). Warming of foods activates thermosensitive molecules in the taste transduction pathway, leading to changes in taste (Ullrich et al. 2005). The bitter taste of the branched-chain amino acids (BCAA)-enriched supplement is significantly improved by prewarming at 60°C compared to that served at 25°C. BCAA is stable at 60°C and warming of food results in an increased calorie intake and improvement of nutritional status in cirrhotic patients with hepatocellular carcinoma (Itou et al. 2009). Texture and appearance of food are also important palatabilities regulating food intake.

TABLE 18.3
Mechanisms of Taste Alteration in Patients with Cancer

Mechanisms
Impairment of sensory receptor cells by anti-cancer therapy
Zinc deficiency
Oral mucositis
Oral infection
Reflux esophagitis
Gastric ulcer
Impairment of peristaltic movement in digestive tract
Impairment of chorda tympani nerve
Changes in tumor necrosis factor-α, interleukin-1β, and interleukin-6
Increased oxidative stress
Cachexia

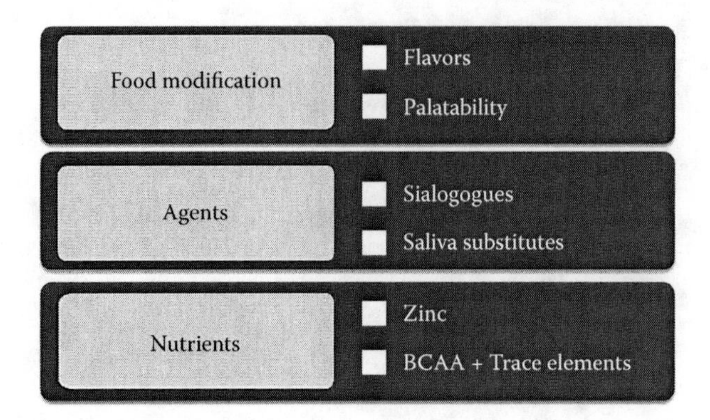

FIGURE 18.2 Therapeutic approach to taste alteration of cancer patients in palliative care. This figure shows a therapeutic approach to taste alteration of cancer patients in palliative care. A holistic approach is recommended in order to alleviate taste alteration.

18.3.2 Agents

18.3.2.1 Sialogogues

Decreased salivary secretion is involved in taste alteration and therefore, sialogogues or saliva substitutes may improve taste alteration. Nizatidine, a histamine H2 receptor antagonist, is known to stimulate salivary secretion. Nizatidine inhibits acetylcholine esterase and subsequently increases acetylcholine, which stimulates muscarinic receptors of salivary glands (Nin et al. 2008). Cevimeline hydrochloride, a muscarinic acetylcholine receptor agonist, increases the salivary flow rate significantly (Vissink et al. 2004). These sialogogues may help patients with preserved salivary gland cells.

Chinese-Japanese herbal medicines are known to stimulate salivary secretion. Byakkokaninjinto increases the expression of aquaporin 5, a regulator of salivary secretion, through activation of muscarinic M3, and stimulates salivary secretion (Yanagi et al. 2008). Bakumondo-to is another Chinese-Japanese herbal medicine, which promotes salivary gland cell proliferation and enlarges the mean size of secretion granules (Kagami et al. 1996). These sialogogues may also have benefit in patients with preserved salivary gland cells.

18.3.2.2 Saliva substitutes

In patients with devastating damage to salivary glands, saliva substitutes are effective for taste alteration. There are now a variety of saliva substitutes available such as gel, carmellose spray, oil, and mucin spray (Momm et al. 2005). Significant benefits of different saliva substitutes on taste alteration are shown in patients treated by radiotherapy for head and neck cancer (Momm et al. 2005). Since palatability differs with each patient and no severe adverse effects of saliva substitutes are reported, testing different saliva substitutes is an effective approach to taste alteration in patients with cancer.

18.3.3 Nutrients

18.3.3.1 Zinc

Zinc is a well-known nutrient associated with taste alteration and zinc supplementation improves taste disorders (Henkin et al. 1976). Although its mechanism remains unclear, zinc plays important roles in the physiology of taste function. Zinc is involved in the synthesis of gustin, a salivary protein regulating taste (Shatzman and Henkin 1981). In patients with cancer, zinc supplementation improves taste disorders in cancer patients treated by chemotherapy (Yamagata et al. 2003). However, it is also reported that zinc does not prevent taste alterations in cancer patients treated by radiotherapy (Halyard et al. 2007). Thus, zinc supplementation does not always improve taste alterations and the effects of zinc on taste may differ with types of cancer, its treatments, or nutritional status.

18.3.3.2 BCAA

BCAA are amino acids that cannot be synthesized endogenously in humans (Kawaguchi, Yamagishi, and Sata 2009). BCAA are constituents of protein and are known to have some relevant pharmacologic properties in muscle-protein synthesis, the immune system, ammonia metabolism, and glucose metabolism (Kawaguchi et al. 2009). Recently, the Department of Digestive Disease Information & Research, Kurume University School of Medicine and Seikatsu Bunkasya Co. Inc. (Tokyo, Japan) developed the BCAA-enriched supplement Aminofeel® (Tokyo, Japan) (Kawaguchi et al. 2007) and found that it improves taste alterations in patients with chronic liver diseases (Nagao et al. 2010). As the supplement contains not only BCAA, but also zinc, the impact of BCAA on alleviation of taste sensitivity remains unclear. However, the effect of zinc on taste improvement is still controversial (Halyard et al. 2007) and BCAA may alleviate taste alteration associated with chronic liver disease. In patients with cancer, decreased serum BCAA levels are frequently seen (Choudry et al. 2006), so BCAA may improve taste alterations in patients with cancer (Kawaguchi et al. 2009). Furthermore, BCAA has an ability to synthesize muscle protein. Moreover, BCAA has the potential to suppress cancer proliferation through improvement of insulin resistance (Kawaguchi et al. 2009). For these reasons, BCAA supplementation is recommended for patients in palliative care.

18.4 CONCLUSION

Taste alteration has a variety of etiologies and therefore the management of taste alteration in palliative care is still challenging. In order to alleviate taste alteration and subsequently improve food intake and quality of life, holistic approaches are needed. In addition, further research into the pathogenesis of and development of new treatments for taste alteration is required.

SUMMARY POINTS

- Since taste alteration is frequently seen in patients with cancer, routine assessment for taste alteration is recommended.
- A variety of etiologies may underlie taste alteration.
- Modification of food is an approach to taste alteration. Use of flavors or warming of food may improve taste alteration.
- Sialogogues and saliva substitutes are useful agents that may have a beneficial effect on taste alteration. Various types of saliva substitutes are now available and it is therefore recommended to test different saliva substitutes.
- Supplementation of zinc may alleviate taste alteration. Aminofeel®, a supplement including BCAA plus trace elements, has the potential to affect taste alteration.

ACKNOWLEDGMENTS

This chapter is based upon work supported in part by a Grant-in-Aid for Young Scientists (B) (No. 19790643 to T.K.), a Grant-in-Aid for Scientific Research (C) (No. 21590865 to M.S.) from the Ministry of Education, Culture, Sports, Science and Technology of Japan, a Health and Labour Sciences Research Grant for Research on Hepatitis from the Ministry of Health, Labour and Welfare of Japan, and a Grant for Cancer Research from the Fukuoka Cancer Society.

LIST OF ABBREVIATION

BCAA Branched-chain amino acids

REFERENCES

Choudry, H. A., M. Pan, A. M. Karinch, and W. W. Souba. (2006). Branched-chain amino acid-enriched nutritional support in surgical and cancer patients. *J Nutr* 136:314S–18S.

Halyard, M. Y., A. Jatoi, J. A. Sloan, J. D. Bearden 3rd, S. A. Vora, P. J. Atherton, E. A. Perez et al. (2007). Does zinc sulfate prevent therapy-induced taste alterations in head and neck cancer patients? Results of phase III double-blind, placebo-controlled trial from the North Central Cancer Treatment Group (N01C4). *Int J Radiat Oncol Biol Phys* 67:1318–22.

Henkin, R. I., P. J. Schecter, W. T. Friedewald, D. L. Demets, and M. Raff. (1976). A double blind study of the effects of zinc sulfate on taste and smell dysfunction. *Am J Med Sci* 272:285–99.

Hong, J. H., P. Omur-Ozbek, B. T. Stanek, A. M. Dietrich, S. E. Duncan, Y. W. Lee, and G. Lesser. (2009). Taste and odor abnormalities in cancer patients. *J Support Oncol* 7:58–65.

Hutton, J. L., V. E. Baracos, and W. V. Wismer. (2007). Chemosensory dysfunction is a primary factor in the evolution of declining nutritional status and quality of life in patients with advanced cancer. *J Pain Symptom Manage* 33:156–65.

Itou, M., T. Kawaguchi, E. Taniguchi, S. Shiraishi, R. Ibi, M. Mutou, T. Okada et al. (2009). Heating improves poor compliance of branched chain amino acids-rich supplementation in patients with liver cirrhosis: A before after pilot study. *Mol Med Report* 2:983–87.

Kagami, H., K. Horie, H. Nishiguchi, T. Shigetomi, and M. Ueda. (1996). Effect of 'bakumondo-to', a Chinese-Japanese herbal medicine, on cultured and dispersed salivary gland cells. *J Ethnopharmacol* 53:89–95.

Kawaguchi, T., E. Taniguchi, M. Itou, J. Akiyoshi, S. Itano, M. Otsuka, S. Iwasaki et al. (2006). Appearance-specific satiety increases appetite and quality of life in patients with metastatic liver tumor: A case report. *Kurume Med J* 53:41–46.

Kawaguchi, T., E. Taniguchi, M. Itou, S. Sumie, T. Oriishi, H. Matsuoka, Y. Nagao, and M. Sata. (2007). Branched-chain amino acids improve insulin resistance in patients with hepatitis C virus-related liver disease: Report of two cases. *Liver Int* 27:1287–92.

Kawaguchi, T., S. Yamagishi, and M. Sata. (2009). Branched-chain amino acids and pigment epithelium-derived factor: Novel therapeutic agents for hepatitis C virus-associated insulin resistance. *Curr Med Chem* 16:4843–57.

Momm, F., N. J. Volegova-Neher, J. Schulte-Monting, and R. Guttenberger. (2005). Different saliva substitutes for treatment of xerostomia following radiotherapy. A prospective crossover study. *Strahlenther Onkol* 181:231–36.

Nagao, Y., H. Matsuoka, T. Kawaguchi, and M. Sata. (2010). Aminofeel® improves the sensitivity to taste in patients with HCV-infected liver disease. *Med Sci Monit* (in press).

Nin, T., M. Umemoto, A. Negoro, S. Miuchi, and M. Sakagami. (2008). Nizatidine enhances salivary secretion in patients with dry mouth. *Auris Nasus Larynx* 35:224–29.

Ottery, F. D. (1994). Cancer cachexia: Prevention, early diagnosis, and management. *Cancer Pract* 2:123–31.

Ravasco, P. (2005). Aspects of taste and compliance in patients with cancer. *Eur J Oncol Nurs* 9 (Suppl 2): S84–91.

Rolls, B. J., M. Hetherington, and V. J. Burley. (1988). Sensory stimulation and energy density in the development of satiety. *Physiol Behav* 44:727–33.

Schiffman, S. S. (2007). Critical illness and changes in sensory perception. *Proc Nutr Soc* 66:331–45.

Shatzman, A. R., and R. I. Henkin. (1981). Gustin concentration changes relative to salivary zinc and taste in humans. *Proc Natl Acad Sci U S A* 78:3867–71.

Smith, P. L., J. C. Smith, and T. A. Houpt. (2010). Interactions of temperature and taste in conditioned aversions. *Physiol Behav* 99:324–33.

Steinbach, S., T. Hummel, C. Bohner, S. Berktold, W. Hundt, M. Kriner, P. Heinrich et al. (2009). Qualitative and quantitative assessment of taste and smell changes in patients undergoing chemotherapy for breast cancer or gynecologic malignancies. *J Clin Oncol* 27:1899–905.

Ullrich, N. D., T. Voets, J. Prenen, R. Vennekens, K. Talavera, G. Droogmans, and B. Nilius. (2005). Comparison of functional properties of the Ca2+-activated cation channels TRPM4 and TRPM5 from mice. *Cell Calcium* 37:267–78.

Vissink, A., F. R. Burlage, F. K. Spijkervet, E. C. Veerman, and A. V. Nieuw Amerongen. (2004). Prevention and treatment of salivary gland hypofunction related to head and neck radiation therapy and chemotherapy. *Support Cancer Ther* 1:111–18.

Wismer, W. V. (2008). Assessing alterations in taste and their impact on cancer care. *Curr Opin Support Palliat Care* 2:282–87.

Yamagata, T., Y. Nakamura, Y. Yamagata, M. Nakanishi, K. Matsunaga, H. Nakanishi, T. Nishimoto, Y. Minakata, M. Mune, and S. Yukawa. (2003). The pilot trial of the prevention of the increase in electrical taste thresholds by zinc containing fluid infusion during chemotherapy to treat primary lung cancer. *J Exp Clin Cancer* Res 22:557–63.

Yanagi, Y., M. Yasuda, K. Hashida, Y. Kadokura, T. Yamamoto, and H. Suzaki. (2008). Mechanism of salivary secretion enhancement by Byakkokaninjinto. *Biol Pharm Bull* 31:431–35.

19 Olfaction in Palliative Care Patients

Arkadi Yakirevitch, Michaela Bercovici, and Yoav P. Talmi

CONTENTS

19.1 INTRODUCTION

Smell and taste play a role in appetite, food choices, and nutrient intake for the following reasons: First, these chemosensory signals prepare the body to digest food by triggering salivary, gastric, pancreatic, and intestinal secretions which are termed cephalic phase responses. Second, they enable us to detect and discriminate between foods in the face of fluctuating nutritional requirements. Third, they enable selection of a nutritious diet. Learned associations between a food's smell and taste and its postingestive effects enable the consumer to modulate food intake in anticipation of its nutritional consequences. Fourth, taste and smell signals initiate, sustain and terminate ingestion, and hence play a major role in the quantity of food that is eaten and the size of meals. Fifth, taste sensations induce feelings of satiety and are primary reinforcers of eating. Thus, chemosensory impairments can alter food choices and intake and subsequently exacerbate disease states (Table 19.1).

Olfactory impairment increases a patient's perception of disability and negatively impacts quality of life. In a 14-year study of approximately 1400 patients, self-reported "satisfaction with life" was inversely related to degree of subjective olfactory loss (Miwa et al. 2001). Heald, Piper, and Schiffman (1998) found that chemosensory distortion, assessed in 207 HIV-infected patients, was associated with decreased quality of life in all measured domains. Medicine specialists in endocrinology, nutrition support services, surgery, and oncology are well aware that severe chemosensory dysfunction is a primary factor in the development of anorexia, malnutrition, and wasting (Hutton, Baracos, and Wisner 2007). Though the majority of research on chemosensory perception in cancer patients has examined the direct effects of anticancer therapies such as radiation and chemotherapy, this symptom is frequently cited among patients with advanced cancer for whom curative therapies have been discontinued in favor of palliative care (Yakirevitch et al. 2006). Hutton et al. found that among palliative care oncological patients, individuals experiencing a greater number of chemosensory abnormalities ingested fewer calories. Chemosensory complaint score was negatively associated with global quality of life and in particular with the physical well-being and anorexia-cachexia-related nutritional well-being (Hutton et al. 2007). In this study, 8% of patients with chemosensory complaints rated their abnormal sense of smell as "severe" or "incapacitating." Additionally, malnutrition frequently contributes to the cause of death in patients with cancer; as many as 20% of patients succumb to progressive nutritional deterioration rather than to the malignancy per se (Ottery 1997).

TABLE 19.1
Features of Olfactory Function

1. Humans can smell 4000–10,000 odors
2. Each odorant activates a unique set of olfactory receptors called a "signature"
3. One thousand genes participate in coding of the odor receptors
4. Olfactory receptor cells are true, bipolar neurons. These are the only neurons capable of regeneration, with an average lifespan of 30 days
5. The anatomical projection of the olfactory pathway to the hypothalamus emphasizes the importance of olfaction in eating and nutrition
6. Olfaction is thought to be a "synthetic" sense: its individual components blend, creating a holistic sensation different from any of the distinct, individual components
7. Any interference with olfaction can have an impact on taste, because up to 80% of the taste of a meal is related to how it smells

19.2 BIOLOGY OF OLFACTION

The sense of smell originates in the superior region of the nasal cavity, where the olfactory epithelium lies. Several important cell types make up this pseudostratified columnar epithelium. At the base is a thin layer of basal cells that divide and differentiate throughout life, regenerating the other cell types. Throughout the epithelium are supporting cells that are believed to play a maintenance role, although their exact function remains unclear. Scattered within the olfactory epithelium are specialized glands known as Bowman's glands that secrete thin, watery mucus that protects the epithelial surface while providing a medium for odorant molecules to act. The majority of cells in this epithelium, however, are the olfactory receptor cells, with an average lifespan of 30 days. Olfactory neurons are capable of regeneration; however, the degree of regeneration depends upon the severity of damage.

Unlike taste receptor cells, olfactory receptor cells are true first-order neurons and collectively make up the first cranial nerve, providing a direct conduit from the olfactory receptor to the central nervous system. From each of these bipolar cells, a dendrite extends apically to the surface of the epithelium, giving rise to an olfactory knob. Long, nonmotile cilia project from these knobs into the nasal cavity, creating a large surface area for odorant molecules to bind to and interact. Within the membranes of these cilia are the olfactory receptor proteins, a diverse family of G-protein-coupled receptors encoded by the largest gene family in the human genome. Odorant molecules dissolve within the nasal mucus and then bind to one of these G-protein-coupled receptors. Activation of the G-protein leads to depolarization of the ciliary membrane. Resulting action potentials travel through slow unmyelinated axons that extend in fascicles through the cribriform plate to the paired olfactory bulbs (Figure 19.1). Within the bulbs, the axons synapse with mitral and tufted cells. These second-order neurons then project ipsilaterally to form the bilateral olfactory tracts. They convey olfactory information to multiple areas of the central nervous system that together comprise the primary olfactory cortex. These areas consist primarily of the piriform cortex, the amygdala, and the rostral entorhinal cortex. From the primary olfactory cortex, higher-order projections extend to form a complex web of connections with other areas of the brain, including the orbitofrontal cortex, thalamus, hypothalamus, basal ganglia, and hippocampus, all of which act together to create the perception of smell. The anatomical projection to the hypothalamus emphasizes the importance of olfaction in eating and nutrition.

Olfaction is generally thought to be a "synthetic" sense: its individual components blend, creating a holistic sensation different from any of the distinct, individual components.

Any interference with olfaction can also have an impact on taste, because up to 80% of the taste of a meal is related to how it smells (Wrobel and Leopold 2004).

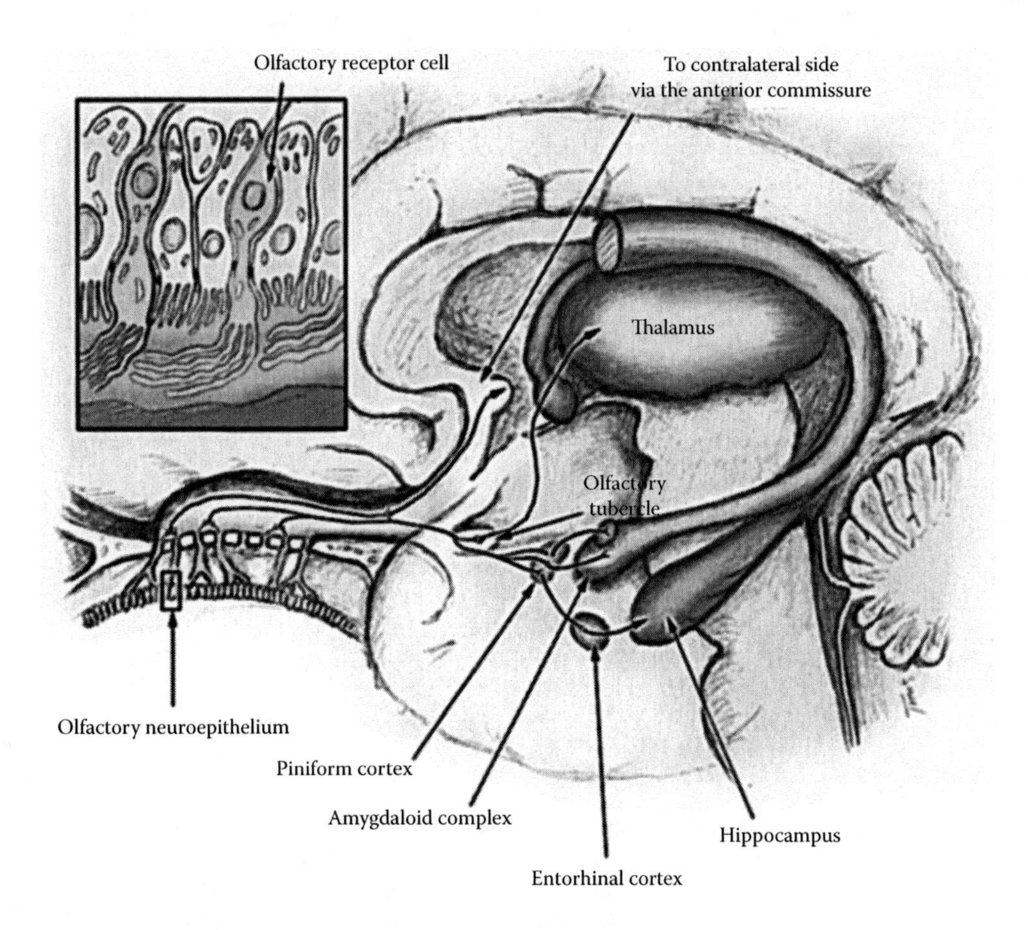

FIGURE 19.1 Olfactory pathway. (Reprinted with permission from eMedicine.com, 2010. Available at: http://emedicine.medscape.com/article/861242-overview.)

19.3 CAUSES OF IMPAIRED OLFACTION

Losses in smell perception result from normal aging, certain disease states (especially cancer, Alzheimer's and Parkinson's disease), medications, viral insult, malnutrition, head trauma, surgical interventions, and environmental exposure (Table 19.2 shows representative medical conditions that affect the senses of taste or smell). As the majority of palliative care patients are elderly individuals, aging has a greater role in chemosensory deterioration in this cohort. Most research suggests that the sense of smell is even more impaired by aging than the sense of taste. Olfactory losses occur at both threshold and suprathreshold levels (Lafreniere and Mann 2009).

Cancer is an example of a chronic medical condition in which patients are vulnerable to taste and smell disorders. Taste and smell changes are found in untreated patients (Ovesen et al. 1991) as well as patients treated with chemotherapy (Bernhardson, Tishelman, and Rutqvist 2009), radiation (Hölscher et al. 2005), and immunotherapy. The data suggest that cancer and its treatment impair the ability to detect the presence of basic tastes, reduce the perceived intensity of suprathreshold concentrations of tastants, and interfere with the ability to discriminate and identify tastes and smells. Furthermore, the data suggest that 50% or more of cancer patients may have impaired taste and smell functioning at some point during the course of their disease and treatment (DeWys and Walters 1975). There appears to be individual variability in the time course of recovery (if any), with the duration of losses ranging from several weeks to 6 months or longer (Ophir, Guterman, and Gross-Isseroff 1988).

TABLE 19.2
Representative Medical Conditions That Affect the Senses of Taste or Smell

Nervous	Alzheimer's disease
	Bell's palsy
	Damage to chorda tympani
	Epilepsy
	Head trauma
	Korsakoff's syndrome
	Multiple sclerosis
	Parkinson's disease
	Tumors and lesions
Nutritional	Cancer
	Chronic renal failure
	Liver disease including cirrhosis
	Niacin (vitamin B3) deficiency
	Vitamin B12 deficiency
	Zinc deficiency
Endocrine	Adrenal cortical insufficiency
	Congenital adrenal hyperplasia
	Panhypopituitarism
	Cushing's syndrome
	Diabetes mellitus
	Hypothyroidism
	Kallman's syndrome
	Pseudohypoparathyroidism
	Turner's syndrome
Local	Allergic rhinitis, atopy, bronchial asthma
	Sinusitis and polyposis
	Xerostomic conditions including Sjogren's syndrome
Viral infections	Acute viral hepatitis
	Influenza-like infections

Source: Data from Schiffman, S. S., and B. G. Graham, *Eur. J. Clin. Nutr.* 54, S54, 2000. With permission.

Possible mechanisms of altered smell in cancer include direct neurotoxic effects on the olfactory epithelium, demyelination of nerve fibers, immunologic inflammatory reactions, or even microvascular injuries. Altered neurotransmitter levels could constitute an additional mechanism leading to chemosensory disorders.

In addition to the direct effects of cancer therapies on the olfactory pathway, any obstruction of airflow by cancer in the nasal cavity or by surgical intervention can have an impact on smelling. Surgery can profoundly alter this sense via a variety of mechanisms, such as resection of portions of the oral or nasal cavity (Biazevic et al. 2008). Oral complications of cancer such as infections (fungal, viral, bacterial), ulcers, drug-induced stomatitis, and dry mouth may also play a role. On the contrary, one should avoid automatically blaming any antineoplastic therapy for chemosensory disorders (as, for example, cisplatinum was not found to cause olfactory deterioration) (Yakirevitch et al. 2005) and should rule out other possible causes.

There are several origins of the food aversions reported by cancer patients. First, impaired taste and smell alter the sensations derived from food. Second, food aversions can be learned during the course of cancer when sensory properties of foods are associated with gastrointestinal distress (e.g., nausea) of therapy (Andrykowski and Otis 1990). Learned aversions and decreased food preferences can persist long after all symptoms of discomfort have subsided.

Cirrhosis of the liver has been reported to be accompanied by olfactory loss. According to the study of Temmel et al. (2005), olfactory function was compromised in 76% of cirrhosis patients. A significant rate of olfactory loss (56%) was also found among the patients with chronic renal failure (Frasnelli et al. 2002).

Drugs in many major pharmacological categories (dopaminergic antagonists, gamma-aminobutyric acid (GABA)-ergic agonists, calcium channel blockers and some orally active local anesthetic, antiarrhythmic drugs) can impair olfactory function (Henkin 1994) and do so more commonly than presently appreciated (Table 19.3 shows some medications that were reported to alter smell and/or taste). Impairment usually affects sensory function at a molecular level by drug inactivation of receptor function through inhibition of tastant/odorant receptor, causing two major behavioral changes:

TABLE 19.3
Medications That Reportedly Alter Smell and/or Taste[a]

Drug Class	Agent
Antianxiety agents	Alprazolam, buspirone, flurazepam
Antibacterials	Ampicillin, azithromycin, ciprofloxacin, clarithromycin, enoxacin, ethambutol,metronidazole, ofloxacin, sulfamethoxazole, ticarcillin, tetracycline
Antidepressants	Amitriptyline, clomipramine, desipramine, doxepin, imipramine, nortriptyline
Antiepileptic drugs	Carbamazepine, phenytoin, topiramate
Antifungals	Griseofulvin, terbinafine
Antihistamines and decongestants	Chlorphenamine, loratadine, pseudoephedrine
Antihypertensives and cardiac medications	Acetazolamide, amiodarone, amiloride, amiodarone, bepridil, betaxolol, captopril, diltiazem, enalapril, hydrochlorothiazide, losartan, nifedipine, nisoldipine, nitroglycerin, propafenone, propranolol, spironolactone, tocainide
Anti-inflammatory agents	Auranofin, beclometasone, budesonide, colchicine, dexamethasone, flunisolide, fluticasone propionate, gold, penicillamine
Antimanic drugs	Lithium
Antimigraine agents	Dihydroergotamine mesilate, naratriptan, rizatriptan, sumatriptan
Antineoplastics	Carboplatin, cyclophosphamide, doxorubicin, fluorouracil, levamisole,methotrexate, tegafur, vincristine
Antiparkinsonian agents	Anticholinergics, levodopa
Antipsychotics	Clozapine, trifluoperazine
Antiviral agents	Acyclovir, amantadine, gancyclovir, interferon, pirodavir, oseltamivir, zaicitabine
Bronchodilators	Bitolterol, pirbuterol
CNS stimulants	Amfetamine, dexamfetamine, methylphenidate
Hypnotics	Eszopiclone, zolpidem
Lipid-lowering agents	Atorvastatin, fluvastatln, lovastatin, pravastatin
Muscle relaxants	Baclofen, dantrolene
Pancreatic enzyme preparations	Pancrelipase
Smoking cessation aids	Nicotine
Thyroid drugs	Carbimazole, levothyroxine sodium and related compounds, propylthiouracil, thiamazole

Source: Data from Doty, R. L. et al., *Drug Safety* 31, 199, 2008 with permission from Wolters Kluwer Pharma Solutions.

[a] The evidence for the involvement of many of these drugs in chemosensory disturbance comes from the Physicians' Desk Reference.

TABLE 19.4
Odor-Related Abnormalities

Anosmia	Absence of odor perception
Hyposmia	Decreased sensitivity to odor perception
Dysosmia	Distorted ability to identify odors
Agnosia	Inability to discriminate perceived odors
Parosmia	Altered odor perception in the presence of another odor
Phantosmia	Odor perception without the presence of any odor

loss of acuity (i.e., hyposmia) and/or distortion of function (i.e., dysosmia) (Table 19.4). These changes can impair appetite and food intake, cause significant lifestyle changes and may require discontinuation of drug administration. Some sleep-inducing agents are associated with taste and, in rare instances, have smell disturbances as potential adverse effects. Zolpidem is listed in the Physicians' Desk Reference as producing "taste perversion" and, more infrequently, "parosmia" (Physicians' Desk Reference 2005). Eszopiclone, a nonbenzodiazepine pyrrolopyrazine derivative of the cyclopyrrolone class, is associated with complaints of "unpleasant taste" (Krystal et al. 2003).

Patients who have had a laryngectomy have a severely reduced sense of smell because they cannot draw air into the nose for detection of odorants because they breathe through the neck. The same applies for every tracheotomized individual. Weaning a patient from tube feeding, obstructive effect of the nasogastric tube should not be overlooked, especially because it is usually placed through the wide side of the nose, dominant also in smell perception.

Among hospice patients who were previous or current smokers, the rate of olfactory function impairment was found to be higher than among nonsmokers (Yakirevitch et al. 2006).

Parosmia is perception of odors that do not really exist. It may or may not be accompanied by decreased olfactory thresholds, and is typically unpleasant and very bothersome. Although the molecular mechanisms leading to parosmia and even the site of the generation (olfactory epithelium, olfactory bulb, and higher central structures) are still unknown, it may be hypothesized that a decrease in the number of olfactory bulb neurons is associated with generation of parosmia (Leopold 2002). A possible mechanism could be the decreased number of olfactory bulb interneurons, resulting in a decrease of lateral inhibition (Mori, Nagao, and Yoshihara 1999). In turn, this may allow olfactory activation to produce an irregular pattern that may result in a "parosmic" sensation.

19.4 PRACTICAL METHODS AND TECHNIQUES

The goals of nutritional intervention in palliative care are to support nutritional status, immune function, body composition, functional status, and quality of life. Understanding and addressing the relationship between abnormal chemosensory function and dietary intake has the potential to improve food enjoyment and nutritional status in palliative care patients. This has been demonstrated in the elderly, for whom the sensory enhancement of foods resulted in increased dietary intake and improved functional status. Recognizing that taste and smell abnormalities are also related to food preference, dietary interventions catering to the unique preferences and chemosensory capacities of palliative care patients may result in improved dietary intake (Hutton et al. 2007). Currently the recommendations include:

- Eating a balanced and nutritious diet with adequate calories
- Avoiding the use of metallic silverware to reduce the risk of metallic taste
- Reducing the consumption of foods that taste metallic or bitter, such as red meat, coffee, or tea, and increasing the consumption of high-protein, mildly flavored foods, such as chicken, fish, dairy products, and eggs
- Serving foods at cold temperature to reduce unpleasant flavors and odors

- Practicing good oral hygiene, including frequent tooth brushing and use of mouthwash
- Using sialogogues (agents that stimulate salivary secretion), such as sugar-free gums or sour-tasting drops
- Using saliva substitutes and lubricating solutions containing mucin and carboxymethylcellulose
- Adding seasonings and spices
- Utilizing flavors

Flavors are mixtures of odorous molecules that can be extracted or blended from natural products, or they can be synthesized based on chromatographic and mass spectrographic analysis of natural products. Flavors in some cases also contain nonvolatile compounds such as amino acid salts (e.g., monosodium glutamate) that induce taste stimulation. Flavors can be added to food prior to, during, or after cooking. For example, simulated beef flavor can be added to beef or beef stock to provide a more intense "beef" sensation. Flavors are analogous to concentrated orange juice or extract of vanilla. Flavor enhancement differs from more traditional methods of increasing odor and taste sensations using spices, herbs, and salt. Spices and herbs contribute different flavors to the food rather than intensify actual food flavors. The studies indicate that flavor-enhanced foods are preferred by frail and sick elderly and can improve immunity, quality of life, and functional status (Schiffman and Warwick 1993).

Enteral artificial highly caloric nutritional supplements have an increasing role in palliative care. It has to be kept in mind that, like parenteral products, they may also suffer from inadequate formulation and chemosensory problems. They often have unpleasant tastes and can cause esophageal reflux, especially in bedridden patients.

When drug therapy is responsible for chemosensory disorders, its termination is commonly associated with termination of taste/smell dysfunction, but occasionally effects persist and require specific therapy to alleviate symptoms.

As noted previously, tracheotomized patients are unable to smell naturally because they cannot draw air into the nose. To overcome this problem a laryngeal bypass with the use of plastic tubing was proposed (Göktas et al. 2008). In addition to this, another method of olfactory rehabilitation described in the literature is "polite yawning." This maneuver involves inhaling through the nose with the teeth apart but the lips closed. Olfactory rehabilitation was reported as successful in up to 83% of laryngectomies with this maneuver (Risberg-Berlin, Möller, and Finizia 2007).

Based on the observation that parosmia is a distorted sense of smell, it can be neutralized with voluntary decrease of olfaction. For example, Müller et al. (2006) opted for a simple nasal clip interrupting ortho- and retronasal olfaction and, thus, reducing parosmia, which promptly increased food intake.

SUMMARY POINTS

- Olfactory dysfunction is an important cause of nutrition problems in palliative care patients.
- Smell disorder may result from normal aging, cancer, organic diseases of the central neural system, medications, viral insult, obstruction or bypass of nasal airflow, and environmental exposure.
- Although this does not address its causes, olfactory dysfunction may be compensated for by sensory enhancement of food and avoiding unpleasant odors.

REFERENCES

Andrykowski, M. A., and M. L. Otis. 1990. Development of learned food aversions in humans: Investigation in a "natural laboratory" of cancer chemotherapy. *Appetite* 14:145–58.

Bernhardson, B. M., C. Tishelman, and L. E. Rutqvist. 2009. Olfactory changes among patients receiving chemotherapy. *Eur J Oncol Nurs* 13:9–15.

Biazevic, M. G., J. L. Antunes, J. Togni, F. P. de Andrade, M. B. de Carvalho, and V. Wünsch-Filho. 2008. Immediate impact of primary surgery on health-related quality of life of hospitalized patients with oral and oropharyngeal cancer. *J Oral Maxillofac Surg* 66:1343–50.

DeWys, W. D., and K. Walters. 1975. Abnormalities of taste sensation in cancer patients. *Cancer* 36:1888–96.

Frasnelli, J. A., A. F. Temmel, C. Quint, R. Oberbauer, and T. Hummel. 2002. Olfactory function in chronic renal failure. *Am J Rhinol* 16:275–79.

Göktas, O., F. Fleiner, C. Paschen, I. Lammert, and T. Schrom. 2008. Rehabilitation of the olfactory sense after laryngectomy: Long-term use of the larynx bypass. *Ear Nose Throat J* 87:528–30.

Heald, A. E., C. F. Pieper, and S. S. Schiffman. 1998. Taste and smell complaints in HIV-infected patients. *AIDS* 12:1667–74.

Henkin, R. I. 1994. Drug-induced taste and smell disorders. Incidence, mechanisms and management related primarily to treatment of sensory receptor dysfunction. *Drug Saf* 11:318–77.

Hölscher, T., A. Seibt, S. Appold, W. Dörr, T. Herrmann, K.-B. Hüttenbrink, and T. Hummel. 2005. Effects of radiotherapy on olfactory function. *Radiother Oncol* 77:157–63.

Hutton, J. L., V. E. Baracos, and W. V. Wismer. 2007. Chemosensory dysfunction is a primary factor in the evolution of declining nutritional status and quality of life in patients with advanced cancer. *J Pain Symptom Manage* 33:156–65.

Krystal, A. D., J. K. Walsh, E. Laska, J. Caron, D. A. Amato, T. C. Wessel, and T. Roth. 2003. Sustained efficacy of eszopiclone over 6 months of nightly treatment: results of a randomized, double-blind, placebo-controlled study in adults with chronic insomnia. *Sleep* 26:793–99.

Lafreniere, D., and N. Mann. 2009. Anosmia: Loss of smell in the elderly. *Otolaryngol Clin North Am* 42:123–31.

Leopold, D. 2002. Distortion of olfactory perception: Diagnosis and treatment. *Chem Senses* 27:611–15.

Miwa, T., M. Furukawa, T. Tsukatani, R. M. Costanzo, L. J. DiNardo, and E. R. Reiter. 2001. Impact of olfactory impairment on quality of life and disability. *Arch Otolaryngol Head Neck Surg* 127:497–503.

Mori, K., H. Nagao, and Y. Yoshihara. 1999. The olfactory bulb: coding and processing of odor molecule information. *Science* 286:711–15.

Müller, A., B. N. Landis, U. Platzbecker, V. Holthoff, J. Frasnelli, and T. Hummel. 2006. Severe chemotherapy-induced parosmia. *Am J Rhinol* 20:485–86.

Ophir, D., A. Guterman, and R. Gross-Isseroff. 1988. Changes in smell acuity induced by radiation exposure of the olfactory mucosa. *Arch Otolaryngol Head Neck Surg* 114:853–55.

Ottery, F. D. 1997. Nutritional oncology: A proactive, integrated approach to the cancer patient. In *Nutrition support: Theory and therapeutic,* eds. S. A. Shikora, and G. L. Blackburn, 395–409. New York, NY: Chapman & Hall.

Ovesen, L., M. Sørensen, J. Hannibal, and L. Allingstrup. 1991. Electrical taste detection thresholds and chemical smell detection thresholds in patients with cancer. *Cancer* 68:2260–65.

Physicians' Desk Reference. 2005. Montvale, NJ: Medical Economics Company, Inc.

Risberg-Berlin, B., R. Y. Möller, and C. Finizia. 2007. Effectiveness of olfactory rehabilitation with the nasal airflow-inducing maneuver after total laryngectomy: one-year follow-up study. *Arch Otolaryngol Head Neck Surg* 133:650–54.

Schiffman, S. S., and Z. S. Warwick. 1993. Effect of flavor enhancement of foods for the elderly on nutritional status: Food intake, biochemical indices, and anthropometric measures. *Physiol Behav* 53:395–402.

Temmel, A. F., S. Pabinger, C. Quint, P. Munda, P. Ferenci, T. Hummel. 2005. Dysfunction of the liver affects the sense of smell. *Wien Klin Wochenschr* 117:26–30.

Wrobel, B. B., and D. A. Leopold. 2004. Clinical assessment of patients with smell and taste disorders. *Otolaryngol Clin North Am* 37:1127–42.

Yakirevitch, A., M. Bercovici, L. Migirov, A. Adunsky, M. R. Pfeffer, J. Kronenberg, Y. P. Talmi. 2006. Olfactory function in oncologic hospice patients. *J Palliat Med* 9:57–60.

Yakirevitch, A., Y. P. Talmi, Y. Baram, R. Weitzen, and M. R. Pfeffer. 2005. Effects of cisplatin on olfactory function in cancer patients. *Br J Cancer* 92:1611–13.

20 Withholding or Withdrawing Nutritional Support at the End-of-Life in Six European Countries*

Hilde M. Buiting, Johannes J. M. van Delden, Judith A. C. Rietjens, Bregje D. Onwuteaka-Philipsen, Johan Bilsen, Susanne Fischer, Rurik Löfmark, Guido Miccinesi, Michael Norup, and Agnes van der Heide

CONTENTS

* Largely reprinted from 'Journal of Pain and Symptom Management,' 34, No 3. Hilde M. Buiting, Johannes J. M. van Delden, Judith A. C. Rietjens, Bregje D. Onwuteaka-Philipsen, Johan Bilsen, Susanne Fischer, Rurik Löfmark, Guido Miccinesi, Michael Rurup, Agnes van der Heide: 'Forgoing artificial nutrition and hydration in patients nearing death in six European countries,' 10 pages, Copyright (2007), with permission from Elsevier.

20.1 INTRODUCTION

In patients nearing death, decisions to withhold or withdraw potentially life-prolonging treatments are frequently made (Bilsen et al. 2009; Seale 2006; van der Heide et al. 2003; van der Heide et al. 2007). Treatments may include high-technology interventions such as dialysis or surgery, but may also concern more basic treatments like the artificial administration of nutrition or hydration (ANH) (Bosshard et al. 2005).

The appropriate use of ANH, especially in patients who cannot express their own wishes anymore (e.g., patients with advanced dementia), continues to be a subject of debate in several countries (Bell et al. 2008; Finucane, Christmas, and Travis 1999). One argument for providing ANH in every case of possible dehydration or malnutrition is that it is a form of basic care that should not be denied to anyone. This perspective is deeply rooted in cultural and religious beliefs and, accordingly, a perspective that probably widely varies across countries (Helman 2000; Pope John Paul II 2004). On the other hand, it is also argued that even basic care can become disproportional under special circumstances (Beauchamp and Childress 2001), such as in terminally ill patients with advanced dementia. Others claim that forgoing ANH is wrong because dying from thirst and hunger is inhumane. Expressed concerns that the patient may starve to death when physicians abstain from ANH have frequently been posed by the attending physicians as well as closely related family members (van der Riet, Brooks, and Ashby 2006). However, there is no clear evidence that forgoing ANH causes discomfort in patients who are in their last phase of life and have no more feelings of hunger or thirst (McCann, Hall, and Groth-Juncker 1994).

Empirical studies on the practice of forgoing ANH in terminally ill patients are often limited to specific clinical settings or countries (McCann et al. 1994; Onwuteaka-Philipsen et al. 2001). More insight into this practice in different settings and countries would contribute to the debate on whether and when providing ANH to severely ill patients should be regarded as disproportionate care.

20.2 NATION-WIDE DEATH CERTIFICATE STUDIES

Between June 2001 and February 2002, nation-wide frequencies and characteristics of the practice of forgoing ANH were studied in Belgium, Denmark, Italy, the Netherlands, Sweden and Switzerland by obtaining random samples of death certificates of deceased persons aged one year or older from death registries to which all deaths are reported (Buiting et al. 2007; van der Heide et al. 2003). All physicians attending a death case—unless the cause of death precluded an end-of-life decision (ELD)—received a written questionnaire. The anonymity of physicians and patients was guaranteed. Questionnaire response percentages were 59% for Belgium, 62% for Denmark, 44% for Italy, 61% for Sweden, 67% for Switzerland and 75% for the Netherlands. The questionnaire focused on characteristics of end-of-life decisions, like the forgoing of ANH that preceded the patient's death. In all studies, ELDs were characterised by whether the act involved an act or omission, the intention of the physician, the effect of the act and the involvement of the patient. ELDs were classified in five categories (Box 20.1). The forgoing of ANH belongs to the fifth category.

BOX 20.1 MEDICAL END-OF-LIFE DECISIONS

1. Euthanasia
   The administration of drugs with the explicit intention of hastening death at the patient's explicit request.
2. Physician-assisted suicide
   The prescription or supply of drugs with the explicit intention to enable the patient to end his or her own life.

3. Ending of life without an explicit patient request
   The administration of drugs with the explicit intention of hastening death without an explicit patient request.
4. Alleviation of pain and symptoms
   In dosages which are large enough to include the hastening of death as a likely or certain side effect.
5. Forgoing potentially life-prolonging treatment
   Withholding or withdrawing medical treatment while taking into account or explicitly intending (potential) hastening of death.

20.2.1 Frequencies of Withholding or Withdrawing ANH in Six West European Countries

The percentage of deaths that were preceded by decisions to withhold or withdraw any potentially life-prolonging treatment varied between 6.3% of all deaths in Italy and 41% of all deaths in Switzerland (Table 20.1). Table 20.1 shows that the rate of forgoing ANH significantly varies between countries: a decision to forgo ANH was made least often in Italy (2.6% of all deaths) and most often in Switzerland (9.9%) and the Netherlands (10.9%). In all countries, ANH was more frequently withheld than withdrawn; this was especially the case for Switzerland (8.5% and 1.7%, respectively). This may in part be due to the fact that forgoing ANH may not always be perceived as explicitly refraining from potentially life-prolonging treatment. The frequency of withholding ANH is more likely to be affected by differences in physicians' awareness of their end-of-life decision-making practices than the frequency of withdrawing ANH, since the latter is more easily perceived as causing death (Farber et al. 2006). However, the difference between all countries in the appreciation of withholding and withdrawing treatment could also be indicative of a real difference in occurrence, which would be consistent with other studies (Le Conte et al. 2004; Yazigi, Riachi, and Dabbar 2005). The relatively high frequency in the Netherlands may be related to the open culture towards end-of-life decision-making there. In the Netherlands, providing ANH to dying patients is often seen as disproportional care: it is frequently considered to only prolong the dying phase and to postpone death (Sheldon 1997). The particularly low percentage of forgoing ANH (2.6%) in Italy is in accordance with the low percentage of decisions to forgo any type of life-prolonging treatment in this country (6.3%). This could be related to the fact that Italy in particular has a strong Catholic tradition and a widespread acceptance of the idea that life is sacred and should be preserved at all costs.

20.2.2 Characteristics of Patients in Whom ANH was Forgone in Six West European Countries

Table 20.2 shows the characteristics of patients in the terminal stage of a disease in whom ANH had been forgone. In all countries, ANH had been forgone in patients in all age groups, but most often in patients who were 80 years or older: percentages for this age group ranged from 1.5% in Italy up to 6.7% in the Netherlands. In all countries, percentages of forgoing ANH were higher among female patients compared to male patients, particularly in Belgium (4.5%), Switzerland (5.9%) and the Netherlands (7.1%). A decision to forgo ANH was most frequently made for patients who died in places other than the hospital, except for Sweden. In Denmark, the Netherlands, Sweden and Switzerland, when place of death could be further distinguished, ANH was most often forgone in nursing homes or homes for the elderly (2.1% in Denmark and up to 5.6% of all deaths in the Netherlands). Decisions to forgo ANH were made relatively often for patients who died from a malignancy or a disease of the nervous system. Furthermore, multiple logistic regression showed

TABLE 20.1
Frequencies of the Decision to Forgo Artificial Nutrition or Hydration (ANH) in Six European Countries (Weighted Percentages)

	Country					
	Belgium	**Denmark**	**Italy**	**Netherlands**	**Sweden**	**Switzerland**
Number of studied deaths	$n = 2950$	$n = 2939$	$n = 2604$	$n = 5384$	$n = 3248$	$n = 3355$
Sudden death	34	33	29	33	30	32
Nonsudden death not preceded by an ELD[a]	27	26	48	23	34	17
Nonsudden death preceded by an ELD	38	41	23	44	36	51
Treatment forgone[b,c]	27	23	6.3	30	22	41
ANH forgone[b] (95% CI)	7.2 (6.4–8.2)	4.7 (4.0–5.6)	2.6 (2.1–3.3)	10.9 (10.1–11.8)	7.0 (6.2–8.0)	9.9 (8.9–10.9)
ANH withheld[b] (95% CI)	5.6 (4.8–6.5)	3.2 (2.6–3.9)	1.6 (1.2–2.2)	8.1 (7.4–8.8)	5.5 (4.8–6.4)	8.5 (7.6–9.5)
ANH withdrawn[b] (95% CI)	2.3 (1.8–2.9)	1.7 (1.3–2.2)	1.2 (0.8–1.7)	3.4 (2.9–3.9)	2.3 (1.8–2.9)	1.7 (1.3–2.2)

Source: Data from *J Pain Symptom Manag.*, 34, Buiting, H. M. et al., Forgoing artificial nutrition or hydration in patients nearing death in six European countries, 305–314, Copyright (2007), with permission from Elsevier.

Note: Physicians may decide to forgo potentially life-prolonging treatment in dying patients; the decision to forgo artificial nutrition or hydration (ANH) is one of these decisions. The frequency of forgoing ANH widely varies across countries: from 2.6% of all deaths in Italy up to 10.9% in the Netherlands. Table 20.1 shows that in all countries physicians more often decided to withhold ANH as compared to withdraw ANH.

[a] End-of-life decisions (ELDs) include: forgoing treatment and use of drugs in (potentially) life-shortening dosages.

[b] Whether or not combined with other ELDs.

[c] "Forgone" indicates withheld or withdrawn.

TABLE 20.2
Determinants of Forgoing Artificial Nutrition or Hydration (ANH) in Six European Countries

	Country											
	Belgium		Denmark		Italy		Netherlands		Sweden		Switzerland	
Studied deaths	$n = 2950$		$n = 2939$		$n = 2604$		$n = 5384$		$n = 3248$		$n = 3355$	
	%[a]	OR (95% CI)[b]	%[a]	OR (95% CI)[b]	%[a]	OR (95% CI)[b]	%[a]	OR (95% CI)[b]	%[a]	OR (95% CI)[b]	%[a]	OR (95% CI)[b]
Age range[c]												
1–64	0.9	1	0.5	1	0.3	1	0.9	1	0.6	1	1.0	1
65–79	2.2	1.1 (0.7–1.8)	1.5	1.6 (0.9–2.9)	0.8	1.2 (0.5–2.7)	3.3	2.4 (1.7–3.3)	2.0	1.5 (0.9–2.6)	2.3	1.4 (0.9–2.1)
80+	4.2	1.5 (1.0–2.4)	2.7	2.2 (1.2–3.9)	1.5	1.6 (0.7–3.6)	6.7	3.1 (2.2–4.2)	4.5	2.0 (1.2–3.4)	6.6	2.3 (1.6–3.5)
Sex[d]												
Male	2.8	1	1.9	1	1.2	1	3.9	1	2.9	1	4.0	1
Female	4.5	1.6 (1.2–2.2)	2.9	1.3 (0.9–1.9)	1.4	1.1 (0.7–1.8)	7.1	1.4 (1.2–1.7)	4.2	1.3 (1.0–1.8)	5.9	1.2 (1.0–1.6)
Place of death[e]												
Hospital	2.7	1	1.6	1	1.0	1	2.4	1	3.5	1	2.9	1
Other places	4.5	1.8 (1.3–2.4)	3.1	1.1 (0.8–1.7)	1.6	1.4 (0.9–2.4)	8.6	1.7 (1.4–2.1)	3.5	0.7 (0.5–0.9)	6.9	1.5 (1.2–2.0)
Cause of death[f,g]												
Cardiovascular	1.0	1	1.0	1	0.4	1	0.8	1	2.6	1	2.1	1
Malignancy	2.7	4.3 (2.8–6.7)	1.6	1.8 (1.1–2.8)	1.4	4.4 (2.2–8.9)	2.5	3.7 (2.5–5.3)	2.2	1.9 (1.3–2.6)	2.9	2.9 (2.1–4.0)
Respiratory	0.6	2.2 (1.2–3.9)	0.3	0.7 (0.3–1.4)	0.1	1.0 (0.2–4.6)	1.0	4.0 (2.6–6.1)	0.3	1.3 (0.6–2.7)	0.7	1.6 (1.0–2.7)
Nervous system[h]	1.7	5.5 (3.4–8.8)	0.9	2.2 (1.3–3.8)	0.2	9.2 (2.9–29.2)	2.1	8.0 (5.5–11.7)	0.2	5.2 (2.0–13.9)	2.6	5.1 (3.6–7.3)
Other	1.2	1.7 (1.0–2.9)	0.9	1.0 (0.6–1.7)	0.6	3.1 (1.4–6.8)	4.5	6.4 (4.5–9.0)	1.8	2.3 (1.6–3.4)	1.6	1.6 (1.1–2.3)

Source: Data from *J Pain Symptom Manag.*, 34, Buiting, H. M. et al., Forgoing artificial nutrition or hydration in patients nearing death in six European countries, 305–314, Copyright (2007), with permission from Elsevier.

Note: This table shows that the frequency of forgoing ANH varies between different patient groups in all countries. Data were analysed univariate (expressed in percentages) and multivariate (expressed in odds ratios (ORs)). The odds ratios indicate whether the chance of forgoing ANH is higher or lower in a particular patient group as compared to the reference group (the group with the odds ratio of 1) even when controlled for other variables in the table. The table, for instance, shows that ANH is most often forgone in patients aged older than 80 years, also when the analysis is corrected for patient's sex and patient's place and cause of death.

[a] Weighted percentages; percentage of patients in whom ANH had been forgone.
[b] Odds ratio, determined using multiple logistic regression analysis.
[c] In 132 cases, information on age was missing.
[d] In 133 cases, information on sex was missing.
[e] In 73 cases, information on place of death was missing.
[f] In 38 cases, information on cause of death was missing.
[g] Cerebrovascular disease is included in cardiovascular diseases for Italy and Sweden and in diseases of the nervous system for Belgium, Denmark, the Netherlands and Switzerland.
[h] Including dementia.

that high age (odds ratio (OR) 1.5–3.1), being female (OR 1.1–1.8) and death from a disease of the nervous system (OR 2.2–9.2) all significantly contributed to the likelihood of forgoing ANH. Apparently, patient-related factors, such as age, gender and diagnosis, appear to be important predictors of forgoing ANH in all six countries and are more often regarded as disproportional care. Higher frequencies of forgoing ANH in elderly patients may be explained by the fact that the patients involved were more seriously ill or had a relatively poor prognosis, and not by age discrimination per se, which has been reported for other ELDs also (van der Heide et al. 2004). Multiple logistic regression analysis for all countries together showed that country as a separate determinant was also significantly associated with forgoing ANH, with relatively high ORs for Sweden (OR 3.0, with Italy as reference country), Switzerland (OR 3.7) and the Netherlands (OR 3.9). The independent effect of country in our study suggests that cultural factors may explain at least part of the variation in the decision to forgo ANH or not.

20.3 COMMUNICATION ABOUT WITHHOLDING OR WITHDRAWING ANH

Decisions to forgo ANH most frequently involved incompetent patients: percentages ranged from about 67% of all cases in Denmark and Switzerland, to 73% in the Netherlands, and 84% or over in Sweden, Belgium and Italy (Table 20.3).

If patients were competent, physicians had discussed the possible hastening of death as a result of the decision to forgo ANH most frequently with the patients themselves in Sweden, Denmark, and the Netherlands, and least frequently in Belgium. The decision to forgo ANH was rarely discussed with incompetent patients themselves, except for the Netherlands. Of all incompetent patients with whom the decision was not discussed, 10% (Sweden) to 22% (Denmark, Switzerland) had in an earlier stage expressed a wish to hasten their end-of-life (not in table). For incompetent patients, relatives were frequently involved in the decision-making process: percentages varied from 63% in Sweden to 83% in Belgium and 91% in the Netherlands. For incompetent patients, the attending physicians frequently involved both relatives and, to a somewhat lesser extent, other caregivers in the decision to forgo ANH. Thus, our results suggest that decisions to forgo ANH are typically based upon ideas and values about medical management in the last phase of life of incompetent patients that are discussed between caregivers and family.

20.4 WITHHOLDING OR WITHDRAWING ANH IN COMBINATION WITH POSSIBLY LIFE-SHORTENING DRUGS TO RELIEVE SYMPTOMS

This study also explored whether patients in whom ANH was forgone received more or less potentially life-shortening drugs than patients in whom other ELDs had been made. We hypothesised that the suffering of terminally ill patients in whom ANH had been forgone may be different from patients in whom ANH had not been forgone. Forgoing ANH was combined with the administration of drugs to relieve symptoms in possibly life-shortening dosages in 52% (Italy) up to 67% (Belgium) of all cases (Table 20.4). Physicians had usually administered opioids (whether or not combined with other types of drugs) in these cases. In all countries, except Belgium, patients in whom ANH was forgone received significantly less drugs to relieve symptoms than other patients for whom other ELDs had been made. This finding may be seen as an indication that forgoing ANH did not induce extra suffering. As such, it confirms the outcomes of other studies that specifically focused on the suffering of patients in whom ANH was forgone. For example, in a prospective, longitudinal, observational study of 178 patients in Dutch nursing homes, Pasman et al. (2005) found no difference in the level of discomfort of patients with dementia who barely ate or drank. A prospective study in a comfort care unit showed similar results: terminally ill patients did not experience hunger and thirst and the administration of ANH played a minor role in the patient's comfort (McCann et al. 1994).

TABLE 20.3
Competence of Patient and Physician's Discussion about the Decision to Forgo Artificial Nutrition or Hydration (ANH)

	Country					
	Belgium	**Denmark**	**Italy**	**Netherlands**	**Sweden**	**Switzerland**
Studied deaths[a]	**n = 131%[b]**	**n = 88%[b]**	**n = 48%[b]**	**n = 465%[b]**	**n = 189%[b]**	**n = 233%[b]**
Discussion with patient and relatives						
Patient was competent (95% CI)[c]	16 (10–23)	33 (24–45)	7.3 (3.2–21)	27 (23–31)	15 (10–21)	33 (27–39)
Discussed with patient	4.0	31	–	17	17	19
Discussed with patient and relatives	55	60	100	79	50	69
Not discussed with patient, but with relatives	21	2.5	–	3.4	12	9.1
Not discussed with patient or relatives	20	6.3	–	0.6	21	2.7
Patient was incompetent (95% CI)[c]	84 (77–90)	67 (55–76)	93 (79–97)	73 (69–77)	85 (79–90)	67 (61–73)
Discussed with patient	–	2.5	1.4	2.1	1	0.9
Discussed with patient and relatives	9.4	7.8	9.4	20	7	13
Not discussed with patient, but with relatives	74	64	67	71	56	61
Not discussed with patient or relatives	17	25	22	7.0	36	25
Discussion with other caregivers[d,e]						
Other physician	29	33	37	43	28	30
Nursing staff	76	64	22	59	60	73
No discussion	18	19	49	19	34	14

Source: Data from *J Pain Symptom Manag.*, 34, Buiting, H. M. et al., Forgoing artificial nutrition or hydration in patients nearing death in six European countries, 305–314, Copyright (2007), with permission from Elsevier.

Note: If patients are incompetent, patients cannot express their own wishes anymore; in such situations the discussion with relatives becomes more important. This table shows that most patients in whom ANH was forgone were incompetent at the time of the decision.

[a] It only concerns patients for whom a decision to forgo ANH had been made (possibly combined with other treatments forgone).

[b] Weighted percentages.

[c] In 46 cases, information about the patient's competence was missing.

[d] Both competent and incompetent patients.

[e] One or more answers are possible.

TABLE 20.4
Decisions to Forgo Artificial Nutrition or Hydration (ANH) and Use of Drugs to Relieve Symptoms in Potentially Life-Shortening Dosages in Six European Countries

	Country					
	Belgium	**Denmark**	**Italy**	**Netherlands**	**Sweden**	**Switzerland**
Number of studied deaths	$n = 2950$[a]	$n = 2939$[a]	$n = 2604$[a]	$n = 5384$[a]	$n = 3248$[a]	$n = 3355$[a]
ANH forgone	7.2 ($n = 252$)	4.7 ($n = 149$)	2.6 ($n = 89$)	10.9 ($n = 712$)	7.0 ($n = 264$)	9.9 ($n = 331$)
Drug administered (95% CI)[b]	67 (61–73)	61[c] (53–69)	52[c] (41–62)	58[c] (55–62)	55[c] (48–61)	62[c] (57–68)
No drug administered (95% CI)	33 (27–39)	39 (31–47)	48 (38–59)	42 (38–46)	45 (39–52)	38 (32–43)
Other ELD[d]	31 ($n = 1099$)	36 ($n = 1206$)	21 ($n = 725$)	33 ($n = 2051$)	29 ($n = 1063$)	41 ($n = 1373$)
Drug administered[e] (95% CI)	73 (70–75)	72[c] (69–75)	88[c] (85–91)	73[c] (70–75)	70[c] (67–73)	69[c] (67–72)
No drug administered (95% CI)	28 (25–30)	28 (25–31)	12 (9–15)	27 (25–30)	30 (27–33)	31 (28–33)
No ELD[d]	62 ($n = 1599$)	59 ($n = 1584$)	77 ($n = 1790$)	57 ($n = 2542$)	65 ($n = 1921$)	49 ($n = 1651$)

Source: Data from *J Pain Symptom Manag.*, 34, Buiting, H. M. et al., Forgoing artificial nutrition or hydration in patients nearing death in six European countries, 305–314, Copyright (2007), with permission from Elsevier.

Note: A frequently expressed concern is that forgoing ANH brings along extra suffering. The patient group in whom ANH is forgone is therefore compared with patients in whom other medical end-of-life decisions have been made. This table shows that patients in whom ANH is forgone did not receive more potentially life-shortening drugs as compared to patients for whom other end-of-life decisions have been made.

[a] Weighted percentages.

[b] In 73 cases, information concerning the type of drug administered was missing (3.1% up to 7.8%).

[c] Difference in the administration of drugs between patients in whom ANH was forgone (whether or not combined with other ELDs) and other patients for whom another ELD had been made, χ^2 test, $p < 0.05$.

[d] End-of-life decisions (ELDs) include: forgoing treatment and use of drugs in (potentially) life-shortening dosages.

[e] In 1368 cases, information concerning the type of drug administered was missing (13% up to 33%).

20.5 INTERNATIONAL DIFFERENCES

In view of the substantial number of deaths that are preceded by decisions to forgo ANH, it can be concluded that providing all patients who are in the terminal stage of a lethal or degenerating disease does not seem to be a widely accepted standard among physicians in Western Europe. Nevertheless, the fact that the frequencies between countries substantially vary suggests that physicians in different countries have different ideas about the appropriateness of making these decisions. It is difficult to verify why physicians consider the practice of ANH differently. It may be related to different healthcare systems. Palliative care, for instance, started in different healthcare settings across countries. It may also be related to different religious beliefs. If cultural differences in end-of-life decision making would result in lower quality of care, this would be problematic. Currently, many efforts are undertaken to develop international comparative quality indicators for end-of-life care. It is very difficult to establish feasible, reliable and valid indicators, and comparing the quality of end-of-life care between countries seems a bridge too far for the time being. However, the standards of health care are comparable between most industrialised countries and it is unlikely that the quality of end-of-life care has an important role in explaining the variance in end-of-life decision making.

20.6 APPLICATIONS TO OTHER AREAS OF TERMINAL OR PALLIATIVE CARE

One of the most important aims of palliative care is to minimise suffering and discomfort. Despite lack of clear evidence that the forgoing of ANH causes discomfort, some people still believe that the forgoing of ANH may contribute to suffering rather than alleviating it (van der Riet et al. 2006). Nevertheless, in actual medical practice the forgoing of ANH often seems routine practice in patients who are terminally ill (Australian Government Department of Health and Ageing 2004; NVVA 1997), especially with regard to artificial nutrition. Withholding nutritional support is generally perceived to enhance patient comfort and is accordingly an appropriate goal for end-of-life care. A country-specific effect in the practice of forgoing ANH is probably more prevalent in specific patient groups. It is for instance plausible that certain clinical situations which are directly related to specific legislation in one country, or are more prone to ethical debates, are more likely to result in a different decision-making process. As mentioned previously, the forgoing of ANH primarily concerns incompetent patients. To study the practice of forgoing ANH between countries for these specific patient groups may be interesting to be able to clarify whether the decision making in these particular areas are primarily culturally and/or medically determined.

20.7 GUIDELINES

In the past decades, a lot of research in the field of palliative care in relation to artificial nutrition or hydration has been performed. For patients suffering from advanced dementia, guidelines in many countries nowadays suggest that administering ANH is disproportionate care. Such guidelines could assist medical professionals in deciding whether to provide ANH to severely ill and demented patients or not.

KEY FACTS IN HOW TO DISTINGUISH FORGOING ARTIFICIAL NUTRITION OR HYDRATION FROM OTHER MEDICAL END-OF-LIFE DECISIONS

- Euthanasia: the administration of drugs with the explicit intention of hastening death at the patient's explicit request.
- Physician-assisted suicide: the prescription or supply of drugs with the explicit intention to enable the patient to end his or her life.
- Ending of life without an explicit patient request: the administration of drugs with the explicit intention of hastening death without an explicit patient request.

- Alleviation of pain and symptoms: the administration of drugs in dosages which are large enough to include hastening of death as a likely or certain side effect.
- Forgoing potentially life-prolonging treatment: withholding or withdrawing medical treatment while taking into account or explicitly intending (potential) hastening of death; forgoing ANH belongs to this category.

Definitions about medical end-of-life decisions may differ between countries. In order to be able to compare frequencies between countries, the same definition should be used. This study used the same definitions in every studied country.

ETHICAL ISSUES

The (non)provision of ANH in terminally ill patients remains a controversial issue. In discussions about ANH it is important to know what ANH exactly embraces for physicians in different countries; e.g., is it tube feeding and hydration that is administered subcutaneously or intravenously? Does it also include spoon feeding? Or do physicians interpret it more narrowly; that is, tube feeding only? In ethical debates such definitions could be important in evaluating whether the decision to forgo ANH may be justified or not. On the other hand, it is argued that the justification for the withdrawal of feeding does not hinge on whether feeding is administered artificially or not. Although complete agreement about the use of ANH seems virtually impossible, clarifying the principles that underlie decisions about ANH in clinical practice is probably an essential first step in optimal end-of-life care.

SUMMARY POINTS

- A substantial number of deaths in Belgium, Denmark, Italy, the Netherlands, Sweden and Switzerland are preceded by a decision to withhold or withdraw artificial nutrition or hydration (ANH). Forgoing ANH is an important aspect of palliative care in all studied West European countries.
- The rate in the forgoing of ANH substantially varies between countries: it is 7.2% in Belgium, 4.7% in Denmark, 2.6% in Italy, 10.9% in the Netherlands, 7.0% in Sweden and 9.9% in Switzerland.
- In all six European countries, age, gender and diagnosis appear to be important factors in the practice of forgoing ANH at the end-of-life.
- The decision making about ANH at the end-of-life is especially difficult because most patients cannot express their own wishes anymore.
- Differences in the forgoing of ANH may be related to country-specific aspects, such as the judicial system, the healthcare system and its religion.

ACKNOWLEDGMENTS

We thank the thousands of physicians in the six countries who provided the data; the national and regional medical associations and other authoritative bodies that supported the study; the national advisory boards for their support; and Caspar WN Looman for his statistical support and advice. We also would like to thank the members of the EURELD consortium (other than the authors): Luc Deliens (Vrije Universiteit Brussel, Brussels, Belgium); Julie van Geluwe, Freddy Mortier (Ghent University, Ghent, Belgium); Annemarie Dencker, Anna Paldam Folker (University of Copenhagen, Copenhagen, Denmark); Riccardo Cecioni, Eugenio Paci (Center for Study and Prevention of Cancer, Florence, Italy); Lorenzo Simonato (University of Padua, Padua, Italy); Silva Franchini (Local Health Authority, Trento, Italy); Alba Carola Finarelli (Regional Department of Health, Bologna, Italy); Paul J. van der Maas (Erasmus MC, Rotterdam, Netherlands); Gerrit van der Wal (Vrije Universiteit Medical Center, Amsterdam, Netherlands); Tore Nilstun (University of Lund, Lund, Sweden); and Georg Bosshard, Karin Faisst and Ueli Zellweger (University of Zurich, Zurich, Switzerland).

LIST OF ABBREVIATIONS

ANH Artificial nutrition or hydration
ELD End-of-life decision
OR Odds ratio

REFERENCES

Australian Government Department of Health and Ageing. 2004. *Guidelines for a palliative approach in residential aged care*. Churchlands: Edith Cowan University.

Beauchamp, T., and J. Childress. 2001. *Principles of biomedical ethics*. New York: Oxford University Press.

Bell, C., E. Somogyi-Zalud, K. Masaki, T. Fortaleza-Dawson, and P. L. Blanchette. 2008. Factors associated with physician decision-making in starting tube feeding. *Journal of Palliative Medicine* 11:915–24.

Bilsen, J., J. Cohen, K. Chambaere, G. Pousset, B. D. Onwuteaka-Philipsen, F. Mortier, and L. Deliens. 2009. Medical end-of-life practices under the euthanasia law in Belgium. *New England Journal of Medicine* 361:1119–21.

Bosshard, G., T. Nilstun, J. Bilsen, M. Norup, G. Miccinesi, J. J. van Delden, K. Faist, and A. van der Heide. 2005. Forgoing treatment at the end-of-life in 6 European countries. *Archives of Internal Medicine* 165:401–7.

Buiting, H. M., J. J. van Delden, J. A. Rietjens, B. D. Onwuteaka-Philipsen, J. Bilsen, S. Fischer, R. Löfmark, G. Miccinesi, M. Norup, and A. van der Heide. 2007. Forgoing artificial nutrition or hydration in patients nearing death in six European countries. *Journal of Pain and Symptom Management* 34:305–14.

Farber, N. J., P. Simpson, T. Salam, V. U. Collier, J. Weiner, and E. G. Boyer. 2006. Physicians' decisions to withhold and withdraw life-sustaining treatment. *Archives of Internal Medicine* 166:560–64.

Finucane, T. E., C. Christmas, and K. Travis. 1999. Tube feeding in patients with advanced dementia: A review of the evidence. *Journal of the American Medical Association* 282:1365–70.

Helman, C. 2000. *Culture, health and illness.* Oxford-England: Butterworth-Heinemann.

Le Conte, P., D. Baron, D. Trewick, M. D. Touze, C. Longo, I. Vial, D. Yatim, and G. Potel. 2004. Withholding and withdrawing life-support therapy in an Emergency Department: Prospective survey. *Intensive Care Medicine* 30:2216–21.

McCann, R. M., W. J. Hall, and A. Groth-Juncker. 1994. Comfort care for terminally ill patients. The appropriate use of nutrition and hydration. *Journal of the American Medical Association* 272:1263–66.

NVVA. 1997. *Prudent medical care. Manual for decision-making concerning patients with dementia in nursing home practice.* Utrecht: NVVA.

Onwuteaka-Philipsen, B. D., H. R. Pasman, A. Kruit, A. van der Heide, M. W. Ribbe, and G. van der Wal. 2001. Withholding or withdrawing artificial administration of food and fluids in nursing-home patients. *Age and Ageing* 30:459–65.

Pasman, H. R., B. D. Onwuteaka-Philipsen, D. M. Kriegsman, M. E. Ooms, M. W. Ribbe, and G. van der Wal. 2005. Discomfort in nursing home patients with severe dementia in whom artificial nutrition or hydration is forgone. *Arch Intern Med* 165 (15): 1729–35.

Pope John Paul II. 2004. Address on life-sustaining treatments and vegetable state: Scientific and ethical dilemmas. Available from: http://www.vatican.va/holy_father/john_paul_ii/speeches/2004/march/ documents/hf_jp-ii_spe_20040320_congress-fiamc_en.html.

Seale, C. 2006. National survey of end-of-life decisions made by UK medical practitioners. *Palliative Medicine* 20:3–10.

Sheldon, T. 1997. Row over force feeding of patients with Alzheimer's disease. *British Medical Journal* 315:7104–327.

van der Heide, A., L. Deliens, K. Faisst, T. Nilstun, M. Norup, E. Paci, G. van der Wal, and P. J. van der Maas. 2003. End-of-life decision-making in six European countries: Descriptive study. *Lancet* 362 (9381): 345–50.

van der Heide, A., B. D. Onwuteaka-Philipsen, M. L. Rurup, H. M. Buiting, J. J. van Delden, J. E. Hanssen-de Wolf, A. G. Janssen, et al. 2007. End-of-life practices in the Netherlands under the Euthanasia Act. *New England Journal of Medicine* 356:1957–65.

van der Heide, A., A. Vrakking, H. van Delden, C. Looman, and P. van der Maas. 2004. Medical and nonmedical determinants of decision making about potentially life-prolonging interventions. *Medical Decision Making* 24:518–24.

Van der Riet, P., D. Brooks, and M. Ashby. 2006. Nutrition and hydration at the end-of-life: Pilot study of a palliative care experience. *Journal of Law and Medicine* 14:182–98.

Yazigi, A., M. Riachi, and G. Dabbar. 2005. Withholding and withdrawal of life-sustaining treatment in a Lebanese intensive care unit: A prospective observational study. *Intensive Care Medicine* 31:562–67.

Section IV

Cancer

21 The Concept of Cachexia-Related Suffering (CRS) in Palliative Cancer Care

R. Oberholzer, D. Blum, and F. Strasser

CONTENTS

21.1 INTRODUCTION

Unintentional weight loss can be caused by a number of disorders. Several of them are treatable and therefore reversible (Rabinovitz 1986). There remains a long list of incurable diseases that are chronically progressive and during the natural trajectory lose their therapeutic options. Among those diseases are advanced cancer, HIV infection with multi-drug-resistant strains, chronic obstructive lung disease, congestive heart failure, neurologic disorders and others.

Although not painful as such, anorexia and cachexia in chronically progressive diseases with insufficiently effective treatment options are troublesome. Patients not only suffer from the physical consequences like fatigue, weakness and reduced physical functioning. Anorexia and cachexia cause a spectrum of negative emotions, which have to be differentiated from proper psychiatric disorders like anxiety and depression. Anorexia and cachexia are unmistakable indications that the underlying disease is not under control and that death is approaching. Naturally food and eating are among the joys of life, which fades away in affected patients. Additionally, anorexia and cachexia may interrupt established social structures when mealtimes no longer are conjoined events. Different cultures underline the importance of social aspects of conjoined mealtimes in various ways. The role as sustainer may be lost when the cook in the family is no longer rewarded by lack of praising the food. These and other psychosocial aspects are known as cachexia-related suffering (CRS). CRS is mainly investigated in advanced cancer disease with manifest cancer cachexia syndrome (CCS). CCS and its consequences are among the most frequent problems of patients with advanced cancer. There is an increasing body of evidence illuminating different aspects and characteristics of CRS in patients, their carers and even healthcare professionals being confronted with CCS in their daily work. There is sufficient evidence to conceptualize CRS. Understanding this concept and the intervention its knowledge opens up may be essential in the successful palliative care management of affected patients and their carers.

21.2 MALNUTRITION

The term malnutrition is usually used for wasting diseases in developing countries, most likely because of assumption of a primary problem of insufficient availability of food. However, even in this population malnutrition often occurs associated with underlying infectious diseases like HIV, tuberculosis and geohelminths. The term malnutrition can also be used for involuntary weight loss in developed countries caused by CCS for instance.

The malnutrition screening index (Kondrup et al. 2003) includes, apart from involuntary loss of weight (cachexia), nutritional intake (in % of normal nutritional intake), body mass index (BMI: body weight [kg]/height [m]^2) and general condition. The index defines one to three points for each of these criteria. In patients older than 70 years, 2 points; in younger ones three points are required for diagnosis (Table 21.1).

21.3 CACHEXIA-RELATED SUFFERING (CRS)

CRS was long underestimated as a significant psychosocial consequence of CCS and includes aspects of distress suffered by patients, carers, partners and even patients' healthcare professionals.

CRS is defined as negative emotions associated with reduced nutritional intake and weight loss (Souter 2005). CRS should correctly be differentiated from eating-related distress (ERD) and weight-loss-related distress (WRD) (Hopkinson, Wright, and Corner 2005). Because these terms are not consistently used in the literature and in clinical praxis, there is to a large extent an overlap between ERD and WRD. In this article we use the term CRS for pragmatic reasons.

TABLE 21.1
Nutritional Risk Assessment

Impaired Nutrition Status	
Mild (1 point per item)	Weight loss >5% in 3 months
	Food intake 50%–75% of normal requirement in preceding week
Moderate (2 points per item)	Weight loss >5% in 2 months
	Body mass index (BMI) 18.5–20.5 AND impaired general condition
	Food intake 25%–50% of normal requirement in preceding week
Severe (3 points per item)	Weight loss >5% in 1 month (≈>15% in 3 months)
	Body mass index (BMI) <18.5 AND impaired general condition
	Food intake 0%–25% of normal requirement in preceding week

In patients >70 years 2 points, <70 years 3 points are required for diagnosis: start nutritional support

Source: Adapted from Kondrup, J. et al. *Clin. Nutr.*, 22, 321, 2003.

There is no agreed medical definition for distress to date. Using the word distress has the potential to mistakenly label patients and to miss those suffering from proper anxiety or depression, psychiatric disorders which need to be treated primarily as such. Therefore CRS might be a more appropriate expression for the matter discussed here.

21.3.1 Prevalence of CRS

CRS may be present in about one third to one half of the patients suffering from loss of appetite and weight loss, whereas 9 out of 10 carers are affected (Hawkins 2000; Hopkinson et al. 2006). Patients of younger age and those located in the community are particularly affected. CRS also affects healthcare workers, although there are no data on frequency (Hopkinson and Corner 2006).

21.3.2 Characteristics of CRS

21.3.2.1 Presentation of CRS

CRS presents comparably in both patients and carers. Emotions like anxiety, anger, feeling upset, bother, concern, frustration and guilt are typically named. Patients may be embarrassed about the visibility of loss of weight (Reid et al. 2009) or feel harassed by their carers. Carers may feel personally rejected and incompetent (McClement, Degner, and Harlos 2004).

There is most likely a continuum between suffering about the inability to eat and weight loss towards proper psychiatric disorders like anxiety and depression. As the treatment of these psychiatric disorders is different, a screening using the Hospital Anxiety and Depressions Scale (HADS), for instance, is of importance.

21.3.2.2 Mechanisms Leading to CRS

Suffering arises when expectations of nutritional intake and weight gain differ significantly from reality. This means measures taken to fight weight loss are not successful (McClement et al. 2004). This occurrence is well known and part of the cause of several common problems in palliative care. This phenomenon was first described by Calman and is therefore known as the Calman gap (see Figure 21.1) (Calman 1984). An underlying lack of knowledge regarding the possible inevitability

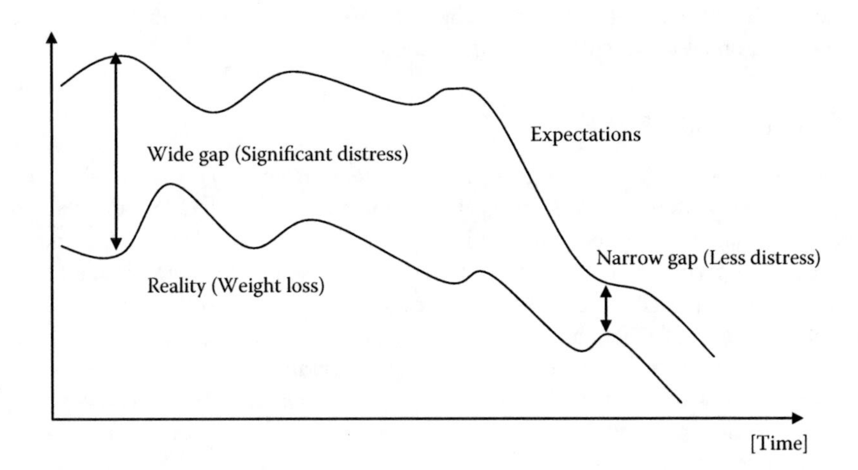

FIGURE 21.1 Calman gap. This figure shows a wide Calman gap causing significant suffering due to high expectations to regain weight and associated physical functioning early in the course of the disease compared to a narrower gap causing less suffering later in the course due to much lower expectations even though weight has decreased further.

of CCS due to the underlying uncontrolled disease may be responsible for inadequate attempts to increase patients' weight.

In *patients* the eating-related symptoms loss of appetite, loss of desire to eat, inability to eat, early satiety, taste changes and food aversion may cause negative emotions (Strasser et al. 2007). Patients may eat almost normally but nevertheless weight decreases. It can be very irritating for patients when they are faced with this incomprehensible independence of eating and weight.

If food intake is limited some patients are suffering from hurting partners. Even well-intended comments and actions from carers aiming to increase nutritional intake might make patients feel guilty. Ongoing attempts to reach the intake targets and centring couples' relationships on food are extreme variants of this same attitude. Healthy eating messages (advice to eat fruit and vegetables) can cause distress if patients feel unable to eat healthy foods.

Carers may overestimate the distress caused by loss of weight compared to other more bothersome symptoms like pain, dyspnoea and weakness (Holden 1991). While carers concentrate on feeding, patients have needs like being listened to, heard and understood, and having their limitations accepted.

As increasing weight loss becomes visible, patients' self-perception is altered and they may isolate themselves socially. Along the trajectory of the disease, patients become weaker and are at risk of losing their independence. Finally, not eating means dying and as patients realize this (Meares 1997), it can cause existential distress.

For *carers*, patients' refusal of food can cause anxiety, guilt, anger and personal rejection. If the refractory nature of treatment of CCS is not understood, carers may put their efforts into keeping the patient alive with eating. Despite a sense of responsibility and willingness to help, there is often uncertainty about the best way to do this. Changing cooking habits, spending a lot of time on preparing food and inability to make the patient eat enough are often observed. For female spouses in particular, the change of their role as food preparer may be a classical situation causing distress, as cooking might have previously been an expression of love. Carers might also seek rewards for their cooking efforts, a sign of good caregiving. Reward in this context could mean that the patient is enjoying the food. Carers may also suffer from lost opportunities to eat together when mealtimes were previously a daily routine. A change in their own eating habits can be observed, which in turn might have an impact on their own weight. Eventually, fear of loss of the beloved one is often present.

Both patients and carers may be distressed when healthcare workers' advice is perceived as inadequate or they don't even acknowledge the weight loss. This leads them to believe that the healthcare workers know little about it, which weakens their confidence.

21.3.3 Reactions to CRS

Reaction patterns are individual and highly variable (Hopkinson 2007). CRS is usually evolving. Depending on personal intellectual resources and communicative skills, CRS can either escalate to the extent of a predominating problem determining the relationship between patient and carer, or it may decrease after a period of adaptation and maturation caused by this new situation. It might be helpful therefore to try and ask oneself whether a reaction is constructive or adverse.

The different patterns of reactions can be summarized as a continuum between self-action and acceptance (Souter 2005). In self-action as well as in acceptance, constructive and adverse reactions can be observed. Waffling, which means being unsure, ambivalence, acting inconsistently and struggling to reconcile tensions are frequently present in those affected. It may offer an entry point for psychosocial interventions.

21.3.3.1 Constructive Reactions

The nature of CCS is, with very few exceptions, progressive and irreversible. Recognizing the terminal nature of the disease and acceptance (Shragge et al. 2007) is the key to relief from CRS.

Incidentally, this reaction is more frequent in patients than in carers. However, having made this step, patients and their carers are able to move the focus of the relationship away from CRS (McClement and Harlos 2008). Instead of focusing on food, carers may find other ways to care, for instance physical care like repositioning, oral care and ambulating. Just being there, giving patients the feeling of not being abandoned, touching, talking about important things and protecting the patient lead to decreased frustration. Carers may feel a sense of solace by respecting patients' autonomy. Nutritional intake activity should be patient driven. Carers should best limit trying to encourage the patient to eat.

Several self-action strategies were detected and described: talking control, promoting self-worth, relationship work and distraction. Promotion of self-worth for instance can be achieved by focussing on what is eaten rather than what is not eaten. In this study, J. Hopkinson presented a model of self-management that offers potential for intervention at the level of individual and contextual difference.

21.3.3.2 Adverse Reactions

When the irreversible nature of CCS is not recognized or not accepted, patients or carers may continue to try to maintain life with increasing food intake. Carers may monitor nutritional intake and even count calories. Adverse reactions beyond encouraging caloric intake include putting pressure on the patient verbally, and non-verbally by distributing food. In very rare extreme situations this may extend to force feeding. Pushing patients to eat can cause pain, nausea, anticipation of emesis and vomiting. Patients may try hard to eat and eat to please their carers. They may hide the full extent of loss of appetite or lie about the amount of food taken. Social withdrawal (McClement et al. 2004) and isolation, pretending to be sleeping or ignoring are known mechanisms with the intent to avoid conflict.

These and other reactions may continue until very late in the course of the disease, hoping that the diagnosis was wrong or there still might be a cure.

21.3.4 Assessment of CRS

A validated assessment tool for CRS is lacking to date. Currently effort is being put into its development. However, a single screening question like: "How much do you feel distressed about your inability to eat?" is sufficient for identification and a simple entry point into the field of CRS. The Functional Assessment of Anorexia/Cachexia Therapy (FAACT) scale also contains certain aspects of CRS and may therefore be helpful for screening purposes (Ribaudo et al. 2001). An adapted version of FAACT is shown in Table 21.2. Auditing or accusing healthcare professionals is an expression of mistrust and may be a sign of underlying CRS.

21.4 APPLICATIONS TO OTHER AREAS OF TERMINAL OR PALLIATIVE CARE

If we try to understand the causes and nature of CCS it might be helpful to review the evolution of the cachexia problem in patients suffering from acquired immunodeficiency syndrome (AIDS). At the time FAACT, the first assessment tool for anorexia/cachexia, was developed in 1993 (Cella, Jacobsen, and Orav 1993), both cancer and AIDS patients were subjects of validating the tool. With the introduction of triple antiretroviral treatment, we witnessed even the most wasted patients gain weight and regain their initial normal level of nutritional status, before they fell sick. This phenomenon makes it obvious that treating the cause is probably the only sustained successful treatment of CCS. According to the short median survival of the investigated patient population, it is obvious that CRS mainly affects patients without effective treatment options. Due to the lack of evidence we can only estimate that patients affected by other chronic progressive diseases known to lead to cachexia like advanced chronic obstructive pulmonary disease (COPD), congestive heart failure and many other terminal situations of diseases might be equally affected. Given the relatively

TABLE 21.2
Adapted FAACT

	Not at All	A Little Bit	Somewhat	Quite a Bit	Very Much
I have a good appetite	0	1	2	3	4
The amount I eat is sufficient to meet my needs	0	1	2	3	4
I am worried about my weight	0	1	2	3	4
I can swallow without difficulties	0	1	2	3	4
Most food tastes unpleasant to me	0	1	2	3	4
My mouth is dry	0	1	2	3	4
My interest in food drops as soon as I try to eat	0	1	2	3	4
When I eat, I seem to get full quickly	0	1	2	3	4
My family or friends are pressuring me to eat	0	1	2	3	4
I have pain in my stomach area	0	1	2	3	4
I am concerned about how thin I look	0	1	2	3	4
I have reduced contacts because I look thin	0	1	2	3	4
Sometimes I feel hungry during the day	0	1	2	3	4
When I think of food I feel hungry	0	1	2	3	4
After having eaten I feel better	0	1	2	3	4

unspecific treatment approach outlined above, we encourage active monitoring for CRS in those patients as well.

Data on CRS are mainly collected from cancer patients from Western Europe and North America. Ethnic minorities were severely underrepresented. The CRS concept can therefore possibly not be generalized. There are no data about CRS from developing countries. There, the problem of malnutrition is very well known. WHO has published many useful guidelines on how to approach those patients, which are based on the different spectrum of causes of malnutrition. Apart from pure lack of nutrition or micronutrients, HIV, tuberculosis and geohelminths are frequently found as underlying infections.

21.5 PRACTICAL METHODS AND TECHNIQUES

Systematic assessment to identify potentially treatable causes of CCS is crucial. However, this is usually done ahead of time when CRS becomes prominent. Nevertheless, it is helpful to use a checklist to systematically search for secondary causes of cachexia, which might be treatable, and weight loss therefore partially reversible (see Table 21.3).

Narrowing the Calman gap by reducing expectations has been shown to significantly reduce suffering.

It is important to be aware that CRS is frequent and it should be assessed for early. Even with a simple screening question like: "Do you suffer from not being able to eat as previously," CRS might be detected and offers the chance for further investigation and interventions. Mitigating CRS with intent to improve quality of life is important in advanced cancer patients lacking reasonable anticancer treatments. Optimization of nutritional intake is no longer the main focus of the therapeutic approach to tackle CCS although for patients this is often perceived as the main mechanism for relieving CRS. However, the two therapeutic approaches are not mutually exclusive and both tracks can be followed in parallel. Table 21.4 summarizes what is currently known about the treatment of CCS and CRS (Hopkinson 2008).

TABLE 21.3
Secondary Causes of Cachexia

- Stomatitis
- Dysgeusia
- Xerostomia
- Affection of the teeth
- Dysphagia
- Heartburn
- Dyspepsia
- Abdominal pain
- Nausea
- Vomiting
- Constipation
- Diarrhoea
- Pain
- Dyspnoea
- Fatigue
- Anxiety
- Social isolation
- Depression
- Drug side effects

Figure 21.2 might help the healthcare professional as a diagnostic and interventional instrument. It is useful to systematically search for the underlying aggravating and alleviating mechanisms leading to CRS of patients and their carers. Meanwhile, the optimization of nutritional intake should continue, possibly with the help of an experienced nutritionist, as the basis of routine palliative care. The assurance that the best efforts at weight control have been made is important for the patient to move to acceptance.

To date we know little about effectiveness of interventions in CRS. Longitudinal trials are underway.

Potential barriers against successful interventions to relieve CRS may be present and it might be useful to aware of them. A lack of knowledge on the part of healthcare professionals is not rare. If they are uncertain, think they can do little or have low expectations of being able to help, they

TABLE 21.4
CRS Interventions

CRS	Addressing, psychosocial support, education, facilitate self-action Examples of probably helpful information Healthy diet has no proven benefit People eat more of the things they enjoy/find easiest to eat People with a small appetite typically find nutritious fluids and soft foods easiest to eat Cold foods, soft foods and fluids can be as nutritious as cooked meals Cancer causes metabolic changes that suppress appetite, making it difficult to eat Disagreements over food are common in families managing CCS, it can be helpful explain to others what is troubling them
Secondary cachexia	Look for and treat nausea, vomiting, stomatitis, oesophagitis, gastroenteritis, constipation, pain, dyspnoea, psychiatric disorder
Primary cachexia	Nutritional counselling (frequent, small, energy- and protein-rich meals), enrichment of food, enteral/parenteral feeding, nutraceuticals (ProSure) Consider progestin (megestrol acetate), corticosteroids, prokinetics (metoclopramide)

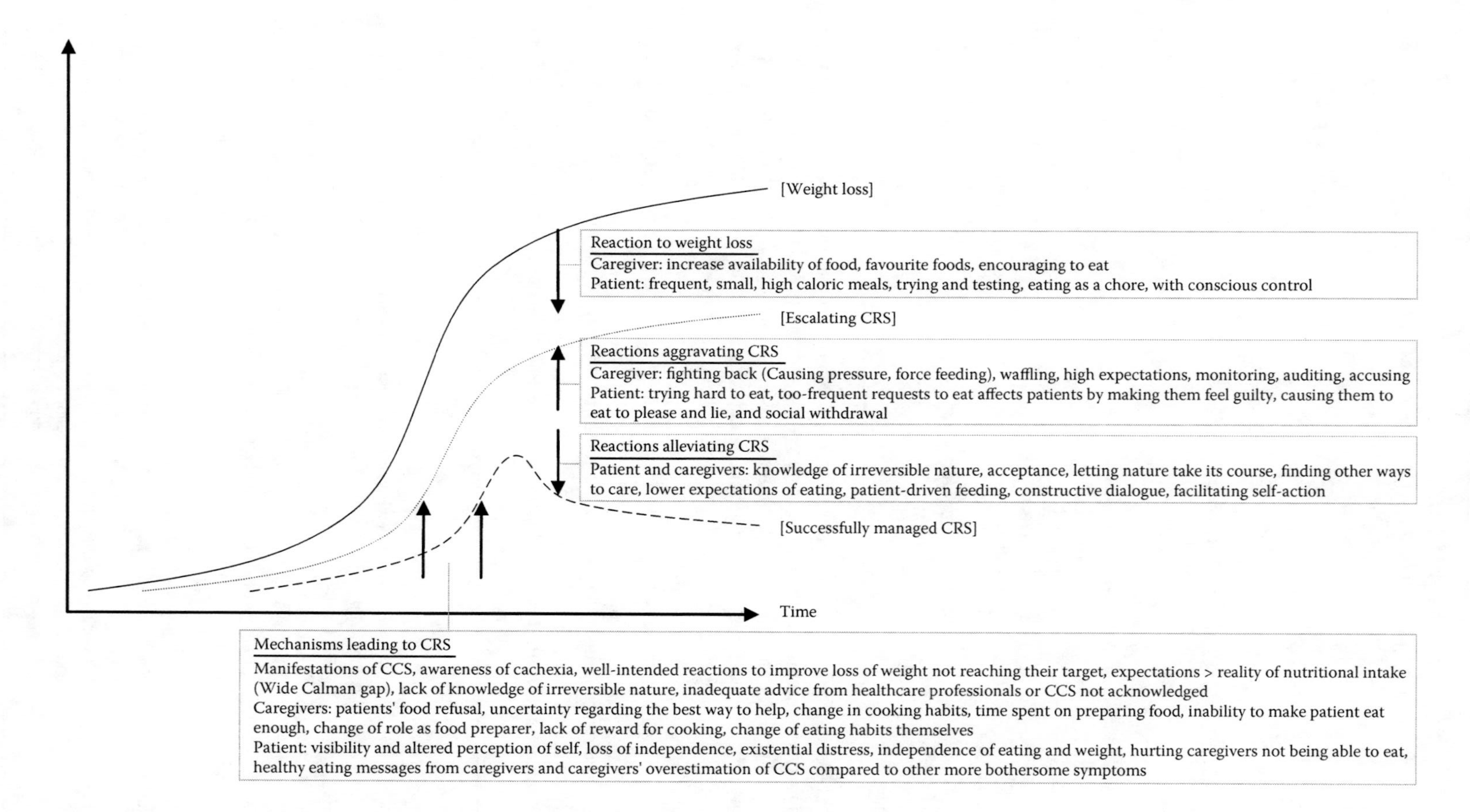

FIGURE 21.2 CRS in practice. Summarized finding of CRS during a single episode of relevant weight loss.

may feel frustrated themselves. Some think it is best not to discuss CRS with patients and carers. Healthcare professional may not know how to respond appropriately and some are scared they could even generate rather than alleviate CRS. There may be concerns about moving people towards acceptance.

KEY POINTS

- Features of cachexia syndrome:
  Unintentional weight loss (cachexia) and loss of appetite (anorexia) can be caused by a number of disorders. Many of them are chronically progressive and lack therapeutic options. Cachexia causing not only physical consequences but negative emotions is called cachexia-related suffering (CRS).
- Features of cachexia-related suffering (CRS):
  CRS was long underestimated as a significant psychosocial consequence of CCS and is defined as negative emotions associated with reduced nutritional intake and weight loss. CRS should correctly be differentiated from eating-related distress (ERD) and weight-loss-related distress (WRD). CRS may be present in about one third to one half of patients suffering from loss of appetite and weight loss, whereas 9 out of 10 carers are affected.
  CRS presents as emotions like anxiety, anger, feeling upset, bother, concern, frustration and guilt.
  Suffering arises when the expectations of nutritional intake and development of weight differ significantly from the reality (known as the Calman gap).
- Features of natural development of CRS:
  Depending on the personal intellectual resources and communicative skills, CRS can either escalate to the extent of a predominating problem determining the relationship of patient and carer or decrease after an episode of adaptation and maturation caused by this new situation.
- Key points of assessment of CRS:
  A single screening question like: "How much do you feel distressed about your inability to eat?" is sufficient to identify and a simple entry point into the field of CRS. The Functional Assessment of Anorexia/Cachexia Therapy (FAACT) scale also contains certain aspects of CRS and may be helpful for screening purposes. There is no validated assessment tool for CRS but work on it is in progress.
- Key points of management of CRS:
  The nature of CCS is, with very few exceptions, progressive and irreversible. Recognizing the terminal nature of the disease and acceptance is the key to relief from CRS. In case the irreversible nature of CCS is not recognized or not accepted, patients or carers may continue to try to maintain life with increasing food intake.
  Systematic assessment, e.g., using a checklist to systematically search for secondary causes of cachexia, which might be treatable and weight loss therefore partially reversible (see Table 21.3), is crucial. Addressing CRS, psychosocial support, education and facilitation of self-action help patients and their carers. Meanwhile, optimizing food intake is ongoing, but no longer a priority of treatment.

ETHICAL ISSUES

Unfortunately CRS is still frequently missed. Even if detected, healthcare professionals are often unable to constructively broach the issue of CRS. Even if there remains no substantial treatment against cancer cachexia, from an ethical point of view it is necessary to openly discuss this truth and the associated psychosocial consequences of weight loss. There is no doubt of the relief of suffering by informing patients as well as their carers appropriately.

SUMMARY POINTS

- Cachexia-related suffering (CRS) was long underestimated as a significant psychosocial consequence of cancer cachexia syndrome (CCS). It is defined as negative emotions associated with reduced nutritional intake and weight loss.
- CRS may be present in about one third to one half of the patients suffering from loss of appetite and weight loss, whereas 9 out of 10 carers are affected.
- Suffering arises when the expectations of nutritional intake and development of weight differ significantly from the reality (also known as the Calman gap). CRS presents as emotions like anxiety, anger, feeling upset, bother, concern, frustration and guilt.
- A single screening question like: "How much do you feel distressed about your inability to eat?" is sufficient to identify CRS.
- The nature of CCS is, with very few exceptions, progressive and irreversible. Recognizing the terminal nature of the disease and acceptance is the key to relief from CRS. Addressing CRS, providing psychosocial support, education and facilitation of self-action help patients and their carers.

ACKNOWLEDGMENTS

Our special thanks go to Jane Hopkinson, science nurse from the Macmillan Research Unit, University of Southampton, United Kingdom, who was substantially involved in the original work which underlies this chapter. We are also grateful to Mr. Daniel Kauffman, librarian at the Cantonal Hospital St. Gallen. Without his contribution of collecting literature, this work would not have been possible. Particularly we thank our patients, as this knowledge and its application comes from conversations with them.

LIST OF ABBREVIATIONS

BMI	Body mass index
CCS	Cancer cachexia syndrome
COPD	Chronic obstructive pulmonary disease
CRP	C-reactive protein
CRS	Cachexia-related suffering
ERD	Eating-related distress
FAACT	Functional Assessment of Anorexia/Cachexia Therapy
HIV	Human immunodeficiency virus
Tb	Tuberculosis
VAS	Visual Analogue Scale
WHO	World Health Organization
WRD	Weight-loss-related distress

REFERENCES

Calman, K. C. 1984. Quality of life in cancer patients – A hypothesis. *Journal of Medical Ethics*, 3:124–27.

Cella, D. F., P. B. Jacobsen, and E. J. Orav. 1993. Quality of life and nutritional well-being: Measurement and relationship. *Oncology* 7:105–11.

Hawkins, C. 2000. Anorexia and anxiety in advanced malignancy: The relative problem. *Journal of Human Nutrition and Dietetics* 13:113–17.

Holden, C. M. 1991. Anorexia in the terminally ill cancer patient: The emotional impact on the patient and the family. *Hospital Journal* 7:73–84.

Hopkinson, J. B., D. N. Wright, J. W. McDonald, and J. L. Corner. 2006. The prevalence of concern about weight loss and change in eating habits in people with advanced cancer. *Journal of Pain and Symptom Management* 32:322–31.

Hopkinson, J. B., D. N. M. Wright, and J. L. Corner. 2005. 'Nothing can be done. These are the words they tell me': Exploring the experiences of weight loss in people with advanced cancer. *ECCO 13 - The European Cancer Conference, Paris, France,* 30 Oct–3 Nov 2005.

Hopkinson, J. B. 2007. How people with advanced cancer manage changing eating habits. *Journal of Advanced Nursing* 59:454–62.

Hopkinson, J. B. 2008. Carers' influence on diets of people with advanced cancer. *Nursing Times* 104:28–29.

Hopkinson, J., and J. Corner. 2006. Helping patients with advanced cancer live with concerns about eating: A challenge for palliative care professionals. *Journal of Pain and Symptom Management* 31:293–305.

Kondrup, J., H. H. Rasmussen, O. Hamberg, and Z. Stanga. 2003. Ad Hoc ESPEN Working Group. Nutritional risk screening (NRS 2002): A new method based on an analysis of controlled clinical trials. *Clinical Nutrition* 22:321–36.

McClement, S. E., L. F. Degner, and M. Harlos. 2004. Family responses to declining intake and weight loss in a terminally ill relative. Part 1: Fighting back. *Journal of Palliative Care* 20:93–100.

McClement, S. E., and M. Harlos. 2008. When advanced cancer patients won't eat: Family responses. *International Journal of Palliative Nursing* 14:182–88.

Meares, C. J. 1997. Primary caregiver perceptions of intake cessation in patients who are terminally Ill., *Oncological Nursing Forum* 24:1751–57.

Rabinovitz, M. 1986. Unintentional weight loss. *Archives of Internal Medicine* 146:186–87.

Reid, J., H. McKenna, D. Fitzsimons, and T. McCance. 2008. The experience of cancer cachexia: A qualitative study of advanced cancer patients and their family members. *International Journal of Nursing Studies* 46:606–16.

Ribaudo, J. M., D. Cella, E. A. Hahn, S. R. Lloyd, N. S. Tchekmedyian, J. Von, and W. T. Leslie. 2001. Re-validation and shortening of the Functional Assessment of Anorexia/Cachexia Therapy (FAACT) questionnaire. *Quality of Life Research* 9:1137–46.

Shragge, J. E., W. V. Wismer, K. L. Olson, and V. E. Baracos. 2007. Shifting to conscious control: psychosocial and dietary management of anorexia by patients with advanced cancer. *Palliative Medicine* 21:227–33.

Souter, J. 2005. Loss of appetite: A poetic exploration of cancer patients' and their carers' experiences. *International Journal of Palliative Nursing* 11:524–32.

Strasser, F., J. Binswanger, T. Cerny, and A. Kesselring. 2007. Fighting a losing battle: Eating-related distress of men with advanced cancer and their female partners. A mixed-methods study. *Palliative Medicine* 21:129–36.

22 An Overview of Gastrointestinal Side Effects in Tumour Therapy: Implications for Nutrition

Sebastian Renger and Frank Mayer

CONTENTS

22.1 INTRODUCTION

Malnutrition is a frequent finding in cancer patients, in particular in advanced stages (Bozzetti et al. 2009). For a variety of tumours, malnutrition is associated with a poor outcome and its pathogenesis is complex. Some metabolic changes are directly cancer-related, e.g., increased liver, muscle protein or carbohydrate turnover and lipolysis. In addition, therapy-related symptoms like anorexia, dysgeusia, nausea, vomiting, constipation, diarrhoea and mucositis add to a reduced uptake of regular food and contribute to malnutrition—with detrimental effects on quality of life, and possibly also on the tolerance of further therapy.

Quality of life is a critical issue for patients suffering from cancer. This is particularly true at a stage of disease that is beyond cure. For many of these patients, modern oncological treatment can prolong survival. However, the patients are treated for long periods of their remaining life span. Even in the era of molecular targeted therapies, the vast majority of patients are still treated with classical cytotoxic drugs. Gastrointestinal side effects—in particular nausea and vomiting—are some of the adverse events feared most by the majority of patients. Sometimes, patients surrender months of survival for a better quality of life (Marín Caro, Laviano, and Pichard 2007). Beyond its nutritional relevance, eating and drinking is an important source of pleasure and part of our social life. The ability to participate in meals with family and friends ensures social contact.

The options for preventing and treating gastrointestinal side effects of tumour therapies have been considerably expanded in recent years. Different societies offer recommendations, which provide guidance for appropriate supportive measures. However, they are usually prepared for the treating physicians, and many patients and their families are very grateful to get some guidance on what they themselves can contribute to the patient's ability to maintain a more or less normal diet. Nutrition is one of the few areas in the care of tumour patients in which the patient or the relatives can significantly contribute. Even though systematic studies are largely lacking, the most frequent gastrointestinal side effects of systemic cancer treatment are briefly reviewed with a particular focus on rational recommendations regarding nutrition. In case side effects cannot be controlled by any of the available means, the potential therapeutic benefits must be critically weighed against the potential side effects (Mayer, Kanz, and Zürcher 2008).

22.2 NAUSEA AND VOMITING

Nausea and vomiting are side effects that the majority of tumour patients are particularly afraid of. Frequent emesis can lead to dehydration, weight loss, metabolic abnormalities and electrolyte imbalance (Roenn 2006). When nauseated, patients reduce their regular food uptake to a minimum in order to avoid vomiting.

Emesis is graded by the frequency of vomiting episodes. Nausea can be judged by the patient only—it is the perception that emesis may occur (ASCO 2006). The classification of chemotherapy-induced nausea and vomiting is divided into three different categories: (1) acute onset, occurring within 24 h of initial administration of chemotherapy, (2) delayed onset, occurring 24 h to several days after initial treatment and (3) anticipatory nausea and vomiting (Jordan, Schmoll, and Aapro 2007) (Table 22.1).

The Common Toxicity Criteria of the National Cancer Institute differentiates five distinct grades of nausea and vomiting ranging from grade 1 (mild) to moderate, severe, life-threatening or disabling and grade 5, defined as a side effect leading to the death of the patient (Smith et al. 2008). Algorithms for prophylaxis and treatment refer to the respective grades.

The emetogenic potential of chemotherapeutic agents is the main risk factor for the occurrence of nausea and vomiting. Combination chemotherapy regimens generally tend to have a higher emetogenic potential than single-agent therapies. For example, cyclophosphamide and doxorubicin are both moderately emetogenic when given as single agents, but the combination of both is highly emetogenic (Grunberg, Osoba, and Hesketh 2005).

Other known risk factors are young age, female gender, low alcohol intake, experience of emesis during pregnancy, impaired quality of life and previous poor experience with chemotherapy (Jordan et al. 2005; Zachariae, Paulsen, and Mehlsen 2007).

22.2.1 PHARMACOLOGICAL THERAPY OF NAUSEA AND VOMITING

5-HT3 receptor antagonists like ondansetron, granisetron or palonosetron are the most effective antiemetics in the prophylaxis of acute nausea and vomiting (Jordan et al. 2005). They are usually

TABLE 22.1
Categories of Chemotherapy-Induced Nausea and Vomiting

Categories	Description
Acute nausea and vomiting	• Within the first 24 h after chemotherapy • Mainly by serotonin (5-HT) release from the enterochromaffin cells
Delayed nausea and vomiting	• 24 h to 5 days after start of chemotherapy • Various mechanisms: mainly substance P-mediated, disruption of the blood–brain barrier, disruption of gastrointestinal motility, adrenal hormones
Anticipatory nausea and vomiting	• Occurrence is possible after 1 cycle of chemotherapy • Involves the element of classic conditioning • In approximately 30% of patients by the fourth treatment cycle after experience of emetic episode(s)

Source: Adapted from Jordan, K., H. J. Schmoll and M. S. Aapro, *Crit. Rev. Oncol. Hematol.* 61, 162, 2007.

combined with corticosteroids, e.g., dexamethasone. Unfavourable effects of 5-HT3 receptor antagonists are usually mild. The most commonly described side effects are headache and constipation. The lowest effective dose for each agent should be used, as higher doses rarely yield additional benefits due to receptor saturation (Jordan et al. 2005). Oral and intravenous application are similarly effective. For chemotherapy administered on consecutive days it is recommended to apply 5-HT3 receptor antagonists (except palonosetrons) daily prior to treatment. The same is recommended for dexamethasone. For delayed emesis, 5-HT3 receptor antagonists are used two to three days beyond the last day of therapy.

Aprepitant belongs to a new group of antiemetics and acts as a neurokinin 1-receptor antagonist. It further reduces the incidence of nausea and vomiting of regimens with an intermediate or high emetogenic potential.

There are various guidelines for the optimal use of antiemetics based on the emetogenic potential of the regimens used (e.g., www.nccn.org and www.mascc.org).

22.2.2 Nutritional Impact of Nausea and Vomiting

22.2.2.1 General Aspects

There are too little data to justify evidence-based recommendations for optimal food choices for patients receiving chemotherapy. Based on personal experience, there is no need for a particular diet, even though most patients will prefer dishes with a low fat content and without red meat. In case of nausea, vomiting or taste disturbances, the individual's favourite dishes should be avoided in order to prevent negative conditioning. Increasing the frequency of meals from three to five and reducing the volume of the individual meal seems helpful. When liquids are better tolerated than solid food, high-caloric beverages should be tested. They can be prepared with salt if the patient has an aversion to sweets.

22.2.2.2 Ginger to Prevent or Reduce Emesis

In traditional medicine, ginger was used to improve appetite or overcome nausea. This effect of ginger was evaluated in a clinical trial. A randomised, double-blind, placebo-controlled trial enrolled

664 patients, most of them women receiving chemotherapy for breast, gastrointestinal or lung cancer. Patients received either placebo or one of three doses of ginger (0.5, 1.0, 1.5 g) for 6 days starting two days before chemotherapy in addition to standard antiemetics. All doses of ginger reduced nausea significantly compared to placebo as measured by the patients on an analogue scale. No significant differences were reported for the side effect emesis (Ryan 2009). A major drawback of the study is the fact that aprepitant was not used, as antagonistic effects were reported in a previous phase II study. Therefore, the antiemetic medication used in the study cannot be considered optimal. The use of ginger can certainly not substitute for an optimal supportive medication. However, patients can be encouraged to use this spice when trying to find meals that are tolerated during chemotherapy.

22.3 MUCOSITIS

Mucositis is a treatment-related complication following chemotherapy and radiotherapy. It can occur in the entire gastrointestinal tract and can be associated with painful erosions and ulceration in the mouth, oesophagus, small bowel and colon (Gibson and Keefe 2006; Keefe 2006).

Oral and gastric mucositis may affect up to 100% of patients undergoing high-dose chemotherapy with haematopoietic stem cell transplantation (HSCT) (Rubenstein, Peterson, and Schubert 2004). In particular, in patients undergoing combined chemotherapy and radiation, mucositis is frequently a painful side effect. It is also a well-recognised toxicity associated with some standard-dose chemotherapy regimens commonly used in cancer treatment (Rubenstein et al. 2004).

The mucosal lesions often start off with small erosions, which become confluent over time. After penetration of the basal membrane, a fibrous pseudomembrane develops covering the ulcer. Any area of the mouth may be affected, but mucositis often occurs in the buccal mucosa, and lateral and ventral tongue and soft palate. The gingiva and dorsal surface are less frequently affected.

The intensity of mucositis is also graded; the two most commonly used scales are the World Health Organization (WHO) (Table 22.2) and the U.S. National Cancer Institute classifications. While the WHO summarises objective (ulceration/erythema), subjective (pain) and functional (ability to eat) aspects into a single value, the National Cancer Institute Common Toxicity Criteria version 3 rates the clinical findings of mucositis (erythema, ulceration) and functional consequences of mucositis in two different scales.

TABLE 22.2
WHO Scoring Criteria for Oral Mucositis

Grade	Description
Grade 0	Normal
Grade 1	Soreness with or without erythema; no ulceration
Grade 2	Ulceration and erythema; patient can swallow a solid diet
Grade 3	Ulceration and erythema; patient cannot swallow a solid diet
Grade 4	Ulceration or pseudomembrane formation of such severity that alimentation not possible

Source: Adapted from Treister, N. and S. Sonis, *Curr. Opin. Otolaryngol. Head Neck Surg.* 15, 123, 2007.

22.3.1 Prevention and Therapy of Mucositis

For prevention and therapy, several guidelines exist, e.g., from the Multinational Association of Supportive Care in Cancer (MASCC), which are updated on a regular basis and available on the internet (www.mascc.org). For prevention, it is recommended to undergo professional dental treatment before starting chemotherapy. Patients should be encouraged to stop smoking as early as possible before any treatment with a high risk for mucositis.

Patients should increase conventional teeth hygiene. Teeth should be brushed after every meal with a soft toothbrush as tolerated—especially in the case of parodontitis or gingivitis.

Once mucositis is evident, patients should use an oral irrigator instead of toothbrushes for dental hygiene. Cryotherapy, or the use of ice chips melting in the mouth, during chemotherapy infusion, may be effective, while therapy with 5-fluorouracil (5-FU) is given due to localised vasoconstriction and restricted diffusion of the cytotoxic agent into the mucosa. However, in protracted infusion schedules, this approach is not feasible. Obviously, the use of ice chips is contraindicated in situations where the drug has to reach the oral mucosa, i.e., oropharyngeal cancer.

In cases of painful mucositis, adequate analgesia is very important. While for mucositis grade 2 local analgetic measures are sufficient, systemic analgesics are needed in more severe cases. Mostly potent opiates or patient-controlled analgesia (PCA) with morphine are applied as the treatment of choice for oral mucositis pain in patients undergoing HSCT (Rubenstein et al. 2004). Morphine sulphate appears to be effective in relatively low doses compared to other opiates and may be easier to use, even in paediatric patients.

Because of the injury of the mucous membrane, the mucosa loses its barrier function and becomes permeable to pathogens. As mucositis usually coincides with neutropenia, the permeation of pathogens may result in neutropenic fever. Therefore an antimycotic agent can be considered for mucositis grade I and II. It is recommended for higher-grade mucositis. In case of neutropenic fever in a patient suffering from mucositis, the empirical antibiotic regimen has to cover the gastrointestinal flora (Link, Böhme, and Cornely 2003).

22.3.2 Nutritional Impact of Mucositis

In patients suffering from mucositis grade 2, pureed foods can be eaten, while for severe mucositis the diet is limited to liquids and infusions. Alcohol, spicy food, nicotine, juice and extremely cold, extremely hot or sharp-edged food should be avoided. Once the white blood counts recover, the mucositis usually resolves within a couple of days. Since the duration of impairment of food uptake is rather predictable, the need for parenteral nutrition can be discussed based on the nutritional status of the patient (Bozzetti 2009). The timing and start of parenteral nutrition is still a matter of debate, especially since many patients are not malnourished at presentation. In the context of HSCT, some institutions start parenteral nutrition directly after grafting and maintain it for 15–20 days. In others, parenteral nutrition is initiated once oral feeding falls below 60%–70% of requirements for three days. Parenteral nutrition is discontinued usually when patients are able to tolerate approximately 50% of their enteral demand (Bozzetti 2009).

In cases of severe mucositis, placement of a nasogastric tube is not considered a reasonable option, as the tube adds to the irritation of the mucus membranes and is poorly tolerated by the patients. However, placement of percutaneous gastrostomy can allow for continued enteral feeding in patients irradiated for head and neck cancer.

22.4 DIARRHOEA

Diarrhoea is a side effect associated with a large number of cytotoxic agents, especially fluorouracil (FU) and irinotecan (CPT-11), and with abdominal or pelvic radiotherapy (RT) (Benson, Ajani, and

Catalano 2004). The "Guidelines for the Treatment of Cancer Treatment-Induced Diarrhea" state that the incidence of chemotherapy-induced diarrhoea associated with modulated FU regimens, single agent CPT-11 and the combination of FU plus CPT-11 has been reported to be as high as 50%–80% of treated patients, and ≥30% of patients may experience grade 3–5 diarrhoea (Benson et al. 2004). The incidence is even higher in high-dose regimens, bolus applications of 5-FU, the use of high doses of leucovorin and combination regimens (e.g., CPT-11 plus bolus FU/leucovorin). Persistent severe diarrhoea may be associated with loss of fluids and electrolytes, resulting in life-threatening dehydration, renal insufficiency and electrolyte imbalances. It may contribute to cardiovascular morbidity, e.g., by increased incidence of thromboembolic events. In addition, it decreases patients' quality of life (Kornblau et al. 2000).

It is important to determine the cause of diarrhoea in patients receiving chemotherapy. Besides the effects of cytostatic agents and radiotherapy, infections, for example with rota- and norovirus and *Clostridium difficile*, may induce complex diarrhoea and may require specific interventions or hygienic measures such as isolation in order to avoid spreading of the disease (Mayer et al. 2008).

22.4.1 Assessment and Early Intervention

From a clinical point of view, the severity of diarrhoea depends on its impact on quality of life (e.g., by interfering with daily life, sleep disturbance, etc.), fluid balance (renal insufficiency, symptomatic arterial hypotension) and metabolic changes (metabolic acidosis due to loss of bicarbonate). Thus, the health impact of diarrhoea not only depends on its intensity but also on the overall condition of the patient. A sound clinical judgement is mandatory in assessing patients suffering from diarrhoea.

Nevertheless, for assessing and comparing side effects in clinical trials, criteria are defined. The most standardised assessment tools are the "National Cancer Institute's (NCI) Common Toxicity Criteria for Grading Severity of Diarrhea."

22.4.2 Nutritional Impact of Diarrhoea

Regardless of the cause of diarrhoea, the aim of dietetic treatment is to reconstitute fluid and electrolytic deficits immediately and to adapt the diet to the gastrointestinal function with reduced adsorptive and digestive capacity. Furthermore, primary or secondary malnourishment should be avoided. As for all types of fluid loss, adequate hydration is of critical importance. Patients should be instructed to drink three or more litres of clear fluid per day. In the outpatient setting, it is recommended to have the weight checked by the patient on a daily basis.

To avoid hyponatraemia and hypokalaemia, the fluids should also contain electrolytes, such as sport drinks or decaffeinated tea. Commercially available variants of the WHO oral rehydration solution can be recommended as an alternative to self-prepared solutions. Rehydration solutions should contain Na+ 90 mmol/l, K+ 20 mmol/l, Cl– 80 mmol/l, HCO_3– (hydrogen carbonate, alternative citrate) 30 mmol/l and glucose 111 mmol/l. It can be prepared by adding 13.5 g glucose, 2.9 g sodium citrate, 2.6 g sodium chloride and 1.5 g potassium chloride to a litre of clear water.

As the absorption of sodium and glucose with the help of sodium-glucose cotransport fluid absorption occurs passively, intestinal absorption is usually functioning, even in the case of severe diarrhoea. Therefore, oral rehydration is frequently possible despite persistent diarrhoea.

Primarily, patients experiencing diarrhoea may try the 'BRAT' diet, consisting of bananas, rice, apple sauce and toast (Richardson and Dobish 2007). When the diarrhoea resolves, other easily digestible foods—like rusks or scrambled eggs—may be added. Patients should avoid spicy, high-fat or high-fibre foods, alcohol and fruit juices, and abandon all lactose-containing products during diarrhoea, and for not less than one week following recovery. Similarly, artificial sweeteners have a laxative effect and should be avoided.

After exclusion of infectious causes, in particular *C. difficile* infection, it is possible to use loperamide at its standard recommended dose. In severe cases, tinctura opii may be more efficient. However, it has to be used with caution in order to avoid development of a paralytic ileus. For chemotherapy-related diarrhoea, subcutaneous application of octreotide has been shown to be effective in randomised trials (Roenn 2006). It imitates natural somatostatin and reduces gastrointestinal fluid secretion.

22.4.2.1 Glutamine for Protection of the Intestinal Mucosa

Glutamine is a non-essential, common amino acid with an important role for the intestinal tract. It is essential for normal intestinal structure and stimulates electrolyte and nutrient absorption in the small intestine (Richardson and Dobish 2007). It is assumed that glutamine protects the intestinal mucosa from chemotherapy-induced damage and improves intestinal absorption. A double-blind, placebo-controlled, randomised trial conducted by the Alberta Cancer Board showed positive results with 6 g of glutamine crystalline powder dissolved in water and dosed three times daily for a sequence of 15 days starting 5 days before the first dose of chemotherapy. The ESPEN guidelines suggest that a dose of 0.6 g/kg/day of glutamine may protect the intestinal mucosa of patients undergoing HSCT. However, the optimal dose of glutamine to be used in this context is not yet established (Bozzetti 2009).

22.4.2.2 Probiotics for Prevention of Diarrhoea

Lactobacillus acidophilus and *bifidobacterium* are nonpathogenic microorganisms—so-called probiotics. They are thought to antagonise disturbances in normal microflora by competitively inhibiting the binding of pathogens to intestinal mucosa. Furthermore, probiotics may activate cell-mediated immunity by stimulating the synthesis of cytokines. Von Bültzingslowen, Adlerberth, and Wold (2003) reported a preclinical study with rats on the safety and efficacy of *Lactobacillus plantarum* in the prevention and treatment of 5-FU-induced diarrhoea. The treatment improved food uptake and body weight in 5-FU-treated rats. The total numbers of facultative anaerobes in the intestine was increased. However, there are still concerns that patients undergoing chemotherapy may be at increased risk of infections resulting from probiotics. Therefore, the widespread use of probiotics in cancer patients undergoing chemotherapy cannot yet be recommended. In case the symptoms persist after haematologic and mucosal recovery, a trial of probiotics may be justified.

22.5 CONSTIPATION

Constipation is a frequent problem for cancer patients and is characterised as an infrequent or difficult passage of stool that leads to an incomplete defecation (American College of Gastroenterology Chronic Constipation Task Force 2005). It affects about 40% of patients undergoing palliative chemotherapy (Roenn 2006).

Decreased mobility and physical activity, dehydration, bowel obstruction, spinal cord compression and medications like opioids and antidepressants add to constipation. Some cytotoxic drugs, in particular vinca alkaloids, have been associated with constipation. However, for many patients its pathogenesis is multifactorial.

22.5.1 Pharmacological Therapy of Constipation

Patients complaining about constipation should receive a digital rectal examination. An abdominal x-ray in an upright position shows the distribution of stool in the colon. In case of impaction, a careful enema is the treatment of choice. It is important to consider contraindications like leukopenia and thrombopenia (Mayer et al. 2008). Besides an enema, stimulating (bisacodyl), salinic (sodium phosphate) and osmotic (glycerin) laxatives are available. They are effective within 24–48 hours.

The primary side effect is flatulence. The contact cathartics (e.g., bisacodyl and docusate) are the most widely used group of laxatives (Roenn 2006).

For patients receiving high doses of opiates, opiate receptor antagonists like methylnaltrexone can provide relief of symptoms. Methylnaltrexone is applied subcutaneously. Bowel movements are induced after a period of about four hours.

The 5HT-3-antagonists used for antiemetic prophylaxis are known to induce constipation in up to 20% of patients. It may be worth switching to an alternative substance if there is a suspected connection to the problem.

22.5.2 Managing Constipation

After exclusion of a mechanic ileus, management of constipation is conservative. It depends on the general condition of the patient, the clinical situation and the presumed pathogenesis of constipation. Medical therapy is frequently necessary, especially initially. For medium-term stool regulation, diet and changing habits play an important role. First of all, contributing factors should be eliminated: fluid intake should be increased to at least two litres a day. Physical activity should be encouraged, if the overall condition of the patient allows it. The medication has to be checked and drugs potentially contributing to constipation should be switched if possible.

22.5.3 Nutritional Impact of Constipation

The diet should contain more dietary fibre (recommendation 30 g/day), because stool quantity rises and the colon transit time is shortened. Dietary fibre and its equivalents (oligofructose, lactulose) reach the large intestine and have an effect on stool quantity and consistency. Water-soluble fibre (e.g., pectin, oligofructose, flaxseed, carbo bean gum) is microbiologically digested to short-chain fatty acids that increase bowel motility. Water-insoluble fibres (cellulose, lignin) are not fermented by bacteria—they bind water and increase the stool volume.

Dietary fibre is found in cereals, vegetables and fruits. The adaptation to a fibre-rich diet should happen slowly because of flatulence and pendulous discomfort. It is important to remember an adequate fluid intake.

22.6 CHANGES IN PERCEPTION OF TASTE AND SMELL

A well-known side effect reported by many patients undergoing chemotherapy is dysgeusia or the loss of taste and smell. It is a common problem in patients after intense chemotherapeutic regimens in the context of a HSCT (Epstein et al. 2002), but is also reported following standard dose treatment. Bone marrow transplant recipients have a high incidence of taste and smell alterations, which is associated with delayed physical recovery, general wasting and decreased quality of life. A study from the University of Tuebingen, Germany, included 181 patients who were treated with HSCT. Indications for HSCT included acute leukaemia, lymphoma, myeloproliferative disease or myelodysplastic syndrome (MDS). The patients received either allogenic or an autologous graft after myeloablative or reduced-intensity conditioning. Seventy-one percent of the patients reported moderate to severe changes in taste perception on a semiquantitative visual analogue scale during the acute phase of HSCT. Changes in taste perception were significantly associated with loss of body weight >5 kg (Federmann, Weidmann, and Blumenstock 2009). A complete recovery at the time of the survey was reported by 29% of the patients; 26% still suffered from ongoing moderate to severe taste alterations. A significant difference in time to recovery with a subjective improvement of symptoms after a median of 60 days (range, 3–365) after autologous HSCT vs. 120 days after allogeneic HSCT was observed. Affected patients can be encouraged, as the side effects will improve over time for the majority of patients.

General guidelines for patients suffering from dysgeusia recommend trying highly aromatic and tart foods like herbs and spices, and oranges, which may have more taste. It is also important to offer fluids with meals to help to remove a bad taste in the mouth. Other possibilities are cold, non-odorous foods (Grant and Byron 2006).

KEY FACTS OF MALNUTRITION

- Nutrition of tumour patients is difficult in many cases.
- Eating habits change during therapy—sometimes caused by the tumour itself, sometimes by therapy-related side effects.
- Malnutrition is a common finding in tumour patients.
- It affects quality of life and survival.
- Malnutrition is defined as an inadvertent and illness-related weight loss that causes:
    - interferences of the immune system
    - increased disease frequency
    - enhanced side effects during tumour therapy
    - insufficient tumour therapy and shorter survival
- For patients suffering from gastrointestinal side effects, recommendations, as given in the text, might be helpful to cope with these situations.

ETHICAL ISSUES

Medical interventions represent a bodily injury, which is justified only if the intervention is indicated, if it is performed according to the standard of care after careful information and informed consent. The optimal treatment of therapy-related adverse events is an integral part of every intervention. Thus, tumour treatment must only be offered by healthcare providers who are able to cope with the side effects. Risks and benefits have to be carefully considered before a treatment is started.

SUMMARY POINTS

- Gastrointestinal side effects are common following systemic chemotherapy. The risk associated with a particular regimen can be predicted based on the choice and dose of agents and combinations used.
- Side effects have an impact on the ability to maintain a regular diet. By contributing to malnutrition, they may adversely affect quality of life and prognosis in tumour patients.
- Both patients and their families are eager to contribute actively to well-being in the field of nutrition. Therefore, they are grateful for guidance and recommendations on how to nourish in case of gastrointestinal side effects of systemic tumour treatment.
- Recommendations regarding nutrition need to be combined with the optimal use of supportive medication in order to prevent or at least ameliorate gastrointestinal side effects.

LIST OF ABBREVIATIONS

ASCO	American Society of Clinical Oncology
BMT	Bone marrow transplantation
CPT-11	Irinotecan
ESPEN	European Society for Clinical Nutrition and Metabolism
FU	Fluorouracil

HSCT	Haematopoietic stem cell transplantation
MASCC	Multinational Association of Supportive Care in Cancer
NCI	National Cancer Institute
PCA	Patient-controlled analgesia
RT	Radiotherapy
WHO	World Health Organization

REFERENCES

American College of Gastroenterology Chronic Constipation Task Force. 2005. An evidence-based approach to the management of chronic constipation in North America. *Am J Gastroenterol* 100:1–4.

American Society of Clinical Oncology (ASCO). 2006. American Society of Clinical Oncology guideline for antiemetics in oncology: Update 2006. *J Clin Oncol* 24:2932–47.

Benson, A. B., 3rd., J. A. Ajani, and R. B. Catalano. 2004. Recommended guidelines for the treatment of cancer treatment-induced diarrhea. *J Clin Oncol* 22:2918–26.

Bozzetti, F., J. Arends, and K. Lundholm. 2009. ESPEN Guidelines on Parenteral Nutrition: Non-surgical oncology. *Clinical Nutrition* 28:445–54.

Epstein, J. B., N. Phillips, J. Parry, M. S. Epstein, T. Nevill, P. Stevenson-Moore. 2002. Quality of life, taste, olfactory and oral function following high-dose chemotherapy and allogeneic hematopoietic cell transplantation. *Bone Marrow Transplant* 30:785–92.

Federmann, B., J. Weidmann, and G. Blumenstock. 2009. Incidence and characterization of taste disturbances after allogeneic or autologous hematopoietic stem cell transplantation using myeloablative or reduced-intensity conditioning. Not published yet.

Gibson, R. J., and D. M. Keefe. 2006. Cancer chemotherapy-induced diarrhoea and constipation: Mechanisms of damage and prevention strategies. *Support Care Cancer* 14:890–900.

Grant, B., and J. Byron. 2006. Nutritional implications of chemotherapy (Chapter 8). In *The clinical guide to oncology nutrition*, 2nd edn., 72–87. American Dietetic Association.

Grunberg, S. M., D. Osoba, P. J. Hesketh. 2005. Evaluation of new antiemetic agents and definition of antineoplastic agent emetogenicity–an update. *Support Care Cancer* 13:80–84.

Jordan, K., C. Kasper, H. J. Schmoll. 2005. Chemotherapy-induced nausea and vomiting: Current and new standards in the antiemetic prophylaxis and treatment. *Eur J Cancer* 41:199–205.

Jordan, K., H. J. Schmoll, and M. S. Aapro. 2007. Comparative activity of antiemetic drugs. *Crit Rev Oncol Hematol* 61:162–75.

Keefe, D. M. K. 2006. Mucositis guidelines: What have they achieved, and where to from here? *Support Care Cancer* 14:489–91.

Kornblau, S., A. B. Benson, R. Catalano, R. E. Champlin, C. Engelking, M. Field, C. Ippoliti, et al. 2000. Management of cancer treatment-related diarrhea. Issues and therapeutic strategies. *J Pain Symptom Manage* 19:118–29.

Link, H., O. A. Böhme, and K. Cornely. 2003. Antimicrobial therapy of unexplained fever in neutropenic patients. *Ann Hematol* 82:105–17.

Marín Caro, M. M., A. Laviano, and C. Pichard. 2007. Impact of nutrition on quality of life during cancer. *Curr Opin Clin Nutr Metab Care* 10:480–87.

Mayer, F., L. Kanz, and G. Zürcher. 2008. Gastrointestinale Nebenwirkungen und Ernährung bei Tumortherapie. *Der Onkologe* 14:58–64.

Richardson, G., and R. Dobish. 2007. Chemotherapy induced diarrhea. *J Oncol Pharm Pract* 13:181–98.

Roenn, J. 2006. Pharmacological management of nutrition impact symptoms associated with cancer (Chapter 15). In *The clinical guide to oncology nutrition*, 2nd edn., 165–79. American Dietetic Association.

Rubenstein, E. B., D. E. Peterson, and M. Schubert. 2004. Clinical practice guidelines for the prevention and treatment of cancer therapy-induced oral and gastrointestinal mucositis. *Cancer* 100 (9 Suppl):2026–46.

Ryan, J. L. 2009. PUBLISH AHEAD OF PRINT: Ginger Provides Significant Reduction of Chemotherapy-induced Nausea. www.asco.org.

Smith, L. C., P. Bertolotti, K. Curran, B. Jenkins, and IMF Nurse Leadership Board. 2008. Gastrointestinal side effects associated with novel therapies in patients with multiple myeloma: Consensus statement of the IMF Nurse Leadership Board. *Clin J Oncol Nurs* 12:37–52.

Treister, N., and S. Sonis. 2007. Mucositis: Biology and management. *Curr Opin Otolaryngol Head Neck Surg* 15:123–29.

Von Bültzingslöwen, I., I. Adlerberth, A. E. Wold. 2003. Oral and intestinal microflora in 5-fluorouracil treated rats, translocation to cervical and mesenteric lymph nodes and effects of probiotic bacteria. *Oral Microbiol Immunol* 18:278–84.

Zachariae, R., K. Paulsen, and M. Mehlsen. 2007. Chemotherapy-induced nausea, vomiting, and fatigue–the role of individual differences related to sensory perception and autonomic reactivity. *Psychother Psychosom* 76:376–84.

23 Nutritional Status and Relationship to Upper Gastrointestinal Symptoms in Patients with Advanced Cancer Receiving Palliative Care

Giacomo Bovio and Tiziana Sappia

CONTENTS

23.1 INTRODUCTION

Malnutrition is our body's reaction to inadequate food intake. The early assessment of malnutrition is particularly important when dealing with subjects at risk such as hospitalized or palliative care patients: an adequate nutritional approach could play a fundamental role in improving their quality of life.

The most evident clinical effects of malnutrition stem from the insufficient supply of protein-energy, although it usually entails a widespread deficiency in all nutrients.

Patients with advanced cancer are often affected by malnutrition and nourishment difficulties. About 80% of these patients show CACS with its characteristic weight loss, anorexia, alterations in metabolism, asthenia, reduced calorie intake, depletion of fat mass and serious muscle catabolism. The pathogenesis of CACS is multifactorial. Key features of CACS are listed in Table 23.1.

Bozzetti and Mariani (2009) have proposed an easy classification based on a combination of body weight (BW) loss (<10% precachexia, >10% cachexia) and the presence/absence of at least one symptom of anorexia, fatigue or early satiation. There is then a further distinction: class 1 = precachexia without symptoms; class 2 = precachexia with symptoms; class 3 = cachexia without symptoms; class 4 = cachexia with symptoms. This method is very simple, making either laboratory investigations or body composition assessment unnecessary.

23.1.1 Malnutrition: Causes and Consequences

All malnutrition events can be ascribed to the following causes:

a. Reduced food intake due to anorexia, nausea, dysphagia, etc.
b. Loss of nutrients due to diarrhoea, malabsorption, vomiting, nephrotic syndrome, haemorrhage.
c. Increased nourishment needs due to surgical operations, sepsis.
d. Alterations in metabolism caused by neoplasia, for example, hypermetabolism.

The lack of nutrients at cellular level causes biochemical damage due to the alteration of the cell enzymatic systems; then functional damage follows, with either general symptoms such as asthenia, anorexia or specific symptoms; in the end the damage becomes anatomical.

Malnutrition has serious consequences for all organs and systems.

TABLE 23.1
Key Features of Cancer Anorexia Cachexia Syndrome

1. It is a complex metabolic syndrome often affecting cancer patients
2. It increases morbidity and mortality
3. It is different from other secondary anorexia cachexia syndromes since it shows an increase in proinflammatory cytokines
4. It alters carbohydrate metabolism (increased gluconeogenesis, glucose intolerance and insulin resistance), lipid metabolism (lipolysis activation, increased lipid mobilizing factor) and protein metabolism (increased turnover and proteolysis, increased acute phase proteins, increased proteolysis-inducing factor)
5. It entails weight loss, anorexia, fatigue and other associated symptoms such as impaired oral intake

23.2 APPLICATION TO OTHER AREAS OF PALLIATIVE CARE

The assessment of nutritional status is relevant for both home and hospital patients. Nutritional screening represents a basic tool to detect malnutrition and enables the setting up of all necessary measures in order to restore a correct nutritional status. Nutritional assessment should be performed at least once a week and this is particularly important for malnourished patients.

The importance of nutritional screening is supported by many articles which state that the correction of malnutrition involves positive effects such as an increase in life expectancy, a reduction in the length of hospitalization, a quicker recovery from ulcers and an improved quality of life.

Nutritional assessment is a prerequisite for taking any nutritional action and carrying out successful monitoring of nutritional parameters, including active control of any nutrition-related symptoms.

23.3 PRACTICAL PROCEDURES AND TECHNIQUES

There are many different parameters involved in nutritional assessment in clinical practice (weight, height, sex, subcutaneous fat thickness, laboratory analysis, etc.). Each parameter, however, does not by itself allow a correct diagnosis.

The clinical practice of the nutritional assessment usually covers the following issues: case history, dietary records, physical examination, anthropometric measurements and laboratory analysis.

23.3.1 Case History

This enables the assessment of the primitive tumour and any metastases, together with other contingent pathology and medical treatments. In palliative care patients, the assessment of appetite is of particular importance and is performed by means of numerical and visual rating scales.

23.3.2 Dietary Records

In order to evaluate food consumption and dietary habits, investigations are carried out by means of a set of recordings made either by qualified personnel or by the patients themselves. Investigation about food intake may cover either a short or a long period of time, possibly using special questionnaires where appropriate.

The main tools are the following (Table 23.2):

a. *The 24-hour food recall.* This is a recording of food and beverage intake over the previous 24 hours; it is a simple and in-depth collection of data, made easy by memory immediacy, yet quite unreliable due to diet variability over time.
b. *Diet diaries.* These involve the collection of data based on specific instructions, made either by the patient or by the caregiver, enabling an assessment of serving size and frequencies. Recordings are to be made either over a week or over three non-consecutive days including one Sunday or public holiday. Quantities should be ascertained with accuracy, making use of adequate scales or identified by serving size defined by common kitchen utensils (spoon, cup, etc.).
c. *Food frequency questionnaires.* These are usually associated with dietary history. They assess food intake over a day, a week or a longer period. They enable the recollection of dietary habits over a long period and can be self-administered by the patient.
d. *Dietary history.* The reconstruction of the patient's dietary history requires an interview in order to collect data about the food intake over the long term; this can also be achieved by means of checklists and with the help of pictures.

TABLE 23.2
Dietary Record Methods

Methods	Advantages	Disadvantages
Diet diary	Permits accurate estimates Accurate method if patient is instructed by professional staff and/or feels deeply motivated	Time consuming for the patient, who must be committed to the task Requires the patient to be instructed Applicable only to educated patients The patient, feeling monitored, might modify his/her dietary habits High incidence of mistakes and/or incomplete data compared to the 24-hour food recall
24-hour food recall	Easy Direct Inexpensive Needs a limited amount of time The subject does not need to be instructed	Since it is based upon a single day, it does not supply sufficient data to compensate for daily, seasonal and festivity variations Overestimates small intakes and underestimates big intakes 10% underestimating food consumption
Scale weighing	Accurate method	Highly time and personnel consuming High financial costs Not applicable when not taking meals at home
Food frequency questionnaires	Fast and practical method A survey considering a long period of time	Diminished accuracy
Dietary history	It gives hints about the patient's overall diet	Overestimating food consumption, particularly micronutrients Time consuming

23.3.3 Physical Examination

This is an evaluation of all those elements which may represent markers of malnutrition: measurement of fat mass and muscle mass, examination of the skin and its annexes, detection of pressure ulcers and oedemas.

23.3.4 Anthropometric Assessment

23.3.4.1 Body Weight

Body weight (BW) is the simplest anthropometric index giving rapid information about a patient's nutritional status. In palliative care units it is not always easy to weigh patients as they are often unable to stand. In this event weighing chairs or hoisting systems are used. Any change in body composition (fat mass, lean body mass, body water) implies a change in BW. When considering this parameter, however, attention should also be given to the actual extent of variation and to its duration in time. An unintentional weight loss >10% over the previous 6 months is considered a sign of malnutrition and cachexia and implies reduced survival.

To make weight independent from height, the use of the BMI (weight in kilograms/height in metres squared) was introduced (Table 23.3).

23.3.4.2 Body Height

The height of patients who are unable to stand can be estimated by measuring their knee height, ulna length or demispan. The patient's height is then estimated by means of formulas and/or tables (Table 23.4).

TABLE 23.3
Weight Classification in Relation to Body Mass Index (BMI)

BMI (kg/m^2)	Weight Classification
<18.5	Underweight
18.5–24.99	Normal weight
25.0–29.99	Overweight
≥30.0	Obese

Source: From Chumlea, W. C., *Anthropometric standardization reference manuals*, Human Kinetics Books, Campaign, 1988.

23.3.4.3 Circumferences

Circumferences reflect nutritional status and body fat distribution. Arm circumference, and waist and hip circumferences are usually measured. Waist and hip circumferences are rarely used in palliative care, whereas they are mostly considered in obese patients.

23.3.5 Laboratory Analysis

Laboratory analysis is also needed when evaluating nutritional status: routine blood tests, urinalysis, nutrient levels, metabolic balances, immunological tests, functional tests.

The comparison of some laboratory data with data obtained from other nutritional investigations supplies important indexes enabling further nutritional assessment (i.e., creatinine/height index).

23.3.5.1 Plasma Proteins

The assessment of low plasma protein levels contributes to the nutritional assessment process since inadequate energy-protein intake may result in decreased synthesis of proteins.

Serum albumin forms a large proportion of plasma proteins and its reduction may be indicative of malnutrition. On account of both its long half-life (about 15–20 days) and its distribution (it is also found in the extracellular space), albumin does not represent an accurate index of malnutrition when malnutrition is not prolonged in time.

Transferrin is a beta globulin for iron ion delivery with a half-life of 8–10 days. Since transferrin values are affected by specific pathological conditions and by iron deficiency, they are not an absolute index of malnutrition.

Prealbumin is a carrier of the thyroid hormone thyroxine, with a half-life of about 2 days, and rapidly reflects malnutrition status by modifying its concentration. Its values may be affected by hyperthyroidism, acute infections and trauma.

Retinol-binding protein has a half-life of about 10 hours and carries vitamin A. It is filtered by glomerulus and reabsorbed by renal tubules, thus increasing its value in the event of renal failure. The reduction in its plasma concentration is a reliable indicator of malnutrition (Table 23.5).

TABLE 23.4
Height Assessment in Bedridden Patients

Estimating Height (cm) from Knee Height: (Chumlea 1988)	
Females	84.88 – (0.24 × age) + (1.83 × knee height)
Males	64.19 – (0.04 × age) + (2.02 × knee height)
Estimating Height (cm) from Demispan: (Bassey 1986)	
Females	(1.35 × demispan) + 60.1
Males	(1.40 × demispan) + 57.8

TABLE 23.5
Plasma Proteins

Protein	Half-Life	Causes of Alterations	Specificity
Transferrin	8 days	↓ Pregnancy, chronic infections, liver cirrhosis etc. ↑ Iron deficiency	Low
Albumin	15–19 days	↓Kwashiorkor, serious organic depletion, malabsorption, liver pathologies, nephropathies, etc.	Low
Prealbumin	1–2 days	Thyroxine availability	Good
Retinol-binding protein	10 hours	Retinol levels:↓protein-energy malnutrition	Good

23.3.5.2 Laboratory Analysis to Assess Muscle Mass

Considering the extent of muscle wasting caused by malnutrition, the collection of creatinuria and 3-methylhistidine is particularly important.

Creatinuria is the end product of skeletal muscle creatinine catabolism. Its values are reliable when renal function is normal and if urine collection occurs after at least 2 days of creatinine-free diet. By matching the subject values with the corresponding sex/age % reference values, the creatinine/height index is obtained.

3-Methylhistidine is an amino acid of the fibrillar proteins; its excretion follows the disruption of these proteins. It is a good indicator of muscle catabolism.

23.3.5.3 Nitrogen Balance

This is the measure of nitrogen output subtracted from nitrogen input, expressed in grams. A negative balance indicates an endogenous protein catabolism. Evaluation is made by distinguishing between mild catabolism, ranging from –5 to –10, moderate –10 to –15, and serious, when >–15. The main input of nitrogen comes from diet proteins. Nitrogen output occurs through the excretion of urine and faeces and via the skin. The event of renal failure requires appropriate value adjustments. Nitrogen output is also affected by protein-losing enteropathy, malabsorption and entero-haemorrhages.

23.3.5.4 Immunological Tests

The association between malnutrition and immune system alterations has been widely ascertained. The principal tests used are total lymphocyte counts, T-helper lymphocyte counts and complement fraction 3. Results must be carefully evaluated since alterations in the immune system may also be due to pathologies such as cirrhosis of the liver, renal failure or drug therapies (steroids, immunosuppressors, etc.).

23.3.5.5 Functional Tests

Appropriate tests may concern the immune system, capillary and red blood cell fragility, prothrombin time, platelet aggregation, thyroid radioiodine uptake, and respiratory and muscle function assessment.

There is the possibility, however, of interferences not strictly related to nutrition.

Biochemical analysis in nutritional assessment also includes vitamins, minerals and trace elements.

Vitamins are detected by analysing blood levels.

Minerals and trace elements are measured in blood and urine.

23.3.6 Nutritional Screening Tools

Subjective Global Assessment (SGA) consists of a questionnaire enabling an easy approach to nutritional assessment. It has a first section dealing with medical history (weight change, dietary intake, gastrointestinal symptoms and functional impairment) and a second section concerning physical examination (loss of subcutaneous fat, muscle wasting, oedema, ascites).

Patients are thus divided into three categories: well nourished, mildly-moderately malnourished, severely malnourished.

Thoresen, Fjeldstad, and Krogstad (2002), in a palliative setting, compared SGA results with results obtained from an objective method and they found a high correlation. SGA can be employed in patients receiving palliative care as an easy tool for nutritional assessment.

The American Society for Parenteral and Enteral Nutrition (ASPEN) guidelines (August, Huhman, and A.S.P.E.N. 2009) for patients receiving anticancer treatment and for those undergoing haematopoietic cell transplantation, recommend Patient-Generated Subjective Global Assessment (PG-SGA), SGA and Nutritional Risk Index (NRI) as nutritional assessment tests. The PG-SGA is an adaptation of the SGA. NRI includes measurement of albumin and data on habitual and measured weight.

Other nutritional assessment methods include Nutritional Risk Screening (NRS) and Malnutrition Universal Screening Tool (MUST). Both consider BMI, unintentional weight loss, food intake, clinical condition and/or administered treatment, and classify the risk of malnutrition (mild, moderate, high).

Mini-Nutritional Assessment (MNA) is applied to the elderly. It entails anthropometric, general, dietary and subjective assessment and classifies patients as "at risk of malnutrition" or "malnourished". This screening tool is not yet in use in palliative care units. A study (Slaviero, Read, and Clarke 2003) conducted in patients with advanced cancer receiving palliative chemotherapy has ascertained an association between baseline history of weight loss, C-reactive protein (CRP) and MNA score.

European Society for Clinical Nutrition and Metabolism (ESPEN) guidelines (Kondrup et al. 2003) recommend MUST, NRS and MNA for the elderly.

Bauer, Capra, and Ferguson (2002) verified that PG-SGA is equally effective compared to SGA when assessing the nutritional status of cancer patients in acute care medical facilities.

23.3.7 Human Body Composition

Body composition is modified by physiological (age, sex and physical activity), pathological and nutritional issues. Malnutrition affects body composition by diminishing fat and fat-free mass. In addition, malnutrition can alter intra- and extracellular volume and its negative impact on the availability of both ATP and creatine phosphate can compromise the sodium-potassium exchange mechanisms and, consequently, the overall balance of electrolytes.

Hence the role of body composition data collection when investigating nutritional status.

23.3.7.1 Body Composition Measurement Techniques

The main body composition measurement techniques are the following: measurement of the thickness of the subcutaneous fat using a body caliper, bioelectrical impedance analysis (BIA), dual-energy x-ray absorptiometry (DEXA), imaging techniques (ultrasound, CT and MRI scans) and total body potassium measurement.

The measurement of the thickness of the subcutaneous fat using a body caliper is an easy, inexpensive and quick method of estimating body fat mass. In clinical practice the following skinfolds are measured: triceps, biceps, iliac crest and subscapular skinfold. The average of three consecutive measurements should be considered.

Durnin and Womersley's (1974) table makes it possible to quantify the total body fat mass from the sum of the four skinfolds.

The triceps skinfold is important since, together with arm circumference, it gives the arm muscle circumference and arm muscle area (Table 23.6).

BIA is a noninvasive technique based upon the principle of electrical conduction being different through the different body districts on account of the different amount of water and electrolytes. It determines total body water, fat-free mass and fat mass.

TABLE 23.6
Anthropometric Equations

BMI (kg/m^2) = BW ((kg)/BH^2)
$\text{AMA}\left(\text{cm}^2\right)=\dfrac{\left[\text{AC}\left(\text{cm}\right)-\left(\text{Tsf}\left(\text{cm}\right)\times\pi\right)\right]^2}{4\times\pi}$
AMC (cm) = AC − 3.14 × Tsf

Note: BMI, body mass index; BW, body weight; BH, body height; AMA, arm muscle area; AC, arm circumference; Tsf, triceps skinfold; AMC, arm muscle circumference.

DEXA considers the body's absorption of photons when irradiated by x-rays at two different energy levels. It is used to evaluate bone mineral density. At present, it is considered as the most reliable body composition assessment technique.

Body potassium evaluates fat-free mass. It is not invasive but it is quite expensive. Potassium assessment is based upon the constant ratio existing between total body potassium and radioactive (40K) potassium.

Imaging techniques, such as CT and MRI scanning, assess body fat mass distribution. Ultrasound scans measure the thickness of subcutaneous fat and visceral fat. These techniques are of limited use in clinical practice due to high costs.

23.4 ASPECTS OF NUTRITIONAL STATUS IN PALLIATIVE CARE

There are not many works at present concerning the nutritional evaluation of palliative care patients. The data mentioned below refer either to specific studies of nutritional evaluation or to studies aimed at evaluating the effectiveness of artificial nutrition and covering palliative care patients too (Table 23.7).

A Norwegian study on 46 patients (Thoresen et al. 2002), comparing SGA adequacy opposed to traditional methods of nutritional assessment in palliative care patients, showed that 24 patients (52%) had a weight loss >10%. Mean BMI was 23 ± 4.9 kg/m^2. Thirteen patients (28%) had a triceps skinfold (Tsf) below the fifth percentile, while 10 patients (22%) had an arm muscle circumference (AMC) below the fifth percentile.

Albumin and prealbumin were below the normal range in 15 (33%) and 35 patients (76%) respectively.

A study on 352 patients with metastatic tumour referrals to a palliative medicine programme detected weight loss in 307 patients, with 71% showing a weight loss >10% compared to healthy state BW (Sarhill, Mahmoud, and Walsh 2003). BMI showed no alterations, probably due to the previous presence of obesity in most patients; 83% of patients had hypophagia. The authors recorded a reduced energy intake (EI) and body composition alterations: 51% of patients showed a reduction in fat mass (measured by Tsf) and 30% had a reduced arm muscle area (AMA). Median albumin was 3.2 g/dl; 66% of patients were hypoalbuminaemic. Of 50 patients, 74% had high CRP.

Hutton, Martin, and Field (2006) recruited 151 patients from a regional cancer centre and palliative care programme; they had a mean EI of 1610 ± 686 kcal/day and a mean EI/kg/BW of 25.1 ± 10. EI <34 kcal/kg/BW/day was assessed in 81% of patients. EI was balanced in proteins (16.3 ± 5.3%; 1 ± 0.4 g/kg BW), carbohydrates (55.0 ± 8.5%) and fat (29.7 ± 7.2%). Mean weight loss was 12.7 ± 14.6%.

Out of 144 palliative care patients on a free diet (Bovio, Bettaglio, and Bonetti 2008), 72/128 patients (56%) reported a weight loss >10%. Tsf and AMA were below the fifth percentile in 23% (33 patients) and in 47% (68 patients) respectively. Mean EI was 1337 ± 578 kcal/day and was lower than

TABLE 23.7
Nutritional Facts in Patients Receiving Palliative Care

Author	Patients	Weight Loss	Body Mass Index (BMI)	Energy Intake	Body Composition	Other
Thoresen et al. 2002	46	52% with weight loss >10%. Mean weight loss 15 ± 12.3%	23 ± 4.9 kg/m²		28% had Tsf <5th percentile. 22% had MAMC <5th percentile	Albumin reduced in 15 pts (33%). Prealbumin reduced in 35 pts (76%)
Sarhill et al. 2003	352	71% of 307 patients with weight loss >10%	Median BMI: 23.6 kg/m²	83% of patients with hypophagia	51% with severe fat deficiency. 30% with significant muscle mass reduction	Increased C-reactive protein in 74%. Median albumin: 3.2 g/dl
Hutton et al. 2006	151	Mean weight loss 12.7 ± 14.6%	23.4 ± 5 kg/m²	1610 ± 686 kcal/day. 25.1 ± 10 kcal/kg/body weight. Proteins 1 ± 0.4 g/kg/day		
Bovio et al. 2008	144	56% with weight loss >10%. Mean weight loss 11.32 ± 11%	22.4 ± 4.2 kg/m²	1337 ± 578 kcal/day. 22.6 ± 11 kcal/kg/body weight. Proteins 0.88 ± 0.4 g/kg/day	23% with Tsf <5th percentile. 47% with arm muscle area <5th percentile	Prealbumin low in 74%. Transferrin low in 74%. Albumin low in 76%. Mean serum albumin 3.1 ± 0.5 g/dl
Orreval et al. 2009	621	51% with weight loss >10%	22 ± 4 kg/m²			68% nutritionally at risk
Ludholm et al. 2004	309	Weight loss 10 ± 1% in nutritional support group and 9 ± 1 in the control group		1686 ± 56 in the nutritional support group and 1774 ± 49 kcal/day in the control group		Mean serum albumin 33 ± 0.4 in nutritional support and 34 ± 0.4 g/l in control group

(continued)

TABLE 23.7 (Continued)
Nutritional Facts in Patients Receiving Palliative Care

Author	Patients	Weight Loss	Body Mass Index (BMI)	Energy Intake	Body Composition	Other
Slaviero et al. 2003	73 patients before palliative chemotherapy	9 patients (12%) with weight loss >10%	6 patients (8%) with BMI<20 kg/m2			9 patients (12%) malnourished and 47 (64%) at nutritional risk. Median albumin and prealbumin were respectively 37.5 g/l and 0.22 mg/l
Pironi et al. 1997	164 patients in home artificial nutrition		19 ± 2.7 kg/m^2 in 13 patients; 20.9 ± 2.6 in 19 patients; 19.5 ± 3.6 in 132 patients			135 patients (82%) with protein energy malnutrition
Bozzetti et al. 2002	69 patients in home parenteral nutrition	56 patients (81%) with weight loss >10%				Median serum albumin: 3.3 g/dl. Median lymphocyte count 1150/mm^3. Median serum transferrin 189 mg/dl.

Note: Results are expressed as mean ± SD. Tsf, triceps skinfold.

calculated mean REE (1347 ± 213). Fifty-two percent of patients (75 patients) had EI lower than their REE. Mean EI/kg/BW was 22.56 ± 11. EI was regularly distributed in proteins (15.4 ± 4.8%; 0.88 ± 0.4 g/kg/BW), carbohydrates (52.4 ± 11.6%) and lipids (28.8 ± 9.3%) but 27% of patients (39 patients) were taking less than 0.6 g/proteins/kg/BW/day. Serum prealbumin, serum transferrin and serum albumin were below normal respectively in 74%, 74%, and 76% of the patients.

Further data on the nutritional assessment of palliative care patients can be found in works on the impact of artificial nutrition on survival, nutritional status and quality of life.

The nutritional risk status and the nutritional support of 621 cancer patients admitted to palliative home care services was investigated by telephone interviews (Orrevall, Tishelman, and Permert 2009): 302/593 patients (51%) had a weight loss >10% compared to healthy state BW. Mean BMI in 596 patients was 22 ± 4 kg/m^2. BMI was <18.5 kg/m^2 in 15% of patients. According to a modified NRS-2002, 419 (68%) patients were at nutritional risk.

In 2004 Ludholm et al. evaluated 309 patients divided into two groups. One group was receiving COX inhibitors and recombinant erythropoietin. The other group, as well as being treated pharmacologically with the same two medications, was also receiving nutritional support. Neither group was being administered any specific cancer therapy due to absence of efficacy. Pretreatment weight loss % was 10 ± 1 in the nutritional support and 9 ± 1 in the control group. EI was 1686 ± 56 in the nutritional support group and 1774 ± 49 kcal in the control group, whereas serum albumin was, respectively, 33 ± 0.4 and 34 ± 0.4 g/l in the nutritional support and in the control group.

Slaviero et al. (2003) considered 73 patients with advanced cancer before palliative chemotherapy treatment with docetaxel and vinorelbine. The aim of the study was to evaluate the relationship between anthropometric, biochemical data and MNA. Nine patients (12%) had weight loss >10% and 6 patients (8%) had BMI <20 kg/m^2. MNA data showed that 9 patients (12%) were malnourished and 47 (64%) were at nutritional risk. Median albumin and prealbumin were 37.5 g/l and 0.22 mg/l respectively.

Pironi, Ruggeri, and Tanneberger (1997) studied 164 patients receiving only palliative care. All patients were administered home artificial nutrition (HAN) (135 by enteral and 29 by parenteral nutrition). The aim of the study was to estimate the utilization rate and to evaluate the efficacy of HAN in preventing death from cachexia and in improving patients' performance status. During the study 18 patients were readmitted to the hospital for palliative radiation or chemotherapy; 135 patients (82%) showed protein-energy malnutrition. Protein-energy malnutrition was diagnosed when BMI was <20 in males and <19 kg/m^2 in females or when there was a weight loss >10% during the previous 6 months.

From this work BMI data can also be collected. BMI, after the first month of HAN, was 19 ± 2.7 kg/m^2 in 13 patients, increasing their Karnofsky Performance Status (KPS) score; 20.9 ± 2.6 kg/m^2 in 19 patients, decreasing their KPS score; and 19.5 ± 3.6 kg/m^2 in 132 patients with unmodified KPS.

Bozzetti, Cozzaglio, and Biganzoli (2002) studied 69 patients to assess the impact of HPN on nutritional status, quality of life and survival. Thirty-six patients (52%) were administered second- or third-line chemotherapy. This study includes data on the nutritional status assessed before the administration of nutritional therapy. In particular, 56 patients (81%) had weight loss >10%; median serum albumin was 3.3 g/dl; lymphocyte count 1150/mm^3 and serum transferrin 189 mg/dl.

23.5 RELATIONSHIP BETWEEN NUTRITIONAL STATUS AND UPPER GASTROINTESTINAL SYMPTOMS

Yavuzsen, Walsh, and Davis (2009) recently conducted a survey by administering to 95 palliative care patients a 22-item questionnaire aimed at assessing the degree of anorexia and the prevalence of other gastrointestinal symptoms. The severity of weight loss did not influence the prevalence of gastrointestinal symptoms; the most severe anorexia emerged in patients with the highest weight loss. Mean ECOG-PS was 1.9 ± 1.1.

Another study (Bovio, Montagna, and Bariani 2009), conducted on 143 palliative care patients with mean ECOG-PS 3.1 ± 0.49, showed an association between the different symptoms of the upper gastrointestinal system and malnutrition parameters. In particular, xerostomia, anorexia and dysphagia for solids had a higher occurrence in patients with EI < REE, whereas dysphagia for liquids mostly affected patients experiencing weight loss.

EI was lower in patients with xerostomia, nausea, dysphagia for liquids and solids, dysgeusia, hypogeusia and vomiting if compared to patients unaffected by these same symptoms. Patients with anorexia, nausea, and dysphagia for solids and liquids showed higher weight loss than patients unaffected by these same symptoms, whereas patients with anorexia and hypogeusia showed a lower BMI.

ETHICAL ISSUES

The nutritional assessment of palliative care patients should be considered whenever the administration of adequate nutritional therapy may result in improved quality of life and performance status. The nutritional assessment of palliative care patients is to be considered ethical and professionally correct even when artificial nutrition is inapplicable.

SUMMARY POINTS

- Palliative care patients are often affected by malnutrition and hypophagia.
- Weight loss, anorexia, alterations in metabolism, asthenia, reduced calorie intake, depletion of fat mass and serious muscle catabolism are the main aspects of malnutrition.
- Nutritional assessment usually covers the following issues: case history, dietary records, physical examination, anthropometric measurements and laboratory analysis.
- The main nutritional screening tools are Subjective Global Assessment, Nutritional Risk Screening, Malnutrition Universal Screening Tool and Mini-Nutritional Assessment.
- There is an association between upper gastrointestinal symptoms and malnutrition parameters.

LIST OF ABBREVIATIONS

AC	Arm circumference
AMA	Arm muscle area
AMC	Arm muscle circumference
ASPEN	American Society for Parenteral and Enteral Nutrition
BIA	Bioelectrical impedance analysis
BW	Body weight
CACS	Cancer Anorexia Cachexia Syndrome
CRP	C-reactive protein
DEXA	Dual energy x-ray absorptiometry
ECOG-PS	Eastern Cooperative Oncology Group Performance Status
EI	Energy intake
ESPEN	European Society for Clinical Nutrition and Metabolism
HAN	Home artificial nutrition
HPN	Home parenteral nutrition
KPS	Karnofsky Performance Status
LMF	Lipid-Mobilizing Factor
MNA	Mini-Nutritional Assessment

MUST	Malnutrition Universal Screening Tool
NRI	Nutritional Risk Index
NRS	Nutritional Risk Screening
PG-SGA	Patient-Generated Subjective Global Assessment
PIF	Proteolysis-inducing factor
REE	Resting Energy Expenditure
SGA	Subjective Global Assessment
Tsf	Triceps skinfold

REFERENCES

August, D. A., M. B. Huhmann, and American Society for Parenteral and Enteral Nutrition (A.S.P.E.N.) Board of Directors. 2009. A.S.P.E.N. clinical guidelines: Nutrition support therapy during adult anticancer treatment and in hematopoietic cell transplantation. *Journal of Parenteral and Enteral Nutrition* 33:472–500.

Bassey, E. J. 1986. Demi-span as a measure of skeletal size. *Annals of Human Biology* 13:499–502.

Bauer, J., S. Capra, and M. Ferguson. 2002. Use of the scored Patient-Generated Subjective Global Assessment (PG-SGA) as a nutrition assessment tool in patients with cancer. *European Journal of Clinical Nutrition* 56:779–85.

Bovio, G., R. Bettaglio, and G. Bonetti. 2008. Evaluation of nutritional status and dietary intake in patients with advanced cancer on palliative care. *Minerva Gastroenterologicae Dietologica* 54:243–50.

Bovio, G., G. Montagna, and C. Bariani. 2009. Upper gastrointestinal symptoms in patients with advanced cancer: Relationship to nutritional and performance status. *Supportive Care in Cancer* 17:1317–24.

Bozzetti, F., L. Cozzaglio, and E. Biganzoli. 2002. Quality of life and length of survival in advanced cancer patients on home parenteral nutrition. *Clinical Nutrition* 21:281–88.

Bozzetti, F., and L. Mariani. 2009. Defining and classifying cancer cachexia: A proposal by the SCRINIO working group. *Journal of Parenteral and Enteral Nutrition* 33:361–67.

Chumlea, W. C. 1988. Methods of nutritional anthropometric assessment for special groups. In *Anthropometric standardization reference manuals*, eds. T. G. Lohman, A. F. Roche, and R. Martorell, 93–95. Campaign: Human Kinetics Books.

Durnin, J. V. G. A., and J. Womersley. 1974. Body fat assessed from total body density and its estimation from skinfold thickness: Measurements on 481 men and women aged from 16 to 72 years. *British Journal of Nutrition* 32:77–97.

Hutton, J. L., L. Martin, and C. J. Field. 2006. Dietary patterns in patients with advanced cancer: Implications for anorexia-cachexia therapy. *American Journal of Clinical Nutrition* 84:1163–70.

Kondrup, J., S. P. Allison, and M. Elia. 2003. ESPEN guidelines for nutrition screening 2002. *Clinical Nutrition* 22:415–21.

Orrevall, Y., C. Tishelman, and J. Permert. 2009. Nutritional support and risk status among cancer patients in palliative home care services. *Supportive Care in Cancer* 17:153–61.

Pironi, L., E. Ruggeri, and S. Tanneberger. 1997. Home artificial nutrition in advanced cancer. *Journal of the Royal Society of Medicine* 90:597–603.

Sarhill, N., F. Mahmoud, and D. Walsh. 2003. Evaluation of nutritional status in advanced metastatic cancer. *Supportive Care in Cancer* 11:652–59.

Slaviero, K. A., J. A. Read, and S. J. Clarke. 2003. Baseline nutritional assessment in advanced cancer patients receiving palliative chemotherapy. *Nutrition and Cancer* 46:148–57.

Thoresen, L., I. Fjeldstad, and K. Krogstad. 2002. Nutritional status of patients with advanced cancer: The value of using the subjective global assessment of nutritional status as a screening tool. *Palliative Medicine* 16:33–42.

Yavuzsen, T., D. Walsh, and M. P. Davis. 2009. Components of the anorexia-cachexia syndrome: Gastrointestinal symptom correlates of cancer anorexia. *Supportive Care in Cancer* 17:1531–41.

24 Nutrition and Palliative Surgery for Head and Neck Cancer

Takeshi Shinozaki and Ryuichi Hayashi

CONTENTS

24.1 INTRODUCTION

24.1.1 ADVANCED HEAD AND NECK CANCER

As head and neck cancer progresses, it may cause airway obstruction, esophageal obstruction, and aspiration. Oncologists evaluate a patient and determine whether any curative treatment is possible, but for some patients curative surgery, radiotherapy, chemotherapy, and other treatments are not indicated. For such patients, the airway might need to be controlled with a tracheostomy tube and nutrition might need to be provided through a gastrostomy tube or a central venous catheter (Vassilopoulos et al. 1998) (Figure 24.1). Percutaneous endoscopic gastrostomy is useful for treating obstructions of the upper digestive tract. For information on tracheostomy and gastrostomy, please refer to pertinent textbooks.

24.1.2 NUTRITION AND QUALITY OF LIFE

Such invasive procedures for controlling the airway and providing nutrition can markedly decrease a patient's quality of life (QOL), and many patients wish to maintain oral intake for as long as possible. Furthermore, conditions that decrease QOL can continue for more than a year when the function of vital organs, such as the lungs and liver, is not impaired. When patients with advanced cancer of the thoracic esophagus have difficulty swallowing, they have been treated with stents, lasers, and an argon plasma coagulator (Bancewicz 1999; Kubba and Krasner 2000). Stent placement in the thoracic esophagus is an established procedure, although complications can occur (Bancewicz 1999; Bethge

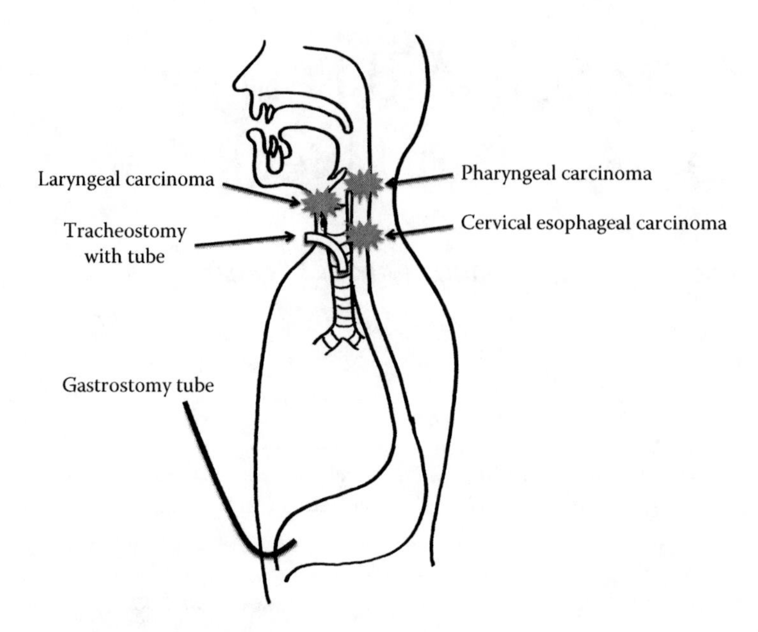

FIGURE 24.1 Problems caused by head and neck cancer. Head and neck cancer causes airway and esophageal obstruction, which may necessitate tracheostomy and gastrostomy.

and Vakil 2001). However, stent placement in the lower pharynx and cervical esophagus is difficult because of anatomical problems (Kubba and Krasner 2000). Bethge and Vakil (2001) reported complications in 5 of 7 cases of stent placement in patients with cancer of the cervical esophagus, and Moses and Wong (2002) found difficulties in the use of self-expanding metal stents in the cervical esophagus, but still suggested that this approach may be useful. Other reports have suggested that palliative surgery may be appropriate for selected patients (Gentile, Cecere, and Elia 1999; Azuren, Go, and Kirkland 1997).

24.2 APPLICATIONS IN OTHER AREAS OF TERMINAL OR PALLIATIVE CARE

The airway takes first priority over other areas. Sedation becomes necessary when the oncologist cannot keep a patient's airway open. The medical staff must consider the negative effects on the airway of dysphagia, aspiration, tracheostomy, and a nasogastric tube.

24.3 PRACTICAL METHODS AND TECHNIQUES

24.3.1 Palliative Surgery

In total pharyngolaryngoesophagectomy (TPLE), after the larynx, hypopharynx, and cervical esophagus have been excised, the food passage is reconstructed with a free jejunum flap, and a permanent tracheostoma is prepared (Figure 24.2). Resection of the larynx permanently disables phonation by means of the vocal cords, but the permanent tracheostoma enables tube-free airway control. The ability to intake food orally is restored by reconstructing a pathway from the pharynx to the upper gastrointestinal tract. Tumor ulceration, bleeding, and foul odors tend to decrease QOL (Azuren et al. 1997). TPLE may control bleeding, pain, and odors from the primary lesion. In contrast, a well-prepared permanent tracheostoma causes no such problems and restoration of oral intake ability maintains the pleasure of eating. Therefore, TPLE markedly improves QOL and increases the chances that the patient can be cared for at home. Many palliative surgeries, such as bypass surgery, have been reported for the treatment of obstruction caused by cancers of the digestive tract.

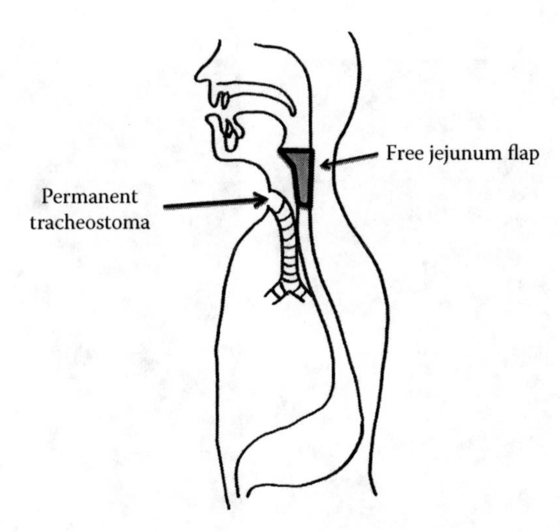

FIGURE 24.2 Diagram of TPLE. The food passage is reconstructed with a free jejunum flap and a permanent tracheostoma is prepared.

24.3.2 Complications and Hospitalization

In our hospital, complications of TPLE were evaluated in 269 patients. Additional operations were performed within 1 month after surgery for 33 patients because of thrombosis or fistulae (12.3%). Six patients (2.2%) died within 1 month after surgery. Balloon dilation was required to treat postoperative stenosis in 27 patients (10.0%). The mean duration of hospitalization was 22.5 days and oral intake started an average of 13.7 days after surgery (Sarukawa, Sakuraba, and Kimata 2006). Feuer, Broadley, and Shepherd (1999) reviewed 22 reports of palliative surgery for obstruction of the lower digestive tract and found mortality rates within 30 days after surgery of 5%–32% (Feuer et al.1999).

24.3.3 Case 1

A 69-year-old man was admitted to our hospital after T4N2cM0 cancer of the cervical esophagus was diagnosed (Figure 24.3). Central venous nutrition was started because the patient had difficulty with oral food intake but wished to see it improve. Because the tumor had invaded a vertebra, we recommended palliative surgery. TPLE aimed at improving oral intake was performed on October 28. Chemotherapy was not administered because of the patient's poor general condition. The operation lasted 11 hours 10 minutes and the volume of blood loss was 727 ml. However, the tumor that had invaded the vertebra could not be completely removed. Oral intake was started on postoperative day (POD) 9 and was maintained for 138 days (Figure 24.4). Bougienage was performed on PODs 44 and 121 to dilate the constriction of the jejunoesophageal anastomosis. Irradiation with 70 Gy was started on POD 21. The patient was satisfied with the results of surgery but died on POD 198 of hyposthenia due to growth of the primary tumor.

24.3.4 Case 2

The patient was a 73-year-old man who visited a physician in September and was found to have cancer of the cervical esophagus. An initial examination at our hospital was performed on October 9. Irradiation (60 Gy) and concomitant chemotherapy with cisplatin and 5-fluorouracil were started, but the cancer continued to progress. Oral intake became impossible on December 12 owing to aspiration, and percutaneous endoscopic gastrostomy was performed on December 27. In March 2002 the patient expressed his wish to regain oral intake ability, but at that time radical surgery was considered impossible because of multiple lymph node metastases. TPLE was performed on May 20 with the

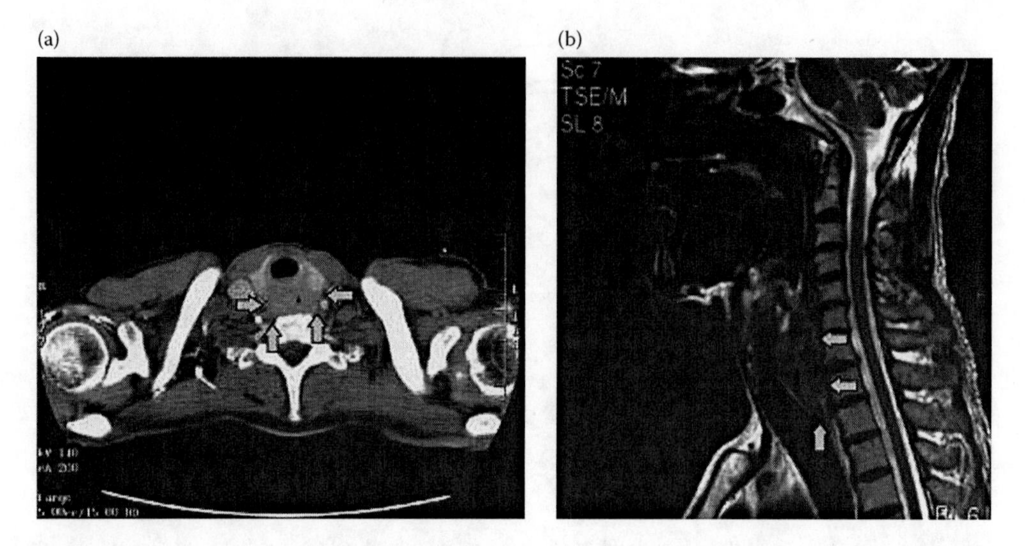

FIGURE 24.3 Enhanced CT (a) and MRI (T2) (b) of patient 1. Cervical esophageal cancer invaded the vertebra. Prevertebral invasion is evaluated, which is not an indication for a curative operation.

aim of restoring oral intake ability. Only the primary lesion was excised; neck dissection was not performed. The operation lasted 5 hours 23 minutes and the volume of blood loss was 240 ml. On the same day, an additional operation was performed to remove an arterial thrombus in the region of anastomosis. Oral intake was started on POD 7 and was maintained for 199 days. Ingestion of steamed rice was possible for a certain period, but the diet mostly consisted of porridge. Because the

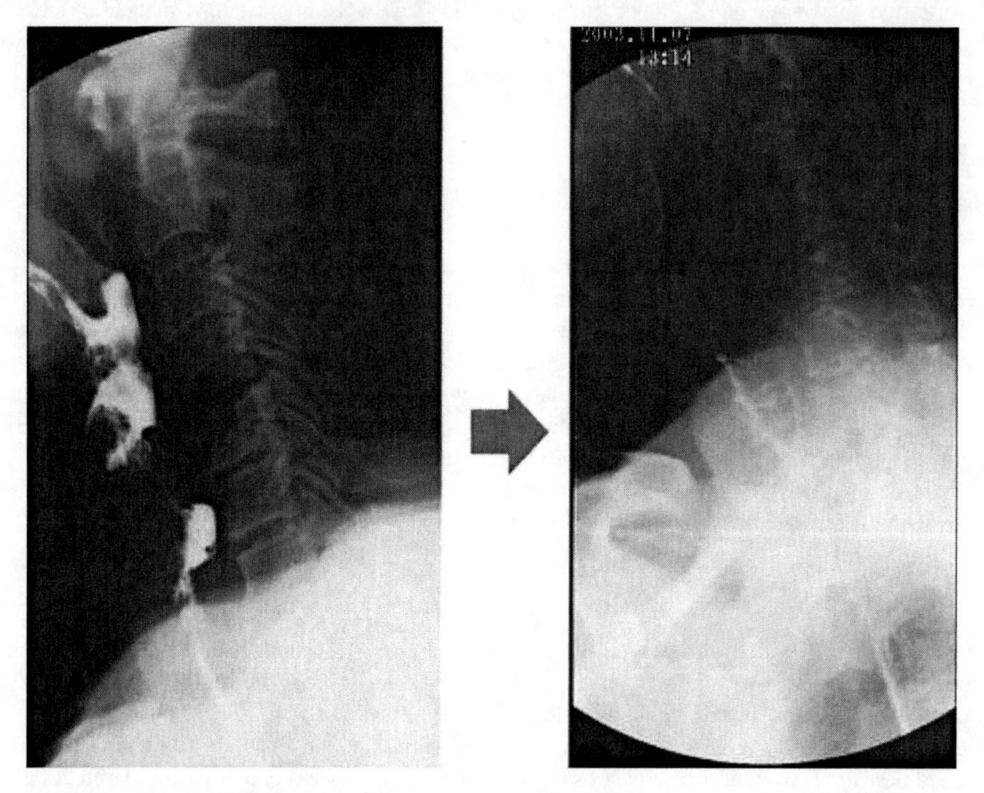

FIGURE 24.4 Videofluoroscopy of patient 1. Pre-operative (left) and post-operative (right) images. Pharyngeal clearance was improved after the operation.

patient could eat his favorite foods after some time, he was satisfied with the results of the surgery. He died on POD 269.

24.3.5 Indication

TPLE is an invasive procedure and deaths may occur in the perioperative period. Of the 269 patients who underwent TPLE at our hospital, 6 (2.2%) died within 1 month. TPLE requires preoperative and postoperative hospital management and has corresponding associated costs (Kubba and Krasner 2000). This has led to doubts regarding the value of TPLE for patients who cannot undergo radical therapy or for patients in the terminal stage of cancer. Some argue that invasive surgery that cannot achieve complete resolution is not recommended. Surgical treatment should aim to improve symptoms, minimize postoperative complications, and shorten the duration of hospitalization. The indications for surgery should be determined on the basis of an overall evaluation of patient satisfaction and potential risks.

The decision to perform palliative therapy may also depend on current trends and local culture. Until a decade ago, inpatients of palliative care wards in Japan who had laryngeal cancer did not receive tracheotomy for airway obstruction, and some Japanese physicians still believe that palliative surgery or chemotherapy should not be performed for patients with advanced cancer. Furthermore, patients who do not want invasive surgery or blood transfusions may not agree to palliative TPLE. Evaluation of QOL is also very difficult because QOL varies between cultures and cannot be measured with a single scale. Thus, the issue of whether to perform palliative surgery requires further consideration of the beliefs and wishes of patients and other persons concerned (Blazeby, Alderson, and Farndon 2000). The proficiency of each medical facility should also be taken into account, because morbidity and mortality rates vary between facilities. Maximizing QOL by minimizing morbidity and mortality rates is the goal of palliative TPLE. Treatment should be performed only after patients have received an adequate explanation of possible complications and have given their informed consent (Vandeweyer, Urbain, and Andry 2000).

Palliative TPLE is not appropriate for all patients with incurable cancer who wish to maintain oral intake. However, QOL was markedly improved following TPLE in the two patients described here. Both patients were satisfied with the outcomes of the surgery.

Palliative TPLE may be appropriate for selected patients, depending on the location and speed of advancement of lesions, their general condition, and living environment, and in accordance with their wishes and religious and personal beliefs (Shinozaki, Hayashi, and Yamazaki 2007).

KEY FACTS OF HEAD AND NECK CANCER

- Head and neck cancer is often accompanied by airway and nutrition problems.
- The airway is controlled with an inserted tracheostomy tube.
- Gastrostomy is useful for treating obstruction of the upper digestive tract.
- These procedures markedly decrease patients' quality of life.
- Palliative surgery may be appropriate for some patients.

ETHICAL ISSUES

As mentioned above, the decision to perform palliative TPLE may also depend on current trends and local culture. Palliative surgery may be appropriate for selected patients on the basis of the location and speed of advancement of lesions, their general condition, and living environment, and in accordance with their wishes and religious and personal beliefs.

SUMMARY POINTS

- As head and neck cancer progresses, it often causes airway and esophageal obstruction, which may necessitate tracheostomy, gastrostomy, or central venous nutrition.
- In TPLE, the food passage is reconstructed with a free jejunum flap and a permanent tracheostoma is prepared.
- Two patients who underwent TPLE were satisfied with the outcomes of the surgery.
- This palliative surgery may be appropriate for selected patients on the basis of the location and speed of advancement of lesions, their general condition, and living environment, in accordance with their wishes and religious and personal beliefs.

LIST OF ABBREVIATIONS

POD Postoperative day
QOL Quality of Life
TPLE Total pharyngolaryngoesophagectomy

REFERENCES

Azuren, D. J., L. S. Go, and M. L. Kirkland. 1997. Palliative gastric transposition following pharyngolaryngoesophagectomy. *Am Surg* 63:410–13.

Bancewicz, J. 1999. Palliation in oesophageal neoplasia. *Ann R Coll Surg Engl* 81:382–86.

Bethge, N., and N. Vakil. 2001. A prospective trial of a new self-expanding plastic stent for malignant esophageal obstruction. *Am J Gastroenterol* 96:1350–54.

Blazeby, J. M., D. Alderson, and J. R. Farndon. 2000. Quality of life in patients with oesophageal cancer. *Rec Results Cancer Res* 155:193–204.

Feuer, D. J., K. E. Broadley, and J. H. Shepherd. 1999. Systematic review of surgery in malignant bowel obstruction in advanced gynecological and gastrointestinal cancer. *Gynecol Oncol* 75:313–22.

Gentile, M., C. Cecere, and S. Elia. 1999. Palliative surgical treatment of thoracic esophageal cancer. *Minerva Chir* 54:835–42.

Kubba, A. K., and N. Krasner. 2000. An update in the palliative management of malignant dysphagia. *Eur J Surg Oncol* 26:116–29.

Moses, F. M., and R. K. Wong. 2002. Stents for esophageal disease. *Curr Treat Options Gastroenterol* 5:63–71.

Sarukawa, S., M. Sakuraba, and Y. Kimata. 2006. Standardization of free jejunum transfer after total pharyngolaryngoesophagectomy. *Laryngoscope* 116:976–81.

Shinozaki, T., R. Hayashi, and M. Yamazaki. 2007. Palliative total pharyngo-laryngo-esophagectomy. *Auris Nasus Larynx* 34:561–64.

Vandeweyer, E., F. C. Urbain, and G. Andry. 2000. Reconstructive surgical techniques after palliative tumor excision. *Rev Med Brux* 21:423–28.

Vassilopoulos, P. P., E. Filopoulos, and N. Kelessis. 1998. Competent gastrostomy for patients with head and neck cancer. *Support Care Cancer* 6:479–81.

25 Total Parenteral Nutrition for Patients with Advanced, Life-Limiting Cancer: Clinical Context, Potential Risks and Benefits, and a Suggested Approach

Amy P. Abernethy and Jane L. Wheeler

CONTENTS

25.1 INTRODUCTION

An array of clinical ambiguities, many with significant ethical and moral charge, plagues end-of-life care. The benefit of providing supplemental nutrition, i.e., additional nutrients beyond that which the patient is able to ingest, represents one such ambiguity. The advanced cancer patient's ability to eat normally is often compromised by tumor burden, chemotherapy, and other treatment regimens. Clinicians, and often families and other caregivers, struggle with the perception that the patient cannot eat in adequate quantity, and with the choice of whether and how to deliver nutritional support. Despite the prevalence of this concern, there is no established protocol delineating the best clinical approach to ensure that advanced cancer patients receive sufficient nutrition. The relationship of nutritional intake to the patient's well-being is not well understood. Nor are there clear recommendations for taking into account the needs of families and caregivers.

Total parenteral nutrition (TPN), the intravenous delivery of nutrients, can alleviate much of the distress surrounding nourishment of patients at the end of life. However, decisions involving the use of this nutritional strategy are complicated by the conflicting nature of the evidence regarding the clinical benefits or detriments of TPN. In assessing whether to provide palliative TPN, clinicians must consider the metabolic changes that affect patients' nutritional needs, the presence of cancer-related anorexia or cachexia, the evidence both for and against providing nutrition at the end of life, family and caregiver concerns, and the moral and ethical issues associated with decisions on TPN at the end of a patient's life.

25.2 METABOLIC CHANGES IN THE PATIENT WITH ADVANCED CANCER

Under normal circumstances, human life is sustained by three metabolic pathways: (1) glucose utilization through glycolysis (gluconeogenesis); (2) fat usage through β-oxidation of fatty acids; and (3) protein synthesis and breakdown, largely via the Krebs cycle and the urea cycle. In times of excess, each pathway adapts according to its own characteristic process: glucose is stored as glycogen; fat is packaged with phosphatidylcholine into very low-, low-, and high-density lipoproteins; and protein is synthesized. In times of need, the body accesses nutrients by breaking down its stores of glycogen, fat, or protein. Fatty acid oxidation is facilitated by carnitine and results in ketone production. Protein degradation, which occurs through several pathways, relies on ubiquitin, cathepsins, and functional proteasomes (Figure 25.1).

The onset of cancer seriously disrupts normal metabolic processes. In cancer patients, the presence of cytokines (primarily tumor necrosis factor-α [TNF-α], interleukin-1 [IL-1], and interleukin-6 [IL-6]) and of certain molecules secreted by tumor cells (such as lipid-mobilizing factor [LMF] and proteolysis-inducing factor [PIF]) results in dramatic metabolic changes (Gadducci et al. 2001; Siddiqui et al. 2006).

First, cancer cells do not follow normal pathways of glucose metabolism. Instead of producing glucose via gluconeogenesis, cancer cells activate the Cori cycle, wherein pyruvate is metabolized to lactate. Because it leads to a drastic decline in ATP production, the Cori cycle substantially compromises metabolic processes. Furthermore, the regeneration of pyruvate necessary to perpetuate the Cori cycle depletes Krebs cycle intermediates, which the body must then regenerate through protein degradation.

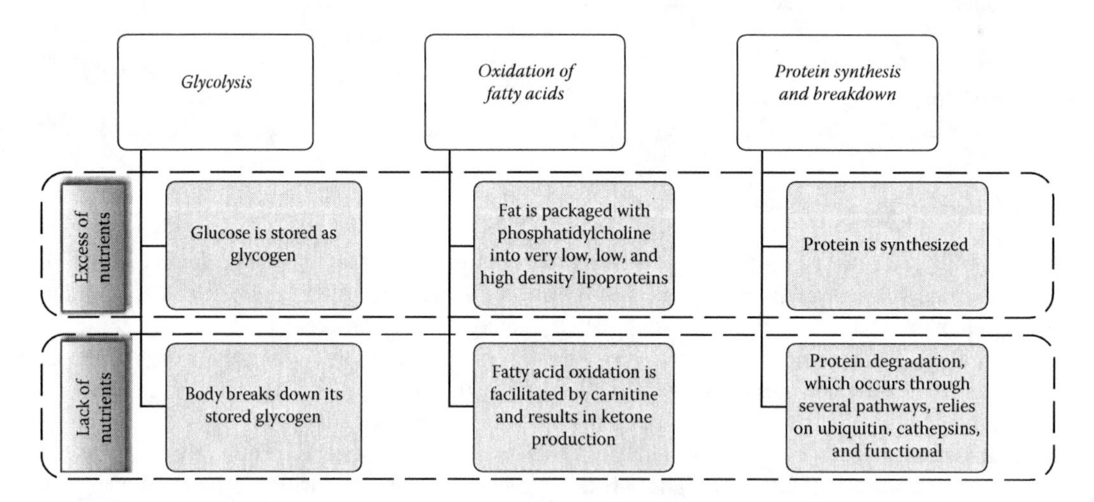

FIGURE 25.1 Outcomes of excess and lack of nutrients.

Cancer also affects the β-oxidation of fatty acids. In a healthy individual, lipolysis is constrained by adequate intake of glucose and the presence of ketones (a by-product of lipolysis). In cancer patients, however, appetite is often suppressed, not only by the cancer itself, but also by nausea, vomiting, and treatment-induced mucositis; the resulting decrease in glucose intake then inhibits fat degradation. Moreover, cytokines and cancer-specific molecules reduce ketone production for each fat molecule, preventing the feedback of ketone production that would normally inhibit lipolysis. Despite their cachexia, cancer patients often present with lower serum ketone levels than do other patients who are equally malnourished. Furthermore, TNF-α and IL-1 down-regulate the lipoprotein lipase, and IL-1 up-regulates hormone-sensitive lipase. Thus, by up-regulating hormone-sensitive lipase, the presence of epinephrine, cortisol, norepinephrine, TNF-α, and IL-1 leads to increased lipolysis. As lipolysis increases and lipoprotein lipase activity decreases, fatty acids are released into the blood, but the peripheral tissues cannot use them; serum triglyceride levels rise (Figure 25.2).

Protein degradation is stimulated not only by the depletion of the Krebs cycle intermediates, but also by TNF-α, IL-1, interferon (IFN), and PIF. These factors increase NF-κB transcription, which in turn activates ubiquitin-dependent proteasomal protein degradation. IL-6 increases cathepsin-stimulated protein degradation.

These metabolic changes are physically apparent to all those who have been involved with a patient in the final stages of cancer. The patient's lack of appetite in conjunction with negative nitrogen balance causes total body weight loss, atrophy of muscle mass, and loss of fat stores. The loss of tissue and of adequate protein stores further impairs the immune system, thereby decreasing the body's ability to heal wounds and to synthesize immunoglobulins (Figure 25.3).

25.3 CANCER ANOREXIA-CACHEXIA SYNDROME

Cachexia, a symptom common among cancer patients, is characterized by loss of appetite, weight, muscle mass, and adipose tissue. Patients with cachexia may experience diminished quality of life, decreased performance status, and in extreme cases, death. More than two-thirds of advanced cancer patients suffer from cachexia and/or anorexia, in a syndrome called cancer-related anorexia-cachexia syndrome (CACS). In evaluating 12 studies enrolling a total of 3047 patients, the Eastern Cooperative Oncology Group (ECOG) found that a loss of greater than 5% of precancer body weight was associated with poorer response to chemotherapy and predicted poor prognosis in cancer

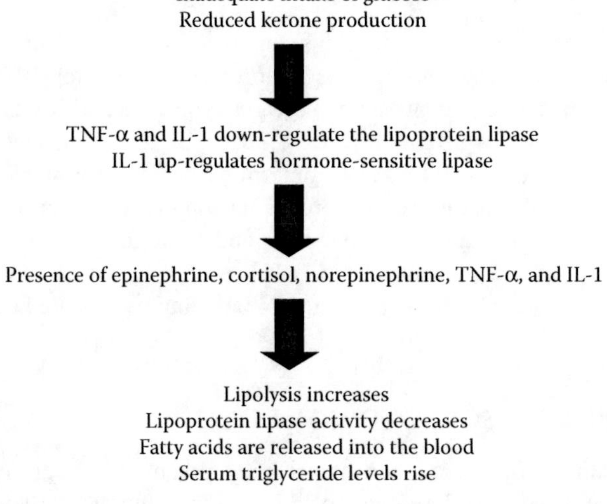

Inadequate intake of glucose
Reduced ketone production

TNF-α and IL-1 down-regulate the lipoprotein lipase
IL-1 up-regulates hormone-sensitive lipase

Presence of epinephrine, cortisol, norepinephrine, TNF-α, and IL-1

Lipolysis increases
Lipoprotein lipase activity decreases
Fatty acids are released into the blood
Serum triglyceride levels rise

FIGURE 25.2 Effect of cancer on metabolism.

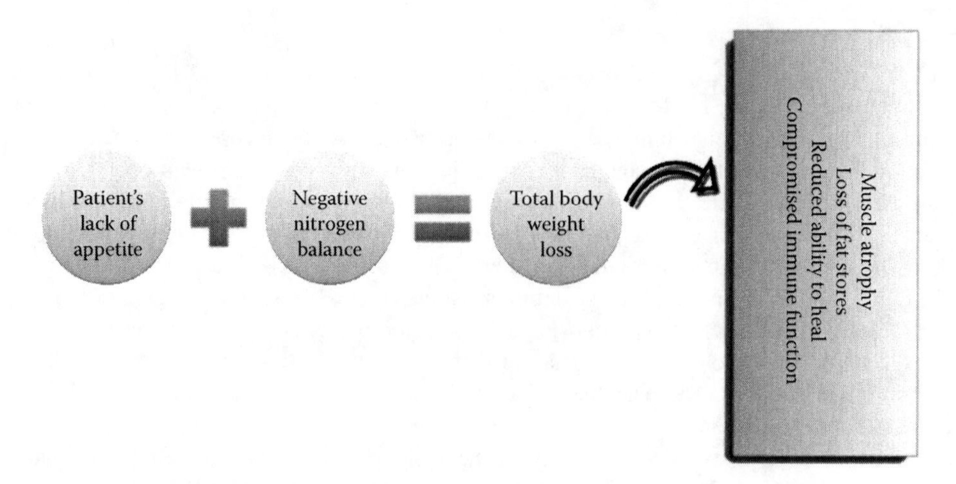

FIGURE 25.3 Metabolic changes in the final stages of cancer.

patients. Loss of greater than 10 kg of normal body weight, which occurs in 40%–70% of patients with advanced solid tumors, accounts for the death of 20%–25% of patients with this degree of weight loss (Hackmayr and Gatzeiner 1992).

In addition to the medical risk it introduces, CACS constitutes a significant source of distress for cancer patients and their families. Issues related to eating—including loss of appetite and of weight—are among the most frequent and prominent factors impairing quality of life for advanced cancer patients and their families. For late-stage cancer patients and their family members, pressure surrounding eating leads to considerable suffering, yet the toll of eating-related disorders such as cachexia and anorexia remains under-recognized in this patient population.

No consistent definition of CACS has been established. In most intervention trials, CACS is defined as a loss of greater than 5% of the patient's precancer body weight. Symptomatic anorexia is not a requirement. Some studies use self-reported weight loss of at least 2.3 kg over the preceding two months or a physician-estimated caloric intake of less than 20 cal/kg of body weight per day. Patients are generally expected to perceive their loss of appetite and/or weight as problematic. The relationship of these definitions to cytokine parameters in CACS remains unclear.

25.4 TOTAL PARENTERAL NUTRITION

TPN, also referred to as intravenous nutrition, first emerged as a clinical strategy in the late 1960s and early 1970s. Although initially developed as a short-term remedy for patients unable to absorb sufficient nutrition (for example, patients with short gut syndrome), TPN has evolved into a long-term treatment strategy as well, with demonstrated efficacy for delivering adequate fat, protein, and glucose to meet the metabolic needs of diverse nonterminal patients for many years, even decades.

Given the dramatic loss of protein and fat stores in terminally ill cancer patients, with the attendant negative effects on the patient's immune system and strength, TPN is a potentially attractive treatment modality in advanced cancer (Table 25.1). However, the question of whether TPN is harmful or helpful to advanced cancer patients continues to be a source of heated debate in the scientific community.

25.5 CLINICAL RISKS ASSOCIATED WITH TPN

Nutritional support with TPN is more labor-intensive and potentially hazardous than enteral nutrition. Certain procedures have been developed to address TPN's unique challenges and to minimize patient risk. Clinical risks and approaches to minimize risk are summarized in Table 25.2.

TABLE 25.1
Key Facts of Total Parenteral Nutrition (TPN)

1. Total parenteral nutrition (TPN), also referred to as intravenous nutrition, emerged as a clinical strategy in the late 1960s/early 1970s
2. TPN initially developed as a short-term remedy for patients unable to absorb sufficient nutrition
3. TPN has evolved into a long-term treatment strategy with demonstrated efficacy for delivering adequate fat, protein, and glucose to meet the metabolic needs of diverse nonterminal patients
4. Given the dramatic loss of protein and fat stores in terminally ill cancer patients, with the attendant negative effects on the patient's immune system and strength, TPN is a potentially attractive treatment adjunct in advanced cancer
5. Whether TPN is harmful or helpful to advanced cancer patients continues to be a source of heated debate

25.6 POTENTIAL NEGATIVE EFFECTS OF TPN

A common perception is that TPN "feeds cancer." The original data behind this statement come from the scientific literature of the 1960s and 1970s, wherein it was reported that laboratory animals on a protein-restricted diet developed fewer spontaneous tumors (Tannenbaum and Silverstone 1953) and fewer carcinogen-induced tumors than did animals fed a normal diet (White 1961). Tumor growth resumed in animals when re-fed after a protein-restricted period. In studies comparing animals that were either protein-restricted, fed ad libitum, or supported with TPN, only the animals with complete protein restriction experienced decreased tumor growth. Feeding (enteral or parenteral) has been associated with increased tumor volume (Steiger et al. 1975) and tumor metastasis (Torosian and Donoway 1991), with tumor volume often increasing in proportion to total body weight. These animal studies suggest that any protein intake, whether enteral or parenteral, causes increased tumor growth and metastasis.

Further, several animal studies also suggest that parenteral nutrition, in particular, leads to increased tumor cell activity. Compared to animals on orally administered diets, animals given TPN developed tumors with increased DNA synthesis and increased mitotic indices (Cameron and

TABLE 25.2
Clinical Risks Associated with TPN

Clinical Risk Associated with TPN	Guidance
Risk of thrombosis: risk of infection	Infuse TPN through a central line near the right atria/superior vena cava junction, ideally via a dedicated access/port
Lysis of red blood cells	Administer TPN in an appropriate volume (≥1.5 l/day)
Dysregulation of blood sugars; treatment-related hyperglycemia	Hyperglycemia may cause significant morbidity and is often aggravated by concomitant therapies (e.g., prednisone)
Immunosuppression	Can be caused by hyperglycemia and effects of TPN infusate
Activation of refeeding syndrome	May arise if the patient has been undernourished for a period of time; associated risks include fatal cardiac arrhythmia, systolic heart failure, respiratory insufficiency, and hematologic derangements
Increased risk for infection	TPN is an excellent culture medium and thus increases the risk of bacteremia
Metabolic and electrolyte abnormalities	Can result if nausea/vomiting, acute renal failure, or liver failure cause imbalances that change potassium, sodium, and protein requirements; amino acid composition must be recalibrated

Pavlat 1976). One study, which measured the release of the tumor markers spermine, spermidine, and putrescene, determined that animals fed via TPN had higher levels of these markers than did either animals on protein-restricted diets or animals fed ad libitum; this effect was most pronounced in animals whose tumor growth had been inhibited by limited blood supply.

Human trials have documented the effect of TPN on cancer mitosis/growth. When compared to gastric tumors resected from patients who had not received TPN, those resected from patients who had received 10 days of preoperative intravenous nutrition had higher rates of thymidine incorporation (Bozzetti et al. 1999), evidence that tumors may grow in the context of TPN administration. The effect of TPN on DNA synthesis is swift: among patients with rectal cancer, preoperative TPN accelerated tumor protein synthesis in only 20 hours (Heys et al. 1991).

Not all information about TPN in this setting is negative. Some investigators have suggested that TPN's effect on DNA synthesis could be harnessed to serve treatment purposes; researchers have first provoked DNA synthesis via TPN, then introduced chemotherapeutic agents that exert their greatest effect by killing cancer cells during DNA synthesis. The ability of TPN to inhibit or prevent weight loss has been exploited during chemotherapy; animal studies have shown that when chemotherapy is given concomitantly with TPN, a positive nitrogen balance can be maintained. Furthermore, simultaneous chemotherapy and TPN can have a selective effect on tumor growth. According to the findings of one study, animals that received TPN followed by methotrexate had smaller tumor volumes than either those given methotrexate and fed ad libitum or those on protein-restricted diets.

Despite these promising data, a prospective trial of TPN conducted in human patients with metastatic colon cancer treated with 5-fluorouracil (5-FU) found that patients not receiving TPN (i.e., controls) had substantially longer survival than patients who received TPN (Nixon et al. 1981). Skeptics have suggested that this survival benefit reflected the fact that more patients with liver metastases were included in the TPN group than in the control group.

A subsequent study of 32 sarcoma patients evaluated nitrogen balance, serum protein levels, and survival in patients with and without TPN. Although patients who received TPN had nearly four times greater protein intake ($g/m^2/day$) than those on an oral diet, and although the former group had a less negative nitrogen balance, their serum protein levels were nearly identical to those fed orally and survival was no different between groups (Shamberger et al. 1984).

A meta-analyses of all the prospective trials of patients receiving concurrent TPN and chemotherapy concluded that TPN conferred no survival benefit and, due to the increased risk of infection, might even be detrimental (Klein and Koretz 1994). However, because much of the prospective data on TPN and chemotherapy in patients with solid tumors were generated more than a decade ago, when chemotherapy and its support protocols differed substantially from current treatment regimens, the validity of such data today is questionable.

25.7 POTENTIAL POSITIVE EFFECTS OF TPN

Few data support the use of TPN in patients with solid tumors. However, while scant, these data emerge from more recent research and may therefore better reflect contemporary supportive care practices in oncology.

Promising early results were reported in a retrospective review of 21 patients with advanced ovarian cancer and malignant obstruction (Abu-Rustum et al. 1997). As determined by their primary treating physicians, eleven patients received TPN. These patients lived 89 days on average, while those who did not receive TPN lived an average of 71 days. Because the study's sample size was small, this difference in survival was not statistically significant. Furthermore, three of the women receiving TPN were newly diagnosed, and two of the three were able to resume oral nutrition again. Results are thus inconclusive.

In a more recent study, partial parenteral nutritional support showed potential benefit for advanced cancer patients. A total of 152 patients with newly diagnosed stage IIIB or stage IV cancer of multiple types were randomized to chemotherapy and enteral nutrition with enteral supplementation, or to chemotherapy and enteral nutrition with 30% parenteral nutrition. Although both groups had similar protein and caloric intake, those who received partial parenteral nutrition had greater survival, quality of life, and appetite than those who received no parenteral support (Shang et al. 2006). A 2009 study found that the majority of home TPN was used to supplement oral intake rather than as the sole source of nutrients (Orrevall et al. 2009).

25.8 APPLICATIONS TO OTHER AREAS OF TERMINAL OR PALLIATIVE CARE

A number of studies have looked at the experience of patients who receive bone marrow transplants and TPN support throughout the transplant period. These patients most often present, or are at risk for, mucositis and graft-versus-host disease—processes which are quite different from cancer cachexia and tumor-related gastrointestinal obstruction associated with end-stage solid tumors. The studies suggest that TPN may be beneficial in the setting of protein malnutrition, myeloablative chemotherapy, and bone marrow transplantation.

In certain non-cancer palliative care scenarios, patients may be candidates for TPN. To warrant consideration, patients should be in good physical and mental condition, have an expected life span of at least three months, and have moderate to good functional status (e.g., Karnofsky Performance Status >50). Relevant patients generally suffer from conditions such as intestinal obstruction, fistulas, or other issues making enteral nutrition impossible. As with cancer patients, the decision regarding TPN should be taken after careful multidisciplinary discussion and communication with the patient and family or caregivers.

25.9 GUIDELINES FOR CLINICAL PRACTICE

25.9.1 Guidelines for Patients with Advanced Cancer

Several professional societies have independently weighed the evidence for and against using TPN for terminally ill cancer patients; universal consensus holds that such treatment is not indicated by the evidence. In 1989, the American College of Physicians stated, "Parenteral nutrition was associated with net harm in cancer patients receiving chemotherapy (more death, less response to treatment, partial or complete)" (American College of Physicians 1989). In 2001, the American Gastroenterology Association concluded that "...[parenteral nutrition] should not be given to patients undergoing chemotherapy or radiation because it increases the risk of complications and impairs the response to treatment; [it] should not be provided to persons with limited life expectancies (<3 months)" (American Gastroenterology Association 2001). In 2002, the American Society for Parenteral and Enteral Nutrition (ASPEN) stated that "nutrition support should not be used routinely as an adjunct to chemotherapy [but may] be appropriate for patients receiving anti-cancer therapy who are moderately/severely malnourished" (ASPEN Board of Directors, the Clinical Guidelines Task Force 2002). The Society also stated that nutritional support is "rarely indicated for terminally ill cancer patients." The European Society for Clinical Nutrition and Metabolism (ESPEN) has issued clinical practice guidelines for parenteral nutrition that grade the evidence and cover outcomes including quality of life.

25.9.2 Additional Factors Influencing the Palliative Use of TPN

Despite the lack of evidence supporting TPN in late-stage cancer, a survey found that the most common diagnosis among home-based patients receiving TPN was cancer. These patients had lower survival rates than all other groups receiving home TPN, except for those with AIDS (Howard et al. 1995). Advanced cancer patients receiving home TPN had an average life expectancy of 2–5 months (August et al. 1991), and many lived no longer than they might have with hydration alone (about 40 days for the malnourished patient). In the minority, however, were some important outliers, patients who had a clear "survival" benefit from TPN; these patients share the common characteristic of good performance status at the time TPN was initiated (Bozzetti et al. 2002).

Clearly, the decision to pursue home TPN in patients with late-stage cancer is influenced by factors other than the evidence base (Figure 25.4). Among these influences, family and societal values about nutrition appear to exert a predominant influence on the decision of whether or not to offer nutritional support at the end of life. In fact, this decision places considerable stress on patients and their families, who often struggle to sort out issues related to eating and nutrition at the end of life. In a qualitative study of 13 advanced cancer patients and 11 of their family members before and after TPN administration, patients described frustration with their inability to eat, and family members described going to great lengths to prepare appetizing meals, only to be disappointed (Orrevall et al. 2004). Both groups experienced mealtime as a time of great worry and desperation, perceived physicians to be concerned about or interested in nutritional issues, and viewed TPN as a positive solution to the "chaos that surrounded mealtime."

In assessing the medical necessity and/or utility of TPN, physicians must not just consider the wishes of the patient and family, but also take into account the variable data regarding the effect of TPN on quality of life among patients with late-stage cancer. Patients requiring home parenteral nutrition tend to begin with a lower quality of life, are more likely to suffer from depression, and experience more psychological problems than do patients not on home TPN. One study found that quality of life improved in only 20%–40% of cancer patients while on home TPN; in the majority, quality of life remained stable until the last one to two months of life, after which quality of life declined (Bozzetti et al. 2002).

Despite declining quality of life, patients and their families may perceive TPN-related benefits that are not apparent to others. In a study of the utility of TPN in patients on home parenteral nutrition, 82% of families believed that TPN was beneficial in most cases, while the nutrition support service felt that it was beneficial in only 50% of these cases (August et al. 1991). One difference of opinion occurred, for example, when a patient received TPN for only 12 days, and during that time was able to be married.

One force swaying families in favor of TPN is the common fear that patients will starve to death or experience thirst or hunger. This worry is largely unfounded; more than 60% of terminally ill cancer patients in hospice therapy never endure thirst or hunger, and those who do find that such symptoms can be alleviated with small sips of water, food, and lubrication to the lips. These

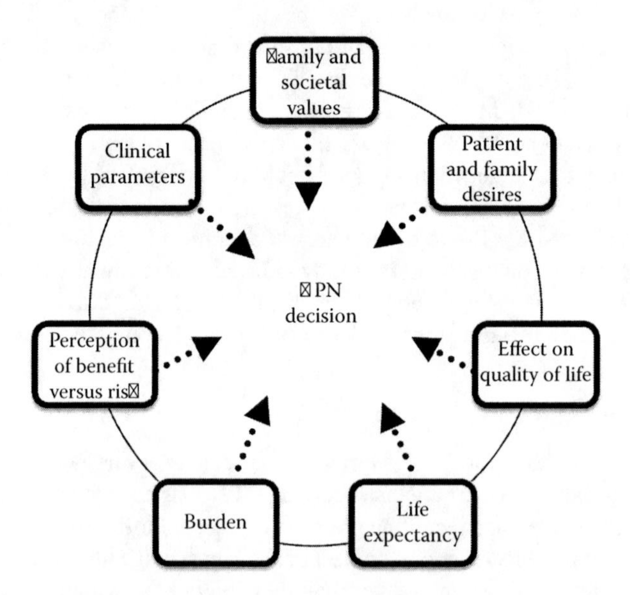

FIGURE 25.4 Factors influencing the palliative use of TPN.

symptoms are more often due to concurrent administration of drugs than to actual dehydration or starvation (McCann, Hall, and Groth-Juncker 1994).

25.9.3 TPN: A Pragmatic Clinical Approach

Before initiating TPN, the attending physician must always discuss its risks and logistics with family members. A typical conversation prior to deciding for or against TPN might address some or all of the decision-making factors presented in Table 25.3.

The additional burden of TPN—both physical and emotional—on both the patient and family can be substantial. Even when the patient is willing to accept these risks and the burden of administering TPN, the family may not be able to adequately support them in this process. In a survey that examined end-of-life wishes among cancer patients and their families, 77% of patients wanted to go home, but their families reported feeling heavily burdened at this time, with more than 60% stating they were overwhelmed, stressed, and sleep-deprived, and 15% suggesting that they themselves had considered suicide. The burden of home TPN on the patient's family must certainly be considered in any decision to administer TPN.

KEY POINTS TO COMMUNICATE TO PATIENTS AND THEIR FAMILIES

- TPN carries several risks, including infection and thrombosis.
- Evidence from research studies do not demonstrate clear benefit from TPN.
- Patients with advanced cancer typically do not experience hunger or thirst related to nutritional deficits, though this is often the reason that TPN is considered.
- It is estimated that up to one-fifth of patients with end-stage cancer who receive TPN will need to be admitted to the hospital for TPN-related complications.
- Patients receiving TPN require frequent laboratory testing.
- Someone (the patient, a family member, or caregiver) must be at home to receive deliveries of TPN, and must be physically able to hang the TPN in a sterile fashion.

TABLE 25.3
Arguments against and for TPN in Advanced Life-Limiting Illness (Supported by Varying Levels of Evidence and/or Perception)

Biological	↑ Tumor growth	Supplement to oral intake
	Metastasis	Inhibition/prevention of weight loss
	↑Tumor cell activity	Longer survival?
	↑Thymidine incorporation	
	Low/no impact on serum protein	
Psychosocial	↑Distress	↑Quality of life
	Logistical burden	↑Appetite
	Expense	Family/caregiver peace of mind
	Appearance of "the end"	Perceived active care
		↓Distress

- If the patient is in a nursing home or in-patient hospice unit, staff in those facilities must be able to support TPN administration, and must be accepting of the practice.

ETHICAL ISSUES

With the emergence of evidence-based medicine, clinical decision-making increasingly relies upon data that support best practices to achieve optimal outcomes. In fields that focus on cure of disease, the application of evidence-based medicine is relatively straightforward. One must: review and critically appraise the evidence, consider which procedures and protocols have demonstrated effectiveness for improving outcomes in patients similar to the one at hand, and refer to evidence-based guidelines in implementing approaches supported by the literature. In the context of palliative and end-of-life care, however, the process is far more ambiguous. Disease-free status, survival, or maintenance of current performance status no longer represent reasonable outcomes. Physicians face difficult, ethically complex considerations as to what could constitute the basis for making decisions in these circumstances. Perhaps the most viable outcome in these situations is quality of life, which itself is a complex indicator and sometimes difficult to measure.

The issue of TPN at the end of life sheds light on the challenges that arise in applying principles of evidence-based medicine to palliative and end-of-life care, as well as on the ethical concerns associated with providing care in this stage of the disease trajectory. Here, clinical decision-making is not necessarily clarified by "evidence," which can be contradictory and can introduce more questions than it answers. In considering whether to use TPN for patients with end-stage cancer, physicians must balance contradictory data about its benefits and its costs, knowing that any choice they make will be only partially supported by the evidence. Under these circumstances, it is a professional and ethical imperative to practice open communication with patients and families.

The TPN controversy also illuminates the important place of non-medical considerations in clinical decision-making, especially at the end of life and in advanced cancer. How does the physician balance a family's desire to see their loved one nourished against the risk of a potentially life-threatening treatment complication? Does a patient's or family's desire for a treatment warrant the treatment, even if it is not medically indicated? If the family's desire for TPN is driven by religious views, does that change the equation? What weight should be given to quality-of-life implications for family members themselves, who experience less distress related to the patient's eating and nutrition when he/she receives TPN?

No simple answers to these questions exist. The best current approach in clinical practice is: (1) at the individual patient level, to communicate openly and frequently with patients and families over the course of decision-making, and care more generally; and (2) at the clinic level, to develop practice guidelines based on the best judgment of the providers involved, with reference to existing evidence and clinical experience.

SUMMARY POINTS

- Nutritional concerns are common among patients with advanced life-limiting cancer and cause considerable distress.
- Metabolic changes, in combination with the side effects of cancer treatment, can result in cancer anorexia-cachexia syndrome (CACS). CACS is associated with an array of burdensome symptoms that impair immune response, erode functional status, and compromise quality of life.
- TPN is a method for delivering nutrition to patients who no longer have the ability to eat normally or sufficiently.
- The use of TPN in terminally ill cancer patients remains controversial due to conflicting evidence regarding its risks and benefits.
- TPN is not currently indicated for patients with end-stage cancer, but clinical experience suggests that it may be warranted for these patients under certain conditions.

LIST OF ABBREVIATIONS

5-FU	5-fluorouracil
CACS	Cancer-related anorexia-cachexia syndrome
IFN	Interferon
IL-1	Interleukin-1
IL-6	Interleukin-6
LMF	Lipid-mobilizing factor
NNS	Nutritional support service
PIF	Proteolysis-inducing factor
TNF-α	Tumor necrosis factor-α
TPN	Total parenteral nutrition

REFERENCES

Abu-Rustum, N. R., R. R. Barakat, E. Venkatraman, and D. Spriggs. Mar 1997. Chemotherapy and total parenteral nutrition for advanced ovarian cancer with bowel obstruction. *Gynecologic Oncology* 64 (3): 493–95.

American College of Physicians. 1 May 1989. Parenteral nutrition in patients receiving cancer chemotherapy. American College of Physicians [see comment]. *Annals of Internal Medicine* 110 (9): 734–36.

American Gastroenterological Association. Oct 2001. American gastroenterological association medical position statement: Parenteral nutrition. *Gastroenterology* 121 (4): 966–69.

August, D. A., D. Thorn, R. L. Fisher, and C. M. Welchek. May–Jun 1991. Home parenteral nutrition for patients with inoperable malignant bowel obstruction [see comment]. *Jpen: Journal of Parenteral & Enteral Nutrition* 15 (3): 323–27.

Bozzetti, F., L. Cozzaglio, E. Biganzoli, G. Chiavenna, M. De Cicco, D. Donati, G. Gilli, S. Percolla, and L. Pironi. Aug 2002. Quality of life and length of survival in advanced cancer patients on home parenteral nutrition [see comment]. *Clinical Nutrition* 21 (4): 281–88.

Bozzetti, F., C. Gavazzi, L. Cozzaglio, A. Costa, P. Spinelli, and G. Viola. May–Jun 1999. Total parenteral nutrition and tumor growth in malnourished patients with gastric cancer. *Tumori* 85 (3): 163–66.

Cameron, I. L., and W. A. Pavlat. Mar 1976. Stimulation of growth of a transplantable hepatoma in rats by parenteral nutrition. *Journal of the National Cancer Institute* 56 (3): 597–602.

A.S.P.E.N. Board of Directors, the Clinical Guidelines Task Force. Jan–Feb 2002. Guidelines for the use of parenteral and enteral nutrition in adult and pediatric patients [erratum appears in *Jpen: Journal of Parenteral & Enteral Nutrition* Mar–Apr 2002;26(2):144]. *Jpen: Journal of Parenteral & Enteral Nutrition* 26 (1 Suppl): 1SA–138SA.

Gadducci, A., S. Cosio, A. Fanucchi, and A. R. Genazzani. Jul–Aug 2001. Malnutrition and cachexia in ovarian cancer patients: Pathophysiology and management. *Anticancer Research* 21 (4B): 2941–47.

Heckmayr, M., and U. Gatzemeier. 1992. Treatment of cancer weight loss in patients with advanced lung cancer. *Oncology* 49 (Suppl 2): 32–34.

Heys, S. D., K. G. M. Park, M. A. McNurlan, E. Milne, O. Eremin, J. Wernerman, R. A. Keenan, and P. J. Garlick. Apr 1991. Stimulation of protein synthesis in human tumours by parenteral nutrition: Evidence for modulation of tumour growth. *British Journal of Surgery* 78 (4): 483–87.

Howard, L., M. Ament, C. R. Fleming, M. Shike, and E. Steiger. Aug 1995. Current use and clinical outcome of home parenteral and enteral nutrition therapies in the United States. *Gastroenterology* 109 (2): 355–65.

Klein, S., and R. L. Koretz. Jun 1994. Nutrition support in patients with cancer: What do the data really show?[comment]. *Nutrition in Clinical Practice* 9 (3): 91–100.

McCann, R.M., W. J. Hall, and A. Groth-Juncker. 26 Oct 1994. Comfort care for terminally ill patients. The appropriate use of nutrition and hydration [see comment]. *Journal of the American Medical Association* 272 (16): 1263–66.

Nixon, D. W., S. Moffitt, D. H. Lawson, J. Ansley, M. J. Lynn, M. H. Kutner, S. B. Heymsfield, M. Wesley, R. Chawla, and D. Rudman. 1981. Total parenteral nutrition as an adjunct to chemotherapy of metastatic colorectal cancer. *Cancer Treatment Reports* 65 (Suppl 5): 121–28.

Orrevall, Y., C. Tishelman, M. K. M. K. Herrington, and J. Permert. Dec 2004. The path from oral nutrition to home parenteral nutrition: A qualitative interview study of the experiences of advanced cancer patients and their families. *Clinical Nutrition* 23 (6): 1280–87.

Orrevall, Y., C. Tishelman, J. Permert, and T. Cederholm. Sep 2009. The use of artificial nutrition among cancer patients enrolled in palliative home care services. *Palliative Medicine* 23 (6): 556–64.

Shamberger, R. C., M. F. Brennan, J. T. Goodgame Jr, S. F. Lowry, M. M. Maher, R. A. Wesley, and P. A. Pizzo. Jul 1984. A prospective, randomized study of adjuvant parenteral nutrition in the treatment of sarcomas: Results of metabolic and survival studies. *Surgery* 96 (1): 1–13.

Shang, E., C. Weiss, S. Post, and G. Kaehler. May–Jun 2006. The influence of early supplementation of parenteral nutrition on quality of life and body composition in patients with advanced cancer. *Jpen: Journal of Parenteral & Enteral Nutrition* 30 (3): 222–30.

Siddiqui, R., D. Pandya, K. Harvey, and G. P. Zaloga. Apr 2006. Nutrition modulation of cachexia/proteolysis. *Nutrition in Clinical Practic* 21 (2): 155–67.

Steiger, E., J. Oram-Smith, E. Miller, L. Kuo, and H. M. Vars. Apr 1975. Effects of nutrition on tumor growth and tolerance to chemotherapy. *Journal of Surgical Research* 18 (4): 455–66.

Tannenbaum, A., and H. Silverstone. 1953. Nutrition in relation to cancer. *Advances in Cancer Research* 1:451–501.

Torosian, M. H., and R. B. Donoway. May 1991. Total parenteral nutrition and tumor metastasis. *Surgery* 109 (5): 597–601.

White, F. R. 1961. The relationship between underfeeding and tumor formation, transplantation, and growth in rats and mice. *Cancer Research* 21:281–90.

26 Vitamin Deficiency in Patients with Terminal Cancer

Renata Gorska and Dominic J. Harrington

CONTENTS

26.1 INTRODUCTION

We are entirely dependent on dietary and other exogenous sources of vitamins to satisfy our requirements. A suboptimal supply of these nutrients disturbs metabolic networks and has a wide variety of repercussions. The first half of the twentieth century was the golden age for the identification and characterisation of vitamins, discoveries that originated from the detailed investigation of pathological changes induced by severe deficient states. Sensitive laboratory-based assays for the direct measurements of vitamin blood levels were subsequently developed, and applied to the further study of vitamins in health and disease. Although the determination of circulatory levels gives a good indication of current body stores/dietary exposure for some vitamins, greater insight can often be gained when these assays are used in combination with functional biomarkers that directly reflect status within target tissues.

26.1.1 Challenges Faced by Patients with Terminal Cancer

In addition to poor dietary intake, surgical and nonsurgical interventions used for the treatment of cancer can induce vitamin deficiencies. The absorption of vitamins is reliant on the gastrointestinal tract; interventions that compromise the functionality of this system diminish bioavailability. Radiation therapy can cause damage to the gastrointestinal mucosa, while chemotherapy regimes may impair epithelial cell function (Figure 26.1). Malabsorption as a consequence of diarrhoea is an added complication associated with chemotherapy (Davila and Bresalier 2008).

In some patients demand for a specific vitamin may exceed an apparently adequate dietary intake. For example, radiation therapy and chemotherapy increase free radical formation, potentially leading to the greater utilisation of vitamins with antioxidant properties (Jonas et al. 2000). Deficient states can also arise through the sequestering of nutrients to support tumour progression.

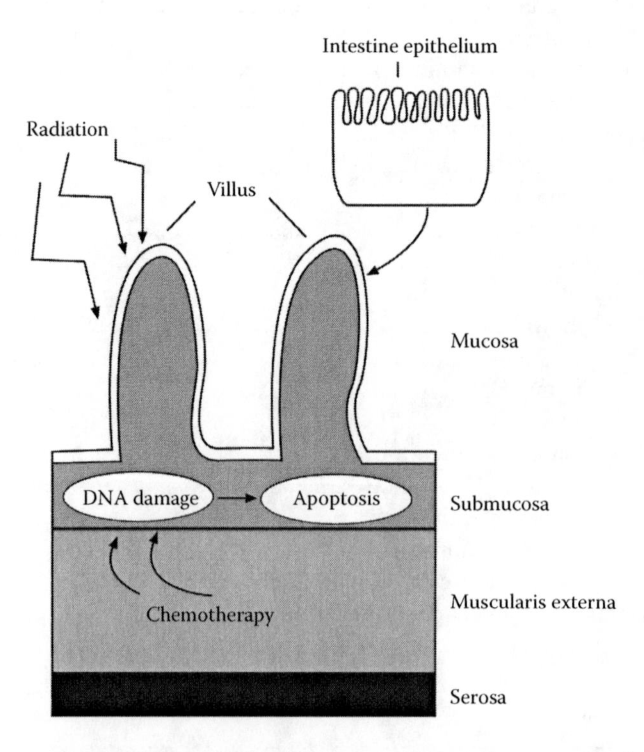

FIGURE 26.1 Structure of the small intestinal wall and effect of chemotherapy and radiation. Chemotherapy and radiation therapy may severely damage the intestinal mucosa, impeding micronutrient absorption.

Drug hepatotoxicity (Davila and Bresalier 2008) provides an additional challenge by impeding the utilisation of some vitamins despite replete tissue stores, leading to the development of functional deficient states.

26.2 FAT-SOLUBLE VITAMINS

Fat-soluble vitamins are absorbed from the proximal intestine and dependent on bile and pancreatic juice secretion for solubilisation (Figure 26.2). Any condition causing the prolonged intestinal malabsorption of fat will lead to a secondary deficiency of fat-soluble vitamins. Deficient states lead to the depletion of tissue stores and are indicated by a decrease in circulatory levels long before pathological changes develop. Sensitive assays for all four fat-soluble vitamin groups are available (Table 26.1).

26.2.1 Vitamin A

Vitamin A is a generic term for compounds with retinol activity, e.g., various aldehyde (retinal), alcohol (retinol) and acid (retinoic acid) forms. The main circulatory form is retinol bound to retinol-binding protein. Vitamin A is required for physiological processes that include vision, maintenance of mucosal barriers, haematopoiesis, bone development and immunocompetence (Ball 2004).

Recently absorbed retinol is transported to hepatic stellate cells for storage as retinyl esters. The mobilisation of these stores to counter dietary restriction or malabsorption is sufficient to maintain circulatory levels and satisfy metabolic demand for several months. The vitamin A status of patients

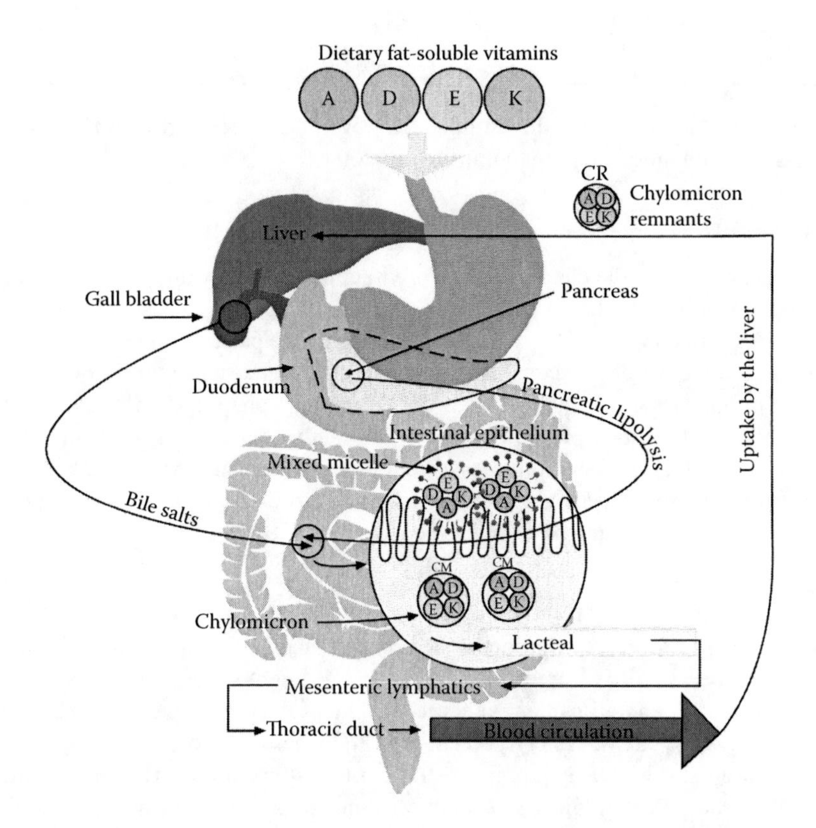

FIGURE 26.2 Absorption of fat-soluble vitamins. Schematic absorption of fat-soluble vitamins.

TABLE 26.1
Fat-Soluble Vitamins

	Major Functions	RDA[a]	Effects of Deficiency	Laboratory Test Available
Vitamin A	Vision, reproduction, growth and development, cellular differentiation, immune function	900 μg/day	Night blindness, keratomalacia, impaired mucus secretion	HPLC (retinol)
Vitamin D	Regulation of calcium and phosphate blood levels, bone mineralisation, control of cell proliferation and differentiation, modulation of immune system	5[b] μg/day	Impaired bone mineralisation, osteomalacia	LC-MS, HPLC, (25-hydroxycholecalciferol, 25-hydroxyergocalciferol), immunoassay, radioassay
Vitamin E	Antioxidant, maintain nervous system	15 mg/day	Neurological disorders, haemolytic anaemia	HPLC (α-tocopherol)
Vitamin K	Coenzyme for a vitamin K-dependent carboxylase, blood coagulation, bone metabolism	120[b] μg/day	Bleeding, osteoporosis, coronary heart disease	HPLC (vitamin K_1), des-carboxy-prothrombin (PIVKA-II), undercarboxylated osteocalcin (uc OC), osteocalcin, urinary vitamin K metabolites, urinary γ-carboxyglutamic acid (Gla)

[a] RDA in adult male (according to the U.S. Food and Nutrition Board).
[b] Nutrient indicate adequate intake (AI) because no RDA can be established.

with terminal cancer has not been widely studied. However, the potential role of vitamin A in cancer prevention has received more attention (Okuno et al. 2004).

26.2.2 Vitamin D

The patient's dependence on the dietary sources of vitamin D to satisfy physiological need is dependent upon the amount of the vitamin that can be synthesised through exposure to sunlight. In turn, production of 25-hydroxy-vitamin D_3 is partly a function of the patient's skin pigmentation (darker pigmentation less effective at northern latitudes) and age, since the thinning of the skin on the elderly patient diminishes epidermal 7-dehydrocolesterol (its precursor) (Holick, Matsuoka, and Wortsman 1989). Brief periods of exposure to bright sunlight generates sufficient vitamin D in white patients, although at northern latitudes even prolonged exposure will bring no benefit during the winter months. The wavelength of light required to convert 7-dehydrocolesterol to previtamin D_3 (290–315 nm, UV-B range) is unable to penetrate glass (Ball 2004).

26.2.3 Vitamin E

Vitamin E is a generic term for a group of tocopherols and tocotrienols. α-Tocopherol is most commonly studied because it is stored by the body and deficient states can be reversed using this vitamin. α-Tocopherol is an antioxidant with a role in the preservation of cell membranes and may protect against oxidative stress. Ninety percent of α-tocopherol is stored in adipose tissue; these reserves are released slowly during dietary restriction to buffer vitamin E status (Blatt, Leonard, and Traber 2001). A decrease in dietary α-tocopherol intake or malabsorption is not reflected by a corresponding decrease in circulatory levels for ~1 month.

Many studies have implicated suboptimal vitamin E status with the development of several cancers. Vitamin E deficiency leads to erythrocyte haemolysis and the development of neurological disorders. Plasma levels of vitamin E were not compromised in male patients with colorectal tumours (Saygili et al. 2003). Of interest however are preclinical data that suggest that tocopherols may influence treatment-related toxicities (Pace et al. 2003).

26.2.4 Vitamin K

Vitamin K is a cofactor for γ-glutamyl carboxylase, which catalyses the post-translational modification of specific peptide-bound glutamate residues into γ-carboxyglutamate in vitamin K-dependent proteins. The liver synthesises seven vitamin K-dependent proteins that have a crucial role in blood coagulation (factors II, VII, IX and X, proteins C, S, and Z). Extrahepatic vitamin K-dependent proteins (osteocalcin, matrix Gla protein, Gas6, and periostin) are implicated in bone formation, mineralisation, regulation and repair. The most abundant forms of vitamin K are phylloquinone (vitamin K_1), which is present in plants and accounts for ~90% of dietary vitamin K intake; and the menaquinones (vitamins K_2), which are of bacterial origin. In the UK, the daily dietary vitamin K reference value is 1 μg/kg, an intake that is regarded as adequate with respect to maintenance of normal coagulation function.

An inadequate supply of vitamin K prevents the optimal γ-carboxylation of vitamin K-dependent proteins. These proteins lack functionality and are referred to as protein-induced by vitamin K absence (PIVKAs). The measurement of PIVKA-II (undercarboxylated factor II) is a functional indicator of vitamin K status, since PIVKA-II is not detectable in the circulation of healthy adults. The prothrombin time (or international normalised ratio [INR]) is a poor indicator of vitamin K status (Suttie 1992).

Hepatic stores of vitamin K_1 are rapidly (<3 days) depleted during dietary restriction (Usui et al. 1990). The susceptibility of patients with cancer to vitamin K deficiency has been highlighted in two studies. In the first, autologous bone marrow transplantation was linked with a rapid fall in circulatory levels of vitamin K_1 and PIVKA-II was detectable within a few days (Elston et al. 1995). In the second study, very low serum vitamin K_1 concentrations were present in a fifth of palliative care patients suggesting poor tissue stores (Harrington et al. 2008). A precarious vitamin K status was confirmed by elevated levels of PIVKA-II in 78% of patients recruited to this study.

26.3 WATER-SOLUBLE VITAMINS

Water-soluble vitamins have a wide array of functions (Table 26.2). With the notable exception of vitamin B_{12}, only limited quantities of water-soluble vitamins are stored within tissue. To facilitate absorption across the enterocytes, vitamin-specific membrane transport processes have evolved within the small intestine (Figure 26.3).

26.3.1 Vitamin C (Ascorbic Acid)

Early signs of vitamin C deficiency include general fatigue, anorexia and depression. Severe deficiency leads to scurvy, which is characterised by capillary bleeding, perifollicular haemorrhage, gingivitis and poor wound healing. Scurvy develops within 1–3 months of absolute dietary vitamin C restriction, when the body pool size falls below 300 mg (normal pool size ~1500 mg).

Low circulatory levels of vitamin C are common in patients with advanced cancer (Saygili et al. 2003) and an association with prognosis has been described (Mayland, Bennett, and Allan 2005). The incidence of vitamin C deficiency in critically ill patients has also been investigated (Schorah et al. 1996; Alexandrescu, Dasanu, and Kauffman 2009).

TABLE 26.2
Water-Soluble Vitamins

	Major Functions	RDA[a]	Effects of Deficiency	Laboratory Test Available
Vitamin B_1 (Thiamine)	Coenzyme in the metabolism of carbohydrates and branched-chain amino acids	1.2 mg/day	Beriberi, Wernicke-Korsakoff syndrome, confusion, cardiac failure, nerve membrane disorder	Thiamine diphosphate, erythrocyte transketolase index (early marker of thiamine deficiency), alpha-keto acids in urine
Vitamin B_2 (Riboflavin)	Coenzyme in numerous redox reactions	1.3 mg/day	No severe specific deficiency syndrome, impacts on vitamin B3, B6, B9, cheilosis, angular stomatitis	Riboflavin, flavin adenin dinucleotide (FAD), flavin mononucleotide (FMN)
Vitamin B_3 (Niacin)	Nicotinamide adenine dinucleotide (NAD) and nicotinamide adenine dinucleotide phosphate (NADP) act as acceptors or donors of electrons for redox reactions	16 mg/day	Pellagra: dermatitis, diarrhoea, dementia	Urinary excretion of N′-methyl-nicotinamide, no reliable blood test available
Vitamin B_5 (Pantothenic acid)	Needed for formation of coenzyme A; is essential for the metabolism of carbohydrates, fats and proteins	5[b] mg/day	No severe specific deficiency syndrome, painful peripheral neuropathy	Calcium-D-pantothenate
Vitamin B_6 (Pyridoxine)	Amino acid metabolism, glycogen phosphorylase (release of glucose from stored glycogen). In brain: synthesis of the neurotransmitter, serotonin from the amino acid, tryptophan, dopamine. Niacin formation: critical reaction in the synthesis of niacin from tryptophan. Hormone function	1.3 mg/day	Irritability, depression, confusion, inflammation of the tongue, sores or ulcers of the mouth, ulcers of the skin at the corners of the mouth	Pyridoxal 5-phosphate (PLP), urinary excretion of 4-pyridoxic acid
Vitamin B_7 (Biotin)	Enzyme cofactor, prosthetic group for four carboxylase enzymes. Synthesis of fatty acids, amino acids and glucose, energy metabolism, excretion metabolism of by-products from protein metabolism, maintenance of healthy hair, toenails and fingernails	30 μg/day	Very rare, hair loss, scaly red rash around the eyes, nose, mouth, and genital area, neurological disorders	Biotin, 3-hydroxyisovaleric acid

Vitamin B_9 (Folate)	One-carbon metabolism of nucleic acids and amino acids	400 µg/day	Megaloblastic anaemia, fatigue, palpitations	Red blood cell folate(s), serum folate(s), homocysteine
Vitamin B_{12} (Cyanocobalamin)	Coenzyme for methionine synthase, coenzyme for metabolism of methylmalonate to succinate (coenzyme L-methylmalonylcoenzyme A mutase)	2.4 µg/day	Pernicious anaemia, food-bound vitamin B_{12} malabsorption	Serum B_{12}, methylmalonic acid (MMA), homocysteine, holotranscobalamin II (TC)
Vitamin C (Ascorbic acid)	Controlling redox potential within cells, hydroxylation reactions, formation of collagen, required to maintain iron in the reduced state, reduces potentially carcinogenic free radicals to nonradical form	90 mg/day	Scurvy, failure of wound healing, anaemia	Ascorbic acid, dehydroascorbic acid, urine dipstick test, ascorbate present in leucocytes

[a] RDA in adult male (according to the U.S. Food and Nutrition Board).

[b] Nutrient indicate adequate intake (AI) because no RDA can be established.

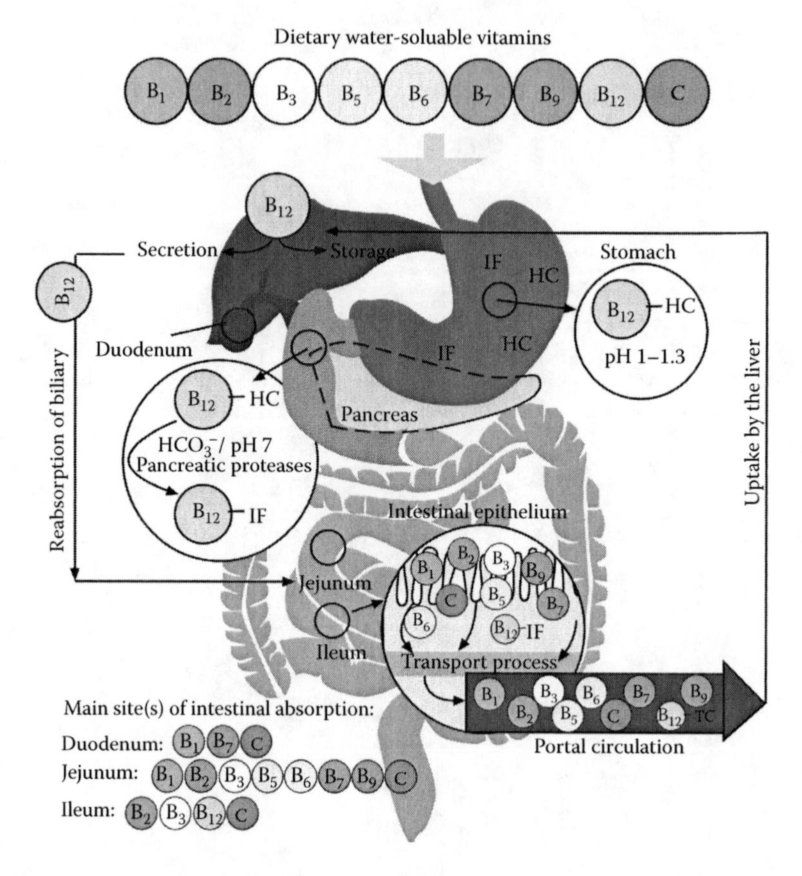

FIGURE 26.3 Absorption of water-soluble vitamins. Schematic absorption of water-soluble vitamins with particular reference to vitamin B_{12}. HC, holohaptocorrin; IF, intrinsic factor; TC, holotranscobalamin II.

26.3.2 Folate (Vitamin B_9)

Folate has an array of biological functions which include the production of purine and pyrimidine nucleotides for DNA synthesis and repair; and the regulation of gene expression through the synthesis of the methyl group donator S-adenosylmethionine (SAM) (Ball 2004).

Patients with advanced cancer develop folate deficiency for several reasons: inadequate dietary intake sustained over a period of 1–4 months; malabsorption; exposure to folate-antagonists; and the sequestering of folate by tumour cells. A deficient state can also be induced through vitamin B_{12} deficiency whereby folate is trapped as methyl derivatives leading to a shortage of nonmethylated forms to support DNA and RNA synthesis (Figure 26.4).

Through its DNA repair function, folate is considered to be protective against the initial development of cancer; however existing tumours are dependent on the availability of folate to support rapid growth and propagation. It is for this reason that folate antagonists are widely used as chemotherapeutic agents to retard tumour cell proliferation.

Folate status is typically assessed by measurement of serum folate levels. This has the disadvantage of only providing an insight into folate intake during the preceding few days. Since the folate content of erythrocytes is fixed at erythropoiesis, red cell-based folate assays reflect mean status over 100–120 days (the time that red cells circulate). Both of these assays report the sum of many different types of folate and are unable to differentiate between the various circulatory forms. Many factors influence the spectrum of folates present in the circulation including common methylenetetrahydrofolate reductase polymorphisms and vitamin B_{12} or B_2 deficiency (Pfeiffer et al. 2004). This can lead to misinterpretation when assays of total folate are utilised.

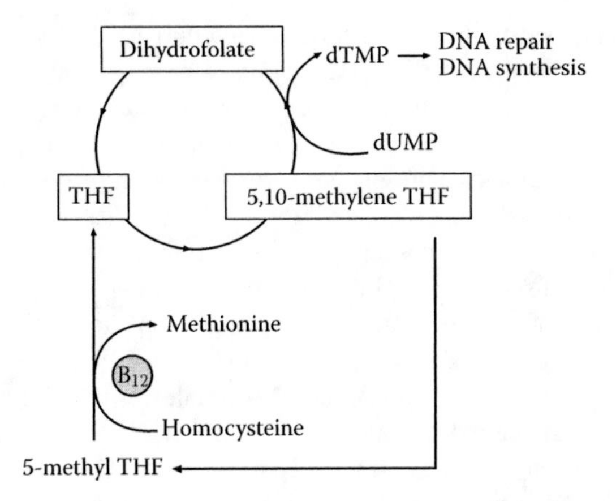

FIGURE 26.4 Interrelation between folate, vitamin B_{12} and homocysteine metabolism. Vitamin B_{12} is required for the conversion of 5 methyl THF to 5,10-methylene THF and the metabolism of homocysteine to methionine. B_{12}, vitamin B_{12}; THF, tetrahydrofolate; dUMP, deoxyuridine monophosphate; dTMP, deoxythymidine monophosphate.

Circulatory levels of homocysteine are a functional marker of folate status. 5-Methyltetrahydrofolate, the most abundant form of folate, is an essential methyl donor for the methionine synthase and vitamin B_{12}-mediated conversion of homocysteine to methionine. Circulatory levels of homocysteine >15 μmol/L are consistent with folate and/or vitamin B_{12} deficiency provided the patient has good renal function (a functional test for vitamin B_{12} status is outlined in section 26.3.3).

The correction of folate deficiency with excessive doses of folic acid, an artificial chemical analogue of folate, is of concern. Unlike the naturally occurring dietary folates, folic acid is fully oxidised and unsubstituted. The conversion of folic acid to its physiological form is dependent on dihydrofolate reductase. When the capacity of this enzyme (~400 μg/d) is exceeded, unmetabolised folic acid accumulates in the circulation (Kelly et al. 1997). Circulatory folic acid is associated with decreased natural killer cytotoxicity (Troen et al. 2006). In addition, the masking of the haematological symptoms of vitamin B_{12} deficiency that may lead to neurological damage is well known.

26.3.3 Vitamin B_{12}

Vitamin B_{12} has the largest and most complicated structure of all the vitamins. In the centre of this structure is a cobalt ion, hence the term cobalamin is used for any compound possessing vitamin B_{12} activity. Vitamin B_{12} is synthesised by microorganisms and enters the food chain in food of animal origin. Deficient states induced by poor dietary intake (i.e., vegetarian or vegan diets) take up to 20 years to manifest. However, clinical deficiencies as a consequence of abnormalities in one of the multiple steps that regulate cobalamin absorption or enterohepatic circulation present more rapidly (~2 years) (Figure 26.3). Ultimately, intestinal uptake of vitamin B_{12} takes place in the ileum by a receptor-mediated process that includes the calcium-dependent binding of a vitamin B_{12}/intrinsic factor complex, whereby this complex is translocated through the enterocytes to the portal circulation and bound to transcobalamin II. The cobalamin-saturated form is referred to as holotranscobalamin II (TC), whereas apo-holotranscobalamin II refers to the unsaturated form (Ermens, Vlasveld, and Lindemans 2003).

The measurement of serum levels of vitamin B_{12} is commonly used as a marker of vitamin B_{12} status. It is often not widely appreciated that circulatory vitamin B_{12} is predominately bound to two proteins and that 'front-line' laboratory assays do not discriminate between these forms. Although

~80% of vitamin B_{12} is carried by haptocorrin (holohaptocorrin, abbreviated as HC), extrahepatic cellular receptors have not been described. TC facilitates receptor-mediated uptake of cobalamin therein to all cells. Circulatory levels of HC decline slowly in response to the onset of a deficient state, typically taking 3–6 years to fall below the lower limit of most assay reference ranges. Circulatory levels of TC fall quickly and give an early indication of deficiency although in assays that cannot discriminate between these two forms this decline is masked by the more abundant HC. Tissue deficiency of vitamin B_{12} is common in patients with serum levels within the reference range and can be revealed using the serum methylmalonic acid assay.

In humans the function of two enzymes are dependent on vitamin B_{12}: methylmalonyl-CoA mutase and methionine synthase. Methylmalonyl-CoA mutase converts methylmalonyl-CoA to succinyl-CoA. When the supply of vitamin B_{12} is suboptimal, this reaction cannot proceed, leading to the increased formation of methylmalonic acid. Circulatory levels of methylmalonic acid are a functional indicator of vitamin B_{12} status with concentrations <271 nmol/L considered to be within the reference range for healthy populations. Methionine synthase is folate mediated and essential for the synthesis of methionine from homocysteine (Section 26.3.2).

In over 50% of patients with hepatocellular carcinoma, elevated levels of HC are found, most likely as a result of diminished clearance by the liver (Ermens et al. 2003). In other cancers, breast, pancreatic, stomach and colon, large increases in both unsaturated TC and HC are occasionally seen. Elevated serum vitamin B_{12} levels and its relation to C-reactive protein have been evaluated as a predictive factor of prognosis (Kelly, White, and Stone 2007). Other studies suggest that carcinoid tumours are associated with the development of pernicious anaemia (Rybalov and Kotler 2002). In patients with advanced colorectal cancer treated with chemotherapy, serum levels of vitamin B_{12}, folate and homocysteine were satisfactory pre- and post-therapy. Interestingly, patients with sub-clinically low vitamin B_{12} prior to treatment had greater survival than patients with higher values (Bystrom et al. 2009).

26.3.4 Vitamin B_6

Pyridoxal and the phosphate ester derivative pyridoxal 5'-phosphate account for 75%–80% of the circulatory forms of vitamin B_6. Pyridoxal 5'-phosphate is required for the release of the steroid hormone-receptor complex from DNA binding to terminate hormone action.

Vitamin B_6 deficiency has been implicated in the development of diseases affected by steroid hormones, including prostate and breast cancers. An inverse association between dietary vitamin B_6 intake and risk of colorectal adenoma or cancer has also been reported (Wei et al. 2005). Few studies have investigated the vitamin B_6 status of terminally ill patients with cancer. No deterioration in status was seen in patients with advanced breast cancer treated with megestrol acetate or tamoxifen (Schrijver et al. 1987).

26.3.5 Thiamine (Vitamin B_1)

Syndromes caused by thiamine deficiency include beriberi and Wernicke-Korsakoff syndrome. Thiamine has two primary functions: alpha-keto acid decarboxylation (carbohydrate metabolism) and transketolation (pentose phosphate pathway).

Thiamine deficiency is well described in patients with advanced cancer (Barbato and Rodriguez 1994). In particular, thiamine deficiency presents in patients with rapidly growing malignancies. To support rapid growth and proliferation, tumour cells require large amounts of energy, which in part is derived from the anaerobic breakdown of glucose to ATP. The pentose phosphate pathway is important in glucose metabolism, with transketolase an integral enzyme for the nonoxidative synthesis of 5-carbon sugars. Thiamine is metabolised to thiamine pyrophosphate, the cofactor of transketolase. The upregulation of transketolase activity during tumour progression has been widely reported.

Transketolase activity is decreased in thiamine deficiency and is used as an early marker of decreasing thiamine status. Thiamine supplementation is common in cancer patients, although concerns have been raised that in some cases this has the propensity to accelerate tumour growth (Comin-Anduix et al. 2001). Macleod (2000) presented a case study of a terminally ill cancer patient who developed thiamine-related Wernicke encephalopathy, despite apparently adequate dietary intake.

26.3.6 Riboflavin (Vitamin B_2)

Riboflavin is a component of coenzymes flavin mononucleotide (FMN) and flavin adenine dinucleotide (FAD), and is involved in the metabolism of several other vitamins (vitamin B_6, niacin, and folate). Interaction between folate and riboflavin in patients with colorectal and cervical cancer showed that increased plasma riboflavin levels were associated with decreased plasma homocysteine levels (Powers 2005).

26.3.7 Niacin (Vitamin B_3)

Niacin (nicotinic acid) deficiency or pellagra is a result of an inadequate dietary intake of niacin or tryptophan. Niacin can be synthesised from tryptophan, a reaction that is reliant on vitamins B_2 and B_6. In the context of cancer, studies on niacin deficiency have focused mainly on the risk of cancer development rather than status in terminally ill patients.

26.3.8 Biotin (Vitamin B_7)

Biotin is a cofactor to many enzymatic reactions involved in metabolism of lipid proteins and carbohydrates. Biotin deficiency is exceedingly rare, but can develop after 3–4 weeks of dietary restriction or through malabsorption.

26.3.9 Pantothenic Acid (Vitamin B_5)

Deficiencies of this vitamin are exceptionally rare and have not been widely studied in cancer patients.

26.4 PRACTICAL METHODS AND TECHNIQUES

26.4.1 Fat-Soluble Vitamins

26.4.1.1 Vitamin A

Retinol is measured in serum/plasma most commonly by HPLC. Typical reference range: 1.4–3.8 μmol/L.

26.4.1.2 Vitamin D

Serum vitamin D_3 + D_2 is predominately measured by competitive immunoassays or methods based on chromatographic separation (HPLC, LC-MS/MS). Typical reference limits: optimal status 75–200 nmol/L; insufficiency 37–75 nmol/L; severe deficiency <37 nmol/L.

26.4.1.3 Vitamin E

α-Tocopherol is most commonly measured in serum/plasma by HPLC. Typical reference range: 11.6–41.8 μmol/L. Levels of α-tocopherol correlate with cholesterol and hence are often expressed as the α-tocopherol-cholesterol ratio (reference range >2.22).

26.4.1.4 Vitamin K

Phylloquinone is measured in serum/plasma by HPLC. Typical reference range: 0.33–3.44 nmol/L. Hepatic functional status is assessed by PIVKA-II measurement by ELISA.

26.4.2 Water-Soluble Vitamins

26.4.2.1 Vitamin C

Vitamin C (ascorbic acid) is measured in plasma by various techniques (e.g., HPLC). Typical reference range: 22–85 μmol/L.

26.4.2.2 Folate

Folate status is assessed by measurement in serum (short-term indicator) and red blood cells (mean status over ~120 days). Typical reference range: serum 7–36 nmol/L, red cell 408–1700 nmol/L. Functional status is partly indicated by homocysteine levels (<15 μmol/L).

26.4.2.3 Vitamin B_{12}

Various methodologies are available: chemical, microbiological or immunoassay. Serum cobalamin concentration is often determined by automated immunoassays. Typical reference range: 250–900 ng/L. Functional status is indicated by serum methylmalonic acid levels (<271 nmol/L).

26.4.2.4 Vitamin B_6

Direct methods include determination of pyridoxal-5'-phosphate in whole blood. Typical reference range: 35.2–110.1 nmol/L) and EDTA plasma measured by HPLC: 14.6–72.9 nmol/L.

26.4.2.5 Thiamine (Vitamin B_1)

Whole blood levels are determined by HPLC. Typical reference range: 66.5–200 nmol/L. Functional status is indicated by erythrocyte transketolase activity.

26.4.2.6 Riboflavin (Vitamin B_2)

Direct methods include the determination of FAD and FMN in whole blood by HPLC. Typical reference range (FAD): 120–160 nmol/L.

26.4.2.7 Niacin (Vitamin B_3)

Urinary excretion of metabolites, N-methyl-nicotinamide and N-methyl-2-pyridone-5-carboxamide is used to assess niacin status. NAD^+ and $NADP^+$ concentrations and their ratio in red blood cells may be sensitive and reliable status indicators. A ratio of erythrocyte NAD to NADP <1.0 may identify subjects at risk of developing deficiency.

26.4.2.8 Biotin (Vitamin B_7)

Biotin is measured in serum/plasma by microbiological methods, avidin-binding assays, determination of biotin excretion and 3-hydroisovaleric acid in urine. Typical serum concentrations: 100–400 μmol/L.

26.4.2.9 Pantothenic Acid (Vitamin B_5)

Typical blood levels: 0.9–1.5 μmol/L. Status can be deduced from urinary pantothenate excretion.

KEY FACTS: VITAMIN DEFICIENCY IN PATIENTS WITH TERMINAL CANCER

- Vitamins are chemically diverse.
- The impact of terminal cancer on status is greater for some vitamins than it is for others.

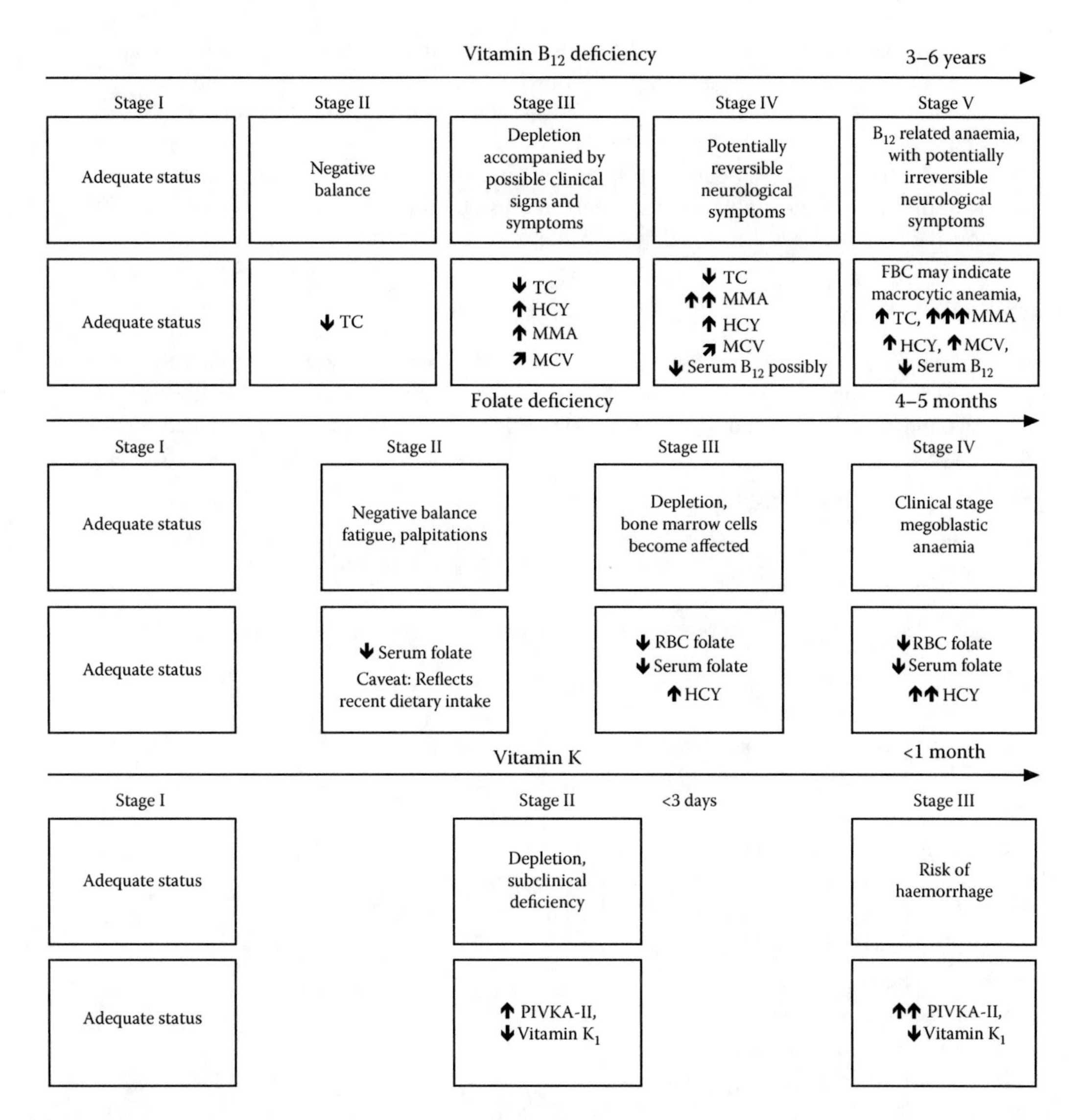

FIGURE 26.5 The stages of B_{12}, folate and vitamin K_1 deficiency. Stages of depletion for vitamin B_{12}, folate and vitamin K. For each vitamin the stages of deficiency are shown and available laboratory tests indicated. FBC, full blood count; HCY, homocysteine; MCV, mean corpuscular volume; MMA, methylmalonic acid; PIVKA-II, des-carboxy-prothrombin; RBC, red blood cell; TC, holotranscobalamin II.

- Deficient states develop at very different rates (from a few days to several years).
- Vitamin status can be monitored with a variety of laboratory-based assays long before pathological changes manifest.
- Stages of vitamin deficiency (B_{12}, folate, vitamin K) are illustrated in Figure 26.5.

SUMMARY POINTS

- Vitamins are required to support many metabolic networks.
- Vitamin deficiencies are common in patients with terminal cancer as a consequence of anorexia, and the use of treatment regimes that induce nausea and a loss of appetite.

- Vitamin deficiencies in patients with terminal cancer can result from surgical interventions, and impaired gastrointestinal function following chemotherapy and radiation therapy.
- Laboratory tests are widely available to identify deficient states and monitor the efficacy of nutritional support.
- A high proportion of patients with terminal cancer are unlikely to maintain an adequate vitamin status without nutritional support. It must, however, be recognised that some vitamins are required for the growth and proliferation of tumour cells.

ACKNOWLEDGMENTS

The authors gratefully acknowledge our colleagues Dr. Martin Shearer, Dr. Agata Sobczyńska-Malefora, Mr. Kieran Voong and Mr. David Card from The Human Nutristasis Unit. We also thank GSTS Pathology and Guy's and St. Thomas' NHS Foundation Trust for their continued support.

LIST OF ABBREVIATIONS

FAD	Flavin adenine dinucleotide
FBC	Full blood count
FMN	Flavin mononucleotide
HC	Holohaptocorrin
HCY	Homocysteine
IF	Intrinsic factor
INR	International normalised ratio
MCV	Mean corpuscular volume
MMA	Methylmalonic acid
NAD	Nicotinamide adenine dinucleotide
NADP	Nicotinamide adenine dinucleotide phosphate
PIVKAs	Protein induced by vitamin K absence (or antagonism)
PIVKA-II	des-Carboxy-prothrombin
RBC	Red blood cell
SAM	S-adenosylmethionine
TC	Holotranscobalamin II
uc OC	Undercarboxylated osteocalcin

REFERENCES

Alexandrescu, D. T., C. A. Dasanu, and C. L. Kauffman. 2009. Acute scurvy during treatment with interleukin-2. *Clinical and Experimental Dermatology* 34:811–14.

Ball, G. F. M. 2004. *Vitamins. Their role in the human body*. Oxford, UK: Blackwell Publishing.

Barbato, M., and P. J. Rodriguez. 1994. Thiamine deficiency in patients admitted to a palliative care unit. *Palliative Medicine* 8:320–24.

Blatt, D. H., S. W. Leonard, and M. G. Traber. 2001. Vitamin E kinetics and the function of tocopherol regulatory proteins. *Nutrition* 17:799–805.

Bystrom, P., K. Bjorkegren, A. Larsson, L. Johansson, and A. Berglund. 2009. Serum vitamin B12 and folate status among patients with chemotherapy treatment for advanced colorectal cancer. *Upsala Journal of Medical Sciences* 114:160–64.

Comin-Anduix, B., J. Boren, S. Martinez, C. Moro, J. J. Centelles, R. Trebukhina, N. Petushok, W. N. P. Lee, L. G. Boros, and M. Cascante. 2001. The effect of thiamine supplementation on tumour proliferation—A metabolic control analysis study. *European Journal of Biochemistry* 268:4177–82.

Davila, M., and R. S. Bresalier. 2008. Gastrointestinal complications of oncologic therapy. *Nature Clinical Practice Gastroenterology & Hepatology* 5:682–96.

Elston, T. N., J. M. Dudley, M. J. Shearer, and S. A. Schey. 1995. Vitamin K prophylaxis in high-dose chemotherapy. *Lancet* 345:1245.

Ermens, A. A. M., L. T. Vlasveld, and J. Lindemans. 2003. Significance of elevated cobalamin (vitamin B12) levels in blood. *Clinical Biochemistry* 36:585–90.

Harrington, D. J., H. Western, C. Seton-Jones, S. Rangarajan, T. Beynon, and M. J. Shearer. 2008. A study of the prevalence of vitamin K deficiency in patients with cancer referred to a hospital palliative care team and its association with abnormal haemostasis. *Journal of Clinical Pathology* 61:537–40.

Holick, M. F., L. Y. Matsuoka, and J. Wortsman. 1989. Age, vitamin-D, and solar ultraviolet. *Lancet* (2) 8671: 1104–5.

Jonas, C. R., A. B. Puckett, D. P. Jones, D. P. Griffith, E. E. Szeszycki, G. F. Bergman, C. E. Furr et al. 2000. Plasma antioxidant status after high-dose chemotherapy: A randomized trial of parenteral nutrition in bone marrow transplantation patients. *American Journal of Clinical Nutrition* 72:181–89.

Kelly, P., J. McPartlin, M. Goggins, D. G. Weir, and J. M. Scott. 1997. Unmetabolized folic acid in serum: Acute studies in subjects consuming fortified food and supplements. *American Journal of Clinical Nutrition* 65:1790–95.

Kelly, L., S. White, and P. C. Stone. 2007. The B-12/CRP index as a simple prognostic indicator in patients with advanced cancer: A confirmatory study. *Annals of Oncology* 18:1395–99.

Macleod, A. D. 2000. Wernicke's encephalopathy and terminal cancer: Case report. *Palliative Medicine* 14:217–18.

Mayland, C. R., M. I. Bennett, and K. Allan. 2005. Vitamin C deficiency in cancer patients. *Palliative Medicine* 19:17–20.

Okuno, M., S. Kojima, R. Matsushima-Nishiwaki, H. Tsurumi, Y. Muto, S. L. Friedman, and H. Moriwaki. 2004. Retinoids in cancer chemoprevention. *Current Cancer Drug Targets* 4:285–98.

Pace, A., A. Savarese, M. Picardo, V. Maresca, U. Pacetti, G. Del Monte, A. Biroccio et al. 2003. Neuroprotective effect of vitamin E supplementation in patients treated with cisplatin chemotherapy. *Journal of Clinical Oncology* 21:927–31.

Pfeiffer, C. M., Z. Fazili, L. Mccoy, M. Zhang, and E. W. Gunter. 2004. Determination of folate vitamers in human serum by stable-isotope-dilution tandem mass spectrometry and comparison with radioassay and microbiologic assay. *Clinical Chemistry* 50:423–32.

Powers, H. J. 2005. Interaction among folate, riboflavin, genotype, and cancer, with reference to colorectal and cervical cancer. *Journal of nutrition* 135:2960S–66S.

Rybalov, S., and D. P. Kotler. 2002. Gastric carcinoids in a patient with pernicious anemia and familial adenomatous polyposis. *Journal of Clinical Gastroenterology* 35:249–52.

Saygili, E. I., D. Konukoglu, C. Papila, and T. Akcay. 2003. Levels of plasma vitamin E, vitamin C, TBARS, and cholesterol in male patients with colorectal tumors. *Biochemistry-Moscow* 68:325–28.

Schorah, C. J., C. Downing, A. Piripitsi, L. Gallivan, A. H. AlHazaa, M. J. Sanderson, and A. Bodenham. 1996. Total vitamin C, ascorbic acid, and dehydroascorbic acid concentrations in plasma of critically ill patients. *American Journal of Clinical Nutrition* 63:760–65.

Schrijver, J., J. Alexieva Figusch, N. van Breederode, and H. A. van Gilse. 1987. Investigations on the Nutritional Status of Advanced Breast Cancer Patients. The Influence of Long-Term Treatment with Megestrol Acetate of Tamoxifen. *Nutrition and Cancer* 10:231–45.

Suttie, J. W. 1992. Vitamin K and human nutrition. *Journal of the American Dietetic Association* 92:585–90.

Troen, A. M., B. Mitchell, B. Sorensen, M. H. Wener, A. Johnston, B. Wood, J. Selhub et al. 2006. Unmetabolized folic acid in plasma is associated with reduced natural killer cell cytotoxicity among postmenopausal women. *Journal of nutrition* 136:189–94.

Usui, Y., H. Tanimura, N. Nishimura, N. Kobayashi, T. Okanoue, and K. Ozawa. 1990. Vitamin K concentrations in the plasma and liver of surgical patients. *American Journal of Clinical Nutrition* 51:846–52.

Wei, E. K., E. Giovannucci, J. Selhub, C. S. Fuchs, S. E. Hankinson, and J. Ma. 2005. Plasma vitamin B-6 and the risk of colorectal cancer and adenoma in women. *Journal of the National Cancer Institute* 97:684–92.

27 Position of Appetite and Nausea in Symptom Clusters in Palliative Radiation Therapy

Janet Nguyen, Martin Leung, Roseanna Presutti, Francesco Caporusso, Lori Holden, and Edward Chow

CONTENTS

27.1 INTRODUCTION

Cancer patients undoubtedly experience a variety of symptoms associated with their pathology and its treatment. A symptom is defined as a "subjective experience reflecting the biopsychosocial functioning, sensations, or cognition of an individual" (Dodd, Miaskowski, and Paul 2001). Symptoms are multidimensional and can include a patient's perception of prevalence, intensity and distress (Chow et al. 2007). Interestingly enough, symptoms associated with a given cancer and its treatment are becoming more and more predictable because symptoms are not presenting themselves in isolation but rather as part of a whole cluster of other associated symptoms, as demonstrated by several longitudinal studies.

Research into symptom clusters in advanced cancer is complicated due to several variables that can confound the symptom experience. Subjective reports of symptom distress can be confounded by long-term experience with the disease, presence of multiple symptoms, duration of disease experience or any other perceptual disorders (Chow et al. 2007; Fan, Hadi, and Chow 2007). The "partial mediation model" (Beck, Dudley, and Brasevick 2005) alludes to the complexity in understanding dynamics of symptom concurrence in advanced cancer. The model explains how two symptoms can influence each other indirectly through effect on a common symptom. For instance, pain could affect sleep and indirectly influence subjective reports of fatigue (Beck et al. 2005).

Analyses of causal factors underlying commonly observed symptoms in advanced cancer could provide the theoretical framework for correlations between symptoms in a cluster. Nausea and vomiting are frequently observed in advanced cancer. While nausea is an unpleasant subjective feeling of wanting to vomit, vomiting is the forceful expulsion of gastric contents (Lagman et al. 2005). Metabolic abnormalities, brain metastases, chemotherapy, radiation therapy (RT), constipation and certain medications (i.e. opioids or antibiotics) can dispose a patient to develop nausea and vomiting (Lagman et al. 2005). Emotional distress (for instance, anxiety and fear) and pain can also stimulate the development of nausea (Lagman et al. 2005). Nausea and vomiting centres in the medulla have been hypothesized to share common afferent neural pathways (Lagman et al. 2005), which may explain their concurrence in advanced cancer patients (Walsh and Rybicki 2006). Prioritization of certain symptoms by patients can increase the possibility of those symptoms being relieved through clinical intervention. This hypothesis was confirmed for some physical symptoms, such as pain and constipation. However symptom prioritization had little influence over the alleviation of subjective symptoms such as nausea, fatigue, physical function, role function and activity (Stromgren et al. 2002).

Symptom clusters may be useful in more quickly identifying and treating the underlying pathology that is to blame for the symptoms that invariably present. The importance of including quality of life (QOL) and symptoms as a component of palliative treatment assessment was emphasized by Tannock (1987), who wrote, "When cure is elusive, it is time to start treating the patient and not the tumor."

27.2 KEY FEATURES OF SYMPTOM CLUSTERS

27.2.1 What Are They?

Symptoms rarely occur in isolation, especially in the case of advanced cancer patients. Past reporting indicates that cancer patients experience an average of 11–13 concurrent symptoms (Chow et al. 2007).

These symptoms are a consequence of the disease, the associated treatment or a combination of the two (Barsevick et al. 2006). They could also have a significant effect on patients' physical, emotional and cognitive sense of well-being.

Systematic attention to the occurrence of multiple symptoms in cancer patients identified the presence of symptom "complexes" or "clusters."

Dodd et al. (2001) were among the first to coin the term symptom clusters in their research in pain, fatigue and sleep disturbances. They described symptom clusters as having the presence of three or more concurrent related symptoms that may or may not have a common aetiology. The suggested strength of these relationships was not specified in the study, nor was the amount of time that all symptoms within a cluster must be present to be considered one.

Kim et al. (2005) described symptom clusters as two or more related symptoms that occur together, form a stable group, and are relatively independent of other clusters. They also described symptom clusters as affecting disease course, treatment, function, QOL or prognosis, all of which differ from the summation of individual symptoms. The available literature additionally suggests that at least 75% of the symptoms within the cluster, including the most prevalent symptom, must be present in order for a patient to be considered as experiencing the cluster.

Additionally, Miaskowski, Dodd, and Lee (2004) defined symptom clusters as sharing a common aetiology in each individual cluster and having a common variance.

27.2.2 Why Are They Useful?

Cancer patients report experiencing multiple symptoms and these predict changes in patient function, treatment failures and post-therapeutic outcomes.

Many of the earlier clinical studies focused on treating the dimensions of individual symptoms and not the multiple symptoms presented by most patients. While studying individual symptoms advanced understanding in isolated symptoms, this may have explained why single symptom treatment did not necessarily improve QOL.

There are new avenues in symptom management and palliative care due to research in symptom clusters, as well as an increased awareness of symptom clusters due to significant research on the influence of concurrent symptoms on patient outcomes.

This research will be valuable in patient cancer treatment, especially in aiding symptom management and increasing the understanding of disease pathophysiology (Walsh and Rybicki 2006).

27.3 TOOLS USED IN SYMPTOM CLUSTER RESEARCH

Thus far, the majority of symptom cluster studies have utilized common assessment tools including the Edmonton Symptom Assessment System (ESAS), M.D. Anderson Symptom Inventory (MDASI), Symptom Distress Scale and Brief Pain Inventory (BPI). For the two studies discussed in detail in this chapter, the ESAS tool was utilized (Table 27.1). In order to elucidate the presence of symptom clusters, patients with metastatic cancer that were referred to an outpatient palliative RT clinic were asked to rate their symptom distress utilizing the ESAS. In addition, patient demographics, cancer history, analgesic consumption and disease status were recorded. Patient demographics recorded included age, sex, inpatient or outpatient status, weight loss of >10% over the past 6 months and Karnofsky performance status. A Principle Component Analysis (PCA) with "varimax rotation" was performed on the nine ESAS symptoms in order to determine interrelationships between symptoms.

27.4 RADIATION-INDUCED NAUSEA/VOMITING

Palliative RT is an established treatment for a variety of malignancies, whether given alone or as a combinatory component with surgery or chemotherapy (Feyer et al. 2005). As palliative interventions are unlikely to lead to prolonged survival and significant tumour regression, QOL and reducing patient symptomatology become a more meaningful end point when compared with the traditional end points, such as survival times and local control. Thus, the therapeutic benefits of treatment must also take into consideration the degree of tolerable side effects (Feyer et al. 2005).

Approximately one-third of patients undergoing RT experience radiation-induced nausea and vomiting (RINV) (Feyer et al. 2005; Wong et al. 2006). There tends to be a distinct pattern of RINV, with an asymptomatic latent period lasting approximately 40–90 minutes, followed by an acute nausea and/or vomiting period of about 6–8 hours. Following the acute period is the recovery period (Tramer et al. 1998). Although these symptoms are usually less severe and less frequent with RT than with chemotherapy, they may still be very distressing for a large

TABLE 27.1
Key Features of ESAS

1. The ESAS is an 11-point scale evaluating 9 frequently observed symptoms with a rating from 0 to 10 (0 = absence of symptom, 10 = worst possible symptom)
2. The 9 symptoms evaluated are pain, fatigue, nausea, depression, anxiety, drowsiness, appetite, sense of well-being and shortness of breath
3. The ESAS tool has been validated in the cancer population

proportion of RT patients. Thus, this can lead to unplanned interruptions in radiation treatment if the symptoms are prolonged and/or severe. In addition, nausea and vomiting persisting through RT may cause dehydration, electrolyte imbalance and malnutrition, further impinging patients' QOL (Feyer et al. 2005).

RINV has been reported to occur more frequently in patients that receive total body or half body irradiation, as well as those that receive radiation to the upper abdomen (Feyer et al. 2005). Other factors that influence radiation-induced emesis are the dose and fractionation given, and patient characteristics (i.e., age, sex, previous nausea and vomiting, etc). Emesis also increases proportionally with irradiation volume, emphasizing the importance of field size (Feyer et al. 2005). Increased severity and duration of nausea or vomiting may lead to loss of appetite and/or weight loss.

27.5 NAUSEA/VOMITING AND APPETITE IN SYMPTOM CLUSTERS IN BONE METASTASES

Bone metastases are a frequent complication of cancer. Breast and prostate carcinomas are the most common to develop metastases to the bone, with an incidence of 75% and 68%, respectively. In addition, lung, thyroid and renal carcinoma develop metastases to bone in about 40% of cases (Chow et al. 2007). Fifty to seventy-five percent of these patients will need treatments using local or systemic therapies. RT has been demonstrated to relieve bone pain in approximately 80% of patients. However, some patients have reported no significant improvement in QOL, and this can be attributed to patients having multiple bone metastases. While pain may be alleviated at one irradiated site, this may cause the unmasking of pain at other bone metastatic sites.

In a study performed by Chow et al. (2007), the primary objective was to study whether bone pain "clusters" with any other symptoms in 518 patients with bone metastases before and after RT. The secondary objective was to compare and contrast the cluster patterns in responders and non-responders to RT (Table 27.2). Three symptom clusters were found using PCA. Cluster 1 included fatigue, pain, drowsiness and poor sense of well-being, cluster 2 consisted of anxiety and depression, and cluster 3 consisted of shortness of breath, nausea and poor appetite. Patients experiencing nausea will usually also have a loss of appetite and not receive adequate nutrition. This further causes weight loss and weakness.

It is important to note that alleviation of pain may have influenced the experience of other symptoms, as there was a difference in symptom clustering between responders and non-responders. We further investigated how RT to bone metastases influenced the dynamics of symptom clusters over time. The mean symptom severity for the majority of the ESAS items significantly decreased over time (baseline to week 12), except for nausea, depression and shortness of breath. Finally the

TABLE 27.2
Key Facts for Classification of Responders and Non-responders to Palliative Radiation for Painful Bone Metastases

1. Responders are patients that have had either a complete response or partial response to radiation therapy
2. A complete response indicates a pain score of 0 out of 10 with no concomitant increase in analgesic intake
3. A partial response means there is (i) a pain score reduction of 2 or more at the treated site on a 0–10 scale without analgesic increase or (ii) an analgesic reduction of 25% or more from baseline without an increase in pain score
4. Non-responders are classified as those with stable disease or those with progression
5. Progression means there is (i) an increase in pain score of 2 or more points above baseline at the treated site with stable analgesic intake or (ii) an increase in analgesic intake of 25% or more from baseline with the pain score remaining stable or at least 1 point above baseline.

clusters were found to fragment during follow-ups conducted 1, 2, 4, 8 and 12 weeks post-RT in both responders and non-responders to RT, alluding to the dynamic nature of symptom clusters (Tables 27.3 and 27.4, Figure 27.1) (Chow et al. 2007).

In the second study, performed by Fan et al. (2007), the authors analyzed 1296 patients with any site of metastasis. The patient population consisted of 64% bone metastases from primary lung, breast and prostate cancer. PCA with varimax rotation was again employed on the nine-symptom ESAS scale. Utilizing Kim et al.'s (2005) definition, three symptom clusters were identified, accounting for 62% of the total variance. Cluster 1 consisted of nausea, lack of appetite, poor sense of well-being and pain. Cluster 2 included fatigue, drowsiness and shortness of breath, and cluster 3 consisted of anxiety and depression. Again, nausea and poor appetite were present in the same symptom cluster.

TABLE 27.3
Summary of Symptom Cluster Changes in Bone Metastases Patients from Baseline by Responders

	Cronbach's Alpha	Symptoms
At Baseline		
Cluster 1	0.77	*Fatigue, drowsiness,* well-being, pain
Cluster 2	0.81	*Anxiety, depression*
Cluster 3	0.61	Nausea, appetite, breathlessness
At Week 1		
Cluster 1	0.75	*Fatigue, drowsiness*, appetite, breathlessness
Cluster 2	0.83	*Anxiety, depression,* well-being
Cluster 3	0.44	Nausea, pain
At Week 2		
Cluster 1	0.81	*Fatigue, drowsiness*, *anxiety, depression*, pain
Cluster 2	0.77	Nausea, appetite, well-being
Cluster 3	—	Breathlessness
At Week 4		
Cluster 1	0.82	*Fatigue, drowsiness*, appetite, breathlessness
Cluster 2	0.90	*anxiety, depression*, well-being
Cluster 3	0.40	Nausea, pain
At Week 8		
Cluster 1	0.87	*Fatigue, drowsiness*, well-being, *anxiety, depression,*
Cluster 2	0.69	Breathlessness, nausea, appetite
Cluster 3	—	Pain
At Week 12		
Cluster 1	0.90	*Fatigue, drowsiness*, nausea, *anxiety, depression, well-being*
Cluster 2	0.58	Breathlessness, appetite
Cluster 3	—	Pain

Source: Reprinted with kind permission from Springer Science+Business Media: *Support Care Cancer*, Symptom clusters in cancer patients with bone metastases, 15, 2007, 1035, Chow, E. et al.
Note: *Italics* indicate symptoms consistently clustering together. Table 27.3 lists the symptom clusters in responders during different follow-up intervals following radiotherapy for painful bone metastases. A higher Cronbach's alpha coefficient = a higher correlation.

TABLE 27.4
Summary of Symptom Cluster Changes in Bone Metastases Patients from Baseline by Non-responders

	Cronbach's Alpha	Symptoms
At Baseline		
Cluster 1	0.77	*Fatigue, drowsiness,* well-being, pain
Cluster 2	0.81	*Anxiety, depression*
Cluster 3	0.61	Nausea, appetite, breathlessness
At Week 1		
Cluster 1	0.69	*Fatigue, drowsiness*, breathlessness
Cluster 2	0.81	*Anxiety, depression,* well-being
Cluster 3	0.65	Nausea, appetite, pain
At Week 2		
Cluster 1	0.75	*Fatigue, drowsiness*
Cluster 2	0.83	*Anxiety, depression,* nausea, appetite, well-being
Cluster 3	0.29	Breathlessness, pain
At Week 4		
Cluster 1	0.65	*Fatigue, drowsiness*, nausea
Cluster 2	0.82	*Anxiety, depression*, well-being, pain
Cluster 3	0.25	Breathlessness, appetite
At Week 8		
Cluster 1	0.73	*Fatigue, drowsiness*, nausea
Cluster 2	0.81	*Anxiety, depression*, well-being, pain, appetite
Cluster 3	—	Breathlessness
At Week 12		
Cluster 1	0.75	Pain, *fatigue, drowsiness*, appetite
Cluster 2	0.85	*Anxiety, depression*, well-being
Cluster 3	0.43	Nausea, breathlessness

Source: Reprinted with kind permission from Springer Science+Business Media: *Support Care Cancer*, Symptom clusters in cancer patients with bone metastases, 15, 2007, 1035, Chow, E. et al.

Note: *Italics* indicate symptoms consistently clustering together. Table 27.4 lists the symptom clusters in non-responders during different follow-up intervals following radiotherapy for painful bone metastases. A higher Cronbach's alpha coefficient = a higher correlation.

27.6 NAUSEA/VOMITING AND APPETITE IN SYMPTOM CLUSTERS IN BRAIN METASTASES

Brain metastases are the most frequent neurological complication related to cancer. Between 20% and 40% of cancer patients will suffer from brain metastases with most having primary lung or breast carcinomas (Langer and Mehta 2005). A rapid deterioration in patient function is usually expected following diagnosis, with potential devastating effects to social, physical and mental capabilities. The optimal management of brain metastases remains controversial. Whole brain radiotherapy (WBRT) in conjunction with steroids has been commonly used in the treatment of most patients, especially those with multiple metastases (Chow et al. 2008). The objective of WBRT is to provide symptomatic relief, to allow for tapering of the dose of corticosteroids and to possibly improve survival. Although many trials have shown that WBRT can reduce neurologic symptoms,

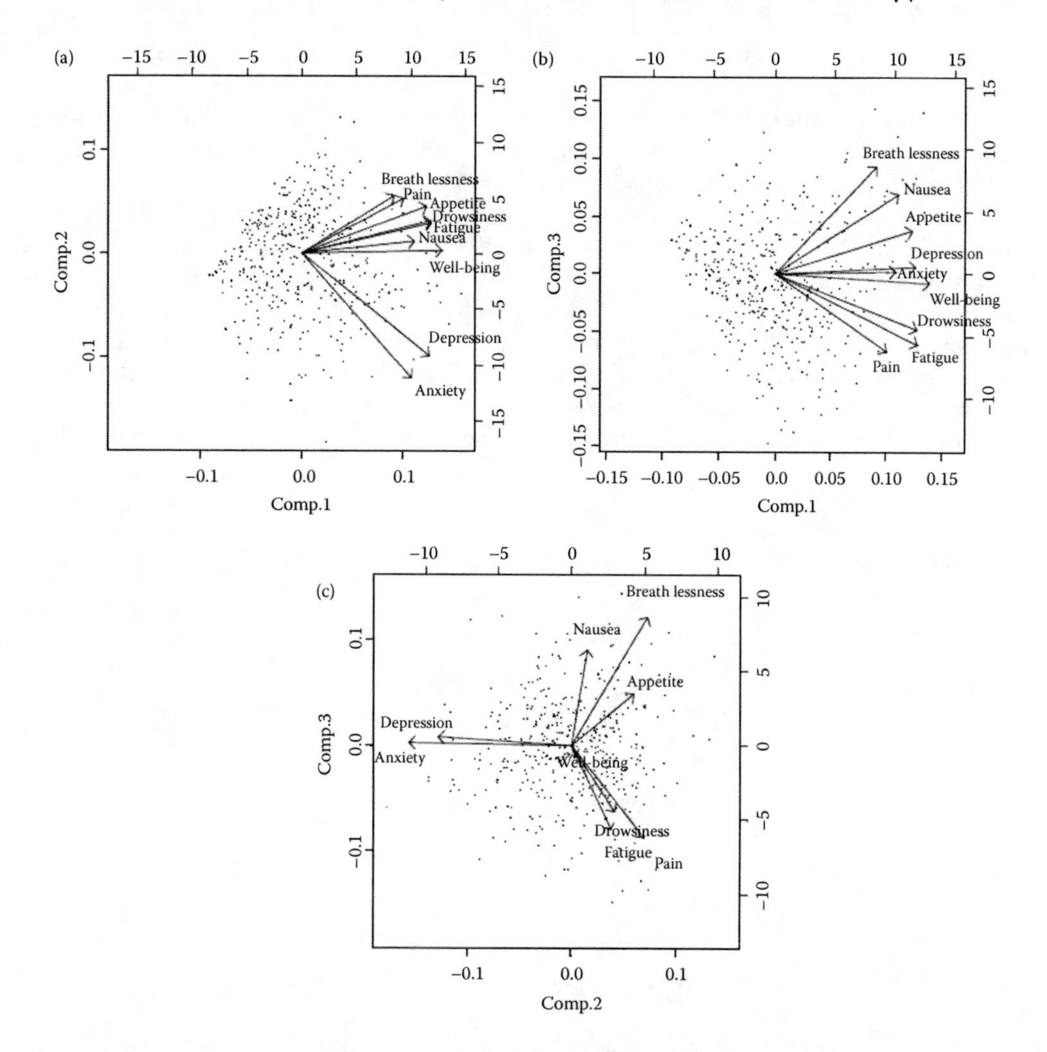

FIGURE 27.1 Biplot among three principal components or clusters in bone metastases patients following radiation therapy. This figure shows the biplot depicting the planes of a three-dimensional model. The arrows of longer length and closer proximity suggest a higher correlation between symptoms. The clusters were represented in all biplots, but were best evidenced in (c) as all three clusters were evident in the biplot between components 2 and 3. Clusters 2 and 3 were clear in the biplots in (a) and in (b). A PCA with varimax rotation was used to transform a number of observed variables into a smaller number of variables (called principal components). (Reprinted with kind permission from Springer Science+Business Media: *Support Care Cancer*, Symptom clusters in cancer patients with bone metastases, 15, 2007, 1035, Chow, E. et al.)

median survival following a diagnosis of brain metastases is generally only 3–6 months (Chow et al. 2008). The true benefits of this type of treatment in performance status and QOL have yet to be fully elucidated. Moreover, there is evidence that WBRT has little effect on symptom control from brain metastases.

27.6.1 Studies Conducted

We examined if symptom clusters in patients with brain metastases existed and whether (if present) they changed following WBRT (Chow et al. 2008). Over a period of 3 years, 170 patients received WBRT. The ESAS was administered at baseline (prior to WBRT), and at 1, 2, 4, 8 and 12 weeks following WBRT. Three symptom clusters were found at baseline, with cluster 1 including fatigue, drowsiness, shortness of breath and pain. Cluster 2 consisted of anxiety and depression, and cluster 3 included nausea, poor appetite and poor sense of well-being (Figure 27.2). Poor appetite, along with fatigue and drowsiness, were also found to have a significant overall trend of increasing symptom distress over time. Those same three symptoms also revealed worse symptom distress scoring at the 12-week follow-up compared with baseline.

A second study, by Hird et al. (2009), explored symptom clusters in cancer patients with brain metastases using the Spitzer Quality of Life Index (SQLI), which assesses QOL based on five domains: activity, daily living, health, support and outlook (scored on a scale from 0 to 2, where 0 is the worst and 2 is the best). Patients also completed a study-made questionnaire consisting of 17 brain metastases-specific symptom items (scored as none, mild, moderate or severe). These 17 items included headache, weakness, memory loss, confusion, dizziness, trouble concentrating, decreased alertness, imbalance problems, seizures, speech difficulty, vision problems, problems with smell, hearing or tingling, numbness, fatigue, personality change, nausea and vomiting

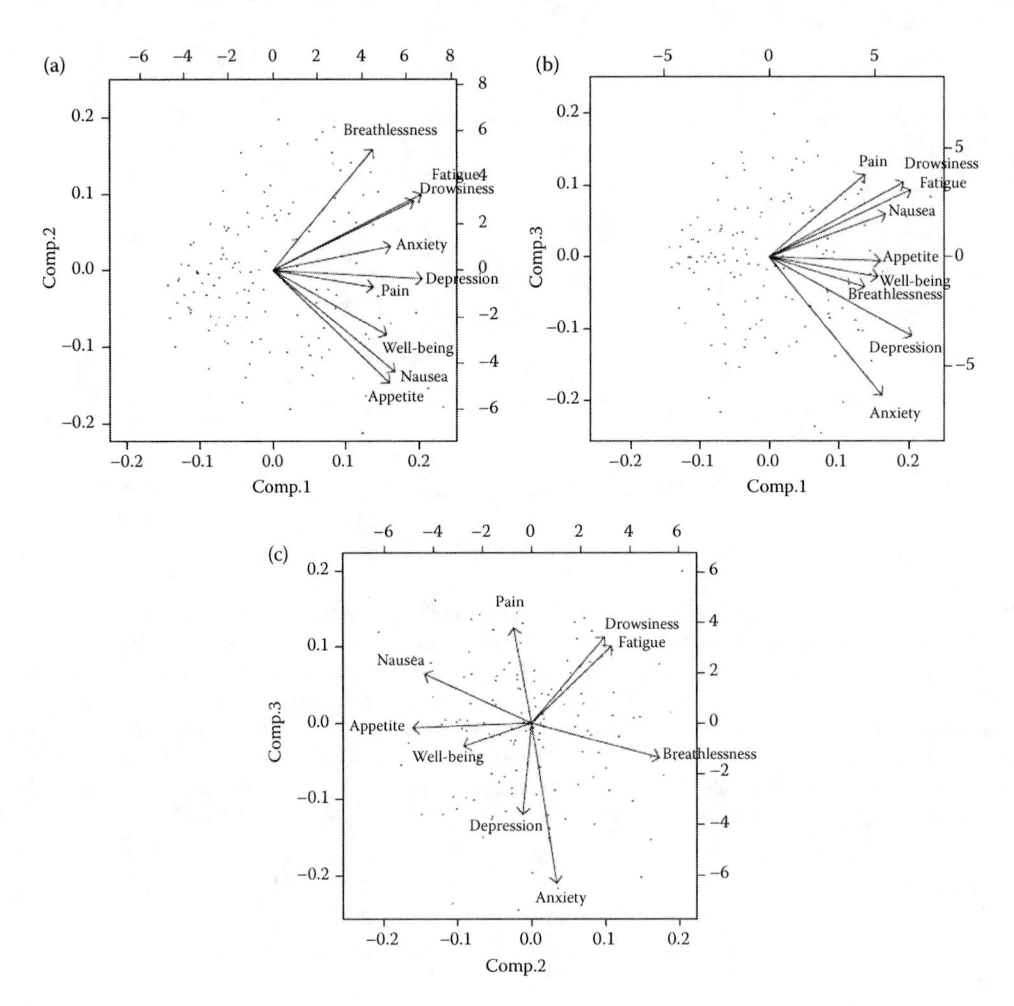

FIGURE 27.2 Biplot among three principal components or clusters in brain metastases patients following whole brain radiation therapy, depicting the planes of a three-dimensional model. This figure shows the biplot depicting the planes of a three-dimensional model. The arrows of longer length and closer proximity suggest a higher correlation between symptoms. Clusters 2 and 3 were clear in the biplots in (a) and (c). All three clusters were evident in the biplot between components 2 and 3 (c). A PCA with varimax rotation was performed. (Reprinted from *J. Clin. Oncol.*, 20, Chow, E. et al., Symptom clusters in cancer patients with brain metastases, 76–82, Copyright (2008), with permission from Elsevier.)

(Hird et al. 2009). Patients in this study completed these two QOL assessments at baseline, and at 1-, 2- and 3-month follow-up following WBRT. Steroid doses were not captured in this study or the previous one.

In this current study, 129 patients participated. Symptom cluster analysis of the 17 brain metastases-specific symptoms using PCA revealed three clusters at baseline. Cluster 1 included trouble concentrating, decreased alertness, confusion, imbalance problems, memory loss, weakness, fatigue, vision problems and problems with smell, hearing or tingling. Cluster 2 consisted of nausea, vomiting, headache and dizziness, and cluster three contained seizures, numbness, speech difficulty and personality change. At baseline, approximately 24% and 21% of patients rated nausea and vomiting, respectively, as mild, moderate or severe. At each follow-up, nausea and vomiting consistently clustered together, although the constituents of each symptom cluster changed over time (Figure 27.3). This study found that by employing an instrument more focused on patients with brain metastases, more symptom clusters were identified.

27.6.2 Study Conclusions

Few studies in this area of research have aimed to find clinically relevant responses, such as QOL outcomes. If WBRT were indeed beneficial in relieving symptoms experienced by patients with brain metastases, the prevalence of a symptom cluster would be expected to diminish. However, this was clearly not the case, as three symptom clusters still appeared at 12 weeks in our study (Chow et al. 2005) (Table 27.5). In fact, the strength of the internal consistencies of the clusters seemed

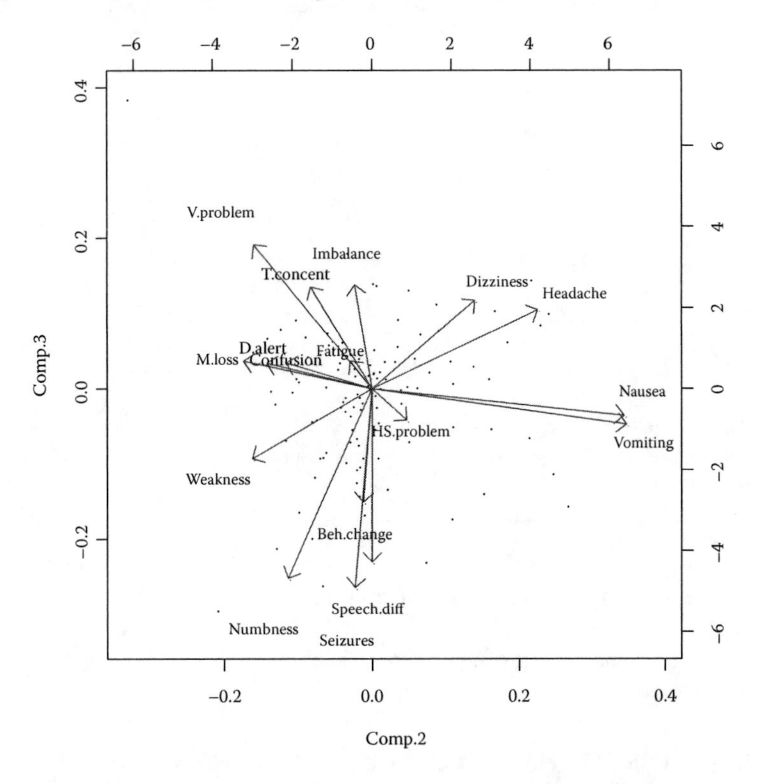

FIGURE 27.3 Biplot among the three clusters in brain metastases patients following whole brain radiation. This figure shows the biplot depicting the planes of a three-dimensional model. The arrows of longer length and closer proximity suggest a higher correlation between symptoms. A PCA with varimax rotation was performed. (Reprinted with kind permission from Springer Science+Business Media: *Support Care Cancer*, Exploration of symptom clusters within cancer patients with brain metastases using the Spitzer Quality of Life Index, 18, 2009, 335, Hird, A. et al.)

TABLE 27.5
Summary of Symptom Cluster Changes from Baseline to Subsequent Follow-ups in Patients with Brain Metastases

	Cronbach's Alpha	Symptoms
At Baseline		
Cluster 1	0.65	*Fatigue, drowsiness,* breathlessness, pain
Cluster 2	0.74	*Anxiety, depression*
Cluster 3	0.61	Nausea, poor appetite, poor sense of well-being
At Week 1		
Cluster 1	0.65	*Fatigue, drowsiness,* breathlessness
Cluster 2	0.78	*Anxiety, depression,* poor sense of well-being, pain
Cluster 3	0.47	Nausea, poor appetite
At Week 2		
Cluster 1	0.66	*Fatigue, drowsiness,* breathlessness, nausea
Cluster 2	0.76	*Anxiety, depression,* poor appetite, poor sense of well-being
Cluster 3	—	Pain
At Week 4		
Cluster 1	0.73	*Fatigue, drowsiness,* poor appetite, breathlessness
Cluster 2	0.82	*Anxiety, depression,* poor sense of well-being, nausea
Cluster 3	—	Pain
At Week 8		
Cluster 1	0.82	*Fatigue, drowsiness,* poor appetite
Cluster 2	0.81	*Anxiety, depression,* poor sense of well-being, pain
Cluster 3	0.59	Nausea, breathlessness
At Week 12		
Cluster 1	0.70	*Fatigue, drowsiness,* pain
Cluster 2	0.78	Poor sense of well-being, nausea, depression
Cluster 3	0.65	Breathlessness, poor appetite, anxiety

Source: Reprinted from *J. Clin. Oncol.*, 20, Chow, E. et al., Symptom clusters in cancer patients with brain metastases, 76–82, Copyright (2008), with permission from Elsevier.

Note: *Italics* indicate symptoms consistently clustering together. Table 27.5 lists the symptom clusters during different follow-up intervals following whole brain radiotherapy for brain metastases. A higher Cronbach's alpha coefficient = a higher correlation between symptoms.

to strengthen during the 12-week period. The shift of symptoms and increase in cluster strength at 12 weeks may be the result of a changing patient population due to attrition, volatility of a symptom experience in each patient, the effect of WBRT or due to the deterioration of the patients. A limitation in investigating the relationship of symptom clusters and WBRT is the absence of a control group in these two studies.

27.7 APPLICATIONS TO OTHER AREAS OF PALLIATIVE CARE

Patients who prioritize certain symptoms report higher initial scores for those symptoms and describe a significantly better treatment outcome than those who do not do so. Palliative care could be focused on relieving the most prioritized symptoms to optimize patient care and increase cost effectiveness in palliative oncology. Recognizing that certain symptoms tend to occur concurrently allows for better management to improve patients' QOL.

27.8 GUIDELINES

As far as clinical practice and pain management strategies are concerned, symptom clusters, much like the expected symptoms of a given syndrome, may be useful in more quickly identifying and treating the underlying pathology that is to blame for the symptoms that invariably present.

Symptoms within a cluster may or may not have the same origin, and symptoms must have stronger relationships within the same cluster than with symptoms in other clusters (Kim et al. 2005). There is still substantial debate concerning a universal working definition of symptom clusters. A lack of consensus on a symptom assessment tool and statistical methodology is a limitation in the extrapolation of findings and generalization of symptom clusters from various studies.

Cancer patients report experiencing multiple symptoms and these predict changes in patient function, treatment failures and post-therapeutic outcomes. They may have an adverse effect on patient outcomes and have synergistic effects as a predictor of patient morbidity. Adoption of objective measures of symptom presence and severity, administered by trained nurses or physicians, could eliminate problems associated with a subjective self-report questionnaire. It is important to recognize cancer symptoms as dynamic constructs, to understand the comprehensive character of the disease process, and potentially improve symptom assessment and management (Kirkova and Walsh 2007).

When the intent of radiation is palliation, the effect that it has on QOL and symptom distress should be considered. Further investigation is warranted to determine the validity of the clusters noted in these two studies. Investigation of symptom clusters in brain metastases should also take into account the steroid dose, given that symptoms such as loss of appetite, lethargy and breathlessness may be directly affected by steroid use.

Symptom clusters in advanced cancer may be specific to the type of cancer, treatment or a combination of both factors. Thus, assessment tools specifically designed and validated for a particular cancer population are preferred over a general questionnaire to ensure the extraction of symptom clusters that are relevant to the specific symptomatology of that cancer. Future research should focus on physiological mechanisms underlying the expression of symptom clusters specific to advanced cancer.

ETHICAL ISSUES

There are currently no ethical issues to be noted. Symptom cluster research focuses on exploring the extent and strength to which symptoms can occur together, and thus capturing how concurrent symptoms may negatively affect patients' QOL.

SUMMARY POINTS

- It is important to monitor how symptom clusters observed in a palliative cancer population change over time, to establish a definite relationship between symptoms within a cluster and to provide information on the effectiveness of management strategies commonly employed to treat or contain the cancer.
- Symptom clusters in advanced cancer may be specific to the type of cancer, treatment or a combination of both factors.
- Radiation-induced nausea/vomiting, which happens in one-third of patients, may impinge on patients' QOL due to problems such as electrolyte imbalances, dehydration, malnutrition, weight loss and weakness.
- Following RT for bone metastases, nausea and loss of appetite tended to cluster together during many of the follow-ups for bone metastases patients.
- Brain metastases patients who received palliative RT had the symptoms of nausea and vomiting consistently clustering together at each follow-up. These were just two of the 17 brain metastases-specific symptoms that consistently remained together, suggesting WBRT was not able to weaken the clusters and perhaps not able to improve QOL.

- Further investigations on the stability of symptom clusters over time would validate the concept of symptom clusters and improve QOL in palliative cancer populations by allowing co-management of various symptoms that form a cluster, and increase the therapeutic benefit for patients.

LIST OF ABBREVIATIONS

BPI	Brief Pain Inventory
ESAS	Edmonton Symptom Assessment System
MDASI	M.D. Anderson Symptom Inventory
PCA	Principle Component Analysis
QOL	Quality of Life
RINV	Radiation-induced nausea and vomiting
RT	Radiation therapy
SQLI	Spitzer Quality of Life Index
WBRT	Whole brain radiotherapy

REFERENCES

Barsevick, A. M., K. Whitmer, L. M. Nail, S. L. Beck, and W. N. Dudley. 2006. Symptom cluster research: Conceptual, design, measurement, and analysis issues. *Journal of Pain and Symptom Management* 31 (1): 85–95.

Beck, S. L., W. N. Dudley, and A. Brasevick. 2005. Pain, sleep disturbance, and fatigue in patients with cancer: Using a mediation model to test a symptom cluster. *Oncology Nursing Forum* 32 (3): 542.

Chow, E., L. Davis, L. Holden, M. Tsao, and C. Danjoux. 2005. Prospective assessment of patient-rated symptoms following whole brain radiotherapy for brain metastases. *Journal of Pain and Symptom Management* 30:18–23.

Chow, E., G. Fan, S. Hadi, and L. Filipczak. 2007. Symptom clusters in cancer patients with bone metastases. *Support Care Cancer* 15 (9): 1035–43.

Chow, E., G. Fan, S. Hadi, J. Wong, A. Kirou-Mauro, and L. Filipczak. 2008. Symptom clusters in cancer patients with brain metastases. *Journal of Clinical Oncology* 20:76–82.

Dodd, M. J., C. Miaskowski, and S. M. Paul. 2001. Symptom clusters and their effect on the functional status of patients with cancer. *Oncology Nursing Forum* 28:465–70.

Fan, G., S. Hadi, and E. Chow. 2007. Symptom clusters in patients with advanced-stage cancer referred for palliative radiation therapy in an outpatient setting. *Support Cancer Therapy* 4:157–62.

Feyer, P. C., E. Maranzano, A. Molassiotis, R. A. Clark-Snow, F. Roila, D. Warr, and I. Olver. 2005. Radiotherapy-induced nausea and vomiting (RINV): Antiemetic guidelines. *Support Care Cancer* 13:122–28.

Hird, A., J. Wong, L. Zhang, M. Tsao, E. Barnes, C. Danjoux, and E. Chow. 2009. Exploration of symptom clusters within cancer patients with brain metastases using the Spitzer Quality of Life Index. *Support Care Cancer* 18:335–42.

Kim, H. J., D. B. McGuire, L. Tulman, and A. M. Barsevick. 2005. Symptom clusters: Concept analysis and clinical implications for cancer nursing. *Cancer Nursing* 28:270–84.

Kirkova, J., and D. Walsh. 2007. Cancer symptom clusters-a dynamic construct. *Support Care Cancer* 15:1011–13.

Lagman, R. L., M. P. Davis, S. B. LeGrand, and D. Walsh. 2005. Common symptoms in advanced cancer. *Surgical Clinics of North America* 85 (2): 237–55.

Langer, C. J., and M. P. Mehta. 2005. Current management of brain metastases, with a focus on systemic options. *Journal of Clinical Oncology* 25:6207–19.

Miaskowski, C., M. Dodd, and K. Lee. 2004. Symptom clusters: The new frontier in symptom management research. *Journal of the National Cancer Institute Monographs* 32:17–21.

Stromgren, A. S., D. Goldschmidt, M. Groenvold, M. A. Petersen, P. T. Jensen, L. Pedersen, L. Hoermann, C. Helleberg, and P. Sjogren. 2002. Self-assessment in cancer patients referred to palliative care: A study of feasibility and symptom epidemiology. *Cancer* 94 (2): 512–17.

Tannock, I. F. 1987. Treating the patient, not just the cancer. *New England Journal of Medicine* 317:1534–35.

Tramer, M. R., D. J. M. Reynolds, N. S. Stoner, R. A. Moore, and H. J. McQuay. 1998. Efficacy of 5-HT3 receptor antagonists in radiotherapy-induced nausea and vomiting: A quantitative systematic review. *European Journal of Cancer* 34 (12): 1836–44.

Walsh, D., and L. Rybicki. 2006. Symptom clustering in advanced cancer. *Support Care Cancer* 14:831–36.

Wong, R. K. S., N. Paul, K. Ding, M. Whitehead, M. Brundage, A. Fyles, D. Wilke et al. 2006. 5-Hydroxytryptamine-3 Receptor Antagonist with or without short-course dexamethasone in the prophylaxis of radiation induced emesis: a placebo-controlled randomized trial of the national cancer institute of Canada clinical trials group (SC19). *American Society of Clinical Oncology* 24:3458–64.

28 Palliative Gastrojejunostomy and the Impact on Nutrition in Cancer

Poornima B. Rao and Jeffrey M. Farma

CONTENTS

28.1 INTRODUCTION

Gastric outlet obstruction (GOO) is typically manifested by the progressive inability to tolerate oral intake over the course of weeks to months. A patient will present with nausea and vomiting that becomes progressively more severe and ultimately results in a complete inability to tolerate anything by mouth.

28.1.1 Acute Presentation of GOO

The development of GOO or proximal gastrointestinal obstruction in a patient with a known background of advanced malignant disease portends a generally poor prognosis. Though reports in the literature have been variable, recent prospective observational studies report a median overall survival of approximately 64 days in patients who develop GOO secondary to unresected primary or metastatic cancer (Schmidt et al. 2009). Given the anticipated short duration of survival following the development of GOO, symptom relief and overall quality of life should be paramount in discussions of treatment options for patients. The performance status of the patient and their capacity to undergo interventional procedures and, as necessary, repeat interventions should be considered. Various palliative surgical techniques have been employed and studied over the past two decades (Nakakura and Warren 2007).

Occasionally, an acute clinical presentation may manifest. Patients present with severe dehydration as well as a hypochloremic, hypokalemic metabolic alkalosis related to chronic and refractory vomiting. The degree of malnutrition present is associated with the duration of obstructive symptoms and etiology of the obstruction. Because of the intimate anatomic associations within the upper gastrointestinal tract, an array of malignancies may cause the symptom complex that typifies GOO based on intrinsic or extrinsic (compressive) obstruction of the upper gastrointestinal tract. These include gastric cancer, gastrointestinal stromal tumors, and the spectrum of periampullary malignancies including pancreatic, ampullary, duodenal, and biliary cancers.

28.1.2 Clinical Presentation

The diagnosis of GOO is predominantly made clinically (Table 28.1). Patient history including concomitant symptoms such as weight loss, jaundice, abdominal pain, and steatorrhea may point to a specific etiology. Additional symptoms include eating restrictions and early satiety, dysphagia to solids and/or liquids, nausea and vomiting, and gastroesophageal reflux. Physical examination may point to a specific malignancy. Presence of a palpable abdominal mass and lymphadenopathy in the periumbilical or supraclavicular region may suggest locally advanced disease, as well as the presence of a gastric succussion splash, and tympani in the left upper quadrant indicative of gastric dilation and stasis of gastric contents.

28.1.3 Diagnostic Evaluation

Diagnostic evaluation should consist of a complete evaluation for intestinal obstruction. Initial imaging studies include a chest x-ray and abdominal films (Figure 28.1). The presence of a large gastric bubble or dilated stomach and the absence of small bowel dilation or pathologic air-fluid levels suggest more proximal obstruction. Occasionally pneumobilia may be detected, indicating duodenal obstruction distal to the ampulla of Vater. A measure of serum electrolytes, creatinine, complete blood count, and coagulation profile should be performed. Intravenous access should be established and intravenous hydration as well as electrolyte replacement should be promptly initiated. Nasogastric decompression and placement of a urinary bladder catheter will permit continual reassessment of fluid resuscitative efforts and determination of ongoing losses.

Ultimately cross-sectional imaging with computed tomography (CT) or magnetic resonance imaging (MRI) should be obtained to confirm the clinical diagnosis and will allow for a more

TABLE 28.1
Gastric Outlet Obstruction

Gastric Outlet Obstruction
Nausea
Vomiting
Abdominal pain
Weight loss
Inability to tolerate oral intake
Dehydration with hypochloremic, hypokalemic metabolic alkalosis
Vitamins A, C, D, E, K, and B12 deficiencies
Steatorrhea

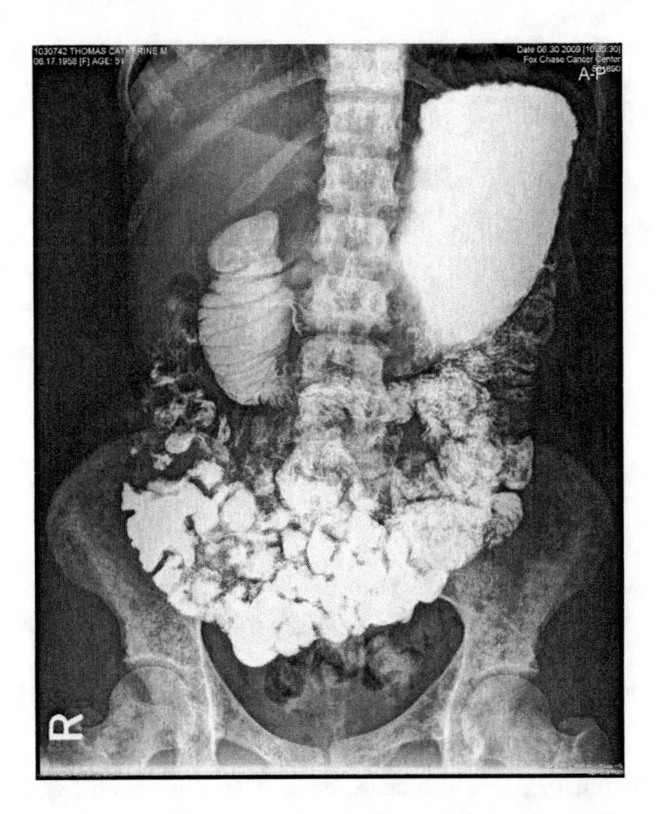

FIGURE 28.1 Upper GI series. UGI series demonstrating markedly distended stomach and proximal duodenum.

accurate determination of the presence of locally advanced or metastatic disease (Figure 28.2). Upper endoscopy will allow for direct intraluminal examination and determination of the presence of intrinsic versus extrinsic compression of the upper intestinal tract as well as the exact location of obstruction. In addition, tissue biopsy for pathological evaluation and ultimately diagnosis can be performed. Clinical context will determine the need for additional testing. A history of prior surgical intervention for upper gastrointestinal cancer, the known presence of recurrent or metastatic disease, or history of additional obstructive symptoms to suggest possibility of multilevel obstructive disease will necessitate additional diagnostic testing (Helton and Fisichella 2007).

28.2 NUTRITIONAL COMPLICATIONS OF GOO

28.2.1 Proximal GOO

Proximal gastrointestinal obstruction results in multiple unique nutritional sequelae. With isolated obstruction at the level of the pylorus, the normal physiologic function of gastric secretion of acid and intrinsic factor will be impaired. The effects of this can be seen with decreased absorption of dietary iron and vitamin C from within the proximal small bowel. In addition, limited intrinsic factor leads to decreased absorption of vitamin B12 (cobalamin) from the terminal ileum downstream, which can lead to fatigue and anemia.

28.2.2 Duodenal and Biliary Obstruction

More distal duodenal obstruction can affect bile salt homeostasis. Though enterohepatic circulation of bile acids may be unaffected by duodenal obstruction, secretion often is, leading

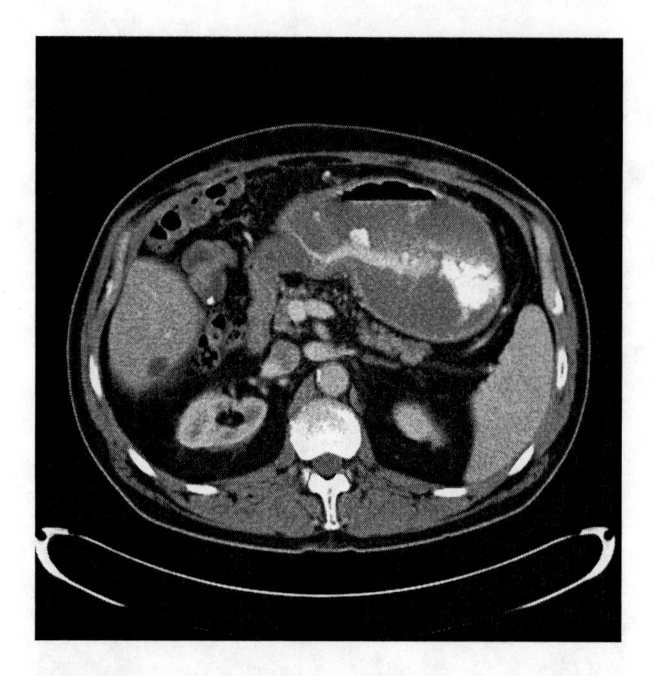

FIGURE 28.2 Gastric outlet obstruction. Computed tomography demonstrated dilated stomach with a narrowed duodenum due to progressive extrahepatic cholangiocarcinoma.

to obstruction of the biliary tree and bile secretion. The result is obstructive jaundice, which has implications for the absorption of dietary fats as well as fat-soluble vitamins. Bile salts are secreted into the duodenum in response to the presence of luminal fatty acids. Once luminal lipolysis has occurred, free long-chain and medium-chain fatty acids and fat-soluble vitamins (vitamin A, E, D, and K) are solubilized by bile salts through the formation of micelles. The absence of bile salt secretion into the intestinal tract compromises this process, leading to fat-soluble vitamin deficiencies as well as fatty acid malabsorption, which results in the collateral effect of secretory diarrhea.

28.2.3 Pancreatic Duct Obstruction

Similarly, isolated pancreatic duct obstruction can lead to a symptom complex of pancreatic insufficiency. The pancreas produces and secretes enzymes essential for the digestion and absorption of carbohydrates, proteins, and fats. Though initiated with exposure to salivary amylase, carbohydrate digestion is propagated through exposure to pancreatic amylase. Pancreatic amylase converts complex carbohydrates into small oligosaccharides, which are presented to the intestinal brush border where the completion of digestion by way of specific disaccharidases occurs. This is followed by both active and passive absorption of the monosaccharide moieties, which are then used for nutrition.

Protein hydrolysis is initiated with mechanical dispersion in the oral cavity and gastric pepsin digestion in the stomach. Within the duodenum, endopeptidases produced by the pancreas hydrolyze bonds within polypeptide chains to permit the generation of oligopeptides. These may be further hydrolyzed into smaller di- or tri-peptides at the intestinal brush border, and then absorbed and utilized for nutrition. Fat absorption requires pancreatic lipase activity to generate free fatty acids from triglyceride moieties, which may then be solubilized and absorbed. Disruption in pancreatic function as a result of ductal obstruction can result in exocrine insufficiency with the consequence of malnutrition related to the inability to appropriately digest and absorb carbohydrates, proteins, and fats.

28.2.4 Nutritional Deficiencies

The obvious nutritional issue as related to gastric outlet and proximal duodenal obstruction is inadequate caloric intake and absorption. More subtle, however, is the progressive development of specific vitamin and mineral deficiencies. Patients with proximal duodenal obstruction often exhibit a profound deficiency in vitamin K that evolves with the progression of biliary obstruction. A significant coagulopathy results from inability to absorb vitamin K due to lack of bile salts within the intestinal lumen. Therefore, the ability to synthesize factors essential to both arms of the coagulation cascade is compromised. Recognition and treatment of this deficiency is essential prior to the performance of any invasive diagnostic or therapeutic procedures (Vander, Sherman, and Luciano 1990).

28.3 SURGICAL TECHNIQUES

Patients with periampullary malignancies are often found to have unresectable disease at the time of diagnosis. Bypass of the area of obstruction is the mainstay of therapy for GOO for the palliation of symptoms. This strategy may employ a combination of percutaneous, endoscopic, and surgical techniques based on the clinical constellation of symptoms.

28.3.1 Gastrojejunostomy

Gastrojejunostomy remains the gold standard for palliation of symptoms of GOO; however, there has been a rapid evolution of bypass technique. Surgical bypass has been traditionally performed through an open technique (Figure 28.3). The precise technique of a surgical gastrojejunostomy has been described with permutations designed to minimize long-term complications associated with the procedure.

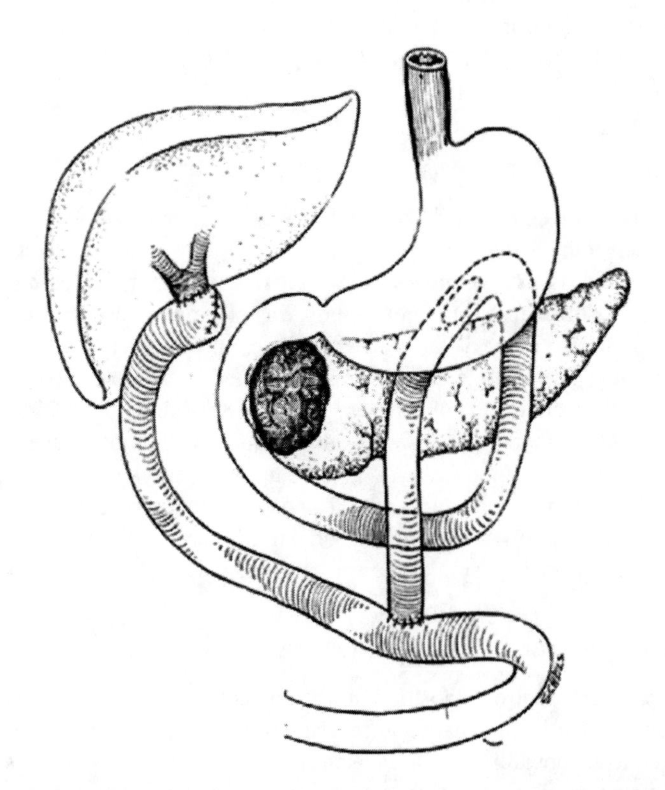

FIGURE 28.3 Schematic of combined gastrojejunostomy and hepaticojejunostomy. (From Scott, N., Garcea, G., Doucas, H. et al., *HPB (Oxford)*, 11, 118, 2009, with permission from Hindawi.)

The results of surgical palliation for GOO are well defined in the literature. The results of a retrospective review reported from the Hopkins group have been validated by other centers in prospective studies. In high-volume centers, surgical biliary and gastric bypass for palliation of symptoms can be accomplished with low operative mortality—typically reported at less than 5%—and with an acceptable morbidity rate of less than 25%. In addition, palliative surgical procedures resulted in improved median survival of 6+ months, compared with the generally accepted dismal prognosis of those who are not palliated (Sohn et al. 1999).

Loop anterior gastrojejunostomy creates an anastomosis between the stomach proximal to the area of obstruction and the antimesenteric aspect of the jejunum 15–25 cm distal to the ligament of Treitz, and thus distal to the level of obstruction. A two-layer hand-sewn side-to-side anastomosis is typically configured to create a luminal diameter of 5–7 cm in length. Described variations of this procedure include retrocolic retrogastric posterior loop gastrojejunostomy, antecolic retrogastric posterior loop gastrojejunostomy, and antecolic antegastric anterior loop gastrojejunostomy. However there is no consensus or data related to outcomes using these different techniques. More recent descriptions detail the use of surgical stapling devices for creation of the anastomosis, as well as using minimally invasive laparoscopic techniques. The bypass procedure does not require functional bowel division. The procedure is well suited for isolated GOO where the biliary and pancreatic duct systems remain patent.

28.3.2 Risks Associated with Gastrojejunostomy

As with any surgical procedure, there are the risks of bleeding, infection, and anastomotic leak. More specific to the gastrojejunostomy procedure are rates of delayed gastric emptying varying with technique and ranging from 2%–31% (Doberneck and Berndt 1987). There is frequent biliopancreatic drainage into the stomach, leading to the possibility of bile reflux-induced gastritis. In addition, because of the direct transit of acidic gastric contents into the more distal and less buffered small bowel, anastomotic ulceration (a marginal ulcer) and bleeding within the efferent jejunal limb can occur (Lillemoe 1998).

28.3.3 Partial Stomach-Partitioning Gastrojejunostomy

Several techniques have evolved in an effort to minimize the anatomic and physiologic consequences of the loop gastrojejunostomy and to limit postoperative symptoms related to the procedure, while at the same time avoiding the risks of a more radical operative resection in the setting of palliative treatment. Partial stomach-partitioning gastrojejunostomy was originally described in Asian series. The technique adds partial division of the distal stomach while maintaining a tunnel of 2–3 cm in diameter along the lesser curvature. The gastrojejunostomy is performed to the stomach that is proximal to the partial transaction (Kaminishi et al. 1997; Arciero et al. 2006; Kubota et al. 2007). The theoretical advantage of the procedure is that it permits preferential emptying of gastric contents through the gastrojejunostomy, thereby minimizing the rate of delayed gastric emptying. This also allows for endoscopic access to the distal stomach and duodenum for potential endoscopic therapeutic maneuvers. In addition, the constant irritation of enteric contents on a tumor mass with the resultant ulceration and bleeding may be minimized by diversion of the enteral stream (Kwon and Lee 2004).

28.3.4 Role of Prophylactic Gastrojejunostomy

The concept of prophylactic gastrojejunostomy in the context of upper gastrointestinal malignancy has been the subject of significant debate and investigation. Initial reports suggested patients with unresectable pancreatic adenocarcinoma, as determined by laparoscopic staging, seldom developed gastroduodenal obstruction that required therapeutic intervention. The rate of obstruction was determined to be less than 20% and as a result, the performance of a laparotomy for creation of a gastrojejunal bypass with the risks associated with both in the context of unresectable cancer was determined to be too great (Espat, Brennan, and Conlon 1999). A recent prospective randomized multicenter trial reports that the performance of a prophylactic gastrojejunostomy in the setting of locally advanced periampullary malignancy provided better surgical palliation and significantly decreased the incidence of GOO in patients (Lillemoe et al.1999). Moreover, additional studies have substantiated the fact that in most cases performance of a prophylactic gastrojejunostomy can be performed without any increase in mortality or morbidity (Van Heek et al. 2003).

Of the patients whose biliary obstruction is treated with surgical bypass, approximately 20%–30% will go on to develop GOO as a result of either local tumor growth or the development of progressive metastatic disease if a gastric bypass is not performed concomitantly (Sohn et al. 1999; Shyr et al. 2000). The recommendation to perform a prophylactic gastrojejunostomy for patients with unresectable upper gastrointestinal malignancy is largely based on reports of several surgical series which suggest that the addition of a gastric bypass to a biliary bypass can be performed without significant impact on overall mortality, morbidity rates, or post-operative length of stay. This finding was validated in a prospective randomized multicenter trial in the Netherlands, providing the basis for the recommendation that in the presence of unresectable periampullary cancer, a gastric bypass should be performed without regard to the presence of obstructive symptoms at the time of presentation (Van Heek et al. 2003).

28.4 BILIARY OBSTRUCTION

Patients with disease known to be unresectable at the time of presentation and whose symptoms are related to biliary obstruction alone are often treated with endoscopic or percutaneous biliary decompressive procedures. Numerous studies have examined the efficacy of nonsurgical approaches to biliary obstruction in comparison to surgical palliative procedures both prospectively and retrospectively. The main advantage of stenting procedures is the ability to use an endoscopic or percutaneous approach with minimal impact to the patient. However, several problems may arise as a result of stent placement with respect to palliation of symptoms. Often, patients are subjected to repeat interventions to maintain stent patency and position, which when compromised can lead to repeat hospitalizations to manage stent-related complications and infections. In a recent retrospective review in the United Kingdom, patients with pancreatic ductal adenocarcinoma who underwent endoscopic stenting of their biliary obstruction were compared to patients who underwent surgical palliation via a double bypass procedure (gastrojejunostomy and hepaticojejunostomy). Though the incidence of procedure-related mortality and morbidity was not significantly different in well-matched groups, their data indicated that the number of readmissions and total length of hospital stay following palliation were significantly greater for patients undergoing endoscopic stenting in comparison to surgical bypass. In addition, the overall survival of patients undergoing surgical bypass was significantly greater than the survival of those undergoing stenting procedures (382 versus 135 days) (Scott et al. 2009). The ultimate conclusion of this and several corroborating studies is that surgical palliation does offer advantages over endoscopic approaches to biliary obstruction. The advantages include a reduction in need for maintenance interventional procedures as well as fewer hospital readmissions following the performance of surgical palliation. In addition, both gastric outlet and biliary obstruction can be addressed at the same operation. The recommendation of surgical bypass needs to be made in the context of patient-associated factors, which include anticipated survival (>6 months), adequate performance status, and patient suitability to tolerate general anesthesia with its associated risks.

28.5 MINIMALLY INVASIVE SURGICAL TECHNIQUES

A more recent advancement in surgical palliation of upper gastrointestinal obstruction has been the utilization of laparoscopic techniques for unresectable advanced upper gastrointestinal malignant disease. The comparison of open versus laparoscopic surgical approaches to palliative gastrojejunostomy has not yet been the subject of randomized controlled analysis, though numerous case-control retrospective analyses have been reported. Recent reports indicate that in expert hands a laparoscopic gastrojejunostomy may be performed without significant difference in mean surgery time, operative blood loss, post-operative length of stay, median time to tolerate a regular diet, and median survival in comparison to an open surgical approach, and may afford the patient early decreased postoperative pain (Guzman et al. 2009; Bergamaschi et al. 1998; Navarra et al. 2006).

28.6 NON-SURGICAL OPTIONS

The most recent development in palliative therapy for GOO has been the employment of self-expanding metal (SEMS) intraluminal stent technology. Comparison between surgical gastrojejunostomy and endoscopic stenting has been the subject of intense review. The techniques have been compared head to head in randomized trials, however patient numbers in all reported series have been small. The general consensus regarding use of stents in the palliation of gastroduodenal obstruction is that endoluminal stenting may be employed with more favorable results in patients with a relatively short life expectancy—those in whom an open or laparoscopic surgical procedure with gastrointestinal anastomosis would be considered too high risk. Patients in whom disease biology and clinical performance would predict a more prolonged life expectancy should be preferentially palliated with a surgical gastrojejunostomy (Jeurnink, van Eijck et al. 2007; Nieveen van Dijkum et al. 2003).

The use of endoluminal stenting procedures to treat malignant GOO is an additional alternative. Endoscopic stenting of obstructive malignant lesions has been the subject of intense analysis including several small randomized clinical trials. An excellent meta-analysis in the Netherlands points out the utility of endoluminal stenting in the palliation of GOO in malignant disease. The findings and recommendations based on 36 case series, 6 case-controlled studies, and 2 randomized clinical trials found little difference between the technical success rate, development of early and late major complications, and symptom control between surgical palliation and endoluminal stenting for palliation of GOO. The endoluminal approach gained an advantage over surgical palliation in initial clinical success rates, the development of minor complications, and shorter length of hospital stay associated with the procedure; however, the recurrence of obstructive symptoms in patients who underwent endoluminal stenting procedures was significantly higher than in those who were palliated with a surgical gastrojejunostomy (Mittal et al. 2004). Overall, mean and symptom-free survival were greater in patients who underwent surgical gastrojejunostomy in comparison to endoluminal placement. The conclusion of the analysis, therefore, is largely based on appropriate application of the approaches to the given patient: Patients with relatively short life expectancy based on disease biology and presentation, poor performance status, and inability to tolerate a major operative procedure may be better suited for endoluminal stenting procedures for palliation, while those with longer life expectancy and better performance status may be best served with a surgical bypass procedure for palliation (Jeurnink, Steyerberg et al. 2007).

Successful palliation of GOO is often reported as restoration of the ability to tolerate oral intake. However, few studies have examined the effect of various interventional procedures on the quality of life in patients with malignant gastrointestinal obstruction by validated instruments. A recent prospective observational study performed at the Memorial Sloan-Kettering Cancer Center examined the effect of endoscopic stenting, surgical bypass, or percutaneous decompressive procedures on quality of life outcomes for patients undergoing palliative treatment of malignant GOO. Two specific instruments were employed to evaluate patient quality of life at baseline, one month and three months after intervention: the European Organization for Research and Treatment of Cancer (EORTC) QLQ-C30 and QLQ-ST022. One quality of life assessment tool has been validated to assess functional, physical, social, and emotional domains. The second is a more specific tool related to quality of life issues specific to gastric cancer including dysphagia, pain, reflux, and eating restriction. Though the study

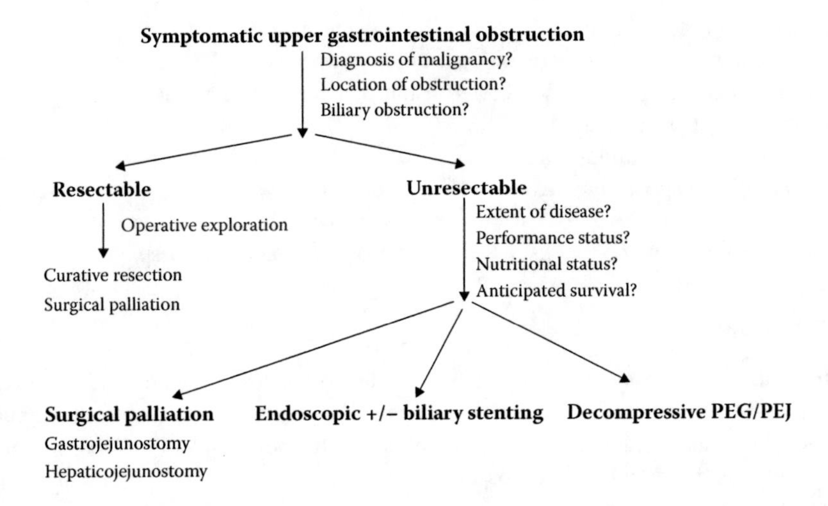

FIGURE 28.4 Decision pathway for evaluation and treatment of gastric outlet obstruction.

size was small, with only 10 of the 50 total patients completing all quality of life surveys, patients undergoing endoscopic stent placement or surgical bypass for palliation of GOO did experience significant improvements in their global health status as well as in symptoms of nausea and vomiting when compared to percutaneous decompressive procedures. There was a significant impairment in physical functioning, as expected, one month after surgical bypass, though all other cancer-related symptoms were unaltered by the interventions. Both endoscopic stent placement and surgical bypass were associated with significant improvements in dysphagia and eating restrictions, relative to decompressive percutaneous procedures. The conclusions reached by the study, again, emphasize the impact of appropriate patient selection for given palliative procedures: Surgical bypass in patients with longer life expectancy, higher performance status, and slower disease progression, while less invasive approaches should be judiciously employed in patients with poor performance status, shorter life expectancy, and more rapidly progressive disease. Highlighted in this analysis is the importance of the recommendation of the physician caring for the patient in determining which line of care a patient will choose to pursue (Schmidt et al. 2009).

28.7 GUIDELINES

On initial presentation of patients with GOO, the mainstay of treatment includes palliation of symptoms, hydration, correction of electrolyte abnormalities, and pain control. Our clinical pathway is demonstrated in Figure 28.4. We utilize endoscopy, radiographic imaging, and biopsy techniques to determine the extent of malignancy, the potential for resection, and the level of gastrointestinal obstruction. If palliation of unresectable malignancy is the mainstay of care we determine the best treatment strategy by evaluating extent of disease, nutritional status, performance status, underlying malignancy, and anticipated survival. Based on all these criteria, and most importantly the patients' and families' specific palliative goals, we then proceed with surgical, endoscopic, or percutaneous treatment options.

ETHICAL ISSUES

As with all interventions, the risks and benefits of the procedure must be fully discussed with the patients and their families. A multidisciplinary approach to these difficult situations helps to facilitate open discussions about reasonable goals of treatment. These treatments need to be individualized to the patient's desires and all the goals of palliation should be discussed and explored to determine the best course of action. If a patient can tolerate surgical intervention, we feel the results may afford the best opportunity to improve their quality of life. This determination is subjective and is based on experience, nutritional reserve, performance status, and estimated life expectancy, all in an attempt to predict operative outcomes.

More concerning ethical dilemmas occur in patients who clinically appear unable to tolerate operative intervention, especially when they have already received palliation with alternative measures. In these patients, a frank discussion needs to proceed balancing the risks and benefits of decompressive gastrostomy and the discussion of end-of-life issues and hospice.

SUMMARY POINTS

- Gastric outlet and biliary obstruction can arise due to upper gastrointestinal malignancies.
- Presentation includes severe nausea, vomiting, dehydration, and abdominal pain with nutritional sequelae related to dehydration, vitamin deficiencies, and malabsorption.
- Treatment must be individualized based on patients' desires and symptoms, performance status, and life expectancy.
- Surgical bypass offers the best option of improved long-term palliation of symptoms in patients who are able to undergo this intervention.
- Newer techniques of gastrojejunostomy and minimally invasive strategies may improve outcomes for surgical palliation.

LIST OF ABBREVIATIONS

CT	Computed tomography
GOO	Gastric outlet obstruction
MRI	Magnetic resonance imaging
NG	Nasogastric tube
PEG	Percutaneous endoscopic gastrostomy
PEJ	Percutaneous endoscopic jejunostomy
SEMS	Self-expanding metal stent

REFERENCES

Arciero, C. A., N. Joseph, J. C. Watson, and J. P. Hoffman. 2006. Partial stomach-partitioning gastrojejunostomy for malignant duodenal obstruction. *The American Journal of Surgery* 191:428–32.

Bergamaschi, R., R. Marvik, J. E. Thorensen, B. Ystgaard, G. Johnsen, and H. E. Myrvold. 1998. Open versus laparoscopic gastrojejunostomy for palliation in advanced pancreatic cancer. *Surgery, Laparoscopy, and Endoscopy* 8 (2): 92–96.

Doberneck, R. C., and G. A. Berndt. 1987. Delayed gastric emptying after palliative gastrojejunostomy for carcinoma of the pancreas. *Archives of Surgery* 122:827–29.

Espat, N. J., M. F. Brennan, and K. C. Conlon. 1999. Patients with laparoscopically staged unresectable pancreatic adenocarcinoma do not require subsequent surgical biliary or gastric bypass. *Journal of the American College of Surgeons* 188:649–55; Discussion 655–57.

Guzman, E. A., A. Dagis, L. Bening, and A. Pigazzi. 2009. Laparoscopic gastrojejunostomy in patients with obstruction of the gastric outlet secondary to advanced malignancies. *American Surgeon* 75:129–32.

Helton, W. S., and P. M. Fisichella. 2007. Intestinal obstruction In *ACS surgery principles and practice*, 6th edn., eds. W. -W. Souba, M. P. Fink, G. J. Jurkovich et al., 514–33. New York: WebMD Professional Publishing.

Jeurnink, S. M., C. H. J. van Eijck, E. W. Steyerberg, E. J. Kuipers, and P. D. Siersema. 2007. Stent versus gastrojejunostomy for palliation of gastric outlet obstruction: A systematic review. *BMC Gastroenterology* 7:18.

Jeurnink, S. M., E. W. Steyerberg, G. Van'T Hof, C. H. van Eijck, E. J. Kuipers, and P. D. Siersema. 2007. Gastrojejunostomy versus stent placement in patients with malignant gastric outlet obstruction: A comparison in 95 patients. *Journal of Surgical Oncology* 96:389–96.

Kaminishi, M., H. Yamaguchi, N. Shimizu, S. Nomura, A. Yoshikawa, M. Hashimota, S. Sakai, and T. Oohara. 1997. Stomach-partitioning gastrojejunostomy for unresectable gastric carcinoma. *Archives of Surgery* 132:184–87.

Kubota, K., J. Kuroda, N. Origuchi, M. Kaminishi, H. Isayama, T. Kawabe, M. Omata and K. Mafune. 2007. Stomach-partitioning gastrojejunostomy for gastroduodenal outlet obstruction. *Archives of Surgery* 142:607–11.

Kwon, J. J., and H. G. Lee. 2004. Gastric partitioning gastrojejunostomy in unresectable distal gastric cancer patients. *World Journal of Surgery* 28:365–68.

Lillemoe, K. D. 1998. Palliative therapy for pancreatic cancer. *Surgical Oncology Clinics of North America* 7:199–216.

Lillemoe, K. D., J. L. Cameron, J. M. Hardacre, T. A. Sohn, P. K. Sauter, J. Coleman et al. 1999. Is prophylactic gastrojejunostomy indicated for unresectable periampullary cancer? A prospective randomized trial. *Annals of Surgery* 230:322–28; Discussion 328–33.

Mittal, A., J. Windsor, J. Woodfield, P. Casey, and M. Lane. 2004. Matched study of three methods for palliation of malignant pyloroduodenal obstruction. *British Journal of Surgery* 91:205–9.

Nakakura, E. K., and R. S. Warren. 2007. Palliative care for patients with advanced pancreatic and biliary cancers. *Surgical Oncology* 16:293–97.

Navarra, G., C. Musolino, A. Venneri, M. L. De Marco, and M. Bartolotta. 2006. Palliative antecolic isoperistaltic gastrojejunostomy: A randomized controlled trial comparing open and laparoscopic approaches. *Surgical Endoscopy* 20:1831–34.

Nieveen van Dijkum, E. J., M. G. Romijn, C. B. Terwee, L. T. de Wit, J. H. van der Meulen, H. S. Lameris, E. A. J. Rauws et al. 2003. Laparoscopic staging and subsequent palliation in patients with peripancreatic carcinoma. *Annals of Surgery* 237:66–73.

Scott, E. N., G. Garcea, H. Doucas, W. P. Steward, A. R. Dennison, and D. P. Berry. 2009. Surgical bypass vs. endoscopic stenting for pancreatic ductal adenocarcinoma. *HPB (Oxford)* 11:118–24.

Schmidt, C., H. Gerdes, W. Hawkins, E. Zucker, Q. Zhou, E. Riedel, D. Jaques et al. 2009. A prospective observational study examining quality of life in patients with malignant gastric outlet obstruction. *The American Journal of Surgery* 198:92–99.

Shyr, Y., C. Su, C. Wu, and W. Lui. 2000. Prospective study of gastric outlet obstruction in unresectable pancreatic adenocarcinoma. *World Journal of Surgery* 24:60–65.

Sohn, T. A., K. D. Lillemoe, J. L. Cameron, J. J. Huang, H. A. Pitt, and C. J. Yeo. 1999. Surgical palliation of unresectable periampullary adenocarcinoma in the 1990s. *Journal of the American College of Surgeons* 188 (6): 658–66.

Vander, A. J., J. H. Sherman, and D. S. Luciano. 1990. *Human physiology*, 5th edn. New York: McGraw-Hill Publishing Company.

Van Heek, N. T., S. M. M. De Castro, C. H. van Eijck, R. C. van Geenen, E. J. Hesselink, P. J. Breslau, T. C. Tran, G. Kazemier, M. R. Visser, O. R. Busch, H. Obertop, and D. J. Gouma. 2003. The need for a prophylactic gastrojejunostomy for unresectable periampullary cancer: A prospective randomized trial with special focus on assessment of quality of life. *Annals of Surgery* 238:894–902; Discussion 902–5.

Section V

Other Conditions

29 Nutritional Support in the Vegetative State: Artificial Nutrition and Hydration in the Limbo between Life and Death

Marco Luchetti and Giuseppe Nattino

CONTENTS

29.1 INTRODUCTION

29.1.1 THE VEGETATIVE STATE

First described by Jennett and Plum (1972), the vegetative state is a clinical setting essentially characterized by vigilance in the absence of consciousness. The criteria for its definition are summarized in Table 29.1.

The vegetative state may be transitory, but it is often protracted. Before pronouncing an adult subject to be in a permanent vegetative state (PVS), at least 3 or up to 12 months must pass, depending on whether the initial insult was traumatic or not, respectively.

TABLE 29.1
Criteria for the Definition of Vegetative State

1. No sign of awareness of self or of surroundings; no capacity of interpersonal interaction
2. Absence of reproducible behavioral response, whether targeted or voluntary, to visual, auditory, tactile, or pain stimuli
3. No understanding of verbal clues
4. Intermittent cycle of periods of wakefulness that alternate with periods of sleep
5. Sufficient conservation of hypothalamus and encephalic brainstem function to allow survival with minimal medical and nursing care
6. Fecal and urinary incontinence
7. At least partial conservation of cranial reflexes

Source: From Multi-Society Task Force on PVS, *N. Engl. J. Med.*, 330, 1499, 1994a.

Assessing PVS remains fraught with problems. The main problem consists in pronouncing the vegetative state permanent, i.e., the formulation of a prognosis. In the document of the Multi-Society Task Force on Medical Aspects of the Persistent Vegetative State published in 1994 (Multi-Society Task Force on PVS 1994b), criteria allowing the recognition of irreversibility with a high degree of clinical certainty were proposed. Although such criteria are precise, the prognostic judgment on the vegetative state is not absolute because it is based on probability. Even more difficult is the prognosis for the so-called minimally conscious state (MCS), which involves the clinical context experienced by some vegetative patients who show signs of a renewed contact with their surroundings. The diagnoses of these consciousness disorders must be predicated on a correct work-up, i.e., allowing prolonged observation with periodic, structured assessments able to document possible clues of environmental contacting which may be initially vague and erratic.

Today a technology race is being run, with increasing in-depth complexity, in the hope of finding the unequivocal answers we do not currently possess. The modern techniques of brain imaging are fascinating and will provide new insights into the cerebral functions of patients in a PVS (Laureys 2004; Schiff 2006), but, however far techniques may progress, technology itself is a source of uncertainty. Similarly to the Achilles and the tortoise paradox, however fast Achilles (technology) may run, the tortoise (the intrinsic uncertainty of the decision process) will always be a short step ahead. Whilst recognizing the probabilistic character of prognosis, we cannot avoid making one or shun responsibility for decisions on the basis of such a prognosis, if necessary.

29.1.2 Nutrition in PVS Patients

In PVS patients, artificial nutrition and hydration (ANH) is always initiated prior to diagnosis, in the first few days following the primary brain insult. It is in this phase that all vital support maneuvers (ANH included), necessary for the organism to overcome the injury and to initiate recovery, are implemented. However, when all fails and the patient's condition stabilizes into PVS, the meaning of ANH changes completely, from being a temporary support measure with a view toward recovery to implying a chronic condition due to the subject's incapacitation to feed him/herself own (Bernat 2006).

The PVS patient, with regard to nutrition and hydration needs, is completely dependent on the care provided by healthcare personnel or family members. In order to maintain adequate nutritional status, all the nutrients must be administered artificially.

Many factors contribute to the survival of PVS patients, but nutritional status is one of the most important. Solid evidence from the scientific literature indicates that PVS patients should be nourished by enteral routes, reserving parenteral nutrition for those rare cases in which the gastrointestinal tract is not viable (Finch 2005; Casarett, Kapo, and Caplan 2005).

Table 29.2 summarizes the key features of the ideal nutritional approach in PVS patients.

TABLE 29.2
Key Features of the Ideal Nutritional Approach in PVS Patients

1. Ability to be maintained for long time
2. Possibility to be managed also in out-of-hospital settings and by individuals with limited healthcare knowledge and skills
3. Ability to meet nutritional needs, respecting the physiology of the digestive system
4. Low incidence of complications
5. Low costs

PVS patients in the community having enteral tube feeding should be supported by a coordinated multidisciplinary team, which includes dietitians, nurses, general practitioners, pharmacists, and other healthcare professionals as appropriate.

29.2 APPLICATIONS TO OTHER AREAS OF TERMINAL OR PALLIATIVE CARE

Though the clinical condition of PVS is peculiar and poses unique ethical problems, the principles of long-term enteral tube feeding that apply to PVS patients are applicable also to several other conditions. In general, enteral tube feeding should be considered in people who are malnourished or at risk of malnutrition and have inadequate or unsafe oral intake and a functional, accessible gastrointestinal tract. Long-term enteral tube feeding is indicated in patients with consciousness disorders (head injury), swallowing disorders (multiple sclerosis, motor neuron disease, Parkinson's disease), anorexia (cancer, liver disease, HIV), upper gastrointestinal obstruction (oropharyngeal or esophageal stricture or tumor), psychological problems (severe depression, anorexia nervosa), and dementia.

29.3 PRACTICAL METHODS AND TECHNIQUES

29.3.1 Energy Expenditure

The individual energy expenditure (EE) is comprised of three main components.

- *Basal metabolic rate (BMR):* the body's EE at rest, without stress and at neutral temperature. In such conditions, about 20% of the EE is due to cerebral metabolism. PVS patients show a decrease of glucose cerebral consumption by 50–60% (Rombeau and Caldwell 1990).
- *Physical activity:* in the PVS patient this is usually negligible with the exception of cases in which diffuse or segmental hypertonus occurs.
- *Specific dynamic action of aliments:* the energy needed to digest, absorb, and process the nutrients introduced with alimentation, which accounts for about 4–5% of the expenditure.

The EE can be measured, for study purposes, by means of indirect calorimetry or, estimated, in daily clinical practice, by means of equations based on parameters such as weight, height, gender, and age. The most commonly used equations are those of Harris-Benedict, of Schofield, and of the World Health Organization (WHO).

EE changes occur when the subject experiences diseases, trauma, and infections, which induce a metabolic stress reaction and, in turn, an increase of energy consumption (Cook, Peppard, and Magnuson 2008). Sedation, myoresolution, fasting, and malnutrition are all conditions that, on the contrary, cause a decrease of the EE.

Many authors have conducted studies in which correction factors are suggested to obtain the EE value starting from the BMR. A set of such correction factors is reported in Table 29.3. The vast majority of clinical studies have been performed on acute patients, so the evidence on the nutritional needs of stable chronic patients is very sparse.

TABLE 29.3
Correction Factors for BEE Calculation

Condition	Correction Factor
Elective surgery	1.10
Complicated surgery	1.25
Trauma	1.2–1.5
Head trauma	1.4
Sepsis	1.5
Severe burn	1.8

Of great interest is a very recent study (McEvoy et al. 2009) showing how, in severe head trauma patients, spontaneously breathing and without sedation, the BMR calculated with either Harris Benedict's or WHO's equations corresponds to the measured value ±10% only in, respectively, 45% and 50% of the cases.

In consideration of these data, it seems advisable, in clinical practice, to initially apply the calculated EE and then proceed by tailoring the intake on the basis of measured body weight, every 10–15 days in the initial recovery phase and every 30 days when the condition is stable.

It is prudent, however, to use closer body-weight monitoring whenever infections or neurovegetative disorders occur.

29.3.2 Nutritional Requirements in PVS Patients

Most enteral feeds come as ready-to-use liquid microbial-free preparations that contain energy, proteins, vitamins, minerals, trace elements, and fluid +/– fiber. A ready-to-use standard feed will usually contain 1 kcal and 0.04 g protein per ml but many other types of enteral feed preparations are available with differing energy, protein ratios, and types of fat or protein.

Immobility leads the patients that survive longer in PVS to a slow but constant wasting of their muscle mass. These patients, in order to maintain their weight, need a progressively lower energy intake. It is not rare to see PVS patients, particularly those with slender body size, who are able to maintain their body weight with an intake of less than 1500 or even 1000 kcal per day. In these cases, since the composition of enteral nutrition (EN) products is set, in order to guarantee a protein intake of 1 g/kg and cover the minimum intake of minerals, micronutrients, and vitamins, it is necessary to give dietary supplements.

The restriction of energy intake may lead to inadequate fluid intake and hence dehydration. The monitoring of daily urine output and its concentration is the most useful guide to adjust the fluid intake to the needs of each single PVS patient. Repeated administration of 100 ml water boluses during the day is able to match the output with the intake, and has the additional advantage of diluting dietary supplements and washing the enteral tube, thus averting the formation of incrustations that may lead to its obstruction and the need to change it.

Patients on long-term EN should be warranted an adequate alimentary fiber intake (25–30 g or 0.5 g/kg per day according to the American Dietetic Association), particularly those who are at high risk of constipation due to immobility or low water intake. For this purpose, the choice of diet should favor products enriched with alimentary fibers or, alternatively, the addition of a dietary supplement should be considered.

29.3.3 Enteral Feeding Routes and Techniques

The gastrostomy tube is the most commonly used route to administer EN to PVS patients. Its placement is generally achieved by means of a percutaneous endoscopic technique (percutaneous endoscopic gastrostomy (PEG)), reserving the surgical technique only for cases where PEG is not feasible.

Jejunostomy, either surgical or percutaneous endoscopic (percutaneous endoscopic jejunostomy (PEJ)), is a viable alternative to gastrostomy in patients with gastroesophageal reflux, and hence at high risk of pulmonary complications due to inhalation, or in those cases where a gastrostomy is not feasible.

Particular gastrostomy tubes are commercially available which have an internal portion long enough to permit the placement of the tip beyond the pylorus, thus allowing the nutrition to be administered in the duodenum or the jejunum.

Naso-gastric and naso-jejunal tubes are indicated only for short-term treatment and in hospitalized patients, since frequent repositioning is needed due to accidental removal, dislocation, and occlusion.

In patients on long-term EN, the administration is usually intermittent, often night-time, so as to leave the day hours for physiotherapy, nursing maneuvers, mobilization, etc. Twenty-four-hour administration is reserved for those patients who cannot tolerate the night-time infusion regimen and need a slow rate of infusion in order to avoid the risk of regurgitation and inhalation. In planning the modality, timing, and rate of EN administration, the need for drug therapies must also be taken into account: e.g., phenytoin must be administered at least 2 hours after EN suspension and at least 2 hours before its start.

Comorbidities may also have an impact on nutritional regimen planning: e.g., diabetic patients may show large changes in blood glucose levels when an intermittent regimen is used.

29.3.4 Complications and Their Prevention

Those who take care of PVS patients having enteral tube feeding should receive training and information on the management of feeding enterostomies, delivery systems, and the regimen, outlining all procedures related to setting up feeds, using feed pumps, the likely risks, and methods for troubleshooting common problems, and be provided with an instruction manual.

Routine and emergency telephone numbers should be provided to contact a healthcare professional who is familiar with the needs and potential problems of people on home enteral tube feeding. The main side effects and complications of enteral tube feeding are described here.

29.3.4.1 Constipation, Impaired Gastrointestinal Motility, and Diarrhea

Immobility, inadequate fluid intake, and lack of dietary fiber are the most frequent factors leading to constipation. If an increase in fluid and fiber intake does not solve the problem, the administration of lactulose and/or the regular use of glycerol enemas may be needed. If patients with impaired gastrointestinal motility are fed enterally, they may develop symptoms of abdominal distension, vomiting, gastroesophageal reflux, pulmonary aspiration, pneumonia, or sepsis. They may also have large gastric aspirates, and impaired fluid and nutritional intakes. The administration of prokinetic agents is used widely to help with these problems by promoting gastric emptying and improving intestinal motility. Metoclopramide and erythromycin appear to be effective in improving gastric motility and may improve tolerance to enteral feeds for a limited period. Diarrhea in patients on EN can have a multifactorial genesis. The commonest causes of diarrhea are too high osmolarity, too high rate of administration, contamination, *Clostridium difficile* infection, hypoalbuminemia, and side effects of drugs or additives (Barrett, Shepherd, and Gibson 2009).

29.3.4.2 Tube Occlusion

Polyurethane tubes do not need to be changed frequently, except when they are damaged or occluded. In order to keep the tube lumen patent, it is mandatory to avoid the formation of feed lumps and incrustations by washing it regularly and particularly soon after the administration, when this is intermittent.

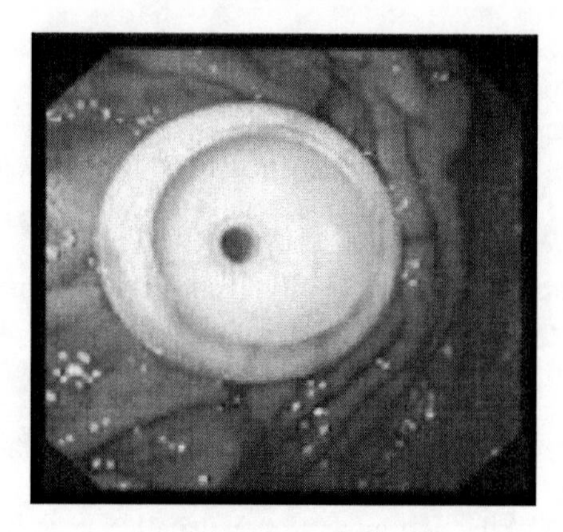

FIGURE 29.1 Soft bumper. The picture shows an endoscopic view of a soft bumper. It has the advantage of a reduced risk of gastric erosions. Only a strong traction can dislodge it, usually during nursing maneuvers.

29.3.4.3 Accidental Tube Removal

Accidental gastrostomy tube removal or dislodgment is usually prevented by the shape of the tube itself. Its intragastric end may be constituted of either a larger portion called a "bumper"—soft (Figure 29.1) or rigid (Figure 29.2)—or, less frequently, an air-filled cuff (Figure 29.3). In the latter case, if the cuff is damaged or the control valve has lost its function, a little traction is sufficient for the tube to pop out. A systematic check of the cuff seal is the only preventive measure. In the case, more frequent, of tubes equipped with a "bumper," only a strong traction can dislodge them. This usually occurs in PVS patients during nursing maneuvers such as making the bed, personal hygiene, mobilization, and physiotherapy. A useful precaution is to give enteral feeds intermittently so as to leave the patient free from nutrition when these maneuvers are carried out.

29.3.4.4 Gastric Sores Due to the Internal Portion of the Tube

This is an often misdiagnosed complication that may lead to gastric erosions and even life-threatening bleeding. It occurs when, during dressing, an excessive pull is applied to the tube securing it too tightly to the skin. The best preventive measure when making the dressing is to rotate the tube clockwise and counterclockwise between thumb and finger, verifying that the rotation is not impaired by excessive traction (Figure 29.4).

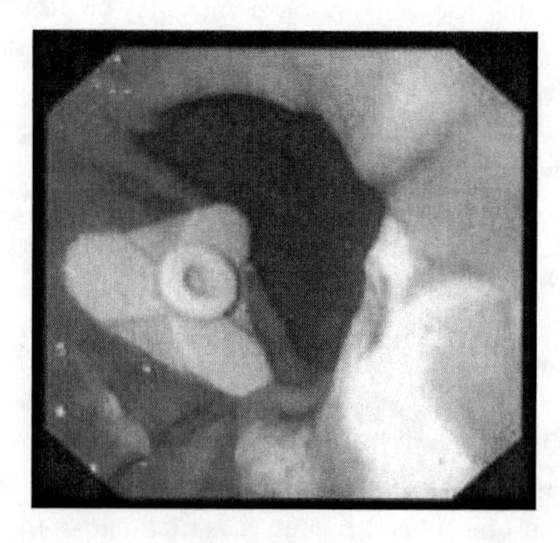

FIGURE 29.2 Rigid bumper. The picture shows an endoscopic view of a rigid bumper. Compared to the soft one, it has an increased risk of gastric erosions. It may be dislodged only by a strong traction.

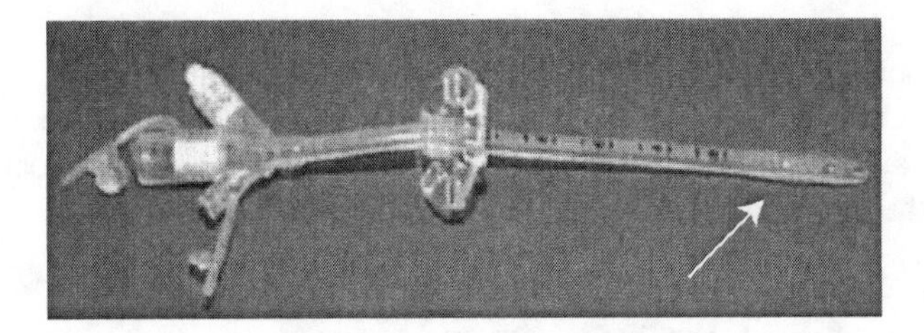

FIGURE 29.3 Tube with air-filled cuff. The picture shows a gastrostomy tube ending with an air-filled cuff (deflated in the picture—white arrow). If the cuff is damaged or the control valve has lost its function, a little traction is sufficient for the tube to pop out.

29.3.4.5 Intestinal Occlusion by Tube Dragging

This is a rare complication, described in few case reports (Ragunath et al. 2004). The inner portion of the tube is progressively dragged by peristaltic waves beyond the pylorus causing occlusion. This can be prevented by simply placing a "marker" on the external part of the tube once it is correctly dressed and checking this marker is always visible.

29.4 ETHICAL ISSUES

Management of patients with consciousness disorders inevitably raises ethical and legal questions about the appropriate degree of life-sustaining treatment.

Nutritional support alone does not reverse or cure a disease or injury, it just enables a patient to meet nutrient needs during curative or palliative therapy. Nutrition support has been demonstrated to be beneficial in competent patients by reducing physical deterioration and improving quality of life. It also seems to prevent the emotional effect of "starving the patient to death" (Fuhrman and Herrmann 2006). However, the available data indicate that it is not beneficial to provide nutrition support for patients with an irreversible or terminal illness (Fine 2006). When the burden of nutrition exceeds the benefits, the patient, surrogate, or healthcare provider can choose to withdraw nutrition support.

29.4.1 Artificial Nutrition and Hydration (ANH): Medical Treatment or Loving Care?

The debate among experts in the last few years has focused on the controversy regarding whether ANH should be considered as a form of medical treatment or of tender loving care, part of a duty

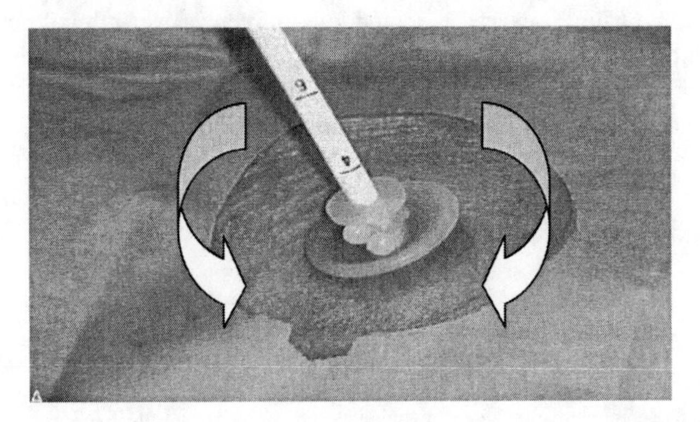

FIGURE 29.4 External view of a gastrostomy tube. The picture shows an external view of a gastrostomy tube. In order to avoid gastric erosions, it must not be pulled strongly or secured too tightly to the skin. This can be prevented, during dressing, by rotating the tube (see arrows) between thumb and finger, verifying the rotation is not impaired by excessive traction.

of solidarity the physician should always carry out (Fine 2006). How this issue is resolved will determine the possibility of the recognition or the denial of the right of the patient to refuse ANH.

In the United States, ANH is considered a medical treatment which the patient may consciously refuse (Casarett et al. 2005). The concept justifying this position is that, among patients in PVS, ANH amounts to the administration of chemical compounds which only physicians can prescribe and control, whereas the recipient cannot be aware of being fed. For this reason, these are excessive medical acts which fail to respect the dignity of the human individual.

In a recent article, Truog and Cochrane (2005) try and change the standpoint, affirming that the justification for withdrawal of ANH does not depend on whether it is administered artificially (i.e., by means of feeding tubes) or naturally (i.e., by mouth). According to their opinion, this distinction is irrelevant, since the decision should be based on the patient's fundamental right to refuse any undesired treatment.

However, decisions concerning nutrition support can be fraught with family conflict. Many families are often reluctant to stop nutrition support for fear of starving their loved one to death, as they perceive nutrition support as food, with its connotations of love, nurturing, and comfort (Planas and Camilo 2002).

29.4.2 Withdrawing ANH

The notion that withdrawing nutrition support contributes to pain and suffering has been widely debated. Positron emission tomography scans have demonstrated that when a patient is in a PVS, the brain areas responsible for pain perception do not function (Finucane, Christmas, and Travis 1999). Some studies of patients who are dying have indicated that thirst and hunger are not a significant problem when patients decide to forgo nutrition support and hydration as long as meticulous mouth care is provided (Ellershaw, Sutcliffe, and Saunders 1995). According to other authors (Bachmann et al. 2003), dehydration does not produce pain or discomfort. In fact, absence of food and beverage intake results in ketosis and release of opioids in the brain, and this, in turn, produces a sense of euphoria and well-being, with no or only a mild sense of hunger or thirst (Mirhosseini, Fainsinger, and Baracos 2005).

Fear of making patients uncomfortable due to thirst encourages clinicians and families to provide fluids to patients when oral intake is declining or artificial nutrition has been discontinued. If hydration is given, the least invasive route should be used. The provision of intravenous hydration can have a negative impact on quality of life by increasing pulmonary secretions, urinary output, nausea, vomiting, and edema (McCallum and Fornari 2006).

Table 29.4 summarizes the key points on ethical issues in ANH of PVS patients.

The Roman Catholic Church exerts a tremendous influence over ethical decisions concerning withdrawing and withholding nutrition support. There are currently two views from the church. The view that ANH is morally optional and may be withdrawn in some patients in PVS has its foundation in the notion that the spiritual life is more important than the physical life. In 1957, Pope Pius XII expressed the view that "Life, health, all temporal activities are in fact subordinated to spiritual ends," and therefore ANH is morally optional when patients can no longer interact with the world around them (Pope Pius XII 2004). The Catholic Bishops of Texas and other Catholic theological

TABLE 29.4
Key Points on Ethical Issues in ANH of PVS Patients

1. Effective communication between clinicians and family on end-of-life issues
2. Decisions based on thoughtful judgments about what a reasonable person would choose
3. Get patients to complete advance directives
4. The wishes of the patient/family should be respected in all healthcare settings

leaders have reiterated that it is acceptable for nutrition support to be withheld or withdrawn from a patient in a persistent vegetative state (McMahon 2004). However, in 2004, Pope John Paul II stated that clinicians are obligated to provide ANH to most patients in a persistent vegetative state. The pope referred to the uncertainty of the vegetative state prognosis and the suffering caused by not feeding and stated that the insertion of feeding tubes and intravenous catheters was not a "medical act" (Pope John Paul II 2004).

29.4.3 Ethical Principles Informing the Decision

What an individual believes versus what his or her religious affiliation teaches may differ. Therefore, healthcare providers must communicate with patients and families to determine preferences. The American Dietetic Association's position paper on providing food and hydration to the terminally ill states: "The patient's expressed desire is the primary guide for determining the extent of nutrition and hydration" (Maillet, Potter, and Heller 2002). The difficulty lies in determining the patient's desires.

Ideally, there should be documentation through advance directives outlining the patient's beliefs, thoughts, and desires concerning care during the final stages of life. However, only 20%–30% of people have advance directives and it is doubtful that all of these individuals review the documents annually as recommended (Campbell, Bizek, and Thill 1999). When the patient is unable to make decisions, a family member becomes a surrogate and is charged with the responsibility of making the decision based on the patient's values, which can be difficult if the patient's values differ from the surrogate's beliefs or if the family disagrees about what to do (Winzelberg, Hanson, and Tulsky 2005).

The prima facie principles that characterize the ethical aspects of clinical medicine are respect for patient autonomy, beneficence, non-maleficence, and justice (Beauchamp and Childress 2001). When caring for patients for whom long-term tube feeding is being considered, clinicians may find these ethical principles at odds with each other.

Effective communication among clinicians, patients, and surrogate decision-makers may help prevent ethical dilemmas (Orr, Marshall, and Osborn 1995). Clinicians should take time to learn about the patient and the patient's values, goals, and beliefs. Despite good communication, clinicians may face ethical dilemmas related to long-term tube feeding that they cannot resolve. In these situations, an ethics consultation may be valuable and, if the issue is still unresolved, referral to court for judicial review may be necessary. Jennett (2002) has reviewed the relevant laws and judicial rulings on patients in PVS and MCS in developed countries.

SUMMARY POINTS

- Artificial nutrition and hydration in PVS is not a temporary support measure but rather a chronic condition.
- PVS patients are completely dependent on the care provided by healthcare personnel or family members.
- The nutritional status is one of the most important factors contributing to the survival of PVS patients.
- PVS patients should be nourished via an enteral route, reserving parenteral nutrition for those conditions in which the gastrointestinal tract is not viable.
- Due to muscle wasting, PVS patients need a progressively lower energy intake over time.
- PEG is the most commonly used route to administer enteral nutrition to PVS patients.
- Jejunostomy is a viable alternative in patients at risk of pulmonary aspiration, or whenever a gastrostomy is not feasible.
- In patients on long-term EN, the administration is usually intermittent, often night-time, so as to leave the day hours for physiotherapy, nursing maneuvers, mobilization, etc.

TABLE 29.5
Key Points to Resolve Ethical Dilemmas on ANH in PVS Patients

1. Clearly express the question of the case
2. Look for relevant guidelines
3. Assess the patient's nutrition status and prognosis
4. Balance the effect of nutrition support vs. no nutrition support
5. Explore the family's feelings about nutrition support
6. Evaluate the different ethical perspectives of the stakeholders
7. Define the key terms: "benefit" or "harm"; "quality of life"; "medical treatment" or "ordinary care"; "futile" treatment
8. Consider all the information and discuss with the stakeholders

- Complications such as constipation, impaired gastrointestinal motility, diarrhea, tube occlusion, accidental tube removal, gastric sores, and intestinal occlusion are possible, and efforts should be made to prevent them.
- We should work towards making the decision process follow an explicit procedure, respecting the diverse moral responsibility of family members, nursing, and medical staff (see Table 29.5).
- The decision to treat aggressively or passively should be made on the basis of reliable information about how the patient would wish to be treated in this condition.

LIST OF ABBREVIATIONS

ANH	Artificial nutrition and hydration
BMR	Basal metabolic rate
EE	Energy expenditure
EN	Enteral nutrition
MCS	Minimally conscious state
PEG	Percutaneous endoscopic gastrostomy
PEJ	Percutaneous endoscopic jejunostomy
PVS	Permanent vegetative state
WHO	World Health Organization

REFERENCES

Bachmann, P., C. Marti-Massoud, M. P. Blanc-Vincent, J. C. Desport, V. Colomb, L. Dieu, D. Kere et al. 2003. Summary version of the standards, options and recommendations for palliative or terminal nutrition in adults with progressive cancer (2001). *Br J Cancer* 89:S107–10.

Barrett, J. S., S. J. Shepherd, and P. R. Gibson. 2009. Strategies to manage gastrointestinal symptoms complicating enteral feeding. *JPEN J Parenter Enteral Nutr* 33:21–26.

Beauchamp, T. L., and J. F. Childress. 2001. *Principles of Biomedical Ethics,* 5th edn. New York, NY: Oxford University Press.

Bernat, J. L. 2006. Chronic disorders of consciousness. *Lancet* 367:1181–92.

Campbell, M. L., K. S. Bizek, and M. Thill. 1999. Patient responses during rapid terminal weaning from mechanical ventilation: A prospective study. *Crit Care Med* 27:73–77.

Casarett, D., J. Kapo, and A. Caplan. 2005. Appropriate use of artificial nutrition and hydration: Fundamental principles and recommendations. *N Engl J Med* 353:2605–12.

Cook, A. M., A. Peppard, and B. Magnuson. 2008. Nutrition considerations in traumatic brain injury. *Nutr Clin Practice* 23:608–20.

Ellershaw, J. E., J. M. Sutcliffe, and M. Saunders. 1995. Dehydration and the dying patient. *J Pain Symptom Manage* 10:192–97.

Finch, H. 2005. Nutrition and hydration for the vegetative state and minimally conscious state patients. *Neuropsychol Rehab* 15:537–47.

Fine, R. L. 2006. Ethical issues in artificial nutrition and hydration. *Nutr Clin Pract* 21:118–25.

Finucane, T. E., C. Christmas, and K. Travis. 1999. Tube feeding in patients with advanced dementia: A review of the evidence. *JAMA* 282:1365–70.

Fuhrman, M. P., and V. M. Herrmann. 2006. Bridging the continuum: Nutrition support in palliative and hospice care. *Nutr Clin Pract* 21:134–41.

Jennett, B., and F. Plum. 1972. Persistent vegetative state after brain damage. A syndrome in search of a name. *Lancet* 1:734–37.

Jennett, B. 2002. *The vegetative state: Medical facts, ethical and legal dilemmas.* Cambridge: Cambridge University Press.

Laureys, S. 2004. Functional imaging in the vegetative state. *Neurorehabilitation* 19:335–41.

Maillet, J. O., R. L. Potter, and L. Heller. 2002. Position of the American Dietetic Association: Ethical and legal issues in nutrition, hydration, and feeding. *J Am Diet Assoc* 102:716–26.

McCallum, P. D., and A. Fornari. 2006. Medical nutrition therapy in palliative care. In *the clinical guide to oncology nutrition,* 2nd edn., eds. L. Elliott, L. L. Molseed, P. D. McCallum, and B. Grant, 201–7. Chicago, Ill: American Dietetic Association.

McEvoy, C. T., G. W. Cran, S. R. Cooke, and I. S. Young. 2009. Resting energy expenditure in non-ventilated, non-sedated patients recovering from serious traumatic brain injury: Comparison of prediction equations with in direct calorimery values. *Clin Nutr* 28:526–32.

McMahon, K. 2004. Should nutrition and hydration be considered medical therapy? *Origins* 33:744–48.

Mirhosseini, N., R. L. Fainsinger, and V. Baracos. 2005. Parenteral nutrition in advanced cancer: Indications and clinical practice guidelines. *J Palliat Care* 8:914–18.

Multi-Society Task Force on PVS. 1994a. Medical aspects of the persistent vegetative state (1). *N Engl J Med* 330:1499–508.

Multi-Society Task Force on PVS. 1994b. Medical aspects of the persistent vegetative state (2). *N Engl J Med* 330:1572–79.

Orr, R. D., P. A. Marshall, and J. Osborn. 1995. Cross-cultural considerations in clinical ethics consultations. *Arch Fam Med* 4:159–64.

Planas, M., and M. E. Camilo. 2002. Artificial nutrition: Dilemmas in decision making. *Clin Nutr* 21:355–61.

Pope John Paul II. 2004. Care for patients in a "permanent" vegetative state. *Origins* 33:737, 739–40.

Pope Pius XII. 2004. The prolongation of life (November 24, 1957). *Origins* 33:750.

Ragunath, K., A. Roberts, S. Senapati, and G. Clark. 2004. Retrograde jejunoduodenal intussusception caused by a migrated percutaneous endoscopic gastrostomy tube. *Dig Dis Sci* 49:1815–17.

Rombeau, J. L., and M. D. Caldwell. 1990. *Enteral and tube feeling,* 2nd edn. Philadelphia, PA: WB Saunders Co.

Schiff, N. D. 2006. Multimodal neuroimaging approaches to disorders of consciousness. *J Head Trauma Rehabil* 21:388–97.

Truog, R. D., and T. I. Cochrane. 2005. Refusal of hydration and nutrition: Irrelevance of the "artificial" vs. "natural" distinction. *Arch Intern Med* 165:2574–76.

Winzelberg, G., L. Hanson, and T. Tulsky. 2005. Beyond autonomy: Diversifying end-of-life decision-making approaches to serve patients and families. *J Am Geriatr Soc* 53:1046–50.

30 Nutrition and Appetite Regulation in Children and Adolescents with End-Stage Renal Failure

Kai-Dietrich Nüsken and Jörg Dötsch

CONTENTS

30.1 INTRODUCTION

The nutritional situation of patients with end-stage renal disease (ESRD) is very heterogeneous. There is no uniform "kidney diet" as the demand for nutrients and fluid varies greatly, depending on age (infants, children, adolescents, adults), current body composition, mode of dialysis, underlying disease, concomitant diseases, and residual diuresis. Many patients show an imbalance of energy homeostasis, characterized by increased energy consumption and a concomitant lack of appetite because of a uremia-induced, disturbed appetite regulation. Acute life-threatening conditions may occur in case of excessive hyperhydration and hyperkalemia. The most important aims of nutritional modifications are prevention of hyperhydration and cachexia, but nowadays also adiposity, electrolyte disorders, disturbed bone metabolism, and cardiovascular complications. In pediatric patients, it is most important to achieve adequate growth and development. Guidelines on nutrition in renal failure, which are based on the best information available at the time of publication, are available from the National Kidney Foundation of the USA (NKF-KDOQI 2000, 2003, 2007, 2009) and the European Dialysis and Transplant Nurses Association/European Renal Care Association (EDTNA/ERCA 2009).

In this chapter the pathophysiological changes of appetite and nutrition in end-stage renal failure will be reviewed with a special focus on children and adolescents.

30.2 APPETITE REGULATION

30.2.1 Normal Appetite Regulation

Hunger, appetite, and satiety are regulated by complex mechanisms including peripheral endocrine and neuronal signals as well as cognition, perception, and learned behavior. The information is mainly integrated at the hypothalamus and brainstem. Under physiological conditions, data about energy consumption and energy availability from currently ingested food as well as energy stores is used to maintain energy homeostasis and body weight. Dysregulation may result either in cachexia or in adiposity. Hunger is a motivational state leading to acquisition and intake of food. Appetite is a similar state, but it emerges without a clear energy deficiency and with a more important role for palatability. Concerning satiety, one has to differentiate between preresorptive and postresorptive satiety. Preresorptive satiety is achieved 10–15 minutes after a meal, before any nutrients have been resorbed, and influences meal size. Mechanisms include signals from stretch and chemo-receptors via the vagal nerve projecting to the brainstem and hormonal anorexigenic signals (Schwartz et al. 2000). Postresorptive satiety is achieved thereafter and is responsible for the interval between two meals. Mechanisms include afferent vagal nerve fibers, triggered both by portal glucosensors and by hepatic sensors of fatty acid oxidation, as well as hormonal signals. An important short- to medium-term regulator is the orexigenic hormone ghrelin (Kojima et al. 1999). A very powerful medium- to long-term regulator is the anorexigenic hormone leptin (Halaas et al. 1995). Ghrelin and leptin have opposing effects on hypothalamic nuclei, which control appetite and energy consumption. In the past, the ventromedial hypothalamus (VMN) was considered the satiety center and the lateral hypothalamus (LHA) was considered the hunger center. However, current research has shown that hypothalamic appetite regulation is more complex.

30.2.2 Dysregulation of Appetite in End-Stage Renal Disease

30.2.2.1 Leptin and Ghrelin (Figure 30.1)

Leptin is a 16.7 kDa peptide hormone that is predominantly produced by adipocytes (Halaas et al. 1995). The anorexigenic effect of leptin was shown in rodents and man. Leptin reaches the hypothalamus via a saturable transport mechanism across the blood-brain barrier and binds to its

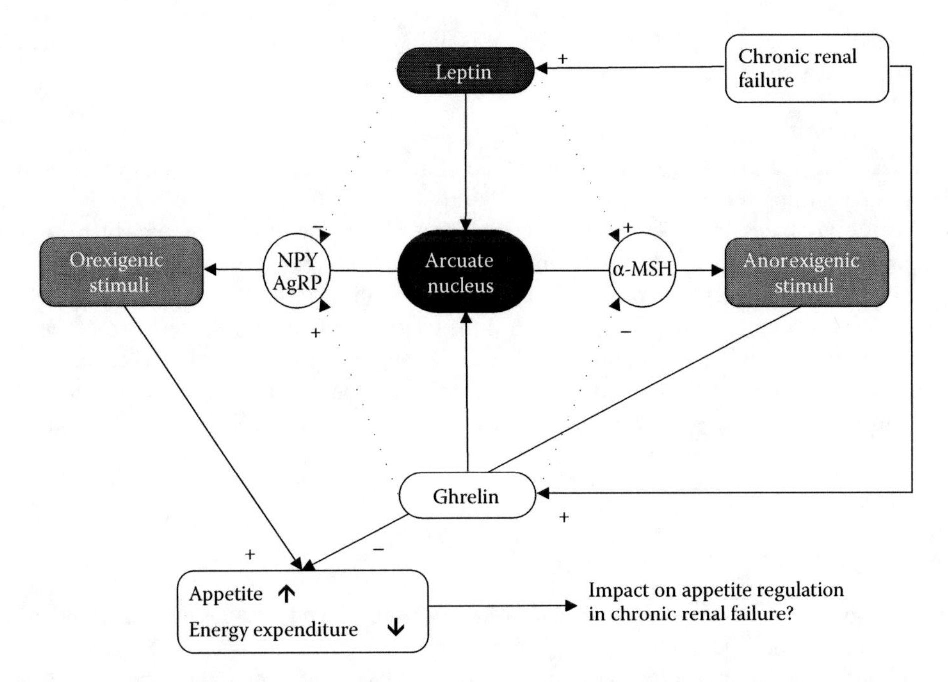

FIGURE 30.1 Postulated regulation of the leptin-ghrelin system in patients with chronic renal failure. NPY, neuropeptide Y; AgRP, agouti-related peptide; α-MSH, alpha-melanocyte-stimulating hormone. (From Dötsch, J. et al., *Pediatr. Nephrol.* 20, 701, 2005. With permission.)

transmembrane receptor mainly in the arcuate nucleus (ARC) and the VMN. Leptin decreases food intake by stimulation of neurons which contain the anorexigenic peptide alpha-melanocyte-stimulating hormone (α-MSH), which then stimulates the melanocortin receptor 4, and by inhibition of neurons which contain the orexigenic peptides neuropeptide Y (NPY) and agouti-related peptide (AgRP). Additionally, leptin increases energy consumption via the paraventricular nucleus by elevating the concentrations of thyrotropin-releasing hormone and corticotropin-releasing hormone. Consequently, leptin induces a negative energy balance. In ESRD, adults and children show elevated circulating leptin concentrations. Leptin is not sufficiently cleared by hemodialysis (HD), but significantly eliminated by peritoneal dialysis (PD) (Dötsch et al. 2005). Leptin knock-out mice (ob/ob mice), which do not have functional leptin, do not show decreased food intake and do not develop uremic loss of body weight after subtotal nephrectomy, but the similarly uremic control group does. This hints at a significant role of hyperleptinemia in uremic inappetence (Cheung et al. 2005).

Ghrelin is a 3.24 kDa peptide hormone that is mainly secreted by the stomach (Kojima et al. 1999). The orexigenic effect of ghrelin was shown in rodents and man. It binds to its receptor mainly in the ARC and LHA. Ghrelin increases food intake by stimulating NPY and AgRP neurons and prevents reduction of food intake mediated by leptin (Nakazato et al. 2001). Fasting and weight loss result in an increase of circulating ghrelin concentrations. Food intake is followed by a 30% decrease of serum ghrelin within 30–60 minutes. In ESRD, ghrelin concentrations are elevated in adults and children (Nüsken et al. 2004) before HD as well as during PD. Ghrelin concentrations decline considerably during HD (Dötsch et al. 2005).

In summary, leptin and ghrelin are antagonists in the context of appetite regulation and may play a role in the development of malnutrition in ESRD. As leptin is not eliminated and ghrelin is significantly cleared by HD, both may contribute to uremic loss of appetite, especially in HD patients. However, it is unclear to what extent both hormones contribute to weight loss of dialysis patients. A therapeutic method to effectively eliminate leptin is not available, although high-flux dialysis filters as well as PD show a certain clearance of leptin. Ghrelin is already elevated in ESRD patients, but does not lead to increased appetite. Therefore, it is unlikely that ghrelin infusions would be effective. Further research is needed to clarify these issues.

30.2.2.2 Uremia

Uremia describes the accumulation of a multitude of substances that are normally excreted by the kidneys. Apart from well-known parameters like urea or creatinine and the hormones depicted above, many substances are unidentified (Chazot 2009). Complications of uremia which contribute to inappetence include nausea, gastric emptying delay, and gastrointestinal ulcers. Consequently, the intake of protein and energy progressively decreases with deteriorating renal function. On the molecular level, amino acid imbalance increases the transport of free tryptophan across the blood-brain barrier, creating a hyperserotoninergic state resulting in activation of the anorexigenic melanocortin receptor 4. Accumulating inflammatory cytokines also suppress appetite. HD supports the inflammatory state because of recurring contact to extrinsic, potentially allergenic surfaces. PD leads to distension of the abdomen and an increased glucose load, which both are satiety signals (Rees and Shaw 2007).

30.3 PROTEIN ENERGY WASTING

Protein energy wasting (PEW) is defined as a loss of somatic and circulating body protein mass and energy reserves (Fouque et al. 2008). PEW is caused by multiple factors, is strongly associated with morbidity and mortality, and has a prevalence of 18%–75% in dialysis patients. PEW is a major risk factor for an adverse outcome for these patients. Protein energy malnutrition (PEM) is an inadequate nutrient intake and an important part of PEW. Further factors contributing to PEW are inflammation, dialysate nutrient losses, metabolic acidosis, and endocrine disorders. Additionally, concomitant diseases affect energy homeostasis. Cachexia is the result of severe PEW.

There are four different criteria to diagnose PEW in adults. First, patients have low serum levels of albumin, prealbumin, or cholesterol. Second, a reduced body mass index (BMI), a reduced percentage of body fat, or an unintended loss of body weight over 3–6 months indicate PEW. Third, a reduced muscle mass and an ongoing reduction of 5% muscle mass in 3 months or 10% in 6 months is pathologic. Last, an inadequate protein or energy intake relative to the individual's nutritional needs (PEM) is an important factor. A common finding when PEM is present is a protein intake less than 0.8 g/kg/d and an energy intake less than 25 kcal/kg/d (Dukkipati and Kopple 2009). In the following the different factors contributing to PEW will be discussed (for PEM see 30.2.2).

30.3.1 Inflammation

Inflammation in ESRD is caused by multiple factors, including uremia, dialysis, and the underlying disease. Inflammation leads to inappetence and increased energy consumption. Patients with a state of inflammation show further elevated leptin serum concentrations. Inflammation is associated with atherosclerosis, muscle wasting, and increased mortality. This combination of symptoms is called the "malnutrition-inflammation atherosclerosis syndrome." Concomitant diseases which are associated with inflammation are infected vascular access sites or catheters, peritonitis, systemic infections, vasculitis, diabetes mellitus, stroke, myocardial infarction, peripheral vascular ischemia, insufficient kidney grafts, impure dialysate, and other factors (Dukkipati and Kopple 2009).

30.3.2 Dialysate Nutrient Losses

Varying amounts of nutrients are lost into the dialysate. The most important among them are amino acids, peptides, proteins, water-soluble vitamins, and minerals. The mode of dialysis significantly affects the amount and type of nutrients lost. HD patients may lose up to 10 g of amino acids during a single dialysis session, but very low amounts of protein because the membranes used preferably eliminate small molecules. However, HD patients may lose a significant amount of proteins due to dialysis-associated blood loss.

PD patients lose about 15 g total protein into the dialysate per day. In severe peritonitis or patients with a high peritoneal transport rate, the protein loss is even higher. Loss of amino acids is about 3.5 g/d. Water-soluble vitamins and electrolytes are lost into dialysate both in HD and PD patients (Dukkipati and Kopple 2009).

30.3.3 Metabolic Acidosis

Acidosis contributes to PEW because it induces protein catabolism (Lim et al. 1998). Especially HD patients are exposed to recurring acidosis before dialysis, whereas PD patients undergo continuous dialysis with sodium bicarbonate-buffered solutions. Tubular bicarbonate loss may occur in patients with residual diuresis.

30.3.4 Endocrine Disorders and Concomitant Diseases

Endocrine disorders contributing to PEW in ESRD patients include resistance to insulin, especially in diabetic patients (Dukkipati and Kopple 2009), as well as resistance to growth hormone and to insulin-like growth factor I, which is of high importance for growth in children (Blum et al. 1991).

30.4 NUTRITION AND DIET

In adults, nutrition affects body weight, body composition, and the development of chronic diseases. In infants, children, and adolescents, nutrition is important for linear growth, neurocognitive development, and sexual development (puberty). Deficits in linear growth and especially neurological development acquired during infancy may persist throughout life. The correct diet is an essential part of the treatment plan in all ESRD patients. Prior to nutritional therapy, the nutritional status, eating behavior, metabolic status, and electrolyte status have to be assessed. Macronutrient (fat, carbohydrate, protein, and fiber), micronutrient (vitamins, minerals), and fluid intake have to be adjusted to the individual needs of a patient. The aims of nutritional therapy are to minimize the sequelae and complications of kidney failure, to maintain normal body composition in adults, and to ensure optimal development in children.

In the following the general aspects of nutrition and diet will be described before the different age groups are discussed in detail.

30.4.1 General Aspects of Nutrition and Diet in End-Stage Renal Failure

30.4.1.1 Calories, Protein, and Body Weight

Cachectic patients are at high risk for complications and death. To maintain not only body weight but a healthy body composition, the supply of energy and protein has to be increased in many HD patients. Patients should weigh themselves every day and keep a diary on body weight and nutritional intake. However, the prevalence of obesity increases even among HD patients, because tasty, high-calorie food is available ubiquitously. Obese patients often show a severely altered body composition, with reduced muscle mass, reduced amount of functional tissues, and a concomitantly high fat mass. These patients represent a high-risk group for cardiovascular complications, which are the major cause of death in HD patients. Achieving and maintaining a healthy body weight by supply of an individually tailored amount of energy, as well as maintaining a healthy body composition and immune system by supply of a sufficient amount of protein is crucial for optimal quality of life (NKF-KDOQI 2000; EDTNA/ERCA 2009).

30.4.1.2 Sodium and Fluids

There are plenty of sodium-rich nutrients in Western diets. Sodium induces thirst, leading to fluid intake and fluid retention. In oligo-anuric patients, excess fluid results in edema of the skin and lungs as well as pleural, pericardial, and abdominal effusions. Furthermore, hypertension is promoted, with the possibility of concomitant cardiac hypertrophy, cardiac insufficiency, vascular damage, cerebral hemorrhage, and death. The patient can recognize sudden weight gain and realize his hyperhydration by daily weighing. The daily amount of sodium and fluid has to be individually determined for each patient. Loss of food palatability due to reduced salt can be compensated for with herbs and spices (NKF-KDOQI 2000; EDTNA/ERCA 2009).

30.4.1.3 Phosphorus and Calcium

Large amounts of phosphorus are typically found in dairy products, nuts, peanuts, legumes, mushrooms, cocoa, cola, meat, and chocolate. Hyperphosphatemia results in secondary hyperparathyroidism and renal osteodystrophy. Calcium-phosphorous crystals accumulate in blood vessels as vascular plaques, and in heart, joints, muscles, and skin, resulting in coronary heart disease, stroke, and other complications. Reduction of nutritional phosphorus is the most important measure to avoid renal osteodystrophy and cardiovascular complications by calcium-phosphorus plaques. Additionally, administration of phosphate-binding medication and vitamin D is recommended (NKF-KDOQI 2000; EDTNA/ERCA 2009). Vitamin D is supplemented by medication containing either cholecalciferol (inactive), 1-hydroxycholecalciferol (activated in the liver) or 1,25-dihydroxycholecalciferol (active vitamin D). Target organs of vitamin D are the intestines, parathyroid, where it suppresses parathormone, bones, and kidney. Adequate calcium phosphate metabolism has to be assessed by regular measurement of parathormone, calcium, phosphate, and bone density.

30.4.1.4 Potassium

Excessive hyperkalemia is a life-threatening condition, because electromechanical dissociation and cardiac arrest may occur. Nutritional potassium reduction is absolutely necessary and life-saving. Large amounts of potassium are typically found in bananas, potatoes, oranges, tomatoes, legumes, certain fruit juices, chocolate, milk, yoghurt, and protein-rich foods (NKF-KDOQI 2000; EDTNA/ERCA 2009).

30.4.1.5 Vitamins and Minerals

Eating a wide variety of foods is recommended to provide the body with vitamins and minerals. As dietary limitations reduce the variety of food and dialysis results in loss of vitamins and minerals, supplementation of vitamins may be necessary. An essential vitamin in kidney failure is vitamin D (NKF-KDOQI 2000; EDTNA/ERCA 2009).

30.4.2 Infants

In contrast to adults, who have to ingest as much energy as they consume to keep energy homeostasis and body weight, children need additional nutrients for growth and development. Birth weight usually doubles within 4–5 months and triples within 12 months. However, energy stores are small, so infants are endangered by fast decompensation in case of nutrient deficiency. In severe renal failure, individually optimized nutrition is key for survival and adequate development. The courses of height, weight, and BMI have to be continuously evaluated by the use of percentile charts. The volume of milk drunk and the drinking pattern have to be recorded. The intake of energy, protein, and electrolytes, especially sodium, potassium, calcium, and phosphorus, has to be calculated. The individual

TABLE 30.1
Equations to Estimate Energy Requirements in Children at Healthy Weights

Age	Estimated Energy Requirement (kcal/d) = Total Energy Expenditure + Energy Deposition
0–3 mo	EER = [89 × weight (kg) – 100] + 175
4–6 mo	EER = [89 × weight (kg) – 100] + 56
7–12 mo	EER = [89 × weight (kg) – 100] + 22
13–35 mo	EER = [89 × weight (kg) – 100] + 20
3–8 y	Boys: EER = 88.5 – 61.9 × age (y) + PA × [26.7 × weight (kg) + 903 × height (m)] + 20
	Girls: EER = 135.3 – 30.8 × age (y) + PA × [10 × weight (kg) + 934 × height (m)] + 20
9–18 y	Boys: EER = 88.5 – 61.9 × age (y) + PA × [26.7 × weight (kg) + 903 × height (m)] + 25
	Girls: EER = 135.3 – 30.8 × age (y) + PA × [10 × weight (kg) + 934 × height (m)] + 25

Source: From National Kidney Foundation – Kidney Disease Outcome Quality Initiative (NKF-KDOQI). *Am. J. Kidney Dis.*, 53, S1, 2009.

Note: EER, estimated energy requirement; mo, months; y, years; PA, physical activity coefficient.

status of protein metabolism, electrolytes, acid-base metabolism, bone metabolism, and hematopoesis has to be assessed by laboratory measurements (Rees and Shaw 2007; NKF-KDOQI 2009).

In most cases, the baseline intake of energy and protein in infants with terminal renal failure is not sufficient. Restoration of normal protein and energy intake plus compensation for dialytic losses is recommended (see Tables 30.1 through 30.4 for dietary recommendations). In case of insufficient weight gain, energy intake has to be adjusted. If oral intake is limited by vomiting or refusal of nutrients, tube feeding should be considered. Sodium has to be supplemented in many patients, especially when kidney dysplasia or urogenital abnormalities are present. Hyperkalemia is often present, but hypokalemia is also possible. Acidosis and dysregulation of calcium-phosphate-metabolism need to be corrected. To treat renal anemia, iron supplementation is needed in addition to erythropoietin. The demand of fluid varies greatly and depends on daily urine volume, course of body weight, presence of edemas, and blood pressure. In most cases, residual diuresis is present, so the fluid volume ingested by breastfeeding (often difficult), infant milk, or as special formula milk is eliminated by the kidney. Electrolyte disorders can often be controlled by modification of intake or excretion, respectively. Vitamins and trace element intake should be normalized (see Table 30.5 for dietary recommendations). In children with dialysis, it is suggested to apply water-soluble vitamin

TABLE 30.2
Physical Activity Coefficients (PA) for Determination of Energy Requirements in Children Aged 3–18 Years

	Level of Physical Activity			
Gender	**Sedentary**	**Low Active**	**Active**	**Very Active**
	Typical activities of daily living (ADL) only	ADL + 30–60 min of daily moderate activity (e.g., walking at 5–7 km/h)	ADL + ≥60 min of daily moderate activity	ADL + ≥60 min of daily moderate activity + an additional 60 min of vigorous activity or 120 min of moderate activity
Boys	1.0	1.13	1.26	1.42
Girls	1.0	1.16	1.31	1.56

Source: From National Kidney Foundation – Kidney Disease Outcome Quality Initiative (NKF-KDOQI). *Am. J. Kidney Dis.*, 53, S1, 2009.

TABLE 30.3
Acceptable Macronutrient Distribution Ranges

Macronutrient	Children 1–3 y	Children 4–18 y
Carbohydrate	45%–65%	45%–65%
Fat	30%–40%	25%–35%
Protein	5%–20%	10%–30%

Source: From National Kidney Foundation – Kidney Disease Outcome Quality Initiative (NKF-KDOQI). *Am. J. Kidney Dis.*, 53, S1, 2009.

supplements. Severe but not excessive uremia is present in many cases. As a result, dialysis often is not needed for survival. In an infant with ESRD, the most important aim of all therapeutic efforts is to achieve survival and adequate development without dialysis whenever possible. Dialysis is difficult and may frequently cause complications. However, dialysis is feasible in the first year of life and inevitably needed in case of conservatively uncontrollable hyperhydration and hyperkalemia, as well as clinical symptoms of uremia including abnormal fatigue and limited consciousness, but also nausea and malnutrition, resulting in persistent failure to thrive.

30.4.3 Children

From the age of 12 months onwards, it is recommended to begin dialysis in all children with ESRD because of a clear benefit for the patient's growth and development. PD is applied in almost all patients up to the age of 10 years. HD is predominantly used in adolescents (see 29.4.3). At the start of dialysis, nutrition has to be adapted (see Tables 30.1 through 30.5 for recommendations). Although they become less uremic after initiation of dialysis, major problems for young children with PD are loss of appetite and nausea because of continuous glucose resorption and distension of the abdomen. A considerable number of patients cannot be nourished orally and need tube feeding. Nutrient loss, especially protein loss to the dialysate because of a high peritoneal surface area, and hyperphosphatemia followed by hyperparathyroidism and renal osteodystrophy are significant issues. Hyperkalemia in PD patients is less common than in HD patients, but still of high relevance because of potentially life-threatening hyperkalemia. Food for the typical patient has to be rich in calories, rich in proteins, low in phosphorus, and low in potassium. Vitamins and trace elements have to be normalized.

TABLE 30.4
Recommended Dietary Protein Intake in Children with End-Stage Renal Failure

	Age	DRI (g/kg/d)	DRI for HD (g/kg/d)[a]	DRI for PD (g/kg/d)[b]
Infants	0–6 mo	1.5	1.6	1.8
	7–12 mo	1.2	1.3	1.5
Children	1–3 y	1.05	1.15	1.3
	4–13 y	0.95	1.05	1.1
Adolescents	14–18 y	0.85	0.95	1.0

Source: From National Kidney Foundation – Kidney Disease Outcome Quality Initiative (NKF-KDOQI). *Am. J. Kidney Dis.*, 53, S1, 2009.

Note: DRI, dietary reference intake; mo, months; y, years.

[a] DRI + 0.1 g/kg/d to compensate for dialytic losses.

[b] DRI + 0.15–0.3 g/kg/d depending on patient age to compensate for peritoneal losses.

TABLE 30.5
Dietary Reference Intake: Recommended Dietary Allowance (RDA) and Adequate Intake (AI)

	Infants		Children		Males		Females	
	0–6 mo	7–12 mo	1–3 y	4–8 y	9–13 y	14–18 y	9–13 y	14–18 y
Vitamin A (μ/d)	400	500	300	400	600	900	600	700
Vitamin C (mg/d)	40	50	15	25	45	75	45	65
Vitamin E (mg/d)	4	5	6	7	11	15	11	15
Vitamin K (μg/d)	2.0	2.5	30	55	60	75	60	75
Thiamin (mg/d)	0.2	0.3	0.5	0.6	0.9	1.2	0.9	1.0
Riboflavin (mg/d)	0.3	0.4	0.5	0.6	0.9	1.3	0.9	1.0
Niacin (mg/d; NE)	2[a]	4	6	8	12	16	12	14
Vitamin B6 (mg/d)	0.1	0.3	0.5	0.6	1.0	1.3	1.0	1.2
Folate (μg/d)	65	80	150	200	300	400	300	400
Vitamin B12 (μg/d)	0.4	0.5	0.9	1.2	1.8	2.4	1.8	2.4
Pantothenic acid (mg/d)	1.7	1.8	2	3	4	5	4	5
Biotin (μg/d)	5	6	8	12	20	25	20	25
Copper (μg/d)	200	220	340	440	700	890	700	890
Selenium (μg/d)	15	20	20	30	40	55	40	55
Zinc (mg/d)	2	3	3	5	8	11	8	9

Source: From National Kidney Foundation – Kidney Disease Outcome Quality Initiative (NKF-KDOQI). *Am. J. Kidney Dis.*, 53, S1, 2009.

Note: RDAs are in bold type; AIs are in ordinary type.

[a] As preformed niacin, not niacin equivalents (NE) for this age group.

30.4.4 Adolescents

Children and adolescents with ESRD who have arm veins sufficient to create an arteriovenous fistula and who are old enough to keep the arm in a steady position for several hours may be offered HD until renal transplantation although PD remains an option. A significant number of the patients are oligo-anuric. However, the major problem with adolescents in puberty is malcompliance. As HD is a discontinuous method, the patients are threatened by decompensation before dialysis. Significant issues are excessive hyperhydration, leading to severe cardiovascular complications, and hyperkalemia resulting in cardiac arrhythmia and arrest. An elevated calcium phosphate product promotes atherosclerosis. Uremic toxins promote inappetence and uremia. Consequently, the patients are trained to assess their state of hydration by weighing and blood pressure measurement, to identify food that contains high amounts of potassium and phosphorus, and to pay attention to a sufficient caloric intake (see Tables 30.1 through 30.5 for dietary recommendations). Fluid intake has to be restricted in oligo-anuric patients; food low in potassium and phosphorus is mandatory for all patients. Because of potential malcompliance, parameters have to be checked frequently and periodic training is necessary.

30.4.5 Adults

Adults with ESRD differ substantially from children and adolescents with this condition. This is a consequence of varying underlying disease (especially the role of diabetes mellitus type 2 has to be mentioned) and different concomitant disease (such as cardiovascular disease). These factors extensively influence nutritional status and diet. Therefore, the situation in adults is beyond the scope of this article.

30.5 APPLICATION TO OTHER AREAS OF TERMINAL OR PALLIATIVE CARE

The majority of patients in palliative care are threatened by kidney failure. Secondary kidney failure may occur in case of reduced kidney perfusion, e.g., in patients with severe cardiac insufficiency or severe dehydration because of insufficient fluid intake or increased fluid loss. Recurrent urinary tract infections, nephrolithiasis, urinary obstructions, proteinuria, diabetes mellitus, arterial hypertension, and cardiovascular disease are major risk factors contributing to kidney failure. Moreover, malignoma may be associated with infiltration of the kidneys or chemotherapy-induced kidney damage.

30.6 PRACTICAL METHODS AND TECHNIQUES

Training of all patients and their parents is mandatory. It has to be clarified unambiguously that dialysis, intake of medication, and adequate intake of fluid, potassium, phosphorus, protein, and energy are essential for development, quality of life, and survival. Therefore, the main educational contents are practical application of dialysis, information on medication, assessment of hydration by weighing and blood pressure measurement, as well as identification, preparation, and intake of appropriate food.

KEY FACTS OF RENAL FAILURE

- The kidneys are required to maintain a stable interior milieu of water and electrolytes, to eliminate toxins, to control blood pressure, to generate red blood cells, and to maintain normal bone density.
- End-stage kidney failure is incompatible with life unless the kidney function is replaced.
- Fluid overload results in high blood pressure, heart failure, and brain bleeding.
- Potassium overload results in cardiac arrest.
- Renal osteodystrophy results in fractures.
- To replace the functions of the kidney, not only dialysis therapy, but also drug therapy and nutritional modifications are vital.
- Nutritional modifications generally include reduction of potassium, reduction of phosphorus, and an individually optimized intake of fluid as well as protein and energy.
- Children with end-stage renal failure additionally show a severe disorder of development.
- An optimal combination of dialysis, drug therapy, and nutrition is life-saving and can largely normalize growth, cognitive development, and sexual development.

ETHICAL ISSUES

In most pediatric patients, ESRD is not a condition of palliative care but maximum therapy is applied. Most patients gain a good quality of life, receive a kidney graft after some years of dialysis, and survive until adulthood. However, in some cases dialysis and transplantation may still be impossible, or maximum therapy may be linked to multiple complications and an extremely poor quality of life. In these cases, consultation of a specialized pediatric ethics committee is desirable to discuss the various options with the parents and, if possible, the patient, and make decisions mutually after careful consideration.

SUMMARY POINTS

- End-stage renal failure substantially interferes with the major regulators of appetite and energy expenditure, namely leptin and ghrelin.
- Loss of appetite, waste of important nutrients by dialysis, and chronic inflammation promote a state of catabolism in end-stage renal failure patients.

- In infants, children, and adolescents the underlying disease and varying age requirements determine the nature of nutritional dysregulation as well as the resulting management of the patients.
- Guidelines on nutrition in renal failure are available from the National Kidney Foundation of the USA and the European Dialysis and Transplant Nurses Association/European Renal Care Association.

LIST OF ABBREVIATIONS

α-MSH	Alpha-melanocyte-stimulating hormone
AgRP	Agouti-related peptide
ARC	Arcuate nucleus
BMI	Body mass index
EDTNA	European Dialysis and Transplant Nurses Association
ERCA	European Renal Care Association
ESRD	End-stage renal disease
HD	Hemodialysis
KDOQI	Kidney Disease Outcomes Quality Initiative
LHA	Lateral hypothalamic area
NKF	National Kidney Foundation
NPY	Neuropeptide Y
PD	Peritoneal dialysis
PEM	Protein energy malnutrition
PEW	Protein energy wasting
VMN	Ventromedial hypothalamus

REFERENCES

Blum, W. F., M. B. Ranke, K. Kietzmann, B. Tönshoff, and O. Mehls. 1991. Growth hormone resistance and inhibition of somatomedin activity by excess of insulin-like growth factor binding protein in uraemia. *Pediatr Nephrol* 5:539–44.

Chazot, C. 2009. Why are chronic kidney disease patients anorexic and what can be done about it? *Semin Nephrol* 29:15–23.

Cheung, W., P. X. Yu, B. M. Little, R. D. Cone, D. L. Marks, and R. H. Mak. 2005. Role of leptin and melanocortin signaling in uremia-associated cachexia. *J Clin Invest* 115:1659–65.

Dötsch, J., K. Nüsken, M. Schroth, W. Rascher, and U. Meissner 2005. Alterations of leptin and ghrelin serum concentrations in renal disease: Simple epiphenomena? *Pediatr Nephrol* 20:701–6.

Dukkipati, R., and J. D. Kopple. 2009. Causes and prevention of protein-energy wasting in chronic kidney failure. *Semin Nephrol* 29:39–49.

EDTNA/ERCA – European Dialysis & Transplant Nurses Association / European Renal Care Association. 2009. European guidelines for the nutritional care of adult renal patients. *EDTNA/ERCA J* 1:22–46.

Fouque, D., K. Kalantar-Zadeh, J. Kopple, N. Cano, P. Chauveau, L. Cuppari, H. Franch, et al. 2008. A proposed nomenclature and diagnostic criteria for protein-energy wasting in acute and chronic kidney disease. *Kidney Int* 73:391–98.

Halaas, J. L., K. S. Gajiwala, M. Maffei, S. L. Cohen, B. T. Chait, D. Rabinowitz, R. L. Lallone, S. K. Burley, and J. M. Friedman. 1995. Weight-reducing effects of the plasma protein encoded by the obese gene. *Science* 269:543–46.

Kojima, M., H. Hosoda, Y. Date, M. Nakazato, H. Matsuo, and K. Kangawa. 1999. Ghrelin is a growth-hormone-releasing acylated peptide from stomach. *Nature* 402:656–60.

Lim, V. S., K. E. Yarasheski, and M. J. Flanigan. 1998. The effect of uraemia, acidosis, and dialysis treatment on protein metabolism: A longitudinal leucine kinetic study. *Nephrol Dial Transplant* 13:1723–30.

Nakazato, M., N. Murakami, Y. Date, M. Kojima, H. Matsuo, K. Kangawa, and S. Matsukura. 2001. A role for ghrelin in the central regulation of feeding. *Nature* 409:194–98.

National Kidney Foundation – Kidney Disease Outcome Quality Initiative (KDOQI). 2000. Clinical practice guideline for nutrition in chronic renal failure. *Am J Kidney Dis* 35:S1–140.

National Kidney Foundation – Kidney Disease Outcome Quality Initiative (KDOQI). 2003. Clinical practice guideline for bone metabolism and disease in chronic kidney disease. *Am J Kidney Dis* 42:S1–202.

National Kidney Foundation – Kidney Disease Outcome Quality Initiative (KDOQI). 2007. KDOQI clinical practice guidelines and clinical practice recommendations for diabetes and chronic kidney disease. *Am J Kidney Dis* 49:S12–154.

National Kidney Foundation – Kidney Disease Outcome Quality Initiative (KDOQI). 2009. Clinical practice guideline for nutrition in children with CKD: 2008 update. *Am J Kidney Dis* 53:S1–123.

Nüsken, K. D., M. Gröschl, M. Rauh, W. Stöhr, W. Rascher, and J. Dötsch. 2004. Effect of renal failure and dialysis on circulating ghrelin concentration in children. *Nephrol Dial Transplant* 19:2156–57.

Rees, L., and V. Shaw. 2007. Nutrition in children with CRF and on dialysis. *Pediatr Nephrol* 22:1689–702.

Schwartz, M. W., S. C. Woods, D. Porte Jr., R. J. Seeley, and D. G. Baskin. 2000. Central nervous system control of food intake. *Nature* 404:661–71.

31 Nutrition in End-Stage Liver Disease

Valentina Medici

CONTENTS

31.1 INTRODUCTION

Malnutrition is a very common manifestation of chronic liver disease, being very frequent in the early phases of cirrhosis and almost universal in end-stage liver disease (ESLD). Malnutrition is characterized by depletion of body fat and proteins, and deficiency of many micronutritients. It is associated with impaired short-term survival and impaired immunocompetence, and it is correlated with the typical manifestations of ESLD, including hepatic encephalopathy, ascites, and hepatorenal syndrome (Pikul et al. 1994). Pre-liver transplant nutritional status is independently associated with the number of infection episodes during the hospital stay (Gunsar et al. 2006). The presence of malnutrition is an independent risk factor for the length of stay in the Intensive Care Unit and the total number of days spent in hospital after liver transplant (Merli et al. 2009). Malnutrition is an often unrecognized complication of ESLD and even the most widely used methods to assess the severity of liver disease such as the Model for End Stage Liver Disease (MELD) and the Child-Pugh scores do not include specific nutritional parameters. The etiologies of malnutrition in all forms of chronic liver disease fall into three general categories: decreased appetite with diminished nutrient intake, inadequate intestinal absorption with increased protein losses, and abnormal metabolism. The clinical evaluation of malnutrition includes history of weight loss of more than 10% of usual weight with the typical depletion of body fat and skeletal muscle mass which is more appreciated in the temporal region of the head and the proximal musculature of the extremities. Other, often unrecognized, manifestations of malnutrition are represented by various types of skin rash (associated with zinc deficiency or vitamins A and C deficiency), glossitis (riboflavin or pyridoxine deficiency), peripheral neuropathy and memory loss (thiamine deficiency), and hyperactive reflexes (magnesium deficiency). The diagnosis and assessment of malnutrition in ESLD is based on the specific measurements of serum levels of micronutrients but more precise nutritional assessment requires the use of specialized testing. Anthropometry is based on the measurement of the mid-arm muscle circumference and triceps skinfold thickness. Bioelectrical impedance analysis compares the electrical conductivity through body fat and body water to determine fat and lean body mass. Nutritional therapy and support play a major role in the management of patients with ESLD and the principle behind the improvement of nutritional status is that it may improve liver function and hence survival.

31.2 PATHOPHYSIOLOGY OF MALNUTRITION IN END-STAGE LIVER DISEASE

ESLD is a systemic condition that is almost universally characterized by malnutrition. Several mechanisms contribute to the development of malnutrition (Table 31.1).

1. *Decreased nutrient intake:* Anorexia, or decreased appetite with inadequate food intake, occurs in as many as two thirds of patients with chronic liver disease. Potential associated mechanisms for anorexia in chronic liver disease include increased circulating tumor necrosis factor-α, interleukin 8, and leptin, each known to diminish appetite and food intake (McCullough et al. 1998). Other factors contributing to reduced food intake include zinc and/or magnesium deficiency with consequent dysgeusia, tense ascites, gastroparesis, and electrolyte imbalances with consequent nausea, vomiting, and early satiety, upper gastrointestinal bleeding, hepatic encephalopathy, and sepsis, dietary management of fluid retention with sodium and water restriction, and carbohydrate restrictions in case of diabetes mellitus.
2. *Decreased intestinal absorption of nutrients:* Adequate biliary and pancreatic secretions are necessary to ensure transport of digestive products across the intestinal epithelium. Cirrhosis is characterized by reduced bile secretion due to decreased hepatic bile synthesis and/or cholestasis with consequent impaired intraduodenal packaging of fat into bile-rich large molecules (micelles), essential for fat absorption (Roggin, Iber, and Linscheer 1972). This mechanism also affects fat-soluble vitamin (A, D, E, and K) absorption. Medications often used in case of ESLD can worsen this process: cholestyramine for example is used for pruritus but it can induce bile salt deficiency. The presence of severe portal hypertension together with frequent small bowel bacterial overgrowth may contribute to leakage of proteins into the intestine (protein-losing enteropathy).

TABLE 31.1
Mechanisms of Malnutrition in End-Stage Liver Disease

Cause	Underlying Mechanism
Decreased intake (anorexia or lack of appetite)	Elevated TNF-α, IL-8, and leptin
Decreased intestinal absorption	Pancreatic insufficiency, cholestasis with reduced bile secretion limiting solubility of fat and vitamins A, D, E, and K prior to uptake
	Portal hypertension with protein-losing enteropathy
	Decreased absorption of folate, thiamine, and disaccharide sugars
Metabolic disturbances	Increased or decreased energy expenditure
	Insulin resistance and reduced glycogen storage
	Decreased protein synthesis and increased breakdown of muscle proteins
	Enhanced utilization of fatty acid for energy

Note: Malnutrition can be caused by several mechanisms including decreased intake or decreased intestinal absorption of nutrients and metabolic problems related to energy utilization.

3. *Metabolic disturbances:* Increased energy expenditure is typical of cirrhosis with unstable inflammatory processes (Greco et al. 1998). Cirrhosis and portal hypertension is characterized by systemic vasodilatation and expanded intravascular blood volume. The direct consequence of this phenomenon is increased heart rate and increased resting energy expenditure. Frequent infections and sepsis can cause further baseline energy expenditure. The hypermetabolic state is also represented by increased muscle breakdown as a source of gluconeogenesis, together with insulin resistance and reduced muscle glycogen storage and metabolism. However, this pattern of energy expenditure is not present in all patients with cirrhosis. The subjects with well compensated, stable cirrhosis are typically hypometabolic and derive about 60% of their energy from fatty acids, similarly to individuals during prolonged starvation (Owen et al. 1983).

31.3 SPECIFIC NUTRIENT DEFICIENCIES IN END-STAGE LIVER DISEASE AND ASSOCIATED CLINICAL FEATURES

Nutrient deficiencies in ESLD include (Table 31.2):

31.3.1 Protein Calorie Malnutrition

Chronic liver disease is associated with disturbances in the metabolism of fats, proteins, and carbohydrates with consequent loss of weight, subcutaneous fat, and skeletal muscle. Various manifestations of protein calorie malnutrition can be identified in up to 100% of patients with advanced alcoholic liver disease (Mendenhall et al. 1984).

31.3.2 Vitamins

Thiamin (dietary deficiency, malabsorption): Wernicke-Korsakoff syndrome characterized by memory loss, unsteady gait, ophthalmoplegia, and peripheral neuropathy, especially in alcoholics.

Vitamin A (malabsorption related to cholestasis): night blindness, follicular rash, and increased risk of cancer development, including hepatocellular carcinoma.

Vitamin D (malabsorption related to cholestasis, reduced exposure to UV lights, and dietary deficiency, treatment with corticosteroids for conditions such as autoimmune hepatitis): osteoporosis and osteomalacia.

Vitamin E (malabsorption related to cholestasis): reduced antioxidant defenses, peripheral neuropathy.

TABLE 31.2
Specific Nutrient Deficiencies and Their Clinical Manifestations

Nutrient Deficiency	Clinical Manifestation
Protein calorie malnutrition	Weight loss, reduced subcutaneous fat, and skeletal muscle
Vitamin B complex	Memory loss, unsteady gait, ophthalmoplegia, peripheral neuropathy
Vitamin A	Night blindness, skin rash, increased risk of cancer
Vitamin D	Osteoporosis and osteomalacia
Vitamin E	Reduced antioxidant defenses
Vitamin K	Increased risk of bleeding
Zinc	Decreased T-cell-mediated immunity, alopecia, encephalopathy
Magnesium	Reduced muscle strength, cardiac arrythmias
Iron	Anemia

Note: Nutrient deficiencies are characterized by specific clinical manifestations.

Vitamin K (malabsorption related to cholestasis, dietary deficiency): increased risk of bleeding.
Folic acid (diet, malabsorption): megaloblastic anemia.

31.3.3 Minerals

Zinc (dietary deficiency, malabsorption, increased urinary excretion due to diuretics): decreased T-cell-mediated immunity, alopecia, acrodermatitis, possible worsened encephalopathy.

Magnesium (dietary deficiency): impaired muscle strength, increased risk of cardiac arrhythmias.

Iron (dietary deficiency, bleeding): microcytic anemia.

31.4 EVALUATION OF NUTRITIONAL STATUS IN END-STAGE LIVER DISEASE

Evaluation of nutritional status in ESLD includes several procedures and techniques (Table 31.3). It has to be noted that conventional methods of nutritional assessment are often confounded by the manifestations of liver failure.

Subjective Global Assessment (SGA): Uses clinical criteria to determine nutritional status without the use of objective measurements. It is more useful than objective measures alone for identifying individuals at nutritional risk because of its ability to take into consideration the multitude of factors influencing the nutritional status (Detsky et al. 1987). The SGA is based on recent weight change, dietary intake, gastrointestinal symptoms (including diarrhea, dysphagia/odynophagia, nausea, vomiting, and anorexia), functional impairment, muscle wasting, subcutaneous fat loss, and edema. The SGA has been shown to be an excellent predictor of outcome in patients undergoing liver transplant (Stephenson et al. 2001).

TABLE 31.3
Measurements of Nutritional Status

Measurement	Measure
Subjective global assessment	Clinical criteria (recent weight change, dietary intake, gastrointestinal symptoms, functional impairment, muscle wasting, subcutaneous fat loss, edema)
Body mass index	Weight (kg)/height $(m)^2$
Anthropometry	Triceps skinfold thickness and mid-arm muscle circumference
Resting energy expenditure	Harris and Benedict equation In men, REE = 66.5 + [13.8 × Wt (kg)] + [5 × Ht (cm)] − [6.755 × A (year)] In women, REE = 655.095 + [9.6 × Wt (kg)] + [1.8 × Ht (cm)] − [4.7 × A (year)] Indirect calorimetry 3.9 VO_2 (inspired) + 1.1 VCO_2 (expired)
Nitrogen balance	Total nitrogen intake is determined from diet, enteral, or parenteral formula consumed by the patient (1 g of nitrogen is represented by 6.25 g of protein) and total nitrogen output is determined by measurements of total nitrogen excreted into urine, stool, and other enteric sources
Bioimpedance analysis	Body fat and fat free mass (FFM), including body cell mass (BCM) and extracellular fluid (ECF)
Urinary creatinine excretion (24 h urine)	Creatinine height index: creatinine excretion measured ÷ creatinine predicted by ideal body weight

Note: Nutritional status can be evaluated by a physical examination but also with more accurate techniques that can provide an objective measurement of the severity of malnutrition.

Body Mass Index (BMI) (weight in kg divided by height in m^2): Campillo et al. (1997) showed that different cut-offs of BMI values can be used as a predictor of malnutrition in patients with various degrees of ascites. In particular, a BMI below 22 in patients without ascites, a BMI below 23 with mild ascites, and below 25 with tense ascites would indicate the presence of malnutrition (Campillo 2006).

Anthropometry: Technique of measuring subcutaneous fat as skinfold thickness using calipers placed on the posterior triceps surface of the upper arm. Muscle mass is estimated from the circumference of the mid upper arm less the product of pi (π, 3.14) and the triceps skinfold thickness. This method can be affected by edema (Heymsfield and Casper 1987). However, mid-arm muscle circumference was found to be an independent predictor of mortality in cirrhosis (Alvares-da-Silva and Reverbel da Silveira 2005). It was also independently associated with survival and improved prognostic accuracy when combined with the Child score (Alberino et al. 2001).

Total Energy Expenditure (TEE) and Resting Energy Expenditure (REE): Energy expenditure (kcal/day) is composed of resting energy expenditure (REE, about 80%), and the remainder as physical exercise and the cost of digestion of the diet. In patients with cirrhosis, total energy expenditure should be measured by indirect calorimetry (Weir 1990). A study on more than 300 cirrhotic patients indicated that the measurement of TEE and REE is essential to distinguish hyper- and hypometabolic patients in order to design a personalized nutritional strategy that can improve morbidity and mortality (Guglielmi et al. 2005).

Nitrogen Balance: Measurement of the nitrogen balance is used to determine if the patient is building (anabolic status) or breaking down (catabolic status) body protein stores before and during nutritional support. In practice, total nitrogen intake can be determined from diet, enteral, or parenteral formula consumed by the patient (where 1 g of nitrogen is represented by 6.25 g of protein), while total nitrogen output is determined by measurements of total nitrogen excreted into urine, stool, and other enteric sources such as fistulous drainage. Several studies have indicated clinical improvements associated with positive nitrogen balance (Soberon et al. 1987). Despite its definite clinical utility, nitrogen balance measurement is normally confined to clinical trials.

Visceral Protein Plasma Concentration (albumin, prealbumin, transferrin, retinol-binding protein): Visceral protein measurement is sensitive to protein calorie malnutrition but is often non-specific in liver disease, where serum levels are affected by abnormal hepatic synthesis and fluid overload.

Handgrip Strength: Hand dynamometry (Alvares-da-Silva and Reverbel da Silveira 2005) is a validated method for nutritional assessment; it is low-cost, simple, and rapid. It allows identification of those patients who are at higher risk of developing complications related to malnutrition and it correlates with poorer clinical outcome (Alvares-da-Silva and Reverbel da Silveira 2005). A limitation of handgrip strength is that subject cooperation is required. Subject cooperation may limit the use of handgrip strength in patients because they are not sufficiently conscious to cooperate or results may not be accurate because of limited efforts by compromised subjects.

Bioimpedance Analysis (BIA): Using electrodes on the dorsal surface of the hands and feet and a weak current, BIA compares the electrical conductivity through body fat (greatest impedance) and body water (least impedance) to determine fat and lean body mass. It is considered a useful method for the quantification of fat and muscle mass in patients without fluid retention and has been used to identify protein calorie malnutrition in compensated cirrhotic patients without significant edema. BIA was shown to correlate with survival in patients with cirrhosis (Selberg and Selberg 2002) but it is in general an impractical method in assessing fluid-overloaded patients.

24-Urinary Excretion of Creatinine: Creatinine is the metabolic product of the skeletal muscle protein creatine, where 18.5 kg of muscle is represented by 1 g of urinary creatinine per day. With stable daily renal function, creatinine excretion correlates well with body cell mass in cirrhosis of various etiologies (Pirlich et al. 1996). Creatinine urinary excretion less than 60% of the normal value (23 mg/kg ideal weight in men and 18 mg/kg ideal weight in women) indicates malnutrition.

31.5 TREATMENT

The rationale for considering nutritional support as part of the comprehensive treatment of the patient with chronic liver disease is based on the high prevalence of malnutrition in this patient population and the concept that improved nutritional status may improve liver function and consequently positively affect survival. Additionally, it is anticipated that maximizing health through improved nutrition may optimize the long-term potential benefits of liver transplantation. The first recommendation is to evaluate the nutritional status and the nutritional needs to determine which approach is most appropriate (oral supplementation, enteral tube feeding, and/or parenteral nutrition). Evaluation of the severity of malnutrition in liver disease requires awareness of the history of appetite and weight change, recognition of the physical signs of malnutrition, and laboratory testing for specific micronutrient deficiencies (Table 31.4 and 31.5).

Patients should be recommended to consume frequent (from 5 to 7) and small meals during the day with one late evening snack and to follow a low-salt diet with a maximum sodium content of 2 g daily. Physicians should avoid prolonged food deprivation, especially during hospitalizations when patients are scheduled to undergo procedures that require fasting. The low sodium diet may be challenging to follow but, with adequate adherence, will minimize use of diuretics and improve fluid retention in patients with cirrhosis.

Patients with cirrhosis should have an intake of 35–40 kcal/kg/day (dry body weight) with a protein intake of up to 1.6 g/kg/day (Nompleggi and Bonkovsky 1994).

Oral Supplementation: When counseling and regular diet are not sufficient to achieve the goal of 35–40 kcal/kg/day, oral nutritional supplements should be considered. A trained dietician should obtain a 3-day diet record in order to determine whether the patient will be able to tolerate oral nutritional supplementation. Oral supplementation with a conventional formula to assure a total intake of 35 kcal and up to 2 g protein/kg body weight is indicated in the non-anorectic patient

TABLE 31.4
Clinical Evaluation of Malnutrition in End-Stage Liver Disease

History
weight loss, loss of appetite, vomiting, diarrhea, decreased energy level
Physical Examination
Loss of subcutaneous fat, skeletal muscle wasting in the temporal areas
Skin rash (flaky paint, hyperfollicular rash)
Glossitis
Ophthalmoplegia
Peripheral neuropathy, ataxic gait, memory loss
Laboratory Tests
Visceral protein plasma concentration (albumin, prealbumin, transferrin, retinol-binding protein)
Vitamin and mineral levels in blood (folate, vitamin B12, iron, vitamins A, D, E, zinc, and magnesium

Note: The evaluation of malnutrition is based on accurate clinical examination and laboratory tests that will assess specific nutrient deficiencies.

TABLE 31.5
Nutritional Support Approaches

Method	Use	Risks and Complications
Oral supplementation	Moderate malnutrition	Inadequate nutrient intake; poor control of nutrient intake
Enteral tube feeding	Moderate to severe malnutrition; encephalopathy	Gastrointestinal bleeding, vomiting, bronchopulmonary aspiration
Parenteral nutrition	Severe malnutrition; liver failure, malabsorption	Sepsis, pneumothorax, excessive fluid load

Note: Nutritional support in end-stage liver disease can be provided by improvement of the oral diet (oral supplementation), by administration of nutrients through tubes positioned in the gastrointestinal tract (enteral tube feeding), or by administration of nutrients through intravenous access (parenteral nutrition).

with compensated cirrhosis and moderate malnutrition. The supplementation of dietary calories at 40 kcal/day and protein 1.5 g/kg/day to severely malnourished cirrhotic patients with alcoholic liver disease for 30 days was well tolerated and improved body fat mass, increased carbohydrate oxidation, and increased body fat storage. These metabolic changes were also paralleled by improved liver function in the subgroup with decompensated liver disease (Child-Pugh class C) (Campillo et al. 1997).

Enteral Tube Feeding: Enteral tube feeding should be considered for patients with ESLD who are typically malnourished and anorectic. This method allows the provision of predetermined and calculated amounts and volumes of calories, protein, electrolytes, and all essential nutrients through a nasogastric or nasoenteric (nasoduodenal or nasojejunal) feeding tube to patients with adequate intestinal absorption (Soberon et al. 1987). Nasoenteric tubes are in general considered a better option but their positioning requires an endoscopic procedure which still limits their application in the normal clinical practice. In patients with ascites and peripheral edema, the use of whole protein and high-energy formulae is recommended. Branched-chain amino acid-enriched formulae are used in patients with hepatic encephalopathy. Pancreatic enzymes should be provided in addition, in particular in case of alcoholic liver disease where pancreatic insufficiency is common. In a randomized trial, patients with alcoholic hepatitis were treated for 4 weeks with a concentrated low-sodium enteral formula providing 35 kcal and 1.25 g protein/kg body weight with equal, approximately 40%, caloric proportions of carbohydrate and fat. Patients were compared to subjects who received conventional hospital diet. Compared to matched control group, patients who received the enteral formula demonstrated improved hepatic encephalopathy and decreased serum bilirubin levels (Kearns et al. 1992). Tube-fed patients demonstrated significantly lower in-hospital mortality compared to a matched control group that received the same amount of calories and protein through an ad libitum oral hospital diet (Cabré et al. 1990). Concerns related to enteral tube feeding in patients with ESLD are represented by gastrointestinal bleeding from esophageal or gastric varices and repeated vomiting with possible bronchopulmonary aspiration.

Percutaneous Feeding Gastrostomy: This procedure consists in the placement of a feeding tube through the skin and the stomach wall, directly into the stomach, and may be indicated in patients with esophageal strictures. However, ascites, impaired coagulation function, and portosystemic collateral circulation associated with portal hypertension limit the use of this procedure in patients with ESLD.

Parenteral Nutrition: Parenteral nutrition support through a catheter positioned in the central vein is the most reasonable approach in the more severely ill and malnourished patients with a greater degree of encephalopathy and fluid retention. Parenterally administered amino acids do not appear to worsen encephalopathy whereas volume and electrolytes can be managed very closely. A meta-analysis of very heterogeneous studies using parenteral nutrition in hepatic coma showed probable improved survival (Naylor et al. 1989). Possible complications of parenteral nutrition are represented by pneumothorax, sepsis, and a supply of an excessive fluid load. However, none of the available studies on parenteral nutrition used detailed measurements of energy and protein requirements and studies comparing parenteral and enteral feeding in ESLD are lacking.

31.6 APPLICATIONS TO OTHER AREAS OF TERMINAL OR PALLIATIVE CARE

1. ESLD is one of the major causes of terminal illness, responsible for 8.8 deaths per 100,000 persons annually in the United States.
2. Severe malnutrition is associated with and can precipitate the typical manifestations of ESLD, including hepatic encephalopathy, ascites, and hepatorenal syndrome. All these complications are very frequently seen in the palliative care setting.
3. Appropriate management of malnutrition will prevent complications of ESLD and improve the quality of life of terminally ill patients.

31.7 PRACTICAL METHODS AND TECHNIQUES

Required nutrient intake in patients with cirrhosis:
Proteins: 1.2–1.6 g/kg/day
Vitamin A: 3000 μg daily
Vitamin D: 50 μg daily
Vitamin K: 120 μg daily
Vitamin E: 1000 mg daily

KEY POINTS OF MALNUTRITION IN END-STAGE LIVER DISEASE

1. Malnutrition is nearly universal in ESLD and is characterized by depletion of body fat, proteins, and many micronutrient deficiencies.
2. The clinical evaluation of malnutrition includes history of significant weight loss and gastrointestinal symptoms; physical examination with particular attention to body weight, muscle mass, and skin; and specialized procedures to measure energy expenditure, skeletal protein mass, and nitrogen balance.
3. The rationale for nutritional support in chronic liver disease includes the prognostic relation between the severity of malnutrition and long-term survival.

ETHICAL ISSUES

The main controversial issue in managing malnourished ESLD patients is represented by the decision to institute parenteral nutrition.

1. Parenteral nutrition is an expensive therapeutic modality that is used to treat patients with intestinal malabsorption. The benefits it offers in terms of life prolongation have to be weighed against its risks and burdens. Ethical issues are implicated in the decisions to administer and, more importantly, to withhold or withdraw parenteral nutrition in patients with ESLD who are not candidates for liver transplantation.
2. The decision to start or withdraw parenteral nutrition should be taken autonomously by the patient but this is not always possible due to encephalopathy in ESLD. This can affect the understanding and participation of the patient in the decision regarding his nutritional support.

3. Nutrition in terminal patients with ESLD should have the only aim to improve the quality of life with the understanding that food has much more significance than simple nutrient provision.

SUMMARY POINTS

- Malnutrition has a very important clinical significance in ESLD and it correlates with the severity of liver disease, survival, and post liver transplant complications.
- The mechanisms leading to malnutrition in ESLD are decreased nutrient intake, decreased intestinal absorption of nutrients, and metabolic disturbances with increased energy expenditure typical of cirrhosis.
- Nutritional status can be assessed by subjective global assessment, body mass index, anthropometry, total energy expenditure, nitrogen balance, visceral protein plasma concentration, handgrip strength, and bioimpedance analysis.
- Adequate nutritional support can improve survival and reduce the risks of complications associated with ESLD. Nutritional support can be provided through oral supplementation, enteral tube feeding, percutaneous gastrostomy, and parenteral nutrition.

LIST OF ABBREVIATION

ESLD End-stage liver disease

REFERENCES

Alberino, F., A. Gatta, P. Amodio, C. Merkel, L. Di Pascoli, G. Boffo, and L. Caregaro. 2001. Nutrition and survival in patients with liver cirrhosis. *Nutrition* 17:445–50.

Alvares-da-Silva, M. R., and T. Reverbel da Silveira. 2005. Comparison between handgrip strength, subjective global assessment and prognostic nutritional index in assessing malnutrition and predicting outcome in cirrhotic outpatients. *Nutrition* 21:113–17.

Cabré, E., F. Gonzalez-Huix, A. Abad-Lacruz, M. Esteve, D. Acero, F. Fernandez-Bañares, X. Xiol, and M. A. Gassull. 1990. Effect of total enteral nutrition on the short-term outcome of severely malnourished cirrhotics. A randomized controlled trial. *Gastroenterology* 98:715–20.

Campillo, B., P. N. Bories, B. Pornin, and M. Devanlay. 1997. Influence of liver failure, ascites, and energy expenditure on the response to oral nutrition in alcoholic liver cirrhosis. *Nutrition* 13:613–21.

Campillo, B. 2006. Validation of body mass index for the diagnosis of malnutrition in patients with liver cirrhosis. *Gastroenterol Clin Biol* 30:1137–43.

Detsky, A. S., J. R. McLaughlin, J. P. Baker, N. Johnston, S. Whittaker, R. A. Mendelson, and K. N. Jeejeebhoy. 1987. What is subjective global assessment of nutritional status? *JPEN* 11:8–13.

Greco, A. V., G. Mingrone, G. Benedetti, E. Capristo, P. A. Tataranni, and G. Gasbarrini. 1998. Daily energy and substrate metabolism in patients with cirrhosis. *Hepatology* 27:346–50.

Guglielmi, F. W., C. Panella, A. Buda, G. Budillon, L. Caregaro, C. Clerici, D. Conte et al. 2005. Nutritional state and energy balance in cirrhotic patients with or without hypermetabolism. Multicentre prospective study by the 'Nutritional Problems in Gastroenterology' Section of the Italian Society of Gastroenterology (SIGE). *Dig Liver Dis* 37:681–88.

Gunsar, F., M. L. Raimondo, S. Jones, N. Terreni, C. Wong, D. Patch, C. Sabin, and A. K. Burroughs. 2006. Nutritional status and prognosis in cirrhotic patients. *Aliment Pharmacol Ther* 24:563–72.

Heymsfield, S. B, and K. Casper. 1987. Anthropometric assessment of the adult hospitalized patient. *J Parenter Enteral Nutr* 11:36S–41S.

Kearns, P. J., H. Young, G. Garcia, T. Blaschke, G. O'Hanlon, M. Rinki, K. Sucher, and P. Gregory. 1992. Accelerated improvement of alcoholic liver disease with enteral nutrition. *Gastroenterology* 102:200–5.

McCullough, A. J., E. Bugianesi, G. Marchesini, and S. C. Kalhan. 1998. Gender-dependent alterations in serum leptin in alcoholic cirrhosis. *Gastroenterology* 115:947–53.

Mendenhall, C. L., S. Anderson, R. E. Weesner, S. J. Goldberg, and K. A. Crolic. 1984. Protein-calorie malnutrition associated with alcoholic hepatitis. Veterans Administration Cooperative Study Group on Alcoholic Hepatitis. *Am J Med* 76:211–22.

Merli, M, M. Giusto, F. Gentili, G. Novelli, G. Ferretti, O. Riggio, S. G. Corradini et al. 2009. Nutritional status: Its influence on the outcome of patients undergoing liver transplantation. *Liver Int* 30:208–14.

Naylor, C. D., K. O'Rourke, A. S. Detsky, and J. P. Baker. 1989. Parenteral nutrition with branched-chain amino acids in hepatic encephalopathy. A meta-analysis. *Gastroenterology* 97:1033–42.

Nompleggi, D, and H. L. Bonkovsky. 1994. Nutritional supplementation in chronic liver disease: An analytical review. *Hepatology* 19:518–33.

Pikul, J, M. D. Sharpe, R. Lowndes, and C. N. Ghent. 1994. Degree of preoperative malnutrition is predictive of postoperative morbidity and mortality in liver transplant recipients. *Transplantation* 57:469–72.

Owen, O. E., V. E. Trapp, G. A. Reichard, Jr, M. A. Mozzoli, J. Moctezuma, P. Paul, C. L. Skutches, and G. Boden. 1983. Nature and quantity of fuels consumed in patients with alcoholic cirrhosis. *J Clin Invest* 72:1821–32.

Pirlich, M., O. Selberg, K. Böker, M. Schwarze, M. J. Müller. 1996. The creatinine approach to estimate skeletal muscle mass in patients with cirrhosis. *Hepatology* 24:1422–27.

Roggin, G. M., F. L. Iber, and W. G. Linscheer. 1972. Intraluminal fat digestion in the chronic alcoholic. *Gut* 13:107–11.

Selberg, O, and D. Selberg. 2002. Norms and correlates of bioimpedance phase angle in healthy human subjects, hospitalized patients, and patients with liver cirrhosis. *Eur J Appl Physiol* 86:509–16.

Soberon, S., M. P. Pauley, R. Duplantier, A. Fan, and C. H. Halsted. 1987. Metabolic effects of enteral formula feeding in alcoholic hepatitis. *Hepatology* 6:1204–9.

Stephenson, G. R., E. W. Moretti, H. El-Moalem, P. A. Clavien, and J. E. Tuttle-Newhall. 2001. Malnutrition in liver transplant patients: Preoperative subjective global assessment is predictive of outcome after liver transplantation. *Transplantation* 27:666–70.

Weir, J. B. 1990. New methods for calculating metabolic rate with special reference to protein metabolism. *Nutrition* 6:213–21.

32 Nutritional Therapy in Amyotrophic Lateral Sclerosis

Katja Kollewe, Sonja Körner, Reinhard Dengler, and Susanne Petri

CONTENTS

32.1 INTRODUCTION

Amyotrophic lateral sclerosis (ALS) is a devastating neurodegenerative disorder. The highest incidence is in adults aged 50–70 years, with men marginally more affected than women, and lies between 2 and 3 per 100,000 adults. The disease is sporadic in 90%–95%, 5%–10% of ALS patients present with the familiar form, and 5%–10% of these have a mutation in the gene coding for superoxide 1 (SOD1). The etiology of the disease remains unclear, even though a variety of pathomechanisms such as glutamate excitotoxicity, oxidative stress, lack of neurotrophic factors, defects in axonal transport, accumulation of intracellular aggregates, and aberrant RNA metabolism have been identified.

Selective loss of upper and lower motor neurons in the primary motor cortex, brainstem, and spinal cord results in rapidly progressive paralysis of skeletal muscles and therefore a decline of motor functions at spinal and bulbar levels. Pelvic sphincters are usually spared. Death usually occurs within 3–5 years, mostly because of respiratory failure, even though longer survival times are observed in a small percentage of patients. Two onset forms are differentiated: the bulbar onset and the limb onset form. It is well known that the limb onset form has a longer survival than the bulbar one (Kollewe et al. 2008).

The patient's nutrition and hydration can be affected in two ways: First, swallowing function can be affected when dysphagia becomes evident. Secondly, due to upper extremity weakness, preparing, cutting, and eating food can become difficult. Moreover, it is known that hypermetabolism leads to weight loss even before dysphagia occurs (Bouteloup et al. 2009). Several studies found that malnutrition and associated weight loss in ALS is an independent negative prognostic factor for survival. Therefore, the nutritional status should be routinely monitored to identify poor dietary intake and malnutrition. When dysphagia progresses and management of dysphagia with modification of food consistency, dietary advice, and special swallowing techniques fails, the necessity of enteral nutrition via PEG or PRG/RIG grows. Data to support the use of PEG tubes are controversial: Some authors have reported prolonged survival (Chio et al. 2002; Mazzini et al. 1995) while others have reported no such effect (Desport et al. 2000; Forbes, Colville, and Swingler 2004; Mitsumoto et al. 2003). However, there are no randomized controlled trials focusing on the use of PEG in ALS patients and Miller et al. conclude that "PEG should be considered for prolonging survival in patients with ALS" in the current update of the practice parameters in the care of the patient with ALS (Miller et al. 2009).

In the following sections, nutrition principles, management of dysphagia, and enteral feeding in ALS patients are described in detail.

32.2 NUTRITION PRINCIPLES IN ALS

Malnutrition and subsequent weight loss are significant and independent negative prognostic indices for survival. Inadequate dietary intake will exacerbate catabolism and atrophies of limb and respiratory muscles. In addition, suboptimal nutrition can weaken the immune system, which contributes to infections, a common cause of death in ALS. The benefits of aggressive and early nutritional therapy can profoundly influence the disease course, quality of life, and survival (Rosenfeld and Ellis 2008).

There is evidence that ALS patients develop a paradoxical state of hypermetabolism, the origin of which has not been fully elucidated to date. Hypotheses include spasticity and fasciculations or increased respiratory work, but increased resting energy expenditure (REE) has also been reported. The cause of that increased REE is unknown but growing evidence points to an important role of impaired mitochondrial function (Bouteloup et al. 2009; Vaisman et al. 2009).

Furthermore, hand and arm weakness (Figure 32.1) can lead to slower eating and render food intake embarrassing for patients. Psychological distress and depression are common in ALS patients and can also lead to decreased food intake. Thus patients can very quickly become deprived of protein, calories, and vitamins as their food and fluid consumption may be restricted already before dysphagia is existent (Kurt et al. 2007).

The management of nutrition necessitates continual assessment and implementation of dietary modification throughout the entire clinical course of the disease. Weight and body mass index

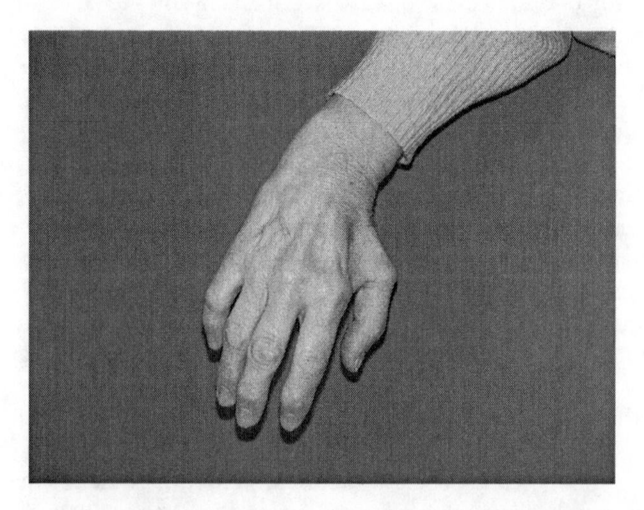

FIGURE 32.1 Hand atrophy. Wasting of the dorsal interosseous muscles. This patient suffered from weakness of both hands. (From Kollewe, K, and Petri, S., *Klinische Neurophysiologie*, 40 (1): 3–14, 2009, with permission from Thieme.)

should be monitored closely. Dietary recall and maintaining a dietary log are very useful, but are difficult for patients to provide, as they often have difficulty speaking and writing and/or overestimate their alimentary intake (Desport et al. 2000).

For patients with hand and arm weakness, physical and occupational therapy is essential. Further feeding assistance like hand braces, altered utensils, mobile arm supports, and modified plates, bowels, and cups should be provided (Rosenfeld and Ellis 2008). Calorically dense and rich meals are recommended for ALS patients already in early disease stages. A well-controlled diet should include enough calories to meet the metabolic needs of the individual and the generation of sufficient fat stores to compensate for the energy lost in muscle mass (Hardiman 2000). This recommendation is supported by a study of Dupuis and colleagues (Dupuis et al. 2008) in which hyperlipidemia was found as a positive prognostic factor for survival in ALS. A dietician experienced in problems associated with neuromuscular diseases should be involved, who can provide alternative high-calorie foods and/or liquids to incorporate into daily meals. Besides an abundant calorie supply, adequate intake of vitamins should be warranted. Especially the supplementation of vitamin D is important, because ALS patients often are deficient in vitamin D due to poor dietary intake and being in a sunlight-deprived state. The physical inactivity further improves the risk of osteoporosis (Heffernan et al. 2004).

Decreased physical mobility and decreased fluid intake often result in constipation. Delayed gastric emptying and delayed colonic transit have been shown in ALS patients (Toepfer et al. 1999). For those patients, high-fiber foods, fruit, and milk of magnesia, and fixed meal times to produce bowel regularity may be helpful. Sometimes osmotic laxatives, bulk-forming laxatives, suppositories, or enemas are necessary (Heffernan et al. 2004).

Self-medication with dietary supplements has become increasingly popular among ALS patients and is used by approximately 80% of them (Miller et al. 2009). Such "nutraceuticals" are supposed to affect proposed mechanisms leading to motor neuron death and are often self-prescribed based on theoretical benefits or anecdotal reports (Rosenfeld and Ellis 2008). Some examples of the numerous dietary supplements are vitamin E, vitamin C, B vitamins, selenium, zinc, genistein, melatonin, creatine, coenzyme Q10, alpha-lipoic acid, L-carnitine, ginseng, and many others (see Table 32.1). Most patients take several supplements simultaneously. There is insufficient evidence of efficacy of individual functional food in the treatment of patients with ALS, so that at present a valid recommendation cannot be given. But high tolerance, safety, relatively low costs, and lack of other effective treatments for ALS explain the continuing use of these dietary supplements by physicians and patients. While until now there has been no substantial clinical trial evidence to support their use, there is no clear contraindication (Orrell, Lane, and Ross 2007). Further studies are needed to evaluate the safety and efficacy of numerous dietary supplements to give appropriate recommendations for their intake.

32.3 MANAGEMENT OF DYSPHAGIA

Dysphagia is an inevitable consequence of cranial motor neuron loss (cranial nerves IX, X, XII) in the pons and medulla. The complaints of eating difficulties can be traced to impairments of mastication, manipulation of food bolus, and deglutition. The appearance of bulbar weakness (Figure 32.2) can occur at any time during the clinical course of ALS and carries an adverse prognostic implication for survival of the patient (Desport et al. 1999). Oropharyngeal weakness affects survival in ALS in two ways. First, it places the patient at continuous risk of aspiration, pneumonia and sepsis. Second, it may curtail the intake of adequate energy. Mealtimes become longer when accompanied by coughing, choking, and drooling. Patients have to eat slowly and eating is transformed to an anxiety-provoking, labor-intensive, tiresome, and time-consuming chore (Golaszewski 2007).

To identify symptoms of dysphagia as early as possible, a careful history should be obtained at each visit. There is no single test to detect dysphagia in patients with ALS. Specific questions regarding the physical manipulation of food and fluid (e.g., frequency of choking, texture of foods, food spillage from the oral cavity), duration of mealtime, and fatigue while eating are essential.

TABLE 32.1
An Overview of Nutritional Supplements and Functional Foods

Nutritional Supplement	Mechanism of Action (Hypothesis)
Selenium	Antioxidants
Vitamin C	Antioxidants
Vitamin A	Antioxidants
Vitamin E	Antioxidants
Curcumin	Antioxidants
Ginseng	Antioxidants
Glutathione	Antioxidants
NAC	Antioxidants
Lipoic acid	Antioxidants/antiglutamate
Green tea	Antioxidants
MAK	Antioxidants
Phytoestrogens	Antioxidants/antiglutamate
Grape seed extract	Antioxidants/antiglutamate
Pycnogenol	Antioxidants/antiglutamate
Creatinin	Antioxidants/antiglutamate/mitochondrial stabilizers
Monohydrate	Antioxidants/antiglutamate/mitochondrial stabilizers
Carnitin	Antioxidants/mitochondrial stabilizers
CoQ10	Antioxidants/mitochondrial stabilizers
Ginkgo biloba	Antioxidants/mitochondrial stabilizers
DHEA	Antiglutamate
Vitamin B12	Other agents
Vitamin B6	Other agents
Folate	Other agents
Zinc	Other agents

Source: Modified from Cameron, A., Rosenfeld, J., *Curr. Opin. Clin. Nutr. Metab. Care*, 5, 631, 2002, with permission from Wolters Kluwer Health..
Note: Nutritional supplements and functional foods with hypothesis of function.

Furthermore, as dehydration often occurs in patients with dysphagia, symptoms of dehydration such as generalized feeling of malaise, decreased urine output, dry mouth, thick mucous, inability to handle pulmonary secretions, and decreased skin turgor should be evaluated at each visit.

Early referrals to speech and language therapists are advocated as they can determine the presence, severity, and nature or pattern of impairment, and the ability of the patient to benefit from direct behavioral treatment to improve the swallowing function. Furthermore they can help the patients to eat more safely and efficiently and impart swallowing techniques to reduce risks of choking and aspiration, such as supraglottic swallowing and postural changes. For example, when the neck is flexed, with the chin down toward the chest, the airway is partially blocked by the epiglottis and the risk of aspiration is decreased (chin tuck maneuver). In addition, patients can be taught to take a breath before swallowing, hold the breath, forcefully exhale, or gently cough after the swallow, then to swallow again (double swallow). This can avoid the quick intake of air prior to coughing, which would suck the aspirated debris deeper into the airway. Finally the environment provided for meals should be free from unnecessary distractions and the patient must avoid talking while eating.

In consultation with a dietician, identification of problem foods, which cause difficulty in swallowing, changes in food consistencies, and feeding strategies can also be made. A pureed diet is probably the universal dysphagia diet. Pureed food requires no chewing, is easy to transport to the pharynx, travels down the pharynx at a slower rate than liquids, and is unlikely to cause permanent obstruction in the lungs if aspirated, thus making it of a safer consistency than liquids or solid food (Heffernan et al. 2004).

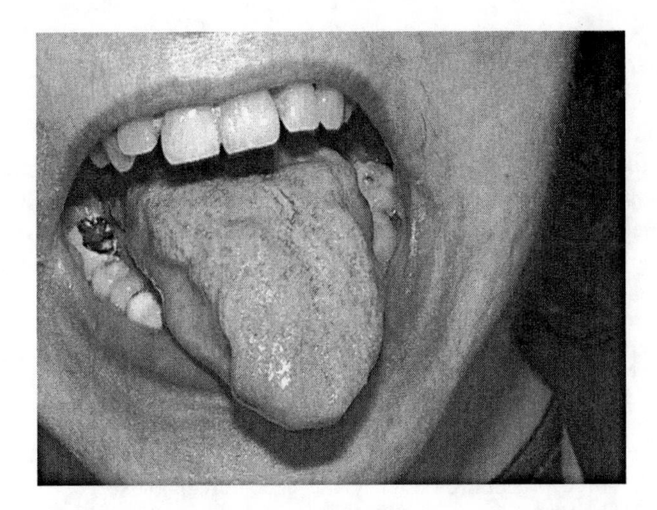

FIGURE 32.2 Tongue atrophy. Tongue atrophy in an ALS patient with bulbar symptoms (dysphagia, dysarthria). (From Kollewe, K, and Petri, S., *Klinische Neurophysiologie*, 40 (1): 3–14, 2009, with permission from Thieme.)

Thin liquids are often seen to spill into the pharynx before the swallow is triggered and are sometimes aspirated, so the use of thicker liquids or the addition of thickeners to liquids is recommended. If patients are restricted to a pureed diet and thick liquids in order to prevent aspiration pneumonia, pulmonary health may benefit but often patients do not consume enough calories because this diet is so unappetizing (Langmore 1999). Hence in some patients a "soft mechanical" diet, which includes meats that are ground or well cooked but require some mastication, may be an alternative. Studies on nursing home residents revealed that many patients are able to swallow food of more solid consistency without complications of pneumonia or weight loss. Patients having difficulty swallowing thin liquids could try to drink carbonated fluids or ice cold fluids before using thickeners to liquids. Mainly in spastic dysphagia due to upper motor neuron loss these techniques can be beneficial. In addition foods that help with liquid ingestion are jello, frozen popsicles, and fruit ice (Andersen et al. 2007) (overview of treatment of weight loss in Table 32.2).

Dependency of feeding and oral care are stronger predictors of pneumonia than dysphagia itself. Thus carers need to be trained to feed patients in a safe way that does not promote aspiration and should also encourage their patients to eat adequate amounts. In addition, intensive oral care should

TABLE 32.2
Treatment of Weight Loss in ALS

Causes of Reduced Food Intake	Treatment
Hand/arm weakness	Physical and occupational therapy
	Hand braces, altered utensils, mobile arm supports, and modified plates, bowls, and cups
	Feeding assistance
Psychological distress/depression	Psychotherapy
	Antidepressants
Bulbar symptoms	Speech and language therapy
	Impart swallowing techniques
	"Soft mechanical" or pureed diet
	Carbonated or ice cold fluids or addition of thickeners to liquids
	Enteral nutrition via PEG or PRG/RIG

Note: Causes of reduced food intake and treatment.

be provided, to avoid gingivitis, excessive plaque, or periodontal disease, which increase amounts of virulent bacteria that are pathogenic to the lungs (Langmore 1999; Langmore et al. 1998).

An effective treatment for sialorrhea (prevalence estimated at 50% of ALS patients), which is associated with aspiration pneumonia, is recommended. First anticholinergic medications should be tried. In patients with medically refractory sialorrhea, botulinum toxin injections into the salivary glands or radiation therapy can be considered (Andersen et al. 2007; Miller et al. 2009).

In summary, an effective dysphagia management program must include advice from a dietician and speech and language therapist as well as attention to the feeding environment and implementation of safe feeding and oral care protocols.

32.4 ENTERAL NUTRITION IN ALS

When dysphagia progresses and the above-mentioned measures become insufficient, the maintenance of enteral nutrition via a gastric tube feeding becomes necessary and surgical interventions must be considered. Three procedures obviate the need for major surgery and general anesthesia: percutaneous endoscopic gastrostomy (PEG), percutaneous radiologic gastrostomy (PRG), and nasogastric tube (NGT) feeding. Data to support the use of PEG tubes are controversial. Some authors reported prolonged survival (Chio et al. 2002; Mazzini et al. 1995) while others reported no such effect (Desport et al. 2000; Forbes et al. 2004; Mitsumoto et al. 2003). A Cochrane review on tube feeding for ALS/motor neuron disease (MND) found no randomized controlled trials comparing the efficacy of enteral tube feeding to those without. Since no such trials have been published so far, all prospective and retrospective controlled studies were reviewed. The authors concluded that at the stage of dysphagia the placing of a PEG may be recommended to maintain adequate nutrition and that, based on controlled prospective cohort studies, an advantage for survival in ALS/MND patients was suggested, but that these conclusions are tentative (Langmore et al. 2006).

32.4.1 Nasogastric Tube in ALS

NGT is a non-invasive procedure that should only be used for short-term feeding in patients who are unfit for either PEG or RIG, as this method presents numerous disadvantages. NGT increases oropharyngeal secretions, can lead to aspiration of tube feeding, can be associated with nasopharyngeal discomfort and pain, and bears the risk of ulceration. However, NGT has also advantages: it can be used if the patient has markedly reduced vital capacity and is not suitable for PEG; it is less invasive and may be replaced in the home environment (Heffernan et al. 2004). If tubes are removed and replaced regularly, it is an adequate short-term option to maintain nutrition for up to several months (Borasio et al. 2001).

32.4.2 Percutaneous Endoscopic Gastrostomy in ALS

PEG is currently the method of choice for enteral nutrition in ALS patients with pronounced dysphagia. Research in the field of permanent gastrostomy has involved PEG almost exclusively. Nevertheless, there are no randomized controlled trials focusing on the use of PEG in ALS patients. PEG is widely available and is one of the most effective means of proactive intervention to stabilize and maintain body weight and hydration (Desport et al. 2000; Heffernan et al. 2004; Miller et al. 2009). PEG insertion is safe and well tolerated, with very low acute and long-term morbidity.

32.4.2.1 Timing of PEG Tube Placement

No consensus on the best timing for PEG placement in ALS patients has been reached to date. It is dependent on weight loss, severity of dysphagia, nutritional status, respiratory function (vital capacity), and general condition of the patient (Table 32.3) (Heffernan et al. 2004; Miller et al. 1999). The current guidelines recommend that PEG insertion should be performed prior to the loss of 5%–10%

TABLE 32.3
Timing of PEG Insertion

Timing of PEG insertion is dependent on
Nutritional status
General condition of the patient
Weight loss
Severity of dysphagia
Respiratory function

Note: Timing of PEG insertion is dependent on several factors.

of body weight and before the forced vital capacity (FVC) falls below 50% of predicted value to minimize the risk of respiratory compromise during the procedure (Andersen et al. 2007; Miller et al. 2009). The reasons for limitations in patients with moderate (FVC 30%–50%) and severe (FVC <30%) dyspnea are not entirely clear but may be related to a further reduction in diaphragm mobility during and after the surgical procedure. During the procedure, mild sedation is required. Therefore, PEG implantation is more hazardous in ALS patients with respiratory impairment. In patients with respiratory impairment with a FVC below 50%, alternatively, a biphasic positive airway pressure mask for continuous non-invasive ventilation during PEG placement can be used (Heffernan et al. 2004; Miller et al. 1999).

Consensus among practitioners suggests the strategy "the earlier, the better" in the course of progressive dysphagia and respiratory insufficiency. This approach allows the patient and the caregivers to use the PEG incrementally.

32.4.2.2 PEG and Aspiration

There is no evidence that PEG reduces the risk of aspiration (Hardiman 2000). PEG does not reduce oropharyngeal secretion or reduce the risk of aspiration of gastric contents. For patients in whom recurrent aspiration is a problem, laryngeal diversion or laryngectomy has been advocated. A meta-analysis of the literature showed a significantly greater risk of aspiration associated with PEG than with PRG. PEG implantation theoretically can further increase the risk of aspiration during and immediately after the procedure. This proposed risk relates to the following purposes: degree of conscious sedation required during PEG implantation; degree of pharyngeal anesthesia required; mechanical stress imposed during endoscopy (Thornton et al. 2002).

32.4.3 Percutaneous Radiologic Gastrostomy/Radiologically Inserted Gastrostomy

This procedure is a newer alternative to PEG in ALS patients. The major advantage of the method is that it needs no or less sedation and can therefore be performed in patients with moderate (FVC 30%–50%) or severe (FVC <30%) respiratory impairment and/or in ALS patients in poor general condition. Non-invasive positive pressure ventilation can be used during PRG/RIG insertion in patients with evidence of respiratory failure. It allows gas exchange to be maintained while lying flat for the PRG/RIG procedure, thereby the risk of carbon dioxide retention and a drop in oxygen saturation is reduced (Lyall et al. 2001). Another advantage is the potentially reduced risk of perioperative aspiration and the avoided risk of oropharyngeal trauma from endoscopy. PRG/RIG may also be undertaken in patients in whom PEG has been unsuccessful (Chio et al. 2004; Thornton et al. 2002). A disadvantage of PRG/RIG can be the smaller caliber of the tube, which bears a greater risk of obstruction. This can be overcome by replacement of the first tube with a greater caliber 15–30 days after insertion.

TABLE 32.4
PEG versus PRG/RIG in ALS Patients with Dysphagia

	Advantages	Disadvantages
PEG	Currently the method of choice in ALS patients Well documented Widely available One of the most effective means of proactive intervention to stabilize and maintain body weight and hydration Insertion safe and well tolerated with very low acute and long-term morbidity	No consensus about the best timing for PEG placement Mild sedation is required during the insertion procedure Limitations in patients with moderate and severe dyspnea Significantly greater risk of aspiration associated with PEG than with PRG
PRG/RIG	Needs no or less sedation Can be performed in patients with moderate or severe respiratory impairment and in patients in poor general condition Non-invasive positive pressure ventilation can be used during insertion Potentially reduced risk of perioperative aspiration Avoided risk of oropharyngeal trauma from endoscopy	Smaller caliber of the tube, with a greater risk of obstruction Requires specialized intervention radiology Not widely available to date Less well documented in ALS patients than PEG

Note: An overview of advantages and disadvantages of PEG in comparison to PRG/RIG.

However, this procedure requires specialized intervention radiology and is therefore not yet widely available and less well documented than PEG (Andersen et al. 2007; Hardiman 2000). In conclusion, with appropriate patient selection, PEG and PRG/RIG implantation are safe procedures with low morbidity and mortality. Survival does not differ significantly between patients undergoing PEG or PRG/RIG (Thornton et al. 2002). Table 32.4 gives an overview of advantages and disadvantages of PEG and PRG/RIG.

32.5 HOME PARENTERAL NUTRITION IN ALS

Literature for home parenteral nutrition (HPN) in ALS is scarce. In one study (Verschueren et al. 2009), 65 patients in later stages of ALS either with HPN or with PEG were observed. The authors concluded that HPN is feasible, safe, and well tolerated, that it can improve quality of life, and that individual survival can be prolonged. Disadvantages of this method are the higher costs, that appropriate training for the caregivers is needed, and the higher infection rates. In ALS patients with severe respiratory insufficiency, HPN can be an alternative to enteral feeding.

ETHICAL ISSUES

Literature on ALS patients' perspectives on enteral feeding is scarce and their views are only mentioned in the population characteristics sections in articles on PEG. Patients may delay gastrostomy due to unfounded perceptions of tube feeding, changes to their body image, and fear of being "nil by mouth." Fear and the added stress to the caregiver are the most commonly expressed worries of the ALS patient (Golaszewski 2007). Two studies showed that patients' attitudes to PEG at baseline were a significant predictor of PEG choice over follow-up. Preferences were unrelated to age, gender, level of education, or severity of disease at baseline (Albert et al. 2001). Patient acceptance of the PEG tube can be greatly improved by telling the patient that they still can eat and drink by mouth (Rosenfeld and Ellis 2008). However, it is also understandable that patients choose to avoid invasive procedures which may prolong their suffering, even though PEG has not conclusively been demonstrated to prolong survival to date (Forbes et al. 2004; Heffernan et al. 2004; Miller et al. 1999). The impact of PEG/RPG/RIG on quality of life is discussed controversially: PEG/PRG/RIG insertion has not been proven to directly improve quality of life. On the contrary, it even may negatively impact the quality of life of patients and carers, when additional support, beyond clinical needs, is lacking. In another study addressing this issue, ALS patients using enteral nutrition expressed feelings of frustration, depression, embarrassment, and role changes within familial relationships. On the other hand, PEG use can preserve time and energy for both patient and caregiver as there is less stress surrounding mealtimes and therefore it can improve quality of life (Golaszewski 2007; Rosenfeld and Ellis 2008). In addition, it can facilitate nursing care in either hospital or home environments because of the simplicity of enteral feeding and the minimal disturbance it causes for the patient (Thornton et al. 2002).

SUMMARY POINTS (MODIFIED ACCORDING TO ANDERSEN ET AL. 2007)

- In general, calorically dense and rich meals are recommended.
- Bulbar dysfunction and nutritional status (body weight, prolonged mealtime) should be routinely monitored at each visit.
- When dysphagia appears, a dietician should be consulted and a speech and language therapist should give advice on swallowing techniques. Caretakers should be trained to feed in a safe way and to assure good oral health to avoid aspiration pneumonia.
- The timing for PEG implantation is based on individual approach, dependent on bulbar symptoms, weight loss (prior to the loss of 5%–10% of body weight), respiratory function (should be above 50%), and patient's general condition. In conclusion, early PEG insertion is highly recommended.
- PRG/RIG is a newer alternative method to PEG, especially in patients with respiratory impairment or in poor general condition.
- PEG and PRG/RIG tubes should have a large diameter (e.g., 18-22 Charriere) in order to prevent tube obstruction.
- NGT can be used for short-term feeding and when PEG or PRG/RIG is not suitable.

LIST OF ABBREVIATIONS

ALS	Amyotrophic lateral sclerosis
BiPAP	Biphasic positive airway pressure
FVC	Forced vital capacity
HPN	Home parenteral nutrition
MND	Motor neuron disease
NGT	Nasogastric tube
PEG	Percutaneous endoscopic gastrostomy
PRG	Percutaneous radiologic gastrostomy
REE	Resting energy expenditure
RIG	Radiologically inserted gastrostomy

REFERENCES

Albert, S. M., P. L. Murphy, M. Del Bene, L. P. Rowland, and H. Mitsumoto. 2001. Incidence and predictors of PEG placement in ALS/MND. *J Neurol Sci* 191:115–19.

Andersen, P. M., G. D. Borasio, R. Dengler, O. Hardiman, K. Kollewe, P. N. Leigh, P. F. Pradat, V. Silani, and B. Tomik. 2007. Good practice in the management of amyotrophic lateral sclerosis: Clinical guidelines. An evidence-based review with good practice points. EALSC Working Group. *Amyotroph Lateral Scler* 8:195–213.

Borasio, G. D., P. J. Shaw, O. Hardiman, A. C. Ludolph, M. L. Sales Luis, and V. Silani. 2001. Standards of palliative care for patients with amyotrophic lateral sclerosis: Results of a European survey. *Amyotroph Lateral Scler Other Motor Neuron Disord* 2:159–64.

Bouteloup, C., J. C. Desport, P. Clavelou, N. Guy, H. Derumeaux-Burel, A. Ferrier, and P. Couratier. 2009. Hypermetabolism in ALS patients: An early and persistent phenomenon. *J Neurol* 256:1236–42.

Cameron, A., and J. Rosenfeld. 2002. Nutritional issues and supplements in amyotrophic lateral sclerosis and other neurodegenerative disorders. *Curr Opin Clin Nutr Metab Care* 5:631–43.

Chio, A., R. Galletti, C. Finocchiaro, D. Righi, M. A. Ruffino, A. Calvo, N. Di Vito, P. Ghiglione, A. A. Terreni, and R. Mutani. 2004. Percutaneous radiological gastrostomy: A safe and effective method of nutritional tube placement in advanced ALS. *J Neurol Neurosurg Psychiatry* 75:645–47.

Chio, A., G. Mora, M. Leone, L. Mazzini, D. Cocito, M. T. Giordana, E. Bottacchi, and R. Mutani. 2002. Early symptom progression rate is related to ALS outcome: A prospective population-based study. *Neurology* 59:99–103.

Desport, J. C., P. M. Preux, C. T. Truong, L. Courat, J. M. Vallat, and P. Couratier. 2000. Nutritional assessment and survival in ALS patients. *Amyotroph Lateral Scler Other Motor Neuron Disord* 1:91–96.

Desport, J. C., P. M. Preux, T. C. Truong, J. M. Vallat, D. Sautereau, and P. Couratier. 1999. Nutritional status is a prognostic factor for survival in ALS patients. *Neurology* 53:1059–63.

Dupuis, L., P. Corcia, A. Fergani, J. L. Gonzalez De Aguilar, D. Bonnefont-Rousselot, R. Bittar, et al. 2008. Dyslipidemia is a protective factor in amyotrophic lateral sclerosis. *Neurology* 70:1004–9.

Forbes, R. B., S. Colville, and R. J. Swingler. 2004. Frequency, timing and outcome of gastrostomy tubes for amyotrophic lateral sclerosis/motor neurone disease–a record linkage study from the Scottish Motor Neurone Disease Register. *J Neurol* 251:813–17.

Golaszewski, A. 2007. Nutrition throughout the course of ALS. *NeuroRehabilitation* 22:431–34.

Hardiman, O. 2000. Symptomatic treatment of respiratory and nutritional failure in amyotrophic lateral sclerosis. *J Neurol* 247:245–51.

Heffernan, C., C. Jenkinson, T. Holmes, G. Feder, R. Kupfer, P. N. Leigh, S. McGowan, A. Rio, and P. Sidhu. 2004. Nutritional management in MND/ALS patients: an evidence based review. *Amyotroph Lateral Scler Other Motor Neuron Disord* 5:72–83.

Kollewe, K, and Petri, S. 2009. Amyotrophe Lateralsklerose. *Klinische Neurophysiologie* 40 (1): 3–14.

Kollewe, K., U. Mauss, K. Krampfl, S. Petri, R. Dengler, and B. Mohammadi. 2008. ALSFRS-R score and its ratio: A useful predictor for ALS-progression. *J Neurol Sci* 275:69–73.

Kurt, A., F. Nijboer, T. Matuz, and A. Kubler. 2007. Depression and anxiety in individuals with amyotrophic lateral sclerosis: Epidemiology and management. *CNS Drugs* 21:279–91.

Langmore, S. E. 1999. Issues in the management of dysphagia. *Folia Phoniatr Logop* 51:220–30.

Langmore, S. E., E. J. Kasarskis, M. L. Manca, and R. K. Olney. 2006. Enteral tube feeding for amyotrophic lateral sclerosis/motor neuron disease. *Cochrane Database Syst Rev* CD004030.

Langmore, S. E., M. S. Terpenning, A. Schork, Y. Chen, J. T. Murray, D. Lopatin, and W. J. Loesche. 1998. Predictors of aspiration pneumonia: How important is dysphagia? *Dysphagia* 13:69–81.

Lyall, R. A., N. Donaldson, M. I. Polkey, P. N. Leigh, and J. Moxham. 2001. Respiratory muscle strength and ventilatory failure in amyotrophic lateral sclerosis. *Brain* 124:2000–13.

Mazzini, L., T. Corra, M. Zaccala, G. Mora, M. Del Piano, and M. Galante. 1995. Percutaneous endoscopic gastrostomy and enteral nutrition in amyotrophic lateral sclerosis. *J Neurol* 242:695–98.

Miller, R. G., C. E. Jackson, E. J. Kasarskis, J. D. England, D. Forshew, W. Johnston, S. Kalra, et al. 2009. Practice parameter update: The care of the patient with amyotrophic lateral sclerosis: Drug, nutritional, and respiratory therapies (an evidence-based review): Report of the Quality Standards Subcommittee of the American Academy of Neurology. *Neurology* 73:1218–26.

Miller, R. G., J. A. Rosenberg, D. F. Gelinas, H. Mitsumoto, D. Newman, R. Sufit, G. D. Borasio, et al. 1999. Practice parameter: The care of the patient with amyotrophic lateral sclerosis (an evidence-based review): Report of the Quality Standards Subcommittee of the American Academy of Neurology: ALS Practice Parameters Task Force. *Neurology* 52:1311–23.

Mitsumoto, H., M. Davidson, D. Moore, N. Gad, M. Brandis, S. Ringel, J. Rosenfeld, et al. 2003. Percutaneous endoscopic gastrostomy (PEG) in patients with ALS and bulbar dysfunction. *Amyotroph Lateral Scler Other Motor Neuron Disord* 4:177–85.

Orrell, R. W., R. J. Lane, and M. Ross. 2007. Antioxidant treatment for amyotrophic lateral sclerosis / motor neuron disease. *Cochrane Database Syst Rev* CD002829.

Rosenfeld, J., and A. Ellis. 2008. Nutrition and dietary supplements in motor neuron disease. *Phys Med Rehabil Clin N Am* 19:573–89.

Thornton, F. J., T. Fotheringham, M. Alexander, O. Hardiman, F. P. McGrath, and M. J. Lee. 2002. Amyotrophic lateral sclerosis: Enteral nutrition provision–endoscopic or radiologic gastrostomy? *Radiology* 224:713–17.

Toepfer, M., C. Folwaczny, A. Klauser, R. L. Riepl, W. Muller-Felber, and D. Pongratz. 1999. Gastrointestinal dysfunction in amyotrophic lateral sclerosis. *Amyotroph Lateral Scler Other Motor Neuron Disord* 1:15–19.

Vaisman, N., M. Lusaus, B. Nefussy, E. Niv, D. Comaneshter, R. Hallack, and V. E. Drory. 2009. Do patients with amyotrophic lateral sclerosis (ALS) have increased energy needs? *J Neurol Sci* 279:26–29.

Verschueren, A., A. Monnier, S. Attarian, D. Lardillier, and J. Pouget. 2009. Enteral and parenteral nutrition in the later stages of ALS: An observational study. *Amyotroph Lateral Scler* 10:42–46.

33 Nutritional Considerations of Palliative Care in Rare Disease: The Motor Disorder Disease Achalasia

Luca Dughera, Paola Cassolino, Michele Chiaverina, and Fabio Cisarò

CONTENTS

33.1 INTRODUCTION

Gastrointestinal motility disorders encompass a wide array of signs and symptoms that can occur anywhere throughout the luminal gastrointestinal tract (Table 33.1). Dysphagia for solids and liquids, regurgitation of undigested food, respiratory complications (nocturnal cough and aspiration), chest pain and weight loss are the main symptoms of achalasia, a rare motor disorder of the oesophagus and lower oesophageal sphincter (LES). Since the first description of achalasia by Sir Thomas Willis in 1674, several theories on the aetiology and pathophysiology have been reported (Boeckxstaens 2007; Farrokhi and Vaezi 2007; Park and Vaezi 2005). Idiopathic (primary) achalasia, most common anywhere but in South America, is a neuromuscular disorder characterized by degenerative changes of the myenteric plexus leading to a loss of peristaltic contractions and impaired LES relaxation in response to swallowing. Primary achalasia is a quite rare disease with an incidence of approximately 1/100,000 and a prevalence rate of 10/100,000. Secondary achalasia shares clinical features with primary achalasia, but there is an identifiable cause. Worldwide, the most common cause of secondary achalasia is *Trypanosoma cruzi* infection, found in Central and South America. When features of achalasia are caused by malignancy or by other infiltrative

TABLE 33.1
Key Facts of Motor Disorder Diseases and Achalasia

- Gastrointestinal motility disorders encompass a wide array of signs and symptoms that can occur anywhere throughout the luminal gastrointestinal tract. GI disorders involving the oesophagus and the stomach are often cause of dysphagia.
- Motility disorders are often chronic in nature and dramatically affect patients' quality of life. These disorders cause a tremendous impact both on the individual patient and on society as a whole.
- The most common gastrointestinal motility disorders are achalasia, non-achalasia oesophageal motility disorders, dyspepsia, gastroparesis, chronic intestinal pseudo-obstruction, irritable bowel syndrome and chronic constipation.
- Achalasia is the classic motility disorder of the oesophagus. The annual incidence of achalasia is estimated at 1/100,000 persons. Clinically, achalasia is characterized by dysphagia, chest pain, regurgitation and aspiration.
- Achalasia is defined manometrically by incomplete relaxation of the LES in combination with aperistalsis of the body of the oesophagus.
- All current forms of treatment for achalasia and other gastrointestinal motility disorders are palliative in nature. Nowadays pharmacologic therapy, other non-surgical therapeutic choices and surgery aim to control symptoms and at best improve QOL.
- Management of malnutrition and inability to nourish is mandatory in all motor disorders involving the upper GI tract and all feasible options must be considered.

diseases such as amyloidosis, the term pseudoachalasia is used. Complications of surgery involving the gastroesophageal junction, such as fundoplication, gastric banding and vagal injury, may lead to pseudoachalasia.

33.2 PATHOPHYSIOLOGY

The coordinated peristaltic wave, which moves the food bolus through the distal oesophagus, depends on excitatory and inhibitory input from local enteric reflexes that originate in the enteric nervous plexus and from extrinsic innervation via the vagus nerve. The peristaltic reflex involves both cholinergic and peptidergic excitatory neurotransmission, resulting in excitation and contraction of both circular and longitudinal muscle proximal to the bolus preceded by aboral relaxation ahead of the bolus. The acetyl cholinesterase inhibitor edrophonium chloride significantly increases LES pressure in patients with achalasia. Botulinum toxin (BTX) is a potent inhibitor of the release of acetylcholine, which reduces LES pressure and improves the "passive" oesophageal emptying by counterbalancing the selective loss of inhibitory neurons in the myenteric plexus. Most studies using BTX or atropine support the concept of preservation of the excitatory, cholinergic innervation to the oesophagus, which implies that the neuronal loss that characterizes achalasia may be selective for inhibitory neurons (Hirano 2006; Kraichely and Farrugia 2006). The hallmark of achalasia is failure of complete LES relaxation. The mechanism of LES relaxation is complex, requiring the coordinated interaction of nerves, smooth muscle, interstitial cells of Cajal (ICC) and neurohormones (Negreanu, Assor, and Mateescu 2008). Aboral relaxation is dependent on what has long been referred to as non-adrenergic, non-cholinergic neurotransmission. A variety of mediators have been proposed, including nitric oxide (NO) and vasoactive intestinal peptide (VIP). Most data now strongly suggest that the major inhibitory neurotransmitter governing relaxation of oesophageal smooth muscle is NO. Loss of VIP- and NO-secreting neurons leads to an imbalance between the excitatory and inhibitory neurons of the myenteric plexus, producing irreversible manometric changes in such patients. Intramuscular ICC have been clearly identified in the LES. ICC have several different functions, serving as pacemakers, generators of a smooth muscle hyperpolarizing factor (carbon monoxide), mechanosensors and mediators of neurotransmission. There is little evidence to suggest a defect in smooth muscle but, together with loss of myenteric neurons, loss of ICC has also been reported (Huizinga, Zarate, and Farrugia 2009; Zarate, Wang, and Tougas 2006).

33.3 CLINICAL PICTURE AND DIAGNOSIS

Achalasia is a progressive disease that appears with symptoms of dysphagia both for liquid and solid foods, regurgitation and chest pain, but also long after meals.

Potential warning signs of dysphagia are listed in Table 33.2. Food collects in the oesophagus: eventually it may pass through the sphincter by the action of gravity and of the weight of the food consumed. Regurgitation in achalasia is very common but it lacks the typical bitter taste of gastroesophageal acid refluxate. Regurgitation may occur during meals, shortly afterwards or hours later, when the patient changes into recumbent position and reports regurgitation of undigested foods. Repeated collection of food causes oesophageal dilation leading to non-cardiac chest pain or to irritation of the mucosa resulting in secondary oesophagitis. Aspiration of food from the oesophagus may lead to pneumonia. More subtle symptoms include slow eating (upon questioning, achalasia patients frequently report being the last to finish their meals, family or friends teasing them to eat up faster, etc.), and the habit of stretching or making side-to-side movements and walking around after meals (to help bolus passage through the aperistaltic oesophagus and across the LES barrier). Patients may also find that standing up during a meal, drinking a glass of water or exhaling hard may help to force food into the stomach. Loss of weight and malnutrition are uncommon but they occur in advanced disease and in elderly patients, so that dietary care is needed.

All patients with dysphagia should undergo upper gastrointestinal endoscopy and radiology to rule out anatomical lesions as the first diagnostic step (Poh and Tutuian 2007). At endoscopy, the LES is strictly closed, even with the help of insufflations of air, but the endoscope can pass this area with gentle pressure. In advanced cases, called "vigorous achalasia," some increased resistance at the gastroesophageal junction is found; the oesophagus may look dilated and hypotonic with retained food in most cases.

Radiological examination may show a typical 'birdbeak' image at the junction, with a dilated oesophageal body, sometimes with an air-fluid level and absence of an intragastric air bubble. Diagnostic certainty is provided only by oesophageal manometric study in over 96% of cases, showing a typical pattern in primary achalasia (Paterson, Goyal, and Habib 2006; Spechler and Castell 2001) (Figures 33.1 and 33.2).

TABLE 33.2
Potential Warning Signs of Achalasic Dysphagia

Coughing/choking during or after eating or drinking
Difficulty chewing/manipulating/controlling food or drink in the mouth
Gurgle voice or altered voice after eating and drinking
Pouching of food in the mouth
Unable to swallow/food sticking in the mouth
Unable to clear own saliva/secretions
Stretching or side-to-side movement during meals
Drooling
Vomiting after meals
Loss of weight
Dehydration
Frequent chest infections

Note: An overview of major and minor signs of dysphagia in achalasia. More subtle symptoms include slow eating (upon questioning, achalasia patients frequently report being the last to finish their meals, family or friends teasing them to eat up faster etc.), and the habit of stretching, making side-to-side movements or walking around after meals.

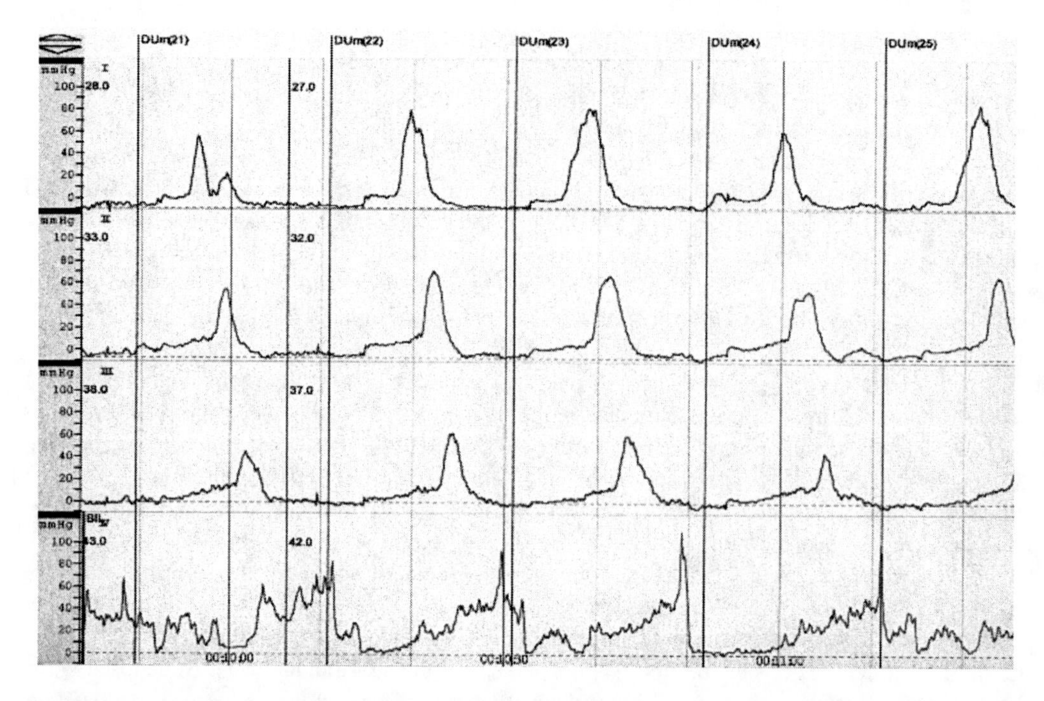

FIGURE 33.1 Normal oesophageal manometry. A normal manometric finding, as defined by Spechler and Castell (2001): basal LES pressure 10–45 mmHg (mid respiratory pressure measured by station pull through technique), LES relaxation with swallow complete (to a level <8 mmHg above gastric pressure). Wave progression peristalsis progressing from UES through LES at a rate of 2–8 cm/s. Distal wave amplitude 30–180 mmHg (average of 10 swallows at two recording sites positioned 3 and 8 cm above the LES). (Personal observation.)

33.4 TREATMENT OPTIONS

33.4.1 Pharmacologic Treatments

The only available drugs are smooth muscle relaxants aimed at reducing LES pressure, such as calcium channel blockers, nitrates and, more recently, phosphodiesterase inhibitors (sidenafil), to be taken usually before meals.

With pharmacologic treatments offering modest, transient improvements at best, endoscopic and surgical treatment options remain the main therapeutic pillars for achalasia. Therefore, they are only indicated in patients not willing or unable to undergo any other procedure, in patients waiting for a more definitive therapy or as supportive treatment for refractory chest pain (Lake and Wong 2006; Pehlivanov and Parisha 2006).

33.4.2 Endoscopic Procedures

Historically, pneumatic dilation (PD) was the first attempt of therapy in oesophageal achalasia (Wong 2004). Modern dilators consist of expanding bags or balloons that forcefully dilate the LES, rupturing muscular fibres. Inpatient vs. ambulatory treatment, sedated vs. unsedated dilatation, fluoroscopic or endoscopic positioning, the dilator system, initial balloon size, speed, pressure, duration and number of dilatations per endoscopic session, and timing of redilatations differ from centre to centre (Annese and Bassotti 2006; Pehlivanov and Parisha 2006). To date the primary modality of endoscopic therapy for achalasia is the injection of BTX into the LES. Injection of 80–100 units of BTX into the LES has been shown to improve symptoms, decrease the LES pressure, improve the oesophageal emptying and increase the LES opening. Overall, BTX is widely demonstrated to be

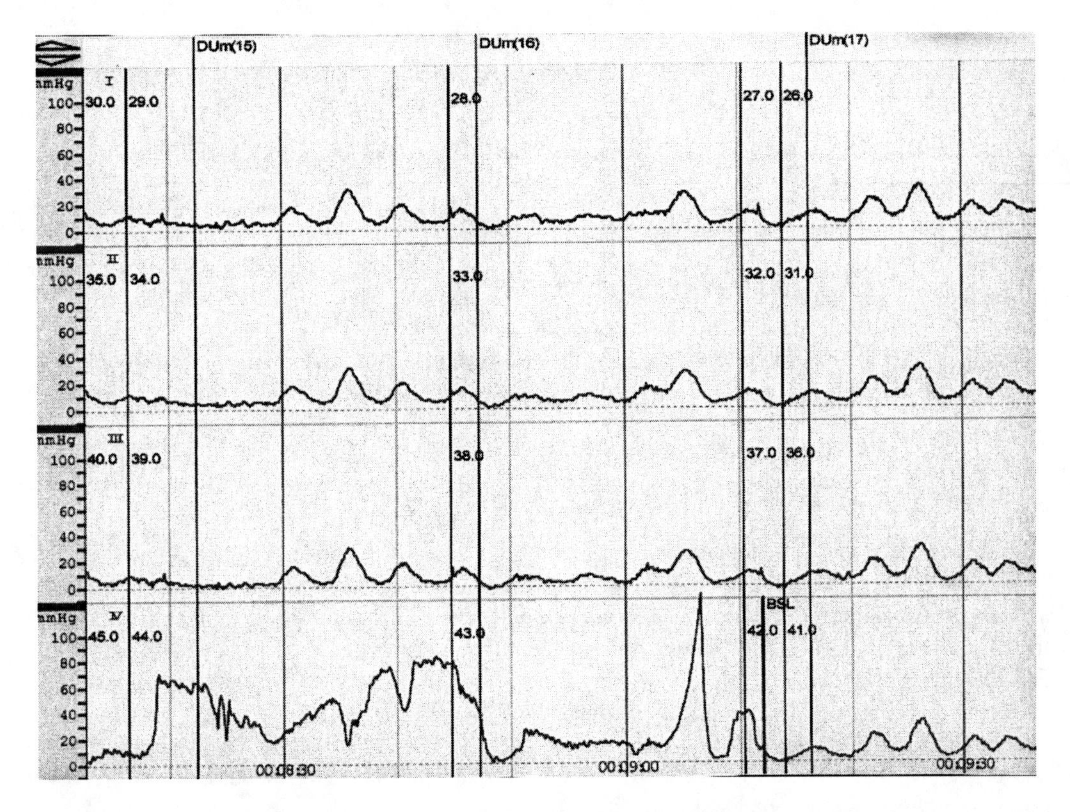

FIGURE 33.2 Oesophageal manometry in achalasia. The manometric features proposed for a diagnosis of classic achalasia are: (1) incomplete relaxation of the LES (defined as a mean swallow induced fall in resting LES pressure to a nadir value >8 mm above gastric pressure) and (2) aperistalsis in the body of the oesophagus characterised either by simultaneous oesophageal contractions with amplitudes <40 mmHg or by no apparent oesophageal contractions. (Personal observation.)

the most effective treatment option in elderly patients, in whom dilation or surgery represent a high-risk procedure, or in patients with comorbid illnesses who are not candidates for PD or myotomy (Dughera, Battaglia, and Maggio 2005).

33.4.3 Surgical Treatment

The feasibility of minimally invasive surgical techniques has dramatically modified the management algorithm, meaning patients are sent for surgery very soon after the initial diagnosis of achalasia. Nowadays the laparoscopic-modified Heller oesophagocardiomyotomy is the standard treatment for patients with achalasia but without prohibitive comorbidities. Perioperative mortality should approach 0% and long-term patient satisfaction exceeds 90%. An antireflux procedure can reduce postoperative heartburn rates by 80% (Herbella, Tineli, and Wilson 2008).

33.5 APPLICATIONS TO OTHER AREAS OF PALLIATIVE CARE

Although some aspects of palliative treatments for achalasia meet the criteria usually applied for the palliative care of dysphagia due to malignancies or to neuromuscular chronic defects, achalasia is not a life-threatening illness. Achalasia per se has a long life expectancy, if complications such as aspiration pneumonia and malnutrition are avoided.

Good quality of life (QOL) preservation must be the primary endpoint in these patients, so treatments that will allow oral nutrition to be maintained must be taken into consideration as a first choice.

The ability to enjoy at least some oral nutrition, especially in public spaces, without spitting saliva or regurgitating should positively influence the maintenance of a social activity, so improving QOL.

33.6 GUIDELINES AND PRACTICAL METHODS AND TECHNIQUES

In the literature, there are very few data concerning the nutritional aspects of achalasia and no specific clinical guidelines have yet been published. However, the management of the patient with achalasia and nutritional problems is very similar to that of patients with swallowing impairments (dysphagia) due to neurological diseases or oesophagogastric cancer (Bower and Martin 2009; Foley, Teasell and Salter 2008; Prosser-Loose and Paterson 2006).

Practical methods and techniques for nasogastric tube insertion, percutaneous endoscopic gastrostomy (PEG) and percutaneous radiologic gastrostomy (PRG) have been fully described in Chapter 16.

33.7 NUTRITIONAL ASPECTS OF ACHALASIA

Initially, loss of weight and malnutrition are uncommon, unless the patient becomes afraid of eating. In more advanced disease and in elderly people, if medical or endoscopic therapies are ineffective and surgical myotomy is not suitable, severe malnutrition may occur and dietary care is needed; the first priority is to decide whether the oral feeding is safe or the alternative routes have to be considered.

Dysphagia is simply defined as any difficulty with swallowing. Normal swallowing consists of four phases: oral preparatory, oral, pharyngeal and oesophageal (Table 33.3). In achalasia both phase 3 and phase 4 are affected: an increased pressure and opening incoordination are often observed in the upper oesophageal sphincter (UES) too.

Oral feeding has important social and psychological significance for patients and their families and should be continued whenever possible. In some patients oral intake is often not adequate even in the absence of significant swallowing difficulties. In mild-moderate achalasia, nutrition is generally poorly affected and, if the family encourages the patient to follow small dietary modifications, loss of weight and malnutrition rarely occur. The effect of achalasia on the diet of patients and their spouses was investigated using a validated questionnaire. The discordance between the diet of the patients and their respective spouses was compared with matched controls. There was no statistically significant difference between the discordance of case couples and control couples. Patients with achalasia and their spouses may eat a quite normal diet (Probert, Spiller, and Atkinson. 1991).

TABLE 33.3
Disruption of the Normal Swallow Process

Stage of Normal Swallow	Affected by	Consequences
Preparatory stage	Reduced range of movement of facial muscles, lip, tongue and jaws. Loss of sight, smell and/or taste	Difficulty in getting food/drink in the mouth and in sealing in the mouth Reduced saliva production
Oral stage	Reduced range of movement of facial muscles, lip, tongue and jaws. Lack of saliva	Difficulty in mastication, in forming and controlling food bolus
Pharyngeal stage	Absence of swallow reflex	Inability to swallow safely Aspiration during swallow
Oesophageal stage	Impaired peristalsis and/or obstruction	Food fails to move into the stomach Aspiration after the swallow

Note: An overview of the pathophysiology of swallowing processes; stages 3 and 4 are usually involved in achalasia.

TABLE 33.4
High-Risk Foods for Achalasia

Stringy fibrous texture e.g., pineapple, runner beans, celery, lettuce
Vegetable and fruit skins (including bean skins) e.g., broad/baked/soya, peas, grapes
Mixed consistency foods, e.g., cereals that do not blend with milk, such as muesli, mince with thin gravy, soup with lumps
Crunchy foods and crumbly items, e.g., toast, flaky pastry, dry biscuits, crisps, bread crust, pie crust, crumble
Hard foods, e.g., boiled and chewy sweets and toffee, nuts and seeds
Husks, e.g., sweet corn and granary bread

Note: In the achalasic patient some foods causing dysphagia must be strictly avoided. Meals have to be consumed slowly and feeding should be avoided when the patient is tired or distracted. Talking while eating also increases the risk of aspiration and patients should be made aware of this.

In some patients, dysphagia may result from poor preparation of the food bolus because of ill-fitting dentures or oral infections due to disease. These causes should be routinely looked for and properly treated. Meals have to be consumed slowly and feeding should be avoided when the patient is tired or distracted (for example while watching television). Talking while eating also increases the risk of aspiration and patients should be made aware of this. Patients must be made aware of potentially high-risk food (Table 33.4). Dysphagia diets are highly individualized. Characteristics of the diet include modification of food texture or fluid viscosity. Food may be chopped, minced or puréed, and fluids may be thickened (Pardoe 1993). Table 33.5 lists food and fluid consistencies

TABLE 33.5
Description of Food and Fluid Consistencies

Consistency	Description
Foods	
Puréed	Thick homogeneous textures, pudding-like consistency
Ground or minced	Easily chewed foods; no coarse textures or raw fruits or vegetables, except for mashed banana
Soft or easy to chew	Soft foods prepared without the use of a blender, meats minced or cut into cubes 1 cm or less, no tough skins, nuts or raw, crispy or stringy foods
Modified general	Soft textures prepared without grinding or chopping, no nuts or crisp foods
Fluids	
Thin	Regular fluids; no changes necessary
Nectar-like	Fluids thin enough to be sipped through a straw or from a cup but thick enough to fall from a tipped spoon slowly
Honey-like	Thick fluids eaten with a spoon, unable to hold their shape, too thick for a straw (e.g., yogurt, honey, tomato sauce)
Spoon-thick	Pudding-like fluids, must be eaten with a spoon (e.g., thickened applesauce, thick milk pudding)

Note: In the achalasic patient the characteristics of the diet include modification of food texture or fluid viscosity. Food may be chopped, minced or puréed and fluids may be thickened.

along with some examples. In general, solid food is assigned to one of four groups, which progress from the easiest to the most difficult to swallow. Special attention should be given to the nutritional adequacy of mechanically altered diets, particularly the puréed form. Regular communication with team members about the patient's changing swallowing capabilities is essential, to verify if the patient needs to progress from a diet of food with normal textures to a dysphagia diet.

The risk of dehydration in achalasic patients is often underestimated, particularly in patients with dysphagia who are receiving all their nutrition by mouth (Finestone, Foley, and Woodbury 2001). The most difficult consistency for these patients is often orally thin fluids such as water. Even when fluids are thickened to ease control, adequate hydration can be a challenge. Fluid requirements should take into account the effects of age, disease and medical treatment.

If a patient is unable to consume food or fluid orally or to consume sufficient quantities of them, or if the risk of aspiration is high, enteral nutrition (tube feeding) should be provided. A careful evaluation of therapeutic options has to be performed: if there is a possibility for surgical myotomy, enteral nutrition will be provisional, considering that for surgery a malnourished patient is always at major risk of postoperative complications. In elderly patients with relevant comorbidities, in which the surgical option is not suitable, the choice for enteral nutrition has to be considered as a definitive therapeutic option.

The direct delivery of nutrients into the stomach or into the jejunum via a feeding tube is frequently used as the sole method of nutritional support of severely dysphagic patients. The use of a gastrostomy tube has to be preferred to naso-oesophageal intubation, even for provisional treatment since nasogastric tube feeding is usually poorly tolerated, extubation by patients is common and the volume of feeds delivered this way is usually not adequate. In one study patients who were fed using a nasogastric tube received 55% of their feeds, whereas those fed with a gastrostomy tube had 93% of their prescribed daily intake (Wilson, Johnson, and Bruce-Lockhart 1990). When nasogastric tube feeding is prescribed, the use of fine-bore tubes is preferred to large-bore ones. However, fine bore tubes are more likely to dislodge, kink or block. Prolonged nasogastric tube feeding is not desirable because it often results in numerous complications and it does not fully protect against aspiration.

In the achalasic patients the option of tube feeding should be offered early after the onset of intractable dysphagia to supplement the oral intake and help maintain the muscle mass. In contrast to what is generally described for the management of dysphagia due to neurological disorders, the use of a PEG is generally impossible for the mechanical resistance due to the enhanced pressure of both UES and LES and the motor disturbances within the oesophageal body that could enhance the risk of complications of the endoscopic procedure. Thus, in the management of dysphagia and malnutrition in achalasia the first choice is the insertion of the feeding tube through a PRG (Given, Hanson, and Lee 2005) rather than a surgical gastrostomy. PRG tube feeding is effective and is usually acceptable to patients and their carers. Long-term complications include tube obstruction and wound infection. In some patients, who are fed via a PRG tube, pulmonary aspiration may occur and intrajejunal feeding has been suggested for these cases. However, technically it is easier to insert a gastric rather than a jejunal feeding tube. An additional advantage is that bolus gastric tube feeding is more physiological, particularly with respect to insulin secretion. Enteral feeding can be started a few hours after the insertion of the feeding tube. The volume of feed is usually restricted in the first 24 hours to one litre and is given at a rate of 50 ml/hour. The volume of feed and the rate of its administration are then gradually increased over the following 3–4 days until the patient's daily nutritional requirements are met (Ney, Weiss, and Kind 2009; Raykher, Russo, and Schattner 2007).

ETHICAL ISSUES

As we said before, achalasia is not a life-threatening illness, and patients have a long life expectancy if complications are avoided. Therefore, if malnutrition occurs or it is impossible to maintain oral nutrition, invasive procedures are needed. In the absence of significant comorbidities the achalasic patient must be considered a fully understanding and self-deciding patient, so, in order to make consent informed, the patient needs to be given enough information to understand the procedures, risks and possible outcomes of the different modalities of enteral feeding.

SUMMARY POINTS

- Achalasia is a quite rare condition affecting both genders at all ages, with a long life expectancy if complications such as aspiration pneumonia and malnutrition are avoided.
- Dysphagia, both for liquid and solid foods, regurgitation, and chest pain, but also long after meals, are the main features of the illness.
- Treatment options include pharmacologic agents, endoscopic procedures or surgery.
- QOL must be a primary endpoint in these patients, so treatment options that allow oral nutrition must be taken into consideration as a first choice.
- Nowadays BTX is the most effective treatment option in elderly patients and in patients with comorbid illnesses who are not candidates for PD or surgical myotomy.
- If malnutrition occurs, delivery of nutrients into the stomach or into the jejunum via a feeding tube is the sole method of nutritional support of severely dysphagic patients.
- The first choice is the insertion of the feeding tube through a PRG, rather than a surgical gastrostomy.

LIST OF ABBREVIATIONS

BTX Botulinum toxin
ICC Interstitial cells of Cajal
LES Lower oesophageal sphincter
NO Nitric oxide
PD Pneumatic dilation
PEG Percutaneous endoscopic gastrostomy
PRG Percutaneous radiologic gastrostomy
QOL Quality of Life
UES Upper oesophageal sphincter
VIP Vasoactive intestinal peptide

REFERENCES

Annese, V., and G. Bassotti. 2006. Non-surgical treatment of oesophageal achalasia. *World J Gastroenterol* 12:5763–66.

Boeckxstaens, G. E. E. 2007. Achalasia. *Best Pract Res Clin Gastroenterol* 21:595–608.

Bower, M. R., and R. C. Martin. 2009. Nutritional management during neo adjuvant therapy for esophageal cancer. *J Surg Oncol* 100:82–87.

Dughera, L., E. Battaglia, and D. Maggio. 2005. Botulinum toxin treatment of oesophageal achalasia in the old old and oldest old: A 1-year follow-up study. *Drugs Aging* 22:779–83.

Farrokhi, F., and M. F. Vaezi. 2007. Idiopathic (primary) achalasia. *Orphanet J Rare Dis* 2:38–46.

Finestone, H. M., N. Foley, and M. G. Woodbury. 2001. Quantifying fluid intake in dysphagic stroke patients: A preliminary comparison of oral and non oral strategies. *Arch Phys Med Rehabil* 82:1744–46.

Foley, N., R. Teasell, and K. Salter. 2008. Dysphagia treatment post stroke: A systematic review of randomised controlled trials. *Age Ageing* 37:258–64.

Herbella, F. A., H. C. Tineli, J. L. Wilson Jr., and J. C. Del Grande. 2008. Surgical treatment of primary esophageal motility disorders. *J Gastrointest Surg* 12:604–8.

Hirano, I. 2006. Pathophysiology of achalasia and diffuse esophageal spasm. *GI Motility online*. doi:10.1038/gimo22.

Huizinga, J. D., N. Zarate, and G. Farrugia. 2009. Physiology, injury, and recovery of interstitial cells of Cajal: Basic and clinical science. *Gastroenterology* 137:1548–56.

Kraichely, R. E., and G. Farrugia. 2006. Achalasia: physiology and etiopathogenesis. *Diseases of the Esophagus* 19:213–23.

Lake, J. M., and R. K. R. Wong. 2006. Review article: the management of achalasia – a comparison of different treatment modalities. *Aliment Pharmacol Ther* 24:909–18.

Given, M. F., J. J. Hanson, and M. J. Lee. 2005. Interventional radiology techniques for provision of enteral feeding. *Cardiovasc Intervent Radiol* 28:692–703.

Negreanu, L. M., P. Assor, and B. Mateescu. 2008. Interstitial cells of Cajal in the gut – A gastroenterologist's point of view. *World J Gastroenterol* 14:6285–88.

Ney, D. M., J. M. Weiss, and A. J. Kind. 2009. Senescent swallowing: Impact, strategies, and interventions. *Nutr Clin Pract* 24:395–413.

Pardoe, E. M. 1993. Development of a multistage diet for dysphagia. *J Am Diet Assoc* 93:568–71.

Park, W., and M. F. Vaezi. 2005. Etiology and pathogenesis of achalasia: The current understanding. *Am J Gastroenterol* 100:1404–14.

Paterson, W. G., R. K. Goyal, and F. I. Habib. 2006. Oesophageal motility disorders. *GI Motility online*. doi:10.1038/gimo20.

Pehlivanov, N., and P. J. Parischa. 2006. Medical and endoscopic management of achalasia. *GI Motility online*. doi:10.1038/gimo52.

Pohl, D. I., and R. Tutuian. 2007. Achalasia: An overview of diagnosis and treatment. *J Gastrointestin Liver Dis* 4:297–303.

Probert, C. S., R. Spiller, and M. Atkinson. 1991. Achalasia and diet: Assessment of the effect of achalasia on the diet of patients and their spouses. *Dysphagia* 6:145–46.

Prosser-Loose, E. J., and P. G. Paterson. 2006. The FOOD Trial Collaboration: Nutritional supplementation strategies and acute stroke outcome. *Nutr Rev* 64:289–94.

Raykher, A., L. Russo, and M. Schattner. 2007. Enteral nutrition support of head and neck cancer patients. *Nutr Clin Pract* 22:68–73.

Spechler, N., and D. Castell. 2001. Classification of oesophageal motility abnormalities. *Gut* 49:145–51.

Wilson, P. S., A. P. Johnson, and F. J. Bruce-Lockhart. 1990. Videofluoroscopy in motor neurone disease prior to crico-pharyngeal myotomy. *Ann R Coll Surg Engl* 72:375–77.

Wong, R. K. 2004. Pneumatic dilation for achalasia. *Am J Gastroenterol* 99:578–80.

Zarate, N., X. Y. Wang, and G. Tougas. 2006. Intramuscular interstitial cells of Cajal associated with mast cells survive nitrergic nerves in achalasia. *Neurogastroenterol Motil* 18:556–68.

Section VI

Pharmacological Aspects

34 Steroid-Induced Side Effects Affecting Diet and Nutrition in Palliative Care: Oral Candidiasis and Other Conditions

Jana Pilkey

CONTENTS

34.1 INTRODUCTION

Corticosteroids are widely used in the practice of palliative care for a variety of reasons. They are useful in decreasing peritumoral edema associated with brain tumors, (Kaal and Vecht 2004) bowel obstructions (Laval et al. 2000), spinal cord compressions (Vecht et al. 1989), superior vena cava syndrome (Rowell and Gleeson 2001), and dyspnea (Bruera and Neumann 1998). They are also used for anorexia, weight loss, general well-being, and fatigue (Bruera and Neumann 1998).

Corticosteroids are used in 30%–60% of palliative patients (Hardy et al. 2001; Nauck et al. 2004; Mercadante, Fulfaro, and Casuccio 2001; Pilkey and Daeninck 2008). In addition, 69%–80% have been on corticosteroids at some point during treatment and 41%–43% are on them at hospice admission (Shafford 2006).

Although the benefits of corticosteroids generally outweigh the risks in palliative care, judicious use is necessary. Nutritionally related adverse effects can be debilitating for patients near the end of their lives, especially if patients are already compromised in their ability to maintain nutritional goals. This chapter will focus on adverse effects that commonly affect diet and nutrition in palliative care.

34.2 ORAL AND ESOPHAGEAL CANDIDIASIS

There is an increased incidence of thrush among patients receiving systemic steroid therapy, although direct causation is difficult to prove (Davies, Brailsford, and Beighton 2006). Steroid therapy leads to decreased humoral immunity, making patients more susceptible to candidal infections (Davies et al. 2006). For palliative patients on systemic corticosteroids, the incidence of thrush seems to be around 30% (Pilkey and Daeninck 2008; Davies, Brailsford, and Beighton 2001).

34.3 RISK FACTORS

Additional risk factors for oropharyngeal and esophageal candidiasis include advanced age, poor Eastern Cooperative Oncology Group (ECOG) score, denture use, xerostomia, and immune suppression. Antibiotics are important in the development of esophageal candidiasis (Davies et al. 2006) and proton pump inhibitors (PPIs) decrease stomach acidity, which normally prohibits candidal infections (Martínez et al. 2002). The greatest risk factor for esophageal candidiasis is oropharyngeal candidiasis. Palliative patients often suffer from many of these risk factors, making this population especially prone to candidal infections.

34.4 PRACTICAL METHODS AND TECHNIQUES

34.4.1 Diagnosis

Diagnosis is usually made on clinical or mycological grounds. Patients will often complain of painful lesions within the mouth or pain on swallowing. However, candidal lesions may also be painless (Davies et al. 2006). Most clinicians are familiar with acute pseudomembranous candidiasis, characterized by white plaques that may cause punctate bleeding when removed. However, there are a variety of clinical presentations, described as a spectrum of disease with four distinct varieties (Axell, Samaranayake, and Reichart 1997). These variations include acute pseudomembranous, acute erythematous, denture stomatitis, and angular cheilitis (Figure 34.1).

Esophageal candidiasis is more difficult to diagnose, but is suspected when oropharyngeal lesions are in place or the patient complains of odynophagia. If undertaken, esophagoscopy may show white plaques, erythematous changes, or ulcerations. Biopsy or culturing *Candida* confirms the diagnosis. Because of the invasiveness of this test, it is usually more appropriate to treat palliative patients based on clinical signs and symptoms alone.

Candida albicans is the most commonly isolated organism. However, non-albicans species are also prevalent and are resistant to treatment with azole-based medication (Davies et al. 2006). This leads to more severe or prolonged infections and the use of multiple and more toxic medications.

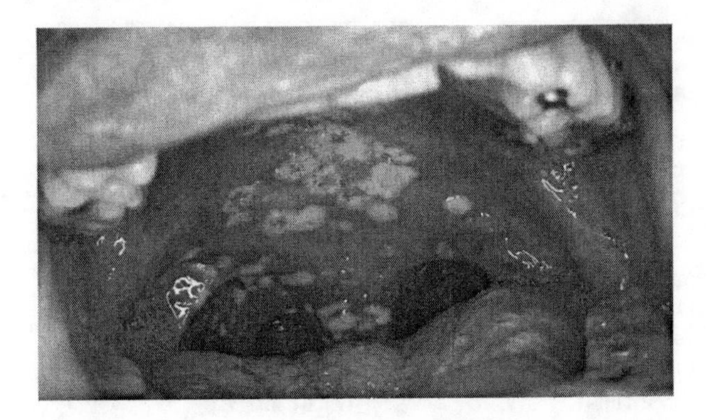

Acute pseudomembranous candidiasis

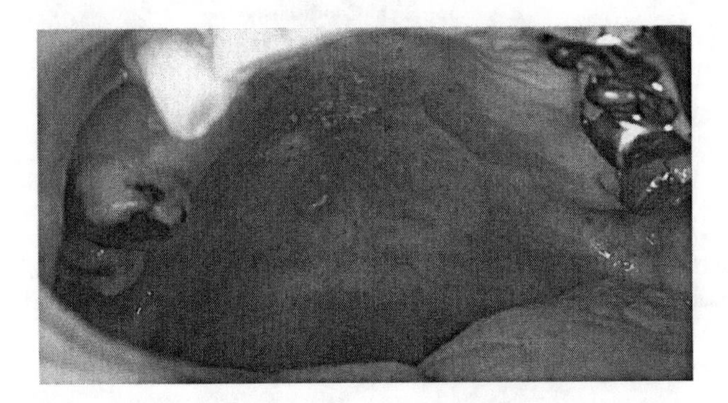

Acute erythematous candidiasis

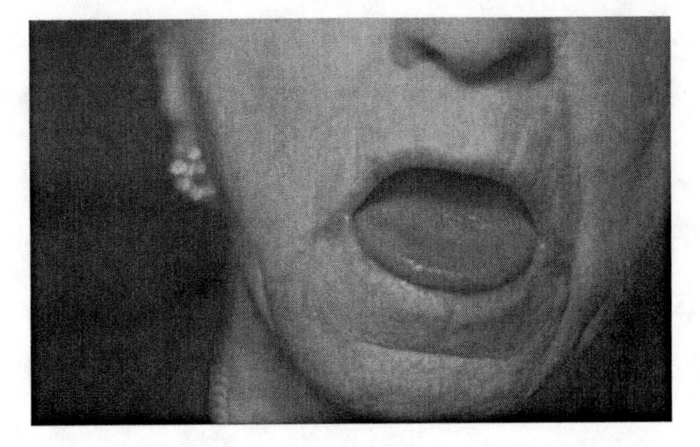

Acute angular cheilitis

FIGURE 34.1 Oral manifestations of candidiasis.

34.4.2 Treatment

Treatment consists of topical or systemic antifungal agents. Topical agents include nystatin, or amphotericin and systemic treatments include clotrimazole, fluconazole, itraconazole, ketoconazole, voriconazole, and echinocandins. Systemic treatment with intravenous amphotericin B is not recommended for palliation due to its significant toxicity and intolerability. Treatment recommendations are given in Table 34.1 (Pappas et al. 2009).

TABLE 34.1
Guidelines for Treatment of Orophayngeal and Esophageal Candidiasis

Oropharyngeal Candidiasis All Treatments are for 7–14 Days			
Mild disease	Clotrimazole 10 mg po 5 times daily	Nystatin suspension 500,000 units swish and swallow 4 times daily	Nystatin pastilles 200,000 units po 4 times daily
Moderate to severe disease	Fluconazole 100–200 mg po/IV once daily		
Refractory disease	Itraconazole solution 200 mg po once daily	Voriconazole 200 mg po/IV twice daily	Amphotericin B suspension 100 mg/ml–1 ml po every 6 hours
Esophageal Candidiasis All Treatments are for 14–21 Days			
First-line	Fluconazole 200–400 mg po/IV once daily		
Refractory	Caspofungin 50 mg IV once daily[a]	Micafungin 150 mg IV once daily[a]	

Source: Adapted and reproduced with permission from the American Infectious Disease Guidelines for the Treatment of Candidiasis 2009. Data published by Dr. Peter Pappas et al in *Clinical Infectious Diseases*; 48; 2009: 503–35. Permission granted by "The University of Chicago Press" © 2009 by the Infectious Diseases Society of America. All rights reserved.

Note: IV, intravenous; po, per os (orally).

[a] In select cases only.

34.4.3 Ethical Issues

Not all diagnostic tests and treatments may be appropriate for every patient. The invasiveness of esophagoscopy may unduly burden a palliative patient and the alternative of empiric treatment with potentially toxic medication, without a confirmed diagnosis, may also be burdensome. More invasive procedures such as esophagoscopy or intravenous antifungals should only be initiated in palliative care after discussions about side effects and goals of care (Table 34.2).

34.5 GASTRITIS AND GASTRODUODENAL ULCERATION

The gastroduodenal mucosal defense system is a complex barrier. Prostaglandins play an integral role in the mucosal defense by stimulating bicarbonate secretion and increasing blood flow.

TABLE 34.2
Key Facts about Candidiasis

1. Candidiasis occurs in about 30% of palliative patients treated with corticosteroids
2. Clinical varieties include: acute pseudomembranous, acute erythematous, denture stomatitis, and angular cheilitis
3. Diagnosis is made on clinical or mycological grounds. Clinically, patients may complain of painful lesions within the mouth or pain on swallowing, but candidiasis may also be painless
4. Treatment of oral or esophageal candidiasis can be achieved topically with nystatin or amphotericin, or systemically with clotrimazole, fluconazole, itraconazole, ketoconazole, voriconazole, and echinocandins
5. Diagnostic procedures and treatment must be tailored to the patient's overall goals of care

Exogenous corticosteroids compromise the barrier by blocking the production of prostaglandins via the cyclooxygenase (COX) pathway (Cryer 2001) (Figure 34.2). Non-steroidal anti-inflammatory drugs (NSAIDS) also block the COX pathway and combining the two medications results in a significant increase in gastrointestinal side effects (Piper et al. 1991).

34.5.1 Incidence

The risk of peptic ulcer disease for people on corticosteroids is twice as high as for the general population, but the risk increases to nearly fifteen times when patients are on both steroids and NSAIDS (Piper et al. 1991). For palliative patients on corticosteroids, the incidence of dyspepsia has been reported as 16% (Hardy et al. 2001) and the incidence of gastrointestinal bleeding as 10% (Mercadante et al. 2001). However, the rate of severe side effects, such as severe dyspepsia or hemorrhage, necessitating withdrawal from corticosteroid therapy was only 4%–5% (Hardy et al. 2001).

34.5.2 Risk Factors

The four risk factors that predict an increased likelihood of developing peptic ulcer disease on corticosteroid therapy are a high steroid dose, previous history of peptic ulcers, advanced cancers, and concurrent NSAID use (Piper et al. 1991).

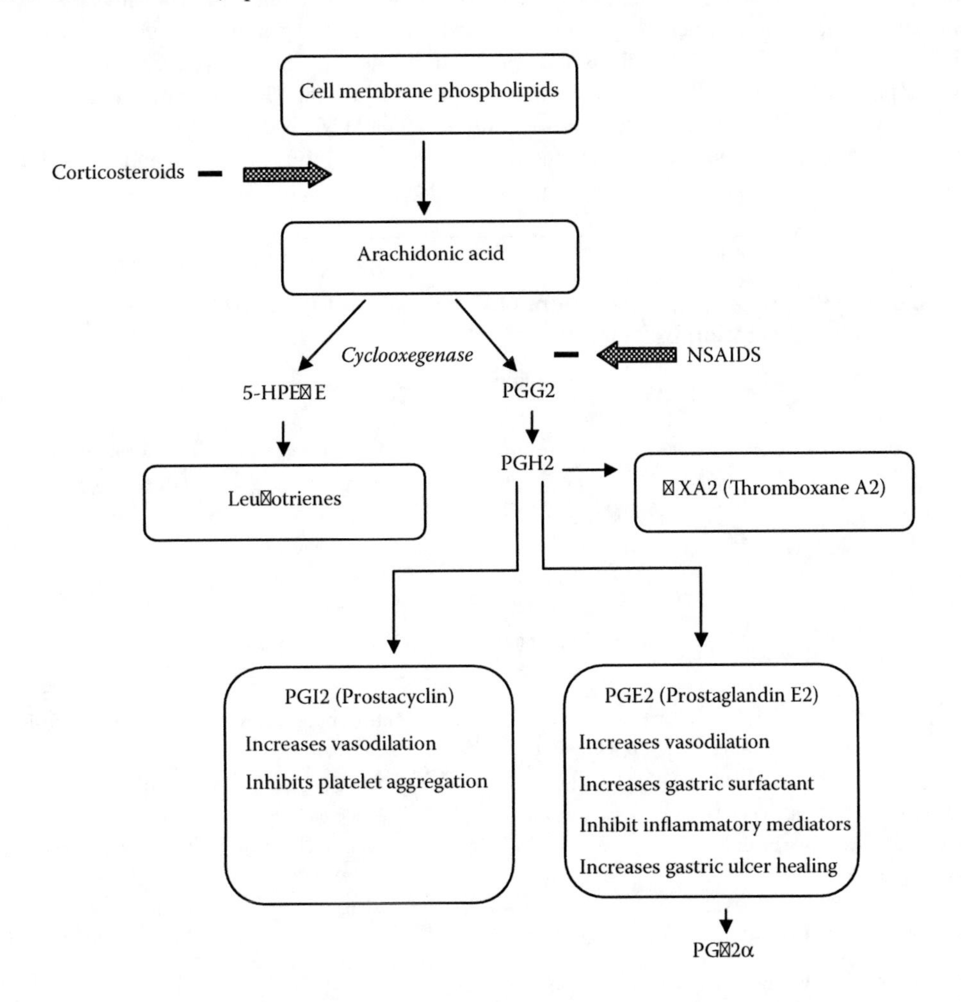

FIGURE 34.2 Corticosteroids and nonsteroidal anti-inflammatory drugs in the cyclooxygenase pathway.

34.6 PRACTICAL METHODS AND TECHNIQUES

34.6.1 Prophylaxis and Treatment

Opinions differ regarding gastroprotection for patients on corticosteroids. Some physicians offer prophylaxis when two or more risk factors are present (Hardy et al. 2001) while others offer prophylaxis almost every time (Mercadante et al. 2001; Pilkey and Daeninck 2008). Clinicians who prescribe corticosteroids should likely, as a minimum, offer gastroprotection to patients who have at least two risk factors, acknowledging that even the use of gastroprotective agents does not guarantee protection for every patient.

There is little evidence to guide optimal prophylaxis or treatment for corticosteroid gastropathy. However, based on extrapolations from the NSAID literature, PPIs are the medication of choice for gastroprotection and treatment, with histamine-2 receptor antagonists (H2As) a second choice for both indications (Leontiadis et al. 2007; Valenzuela et al. 1991).

The newer PPIs (rabeprazole, pantoprazole and lansoprazole) have been shown to be more effective at healing ulcers than omeprazole (Salas, Ward, and Carol 2002) but there has been no definite improvement in mortality, re-bleeding or surgical intervention shown between the oral and intravenous routes of these drugs (Leontiadis et al. 2007).

Therefore, the oral route is appropriate in most palliative patients wanting treatment, unless it is compromised. If there is no oral route, bolus intravenous (IV) PPIs can be initiated, if treatment is desired. Continuous IV infusions are likely only appropriate in select circumstances and endoscopic interventions should be considered on an individual basis after frank discussions are had with patient and family.

When patients near the end-of-life and can no longer swallow, the PPI can be discontinued, given parenterally, or switched to a parenteral H2A. Ranitidine (an H2A) is especially useful in palliative care, due to its ability to be given subcutaneously. An approach to prophylaxis and medical treatment of steroid-induced gastropathy in palliative care is given in Table 34.3.

TABLE 34.3
Agents for the Prophylaxis and Treatment of Corticosteroid-Induced Gastritis and Gastroduodenal Ulceration in Palliative Patients

Prophylaxis

	Oral Dosing	Subcutaneous Dosing	Intravenous Dosing
Pantoprazole	20 mg od	Unknown	20 mg od
Lansoprazole	15 mg od	Unknown	30 mg od
Rabeprazole	20 mg od	Unknown	20 mg od
Esomeprazole	20 mg od	Unknown	20 mg od
Omeprazole	20 mg od	Unknown	20 mg od
Ranitidine	150 mg bid	50 mg tid	50 mg tid

Treatment

	Oral Dosing	Subcutaneous Dosing	Intravenous Bolus Dosing	Intravenous Infusion Dosing
Pantoprazole	20 mg od or bid	Unknown	40 mg od or bid	80 mg bolus then 8 mg/h
Lansoprazole	15–30 mg od	Unknown	30 mg od or bid	90 mg bolus then 9 mg/h
Rabeprazole	20 mg od or bid	Unknown	20 mg od or bid	80 mg bolus then 8 mg/h
Esomeprazole	20–40 mg od	Unknown	20–40 mg od	80 mg bolus then 8 mg/h
Omeprazole	20 mg od or bid	Unknown	20 mg tid	80 mg bolus then 8 mg/h
Ranitidine	150 mg bid	50 mg tid	50 mg tid	50 mg then 0.25 mg/kg/h

Note: od, once daily; bid, twice daily; tid, three times daily.

TABLE 34.4
Key Facts about Steroid-Induced Gastropathy

1. Exogenous corticosteroids block the production of prostaglandins via the cyclooxygenase pathway. This pathway is also shared by non-steroidal anti-inflammatory drugs (NSAIDs)
2. The incidence of dyspepsia for palliative patients on corticosteroids is 16%, with severe symptoms such as gastrointestinal bleeding or severe dyspepsia occurring in 4%–10%
3. Prophylaxis with a PPI or H2A should be considered in all cases and implemented if patients have two or more of the following: a high steroid dose, a previous history of peptic ulcers, advanced cancer, or concurrent NSAID use
4. Treat steroid-induced gastrointestinal side effects with a PPI (as a first-line agent) or with a H2A (as a second-line agent)
5. The oral route is preferred for treatment but if it is compromised, bolus PPIs may be given intravenously and bolus ranitidine may be given intravenously or subcutaneously
6. Endoscopy may be appropriate in certain circumstances, depending on the patient's goals of care

34.6.2 Ethical Issues

The recommendations for gastroprotection are based on expert opinion. However, the number of patients needing to withdraw steroid therapy because of a serious side effect was only 4%–5% (Hardy et al. 2001). One wonders if the high rate of gastroprotection is more related to the fear of not wanting to have the patient die from a treatment-related death or a "bad death" from bleeding, as opposed to a more "natural" or "good death" from another cause (Table 34.4).

It is possible that our own fears or judgments may be resulting in an increased burden of treatment for some patients. When gastroprophylaxis is undertaken for patients on steroid therapy, clinicians should have a clear understanding of the risks and benefits involved and why they feel they are prescribing the medications.

34.7 IMPAIRED GLUCOSE METABOLISM

Corticosteroids activate enzymes that promote gluconeogenesis, insulin resistance, redistribution of adipose tissue, and suppression of insulin release (Vegiopoulos and Herzig 2007). All of these effects combine to induce a state of relative insulin resistance (Oyer, Shah, and Bettenhausen 2006) (Figure 34.3).

34.7.1 Monitoring

End-of-life healthcare providers and endocrinologists recommend regular glucose monitoring when corticosteroids are used, but do not agree on the frequency or monitoring system (Quinn, Hudson, and Dunning 2006). If monitoring is desired, the aim should be a blood sugar level between 10 and 20 mmol/L (McCoubrie et al. 2005). This allows most patients to be free of the symptoms of hyperglycemia while avoiding the dangers of hypoglycemia.

34.7.2 Practical Methods and Techniques

In healthier populations, the first steps of managing diabetes may consist of diet and exercise modulations. However, if the patient has anorexia or cachexia, limiting food choices is not desirable and fatigue may limit exercise tolerance. Furthermore, whether or not to treat steroid diabetes in palliative care depends on symptoms and prognosis rather than numbers alone. If the patient has weeks or months to live, treatment may be appropriate. If they are unconscious, discussions should be had, and consideration given to stopping all hypoglycemic agents and blood sugar monitoring.

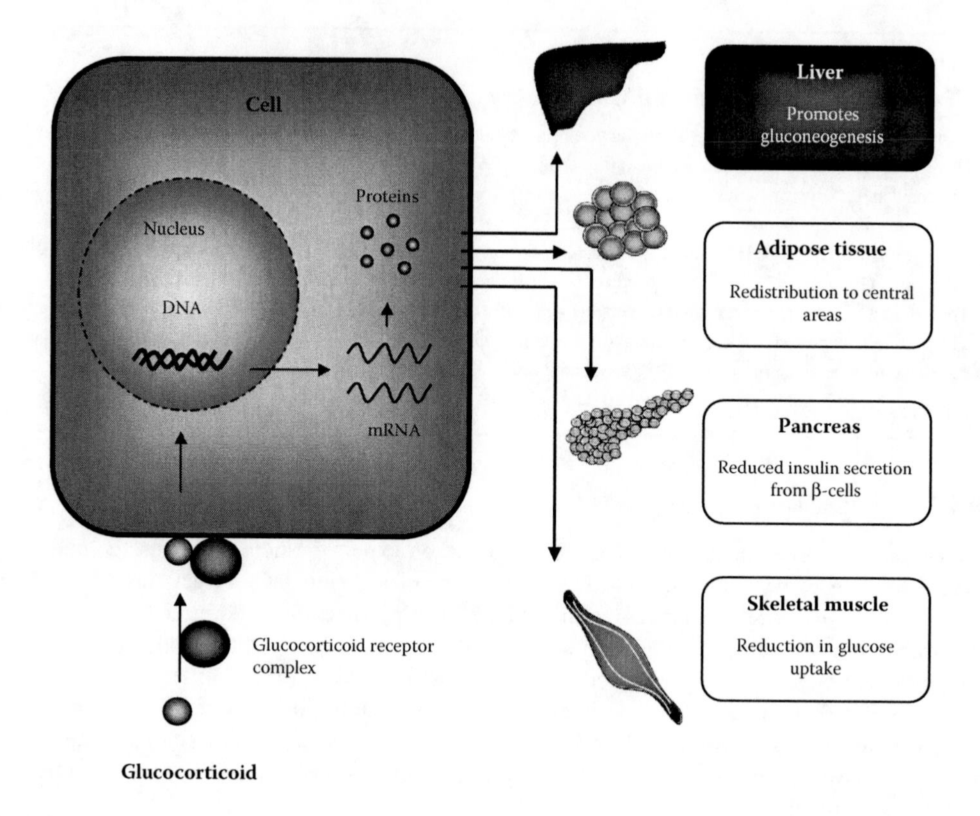

FIGURE 34.3 Glucocorticoids and impaired glucose metabolism.

An approach to steroid diabetes in palliative care is given in Table 34.5. The table gives starting doses for patients who have not previously been on hypoglycemic agents. These doses may not apply to all patients and the appropriate dose for each patient depends on his/her previous hypoglycemic requirements and body composition. Regardless of the starting point, titration is often required and titration necessitates the use of monitoring.

34.7.2.1 Oral Agents

Oral agents are less useful and more prone to cause side effects in the palliative population. Metformin is not recommended because of its propensity to cause lactic acidosis in patients with renal disease (Oyer et al. 2006; McCoubrie et al. 2005), while thiazolidinediones may lead to problems with fluid retention and heart failure (Oyer et al. 2006).

Oral secretagogs stimulate insulin release and must be used with caution because of the significant risk of hypoglycemia. This is especially worrisome if the medication is long-acting and oral intake is variable or decreasing. If an oral secretagog is desired, there may be a role for nataglinide, repaglinide, or gliclazide if used cautiously (Oyer et al. 2006; McCoubrie et al. 2005).

34.7.2.2 Insulin

In the steroid diabetic, glucose levels are highest during the day and normalize overnight (Oyer et al. 2006). Basal insulin should be given in the morning and the insulin chosen should peak during the day. For these reasons, neutral protamine Hagedorn (NPH) insulin has an advantage because the duration of action is shorter and it is less likely to cause nocturnal hypoglycemia (Oyer et al. 2006).

If prandial insulin is required, regular or analog insulin may be used. These agents are ideally titrated to the glucose level two hours postprandially or just prior to the next meal (Quinn et al.

TABLE 34.5
Management of Steroid-Induced Diabetes in Palliative Care

	Monitoring		
	Ideal Blood Glucose	10–20 mmol/L	
	Pharmacologic Management		
	Wean steroids if possible		
	Treat only if patient conscious and desiring treatment		
	Best Oral Hypoglycemic Agents[a]		
Name	**Class**	**Starting Doses**	**Advantages**
Nataglinide	Insulin secretagog	60–120 mg preprandial	Short actingWell tolerated in renal & hepatic failure
Repaglinide	Insulin secretagog	0.5–1 mg preprandial	Short acting
Gliclazide	SulphonylureaInsulin secretagog	80 mg in morning	Well tolerated in mild-moderate renal failure
	Best Basal Insulins		
Name	**Class**	**Starting Doses**	**Advantages**
NPH	Basal insulin	10 units in morning	Peaks during the day
Glargine/Detemir	Basal insulin	10 units in morning	More consistent levels over 24 hours
	Best Prandial Insulins		
Name	**Class**	**Starting Doses**	**Advantages**
Lispro/Aspart/Glulisine	Rapid-acting analog insulin	5 units immediately pre- or postprandial	Flexibility if unsure of oral intake
Regular	Human short-acting insulin	5 units 30–45 min preprandial	Fuller coverage between meals

Source: Based on recommendations from Oyer et al. (2006), McCoubrie et al. (2005), and Quinn et al. (2006).

[a] Use oral hypoglycemic agents cautiously and only in patients with a reliable oral intake.

2006). However, in palliative patients the burden of multiple injections and repeated monitoring must be considered and adjusted to meet the patients' goals of care.

For both oral agents and insulin, it is important to recognize that doses will likely need to be decreased, and sometimes stopped completely, as the patient consumes less orally or treatment with steroids is discontinued (Table 34.6).

TABLE 34.6
Key Facts about Steroid-Induced Diabetes

1. Corticosteroids induce a state of relative insulin resistance
2. Most experts recommend monitoring blood sugar levels in palliative patients prescribed corticosteroids
3. When monitoring and treating steroid-induced diabetes in palliative care, aim for a blood glucose level between 10 and 20 mmol/L to avoid the dangers of hypoglycemia
4. Limiting food choices is not appropriate in palliative care
5. Monitoring and treatment often depends on symptoms and prognosis. If a patient isunconscious, consideration should be given to stopping hypoglycemic agents and blood sugar monitoring
6. If treatment is desired, insulin is the most appropriate agent

34.7.3 Ethics and Diabetic Management in the Dying

The decision to treat diabetes in an unconscious dying patient may be a difficult one. It is unknown whether dying patients experience symptoms attributable to hyperglycemia. Invasive monitoring of blood sugar and administering insulin injections may be uncomfortable and inappropriate for patients in the terminal phase. If we believe the unconscious palliative patient cannot feel symptoms of thirst, polyuria, or altered mental state, interventions to lower glucose levels may not be appropriate.

34.7.4 Hiccups

Hiccups have also been associated with corticosteroids in palliative care. Case reports of hiccups occurring after the administration of corticosteroids have been published (Vazquez 1993; Cersosimo and Burphy 1998) and corticosteroids are one of the most common medications associated with hiccups (Thompson and Landry 1997). Hiccups cause significant morbidity by negatively affecting the amount of nutrition palliative patients can ingest (Smith and Busracamwongs 2003).

Hiccups are involuntary diaphragmatic spasms that occur through a reflex arc (Dickerman et al. 2003). Steroids are thought to lower the threshold for synaptic transmission in the midbrain and directly stimulate the afferent or efferent limb (Dickerman et al. 2003) (Figure 34.4).

For hiccups thought to be caused by steroids, the treatment should first be withdrawal of the offending drug. Should this not be possible, treatment can be undertaken with one of the following medications:

- Baclofen or valproic acid, which work via GABA to activate inhibitory neurotransmitters
- Chlorpromazine or haloperidol, which act by antagonizing dopamine in the hypothalamus

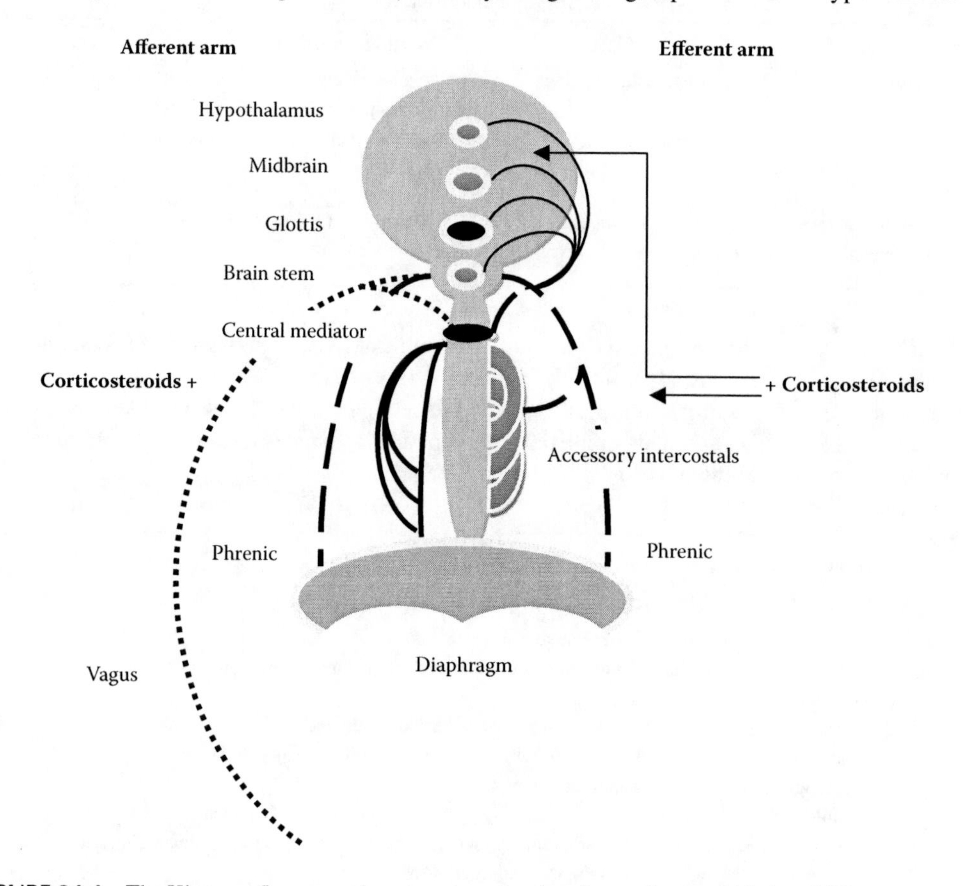

FIGURE 34.4 The Hiccup reflex arc and proposed mechanism for corticosteroid induced Hiccups.

- Metoclopramide or cisapride, which act by enhancing stomach emptying, thereby reducing esophageal contractions

Should these medications not work alone, combinations may be helpful (Smith and Busracamwongs 2003).

34.8 APPLICATIONS TO OTHER AREAS OF PALLIATIVE CARE

This chapter has focussed on diagnosing and treating the side effects of corticosteroids that may impact on nutrition and diet at the end-of-life. Although these side effects are more common in patients on steroids, they are also very common in palliative patients in general.

Candidiasis is common in HIV/AIDS, leukemia, and advanced malignancy even without the use of steroids. Diagnosis and treatment in these populations do not vary significantly from the recommendations given above. However, in the more severely immune-compromised host, the clinician must be aware of the greater possibility of dissemination to a more serious systemic fungemia and the possibility of more toxic treatment. Discussions regarding diagnosis and treatment with patients or families should reflect this difference.

Gastrointestinal (GI) symptoms are also common in palliative patients who have not been prescribed corticosteroids. They are particularly relevant for patients with cancers of the gastrointestinal tract and hepatic failure. Dyspepsia and upper GI hemorrhage, thought to be secondary to gastritis or peptic ulceration, will have a similar approach to that described above, with a focus on treatment with PPIs. Lower GI bleeding or upper GI bleeding thought to be secondary to esophageal varices require different treatments and interventions.

The recommendations in the sections on impaired glucose tolerance and hiccups are more general and may be applied to palliative patients not on steroids who also have these conditions.

SUMMARY POINTS

- Corticosteroids are powerful tools in palliative care and can greatly improve quality of life
- Corticosteroids have significant side effects that can impact diet and nutrition
- Candidiasis occurs in about 30% of palliative patients treated with corticosteroids.
- Treatment of oral or esophageal candidiasis can be achieved topically with nystatin or amphotericin, or systemically with clotrimazole, fluconazole, itraconazole, ketoconazole, voriconazole, and echinocandins.
- The incidence of dyspepsia for palliative patients on corticosteroids is 16% and symptoms of GI bleeding or severe dyspepsia occur in 4%–10%.
- Prophylaxis with a PPI or H2A should be considered in all cases and implemented if patients have two or more of the following: a high steroid dose, a previous history of peptic ulcers, advanced cancer, or concurrent NSAID use.
- Steroid-induced gastrointestinal side effects should be treated with a PPI (first-line agent) or with a H2A (second-line agent).
- Corticosteroids induce a state of relative insulin resistance.
- When monitoring and treating steroid-induced diabetes in palliative care, aim for a blood glucose level between 10 and 20 mmol/L.
- Insulin is the most appropriate agent for treating steroid-induced diabetes in palliative care.
- Corticosteroids predispose to hiccups, which can be treated with baclofen, valproic acid, chlorpromazine, haloperidol, metoclopramide, or cisapride alone or in combination.

ACKNOWLEDGMENTS

We wish to acknowledge the Center for Disease Control (CDC) for the use of their pictures in Figure 34.1. We also wish to acknowledge Dr. Pappas and *Clinical Infectious Diseases* for permission to use the guidelines for the treatment of candidiasis, which are presented, with minor modifications, in Table 34.1.

LIST OF ABBREVIATIONS

PPI	Proton pump inhibitor
NSAID	Non-steroidal anti-inflammatory drug
ECOG	Eastern Cooperative Oncology Group
COX	Cyclooxygenase
H2A	Histamine-2 receptor antagonist
IV	Intravenous

REFERENCES

Axell, T., P. Samaranayake, and O. Reichart. 1997. A proposal for reclassification of oral candidosis. *Oral Surgery Oral Medicine Oral Pathology* 84:111–12.

Bruera, E., and C. Neumann. 1998. Management of specific symptom complexes in patients receiving palliative care. *Canadian Medical Association Journal* 158:1717–26.

Cersosimo, R., and M. Burphy. 1998. Hiccups with high-dose dexamethasone administration – a case report. *Cancer* 82:412–14.

Cryer, B. 2001. Mucosal defense and repair role of prostaglandins in the stomach and duodenum. *Gastroenterology Clinics of North America* 30:877–94.

Davies, A., S. Brailsford, and D. Beighton. 2001. Corticosteroids and oral candidosis. *Palliative Medicine* 15:521.

Davies, A., S. Brailsofrd, and D. Beighton. 2006. Oral candidosis in patients with advanced cancer. *Oral Oncology* 42:698–702.

Dickerman, R., C. Overby, M. Eisenber, P. Hollis, and M. Levine. 2003. The steroid-responsive hiccup reflex arc: Competitive binding to the corticosteroid receptor? *Neuro Endocrinology Letters* 24:167–69.

Hardy, J., E. Ress, J. Ling, R. Burman, D. Feuer, K. Broadley, and P. Stone. 2001. A Prospective survey of the use of dexamethasone on a palliative care unit. *Palliative Medicine* 15:3–8.

Kaal, E., and C. Vecht. 2004. The management of brain edema in brain tumors. *Current Opinion in Oncology* 16:593–600.

Laval, G., J. Girardier, J. Lassauniere, B. Leduc, C. Haond, and R. Schaerer. 2000. The use of steroids in the management of inoperable intestinal obstruction in terminal cancer patients: Do they remove the obstruction? *Palliative Medicine* 14:3–10.

Leontiadis, G., A. Sreedharan, S. Dorward, P. Barton, C. Howden, M. Orhewere, J. Gisbert et al. 2007. Systematic reviews of the clinical effectiveness and cost-effectiveness of proton pump inhibitors in acute upper gastrointestinal bleeding. *Health Technology Assessment* 11:1–164.

Martínez, M., J. López-Ribot, W. Kirkpatrick, S. Bachmann, S. Perea, M. Ruesga, and T. Patterson. 2002. Heterogeneous mechanisms of azole resistance in Candida albicans clinical isolates from an HIV-infected patient on continuous fluconazole therapy for oropharyngeal candidosis. *Journal of Antimicrobial Chemotherapy* 49: 515–24.

McCoubrie, R., C. Jeffrey, C. Paton, and L. Dawes. 2005. Managing diabetes mellitus in patients with advanced cancer: A case note audit and guidelines. *European Journal of Cancer Care* 14:244–48.

Mercadante, S., F. Fulfaro, and A. Casuccio. 2001. The use of corticosteroids in home palliative care. *Supportive Care in Cancer* 9:386–89.

Nauck, F., C. Ostgathe, E. Klaschik, C. Bausewein, M. Fuchs, G. Lindena, K. Neuwohner, D. Schulenber, L. Radbruch, and the Working Group on the Core Documentation for Palliative Care Units in Germany. 2004. Drugs in palliative care: Results from a representative survey in Germany. *Palliative Medicine* 18:100–7.

Oyer, D., A. Shah, and S. Bettenhausen. 2006. How to manage steroid diabetes in the patient with cancer. *Journal of Supportive Oncology* 4:479–83.

Pappas, P., C. Kauffman, D. Andes, D. Benjamin, T. Calandra, J. Edwards, S. Filler et al. 2009. Clinical practice guidelines for the management of candidiasis: 2009 update by the Infectious Diseases Society of America. *Clinical Infectious Diseases* 48:503–35.

Pilkey, J., and P. Daeninck. 2008. A retrospective analysis of dexamethasone use on a Canadian palliative care unit. *Progress in Palliative Care* 16:63–68.

Piper, J., A. Wayne, J. Daugherty, and M. Griffin. 1991. Corticosteroid use and peptic ulcer disease: Role of nonsteroidal anti-inflammatory drugs. *Annals of Internal Medicine* 114:735–40.

Quinn, K., P. Hudson, and T. Dunning. 2006. Diabetes management in patients receiving palliative care. *Journal of Pain and Symptom Management* 32:275–86.

Rowell, N., and F. Gleeson. 2001. *Steroids, radiotherapy, chemotherapy and stents for the superior vena caval obstruction in carcinoma of the bronchus. Cochrane Database Syst Rev.*, 4, CD001316.

Salas, M., A. Ward, and J. Carol. 2002. Are Proton Pump Inhibitors the first choice for acute treatment of gastic ulcers? A meta analysis of randomized clinical trials. *BMC Gastroenterology* 2:17.

Shafford, E. 2006. Is corticosteroid prescribing appropriate in palliative care. *European Journal of Palliative Care* 13:202–4.

Smith, H., and A. Busracamwongs. 2003. Management of hiccups in the palliative care population. *American Journal of Hospice and Palliative Care* 20:149–53.

Thompson, D., and J. Landry. 1997. Drug-induced hiccups. *Annals of Pharmacotherapy* 31:367–69.

Valenzuela, J., R. Berlin, W. Snape, T. Johnson, B. Hirschowitz, J. Colon-Pagan, R. Morse et al. 1991. U.S. experience with omeprazole in duodenal ulcer – multicenter double-blind comparative study with ranitidine. *Digestive Diseases and Sciences* 36:761–68.

Vazquez, J. 1993. Persistent hiccups as a side effect of dexamethasone. *Human and Experimental Toxicology* 12:52.

Vecht, C., H. Haaxma-Reiche, W. Van Putten, M. de Visser, E. Vries, and A. Twijnstra. 1989. Initial bolus of conventional versus high-dose dexamethasone in metastatic spinal cord compression. *Neurology* 39:1255–57.

Vegiopoulos, A., and S. Herzig. 2007. Glucocorticoids, metabolism and metabolic diseases. *Molecular and Cellular Endocrinology* 275:43–61.

35 Appetite Stimulant Use in the Palliative Care of Cystic Fibrosis

Samya Z. Nasr and Darcie D. Streetman

CONTENTS

35.1 INTRODUCTION

Cystic fibrosis (CF) affects approximately 30,000 patients in the United States (Table 35.1). The nutritional goal for CF patients is to achieve normal growth and development. Evidence has shown that lung function is associated with nutritional status in CF and that nutritional status is an independent predictor of survival. Ten percent of CF patients are below the 10th percentile for height and weight (CF Foundation 2008).

Good nutritional status is dependent on the consumption of adequate nutrients, which is driven by complex, interrelated factors such as physical hunger, appetite, food-related behaviors, emotions, knowledge, and beliefs (Table 35.2). Diagnosing the cause of an individual's malnutrition requires careful, multidisciplinary history taking, physical examination, and overall patient/family assessment (Table 35.3).

Appetite stimulants (AS), although efficacious in treating malnutrition in CF, should only be prescribed if decreased food intake secondary to inadequate appetite is the principal cause of the malnutrition and all other contributing factors have been assessed, ruled out, or treated.

TABLE 35.1
Key Features of Cystic Fibrosis (CF)

1. CF is described in 1938 by Dr. Dorothy Anderson
2. It affects Caucasian more than other ethnic groups
3. It affects the lungs, pancreas, digestive tract, and sweat glands
4. It results in gradual deterioration of lung function and failure to thrive
5. Median survival age is over 37 years
6. Patients need more calories to be able to gain weight and prevent pulmonary deterioration
7. By improving nutrition, lung function will probably improve

Note: This table lists the key facts of CF and the need for increasing caloric intake.

35.2 APPETITE STIMULANTS

35.2.1 Megestrol Acetate (MA)

Megestrol acetate (MA) (Megace®) is a synthetic, orally active derivative of progesterone. One of the side effects of MA is appetite stimulation and weight gain. The mechanism of action has not been established. It has been postulated that the effect is partly mediated by neuropeptide Y, a potent central AS. Another speculation of its mechanism of action is that it is a potent inducer of adipocyte differentiation in 3T3-L1 cells in vitro, raising the possibility that it stimulates the conversion of fibroblasts to adipocytes, thereby blocking or reversing the effect of tumor necrosis factor on lipocyte differentiation (Loprinzi, Johnson, and Jensen 1992). It has been used successfully as an AS in adult patients with cancer and acquired immunodeficiency syndrome (AIDS) (Strang 1997).

MA has been used in CF to treat anorexia and weight loss (Eubanks et al. 2002; Marchand et al. 2000; Nasr et al. 1999). In a case report, four patients, ages 10–18.5 years, with severe CF lung disease, anorexia, and weight loss received MA at a dose of 400–800 mg daily and duration of use was

TABLE 35.2
Issues Contributing to Poor Appetite or Poor Food Intake

CF Related		Can Occur in People with CF	
Acute illness, pulmonary exacerbation, inflammation, increased cytokines	Poor gastric emptying and/or gastroesophageal reflux	Depression, anxiety, stress, or sadness	Eating disorder or disordered eating behaviors
Distal intestinal obstructive syndrome (DIOS) or constipation leading to abdominal pain and nausea	Nasal polyps which may impair taste or the ability to eat and breathe comfortably at the same time	Inflammatory bowel disease	Appetite neurotransmitter abnormality (ghrelin, peptide Y, leptin, insulin)
Avoidance of foods mistakenly thought to be "bad" for CF ("carbohydrates causing CF-related diabetes," "fats causing abdominal pain," "milk/milk products causing secretions" etc.)	Sinusitis which may be associated with pain with chewing, or altered taste	Medications (some antidepressants or attention deficit hyperactivity disorder (ADHD) medications)	Economic or access issues
Burden of therapies on time and energy to prepare and eat nutritious foods		Abdominal pain, bloating or other symptoms of malabsorption	

Source: Adapted from Nasr, S. Z., and D. Drury: Appetite stimulants use in cystic fibrosis. *Ped. Pulmonol.* 2008. 43:209–19. Copyright Wiley-VCH Verlag GmbH & Co. KGaA. Reproduced with permission.
Note: The table focuses on the issues contributing to poor appetite or poor intake.

TABLE 35.3
Work-up Strategies for Malnutrition in Cystic Fibrosis

	Symptoms	Information, Tests, and Possible Intervention Strategies
Appetite	Decreased food intake	Diet history, food records History of events leading to poor appetite: Temporal onset Symptoms at the time of onset Emotional/social/financial coexisting issues Behavioral issues around eating Observe mealtime interactions
	Early satiety	Gastric motility study
	Avoidance of high-energy foods	Body satisfaction, desired body weight, eating attitudes, purging behaviors (i.e., non-compliance to enzymes to lose weight)
Absorption/ digestion	Abdominal pain Gas Bloating Frequent, foul stools Visible oil loss	72-hour fecal fat coefficient of dietary fat intake Enzyme history: List of foods or beverages with which enzymes are not taken Information on when and how enzymes are taken Reported compliance to prescribed enzymes Low intestinal pH resulting in poor enzyme bioactivity: good compliance to enzymes reported and observed; enzyme dose 1000–2500 IU lipase/kg/meal minimal response to enzyme dose adjustments in recent past acid suppression or acid blocker therapies may be beneficial
	Stool mass palpitated	Abdominal x-ray; DIOS history
	Refractory symptoms	Rule out other GI processes common in CF: bacterial overgrowth, constipation, intussusceptions, CF-related liver disease, and/or the coexistence of lactose intolerance, celiac disease, etc
Metabolism	Growth failure or unintentional weight loss	Oral glucose tolerance test to rule out glucosuric energy losses
	Increased respiratory symptoms leading to elevated energy requirements	Aggressive respiratory and physio- therapies
	Use of systemic and/or inhaled corticosteroids	Linear height more affected than body weight or body mass index; bone age delay
	Hyponatremia	Recurrent hyponatremia or hyponatremic dehydration

Source: Adapted from Nasr, S. Z., and D. Drury: Appetite stimulants use in cystic fibrosis. *Ped. Pulmonol.* 2008. 43:209–19. Copyright Wiley-VCH Verlag GmbH & Co. KGaA. Reproduced with permission.

Note: The table provides a framework for malnutrition in CF. Issues listed should be addressed carefully.

6–15 months. Patients' appetite improved, with an increase in mean weight for age percentile from <5th percentile to 25th after 6 months of therapy. Quality of life improved (Nasr et al. 1999). Side effects were not reported in this report. A randomized, double-blind, placebo-controlled, crossover study of MA in 12 malnourished children with CF was conducted over a 12-week period, followed by a 12-week washout period, then the alternative treatment. The age range was 21 months to 10.4 years. Weight Z-score, body fat, and lean body mass (LBM) increased, and pulmonary function improved in patients given MA. There was little change in linear growth during MA therapy. Side effects included glucosuria, insomnia, hyperactivity, and irritability (Marchand et al. 2000). Another randomized, double-blind, placebo-controlled study was conducted on 17 CF patients age 6 years and above. MA dose used was 7.5–15 mg/kg/day. The study duration was 6 months. The treatment group had a significant increase in weight-for-age Z-score and reached 100% of their ideal body weight within 3 months of therapy. Weight gain included both fat and fat-free mass as measured by dual energy X-ray absorptiometry (DXA). Pulmonary function improved in the treatment group. Reversible adrenal suppression was observed in most of the patients who received MA. Some patients suffered from insomnia and moodiness while on MA (Eubanks et al. 2002). MA was also reported to cause testicular failure in CF patients and impotence in HIV-infected patients. It is known to cause glucocorticoid-like activity leading to Cushing Syndrome and adrenal insufficiency (Eubanks et al. 2002; Loprinzi et al. 1992; Marchand et al. 2000).

35.2.2 Cyproheptadine Hydrochloride (CH)

Cyproheptadine hydrochloride (CH) (Periactin®) is a first-generation antihistamine which is both a histamine and serotonin antagonist. It also has a secondary effect on appetite stimulation. The mechanism of action is unknown but it is not due to hypoglycemic-induced hyperphagia, as evidenced by normal glucose tolerance testing and normal insulin levels. Also, it is not due to an increase in endogenous growth hormone (GH). CH was shown to be an effective AS in studies of asthmatic children (Homnick et al. 2005) and in other diseases. Both MA and CH were found to be beneficial in HIV.

A 12-week, randomized, double-blind, controlled study of CH versus placebo was conducted in 18 CF patients. The dose was 4 mg QID over a 3-month period. Sixteen patients completed the study. Subjects in the CH group showed significant increase in weight, height, body mass index (BMI) percentiles, ideal body weight/height, weight for age Z-scores, and fat and fat-free mass versus the placebo group. There were no differences in antibiotic use or spirometric measures between the two groups. Transient mild sedation occurred in the CH group. A follow-up study was conducted to evaluate the long-term use of CH (Homnick et al. 2005). Sixteen CF patients enrolled in and 12 completed a 9-month open-label trial following the completion of the double-blind study. Subjects who had changed from placebo to CH gained weight significantly over 3–6 months and those continuing on CH generally maintained previously gained weight. There were some improvements, not statistically significant, in selected spirometric measures and side effects were mild.

35.2.3 Dronobinal (Marinol®)

Dronabinol (Marinol®) is an oral form of delta-9-tetrahydrocannabinol dissolved in sesame oil in soft gelatin capsules. It is the principal psychoactive substance present in marijuana. It is utilized as an alternative to smoked marijuana for AIDS wasting syndrome and nausea following chemotherapy. An important gap in the knowledge base about dronabinol has been an accurate assessment of its abuse potential. A number of studies cite the use of marijuana for treatment of cancer-related anorexia, nausea, vomiting, pain, and mood disorders. There is no evidence of abuse or diversion of dronabinol. There is no street market or value for dronabinol. Furthermore, it doesn't provide effects that are considered desirable in a drug of abuse. The onset of action is slow, and its effects are dysphoric and unappealing (Calhoun, Galloway, and Smith 1998).

A long-term study of dronabinol was conducted in 94 late-stage AIDS patients who had previously participated in a 6-week double-blind placebo-controlled study. The long-term use of dronabinol resulted in consistent increase in appetite with trends toward weight stabilization and modest weight gain. In addition, the data from this study suggested that it may be administered long term in this patient population without development of tolerance to the therapeutic effect. Few patients developed adverse events, including anxiety, confusion, euphoria, and somnolence (Beal et al. 1997).

It has been proposed to administer dronabinol to adolescent and adult CF patients to alleviate malnutrition and help treat wasting (Fride 2002). It was utilized in 11 CF patients with severe nutritional deficiencies who had failed conventional interventions of nutritional counseling and high-calorie supplements. Patients receiving dronabinol had a significant improvement in weight during the treatment period ($p = 0.03$). Side effects were euphoria, hallucinations, and lethargy. All side effects responded to lowering the dosage. No patients stopped the medication due to side effects (Anstead et al. 2003).

35.2.4 Antipsychotic/Antidepressant Agents

35.2.4.1 Antipsychotic Drugs

Excessive body weight gain (BWG) is a common side effect of some typical and atypical antipsychotic drugs (APDs). Weight gain is linked to a decreased metabolic rate, increased caloric intake, and decreased physical activity. It is generally believed that there are multiple mechanisms by which APDs induce weight gain, but their precise nature remains unknown. Weight gain may be a multifactorial process, involving serotonergic, histaminergic, and/or adrenergic neurotransmission. APDs achieve their therapeutic effects by modulating the activity of these neural pathways. Weight gain may also be due to the blockade of certain receptors, for example, 5-HT2c, that modulate appetite and body weight. APDs vary in their propensity to cause weight change with long-term treatment. The largest weight gains are associated with clozapine and olanzapine, and the smallest with quetiapine and ziprasidone. Risperidone is associated with modest weight gain that is not dose related. However, clozapine and olanzapine appear to display a high propensity to induce glucose dysregulation and dyslipidemia. Insulin secretion is preserved and thus high serum insulin levels are observed; there appears to be peripheral insulin resistance, which leads to glucose intolerance and type 2 diabetes mellitus (DM). Sudden BWG, insulin resistance, increased appetite, and related endocrine changes also may be involved in the development of glucose intolerance and dyslipidemia in predisposed individuals. Patients' blood glucose and lipids should be monitored before treatment and at regular intervals (Baptista et al. 2002).

The use of olanzapine in an 18-year-old female with CF and severe body dysmorphism led to a significant increase in body weight. This observation led to an open-label trial of low-dose olanzapine therapy in a group of 12 adults with severe CF disease that had been losing weight despite maximal conventional therapy. When compared to baseline, change in BMI after 6 months of therapy was statistically significant ($p = 0.01$, Wilcoxon sign-rank test) (Ross et al. 2005).

35.2.4.2 Antidepressants

Psychological functioning has been assessed in both children and adults with CF, but the results have been variable. The prevalence of psychological and psychosocial dysfunction of people with CF is associated with worsening disease severity and lack of social support. Antidepressants have been used, in addition to other psychosocial interventions, to treat depression in CF patients (Elgudin, Kishan, and Howe 2004).

In addition, antidepressants have been used as AS. All antidepressants have side effects, including appetite dysregulation. The non-adrenergic and specific serotonergic antidepressants block the 5-HT2C receptor (one of the serotonin receptors). Blockage of this receptor may lead to an increase in appetite. They also block the 5-HT3 (another serotonin receptor), which is the main site of action for nausea and occasional emesis. These two symptoms are usually associated with decreased appetite and failure to gain adequate weight in patients with severe CF disease (Boas et al. 2000).

Mirtazapine (Remeron®) is a noradrenergic and specific serotonergic antidepressant (NaSSA). It also has an antihistamine effect. The tolerability and safety profile reflects a unique pharmacological profile. It is well tolerated and shows particular benefits over other antidepressants in terms of antianxiolytic effects, sleep improvement, and gastrointestinal side effects. Its main side effect is weight gain (Boas et al. 2000; Sykes et al. 2006).

Mirtazapine has been used as an AS in two studies of malnourished CF patients (Boas et al. 2000; Sykes et al. 2006). The first study was a pilot study of five patients age 14–19 years with mean FEV1 of 41.4% with growth failure. All subjects demonstrated an increase in weight (5.8 kg, $p < 0.01$), body fat (13.9–21.8 kg, $p < 0.01$), and weight gain velocity (–3.9 before starting treatment vs. 27.4 kg/year after treatment, $p < 0.05$). All subjects reported mild sedation, dry mouth, increased thirst, and increased appetite. None of the subjects felt these symptoms justified stopping the medication (Boas et al. 2000). The second study was a retrospective study. Six patients were enrolled. Age range was 10–17 years at the start of therapy. All patients had an increase in BMI percentile for age (mean 10.3%, median 8%, and range 2%–25%). Adverse effects were limited to somnolence (Sykes et al. 2006).

35.2.5 Recombinant Human Growth Hormone (rhGH)

Recombinant human growth hormone (rhGH) has been approved by the Food and Drug Administration for use in treating AIDS-associated wasting. GH is a potent anabolic agent that has been used in the posttraumatic state to reduce nitrogen loss. The nitrogen retention induced by GH is associated with increased whole-body protein synthesis and LBM. Human GH is a single polypeptide chain composed of 191 amino acids (molecular weight 22 kDa) and coded on chromosome 17. Secreted by the somatotrophs of the anterior pituitary gland, GH promotes protein synthesis and fat utilization, and decreases glucose oxidation. GH stimulates the production of insulin-like growth factor (IGF-I) in the liver and other organs (muscle, bone, adipose tissue) (Windisch, Papatheofanis, and Matuszewski 1998).

The recommended dosage of rhGH is 4–6 mg administered by subcutaneous injection daily. It offers a more expensive alternative, approximately 10–15 times the cost, to AS such as MA and dronabinol. The adverse effects associated with rhGH therapy include mild edema and arthralgias, carpal tunnel syndrome, gynecomastia, insulin resistance, and glucose intolerance. Nonetheless, treatment has generally been well tolerated. In children, using rhGH for long-term replacement can lead to irreversible adverse effects such as slipped capital femoral epiphysis, acromegaly, and leukemia (Windisch et al. 1998).

Previous studies have documented that patients with CF have a delay in attainment of pubertal maturation. A poor correlation was found between weight gain and linear growth. This study concluded that nutritional supplementation alone may not be the best means for improving short stature in CF (Hardin 2002).

Several studies have documented the safety and efficacy of GH in improving growth and clinical status in CF patients (Hardin et al. 2006; Hardin et al. 2005). A 1-year randomized controlled trial to test the effect of GH on the clinical status of CF children was conducted. Nineteen prepubertal children were recruited. The GH treatment group had significantly greater height, height velocity, weight, weight velocity, and change in lean tissue mass. There was also significant improvement in delta forced vital capacity (FVC) compared with the year before the study; respiratory muscle strength also improved. The number of hospitalizations and outpatient intravenous antibiotic courses significantly decreased. A multicenter, randomized, controlled trial that included 61 prepubertal CF patients confirmed the results of this study. The study duration was 1 year.

GH was reported to enhance nutrition and growth in CF children receiving enteral nutrition (Hardin et al. 2005). GH safely improved height, body weight, bone mineralization, and clinical status in pubertal and adult CF patients with mild to moderate pulmonary disease.

A multicenter, randomized, double-blind, placebo-controlled trial was conducted to evaluate the metabolic and respiratory effects of GH in 63 CF children (bone age 8–18 years). The study concluded that GH therapy had positive metabolic effects but did not improve lung function in CF patients (Schnabel et al. 2007).

35.2.6 Anabolic Androgenic Steroids (AAS)

Since anabolic androgenic steroids (AAS) are derivatives or structural modifications of the parent steroid hormone testosterone, they exhibit both anabolic and androgenic activities. Anabolic effects are the promotion of protein synthesis, nitrogen retention, and skeletal muscle growth. Androgenic effects are the development and maintenance of primary and secondary sexual characteristics in males. In females, androgenic effects are evident as male pattern baldness, deepened voice, clitoromegaly, and growth of facial hair. Oxandrolone has marked anabolic activity and few androgenic effects (ratio 10:1) in comparison with testosterone and methyl-testosterone. Oxandrolone is the only AAS that is U.S. FDA-approved for restitution of weight loss after severe trauma, extensive surgery, chronic infections, malnutrition due to alcoholic cirrhosis, and Duchenne or Becker muscular dystrophy. Statistically significant improvements were reported in the areas of body composition, recovery, muscle strength, and function, and/or functional status. Oxandrolone is used in acute catabolic disorders (e.g., burn injury and acute multiple trauma). It is also used in chronic catabolic disorders, for example, moderate to severe alcoholic hepatitis, chronic obstructive pulmonary disease (COPD), and Crohn's disease. It has been used also in wasting associated with HIV/AIDS. Adverse effects include hepatic dysfunction (increased transaminase levels) and androgenic effects (alopecia, hirsutism, deep voice, and clitoromegaly in girls and women) (Orr and singh 2004). It has not been studied in CF patients.

Prednisone has been studied in CF patients with mild-moderate pulmonary disease to assess its effect on the pulmonary inflammatory process (Auerbach et al. 1985). The study was a 4-year, double-blind, placebo-controlled trial of alternate-day prednisone (2 mg/kg) in 45 CF patients. The patients in the prednisone group showed better growth and pulmonary function and less morbidity compared with those in the placebo group. No complications were reported. Because of this observation, the United States Cystic Fibrosis Foundation sponsored a multicenter, double-blind, placebo-controlled trial of alternate-day prednisone at a dose of 2 mg/kg (high dose), 1 mg/kg (low-dose), or placebo every other day for 4 years. Two hundred and eighty-five patients from 15 CF centers were enrolled in the study from 1986 to 1987. An interim safety analysis was done with mean duration in the study of 33.9 months for the high-dose, 35.3 months for the low-dose, and 36.8 months for the placebo groups. This analysis revealed increased frequency of cataracts, growth retardation, and glucose abnormalities among patients in the high-dose group.

In view of these results, it was recommended by the study ombudsman and a special advisory panel that the study drug be discontinued for all patients in the high-dose prednisone group. At the end of the study, there was significant improvement in the 1 mg group compared to placebo in FVC ($p < 0.025$) in patients colonized with *Pseudomonas aeruginosa* at baseline (Eigen et al. 1995). In addition, there was significant improvement in predicted forced expiratory volume in 1 sec (FEV_1) in the 1 mg/kg group compared to placebo ($p < 0.02$) and reduction in serum IgG concentrations (1 mg/kg vs. placebo, $p < 0.007$; 2 mg/kg vs. placebo, $p < 0.003$). From 6 months onward, height Z-scores fell in the 2 mg/kg group compared to placebo ($p < 0.001$). For the 1 mg/kg group, height Z-scores was lower at 24 months. An excess of abnormalities in glucose metabolism was seen in the 2 mg/kg group compared with the placebo group ($p < 0.005$) (Eigen et al. 1995).

35.3 APPLICATIONS TO OTHER AREAS OF TERMINAL OR PALLIATIVE CARE

Weight loss and malnutrition occur frequently in other terminal diseases and, as with CF, it is important to identify and correct underlying issues before initiating drug therapy aimed solely at increasing appetite and/or weight gain. Much of the data supporting their use originates in diseases other than CF (Beal et al. 1997; Loprinzi et al. 1992; Strang 1997; Windisch et al. 1998). Megestrol has been shown to increase appetite, decrease nausea, and improve general sense of well-being in cancer patients and AIDS patients (Loprinzi et al. 1992; Strang 1997). The appetite stimulation effects of cyproheptadine were originally discovered in asthmatic patients who were prescribed the drug for the antihistamine properties. Today, cyproheptadine is used less as an antihistamine and more as an AS in other disease states (Homnick et al. 2005). The cannabanoids have been used in cancer-related illness since the 1970s for anorexia, nausea, vomiting, pain, and mood elevation, however, a legal pharmaceutical formulation was not available until the 1980s (Calhoun et al. 1998). In fact, dronabinol is only FDA-approved for use in anorexia in AIDS patients and for treating nausea and vomiting due to cancer chemotherapy, but has since been applied off-label to other illnesses (Anstead et al. 2003; Beal et al. 1997; Fride 2002). rhGH has been used in AIDS-associated wasting and in the posttraumatic state, however is not widely studied in other terminal illnesses. Anabolic

TABLE 35.4
Summary of Appetite Stimulants in CF

Drug	Dosage	Side Effects
Megestrol acetate (MA)	400–800 mg/day or 7.5–15 mg/kg/day orally	Glucosuria, insomnia, hyperactivity, irritability, reversible adrenal suppression
Cyproheptadine hydrochloride (CH)	4 mg BID - QID or 0.5 mg/kg/day orally	Transient mild sedation
Dronabinal (Marinol®)	2.5 mg qd – 5 mg BID, PO	Anxiety, confusion, euphoria, somnolence
Antipsychotic		
Olanzapine	5–20 mg qd orally	Liver dysfunction, sleepiness, hyperglycemia
Risperidone	0.5–5 mg qd orally	Glucose dysregulation, dyslipidemia
Antidepressants		
Mirtazapine (Remeron®)	15 mg qd orally	Mild sedation, dry mouth somnolence
Recombinant human growth hormone (rhGH)	4 – qd SC injection	Mild edema, arthralgia, carpal tunnel syndrome, gynecomastia, insulin resistance, glucose intolerance. In children, slipped capital femoral epiphysis acromegaly, leukemia
Anabolic androgenic steroids (AAS) Oxandrolone	0.1 mg/kg/day BID, orally	Hepatic dysfunction, androgenic effects in females (alopecia, hirsutism, deep voice, clitoromegaly), development of primary and secondary sexual features in males. Not studied in CF

Source: Adapted from Nasr, S. Z., and D. Drury: Appetite stimulants use in cystic fibrosis. *Ped. Pulmonol.* 2008. 43:209–19. Copyright Wiley-VCH Verlag GmbH & Co. KGaA. Reproduced with permission.

Note: It provides a summary of appetite stimulants used in CF.

steroids have been widely utilized in many other chronic diseases. Anorexia and weight issues are not unique to CF patients, and most of the agents used in CF for appetite stimulation have been shown to be useful in other terminal illnesses.

ETHICAL ISSUES

The ethical issues surrounding appetite stimulation in CF are minimal. The biggest concern is that appetite stimulation is frequently a side effect of the drug, rather than the FDA-approved indication. For example, cyproheptadine is indicated for use as an antihistamine, the antidepressants are indicated for depression and related disorders, and antipsychotics are indicated for psychiatric illness. Although megestrol suspension is indicated for anorexia, cachexia, and weight loss in AIDS patients, the tablets are indicated for palliative treatment in breast or endometrial cancer, which was the originally studied use. No medication is without the potential for adverse effects. Megestrol can cause reversible adrenal suppression/failure, testicular failure, and impotence (Eubanks et al. 2002; Loprinzi et al. 1992; Marchand et al. 2000). Dronabinol has the potential for abuse, however to date there is minimal evidence of abuse or diversion and it is not thought to possess any street value (Calhoun et al. 1998). Antipsychotics may cause insulin resistance, glucose dysregulation, and dyslipidemia (Baptista et al. 2002; Ross et al. 2005). Additionally, there may be a social stigma that surrounds use of these agents. It is important to discuss the potential adverse effects of these agents with patients and families so they can participate in the risk versus benefit decision to start any of these agents.

SUMMARY POINTS

- Appetite stimulants (AS) can help increase caloric intake and improve weight gain.
- Table 35.4 shows a summary of the AS discussed.
- Etiology of weight loss should be identified and addressed before AS can be offered.

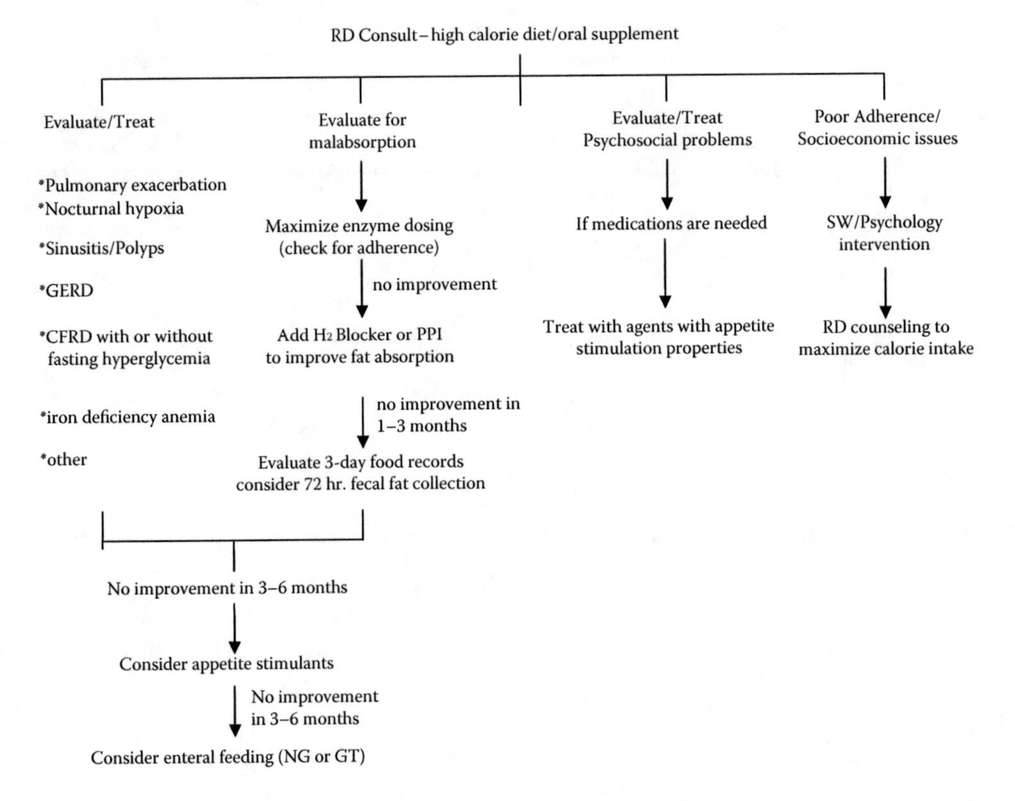

FIGURE 35.1 Algorithm for Cystic Fibrosis Patients at Nutritional Risk (BMI percentile ≤25% or poor weight gain for 3 months). It provides a framework to address workup for patients at nutritional risk. (Adapted from Nasr, S. Z., and D. Drury: Appetite stimulants use in cystic fibrosis. *Ped. Pulmonol.* 2008. 43:209–19. Copyright Wiley-VCH Verlag GmbH & Co. KGaA. Reproduced with permission.)

- Choice of AS should be made according to the physician's experience, patient age and preference, severity of disease, and side effects.
- Figure 35.1 shows an algorithm of workup and intervention for CF patients.

LIST OF ABBREVIATIONS

AAS Anabolic androgenic steroids
APDs Antipsychotic drugs
BMI Body mass index
BWG Body weight gain
CF Cystic fibrosis
CH Cyproheptadine hydrochloride
LBM Lean body mass
MA Megestrol acetate
rhGH Recombinant human growth hormone

REFERENCES

Anstead, M. I., R. J. Kuhn, D. Martyn, L. Craigmyle, and J. F. Kanga. 2003. Dronabinol, an effective and safe appetite stimulant in cystic fibrosis. *Pediatr Pulmonol* 36:343.

Auerbach, H. S., M. Williams, J. A. Kirkpatrick, and H. R. Colten. 1985. Alternate-day prednisone reduces morbidity and improves pulmonary function in cystic fibrosis. *Lancet* 2:686–88.

Baptista, T., N. M. K. N. Y. Kin, S. Beaulieu, and E. A. de Baptista. 2002. Obesity and related metabolic abnormalities during antipsychotic drug administration: mechanisms, management and research perspectives. *Pharmacopsychiatry* 35:205–19.

Beal, J. E., R. Olson, L. Lefkowitz, L. Laubenstein, P. Bellman, B. Yangco, J. O. Morales, R. Murphy, W. Powderly, T.F. Plasse, K.W. Mosdell, and K.V. Shepard. 1997. Long-term efficacy and safety of dronabinol for acquired immunodeficiency syndrome-associated anorexia. *J Pain Symptom Manage* 14:7–14.

Boas, S. R., S. A. McColley, M. J. Danduran, and J. Young. 2000. The role of mirtazapine as an appetite stimulant in malnourished individuals with CF. *Ped Pulmonol* 30:325.

Calhoun, S. R., G. P. Galloway, and D. E. Smith. 1998. Abuse potential of dronabinol (marinol®). *J Psychoactive Drugs* 30:187–95.

Cystic Fibrosis Foundation. 2008. *Cystic Fibrosis Foundation, patient registry 2003*. Bethesda, MD: Cystic Fibrosis Foundation.

Eigen, H., B. J. Rosenstein, S. FitzSimmons, and D. V. Schidlow. 1995. A multicenter study of alternate-day prednisone therapy in patients with cystic fibrosis. Cystic fibrosis foundation prednisone trial group. *J Pediatr* 126:515–23.

Elgudin, L., S. Kishan, and D. Howe. 2004. Depression in children and adolescents with cystic fibrosis: Case studies. *Int J Psychiatry Med* 34:391–97.

Eubanks, V., N. Koppersmith, N. Wooldridge, et al. 2002. Effects of megestrol acetate on weight gain, body composition, and pulmonary function in patients with cystic fibrosis. *J Pediatr* 140:439–44.

Fride, E. 2002. Cannabinoids and cystic fibrosis: A novel approach to etiology and therapy. *J Cannabis Ther* 2:59–71.

Hardin, D. S. 2002. Growth problems and growth hormone treatment in children with cystic fibrosis. *J Pediatr Endocrinol Metabolism* 15:731–35.

Hardin, D. S., B. Adams-Huet, D. Brown, B. Chatfield, M. Dyson, T. Ferkol, M. Howenstine, C. Prestidge, F. Royce, J. Rice, D.K. Seilheimer, J. Steelman, and R. Shepherds. 2006. Growth hormone treatment improves growth and clinical status in prepubertal children with cystic fibrosis: Results of a multicenter randomized controlled trial. *J Clin Endocrinol Metab* 91:4925–29.

Hardin, D. S., J. Rice, C. Ahn, et al. 2005. Growth hormone treatment enhances nutrition and growth in children with cystic fibrosis receiving enteral nutrition. *J Pediatr* 146:324–28.

Homnick, D. N., J. H. Marks, K. L. Hare, and S. K. Bonnema. 2005. Long-term trial of cyproheptadine as an appetite stimulant in cystic fibrosis. *Pediatr Pulmonol* 40:251–56.

Loprinzi, C. L., P. A. Johnson, and M. Jensen. 1992. Megestrol acetate for anorexia and cachexia. *Oncology* 49:46–49.

Marchand, V., S. S. Baker, T. J. Stark, and R. D. Baker. 2000. Randomized, double-blind, placebo-controlled pilot trial of megestrol acetate in malnourished children with cystic fibrosis. *J Pediatr Gastroenterol Nutr* 31:264–69.

Nasr, S. Z., and D. Drury. 2008. Appetite stimulants use in cystic fibrosis. *Pediatr Pulmonol* 43:209–19.

Nasr, S. Z., M. E. Hurwitz, R. W. Brown, M. Elghoroury, and D. Rosen. 1999. Treatment of anorexia and weight loss with megestrol acetate in patients with cystic fibrosis. *Pediatr Pulmonol* 28:380–82.

Orr, R., and M. F. Singh. 2004. The anabolic androgenic steroid oxandrolone in the treatment of wasting and catabolic disorders. *Drugs* 64:725–50.

Ross, E., S. Davidson, S. Sriram, S. Hempsey, Y. Jane, K. Margaret, and S. Bicknell. 2005. Weight gain associated with low dose olanzapine therapy in severely underweight adults with cystic fibrosis. *Pediatr Pulmonol* 40:350.

Schnabel, D., C. Grasemann, D. Staab, H. Wollmann, and F. Ratjen. 2007. A multicenter, randomized, double-blind, placebo-controlled trial to evaluate the metabolic and respiratory effects of growth hormone in children with cystic fibrosis. *Pediatrics* e1230–38.

Strang, P. 1997. The effect of megestrol acetate on anorexia, weight loss and cachexia in cancer and AIDS patients. *Anticanc Res* 17:657–62.

Sykes, R., F. Kittel, M. Marcus, E. Tarter, and M. Schroth. 2006. Mirtazapine for appetite stimulation in children with cystic fibrosis. *Ped Pulmonol* 40:389.

Windisch, P. A., F. J. Papatheofanis, and K. A. Matuszewski. 1998. Recombinant human growth hormone for AIDS-associated wasting. *Ann Pharmacother* 32:437–45.

36 Warfarin–Nutrition Interactions in the Hospice and Palliative Care Setting

Jeffrey L. Spiess

CONTENTS

36.1 INTRODUCTION

Ed Carlson was fed up. February 1933 in Wisconsin was bitterly cold. His dairy cows were dying, bleeding to death because of hemorrhagic sweet clover disease. What was killing his cows was the very thing that should be keeping them alive through the winter—the sweet clover hay that he was feeding them.

Mr. Carlson took matters in his own hands, or more correctly, his own truck. He loaded a dead heifer, about 100 pounds of the sweet clover hay, and a can of non-clotting cow blood. He drove nearly 200 miles through the snow to Madison to seek out the state veterinarian. That office was closed, but chance brought him in contact with Professor Karl Paul Link in the Department of Biochemistry at the University of Wisconsin. Mr. Carlson's disaster provided the spark that led to the discovery and development of a group of chemicals whose anticoagulant properties gave way to a myriad of uses (Link 1959).

The offending agent in the spoiled sweet clover hay was dicoumarol. When the hay was improperly cured, the coumarin it contained was oxidized and then two of the oxidized molecules were coupled to form the dicoumarol. It had been previously shown in cows with hemorrhagic sweet clover disease that the level of the critical clotting protein prothrombin was markedly reduced. Dicoumarol produced the same effect. Vitamin K could reverse the effect in animals as long as it was given early enough. By 1941 dicoumarol was being used as an anticoagulant in various clinical situations, and numerous other coumarin derivatives began to be synthesized and tested. One of the derivatives appeared particularly active and was also quite water soluble, making it practical for oral administration. In 1948 this agent was developed for rodent control under the auspices of the Wisconsin Alumni Research Foundation and the name chosen for it honored this funding source; it was called warfarin.

Dicoumarol and its derivatives have been commonly used as clinical anticoagulants since their development. In the United States, warfarin is overwhelmingly the most commonly used of these agents. For the remainder of this chapter the terms "warfarin" and "vitamin K antagonists (VKA)" are used interchangeably.

36.2 THE COAGULATION CASCADE

In order to understand the anticoagulant effect of VKAs, a brief review of blood clotting is in order. After an injury, the first line of defense against bleeding is elasticity of the skin and contraction of the smooth muscles of the blood vessel walls, as the body tries to minimize the amount of blood being lost. Over the next several minutes, blood platelets clump together to form a plug in the vessel wall. Concurrent with that is the activation of a cascade of chemical reactions involving molecules (clotting factors) from the lining cells of the vessel wall, the platelets, and the circulating plasma. This cascade produces a solid clot comprised of the structural protein fibrin.

Clotting factors normally circulate in an inactive form. On stimulation by injury or disease, they are converted to active enzymes in a sequential cascading fashion during which one activated factor

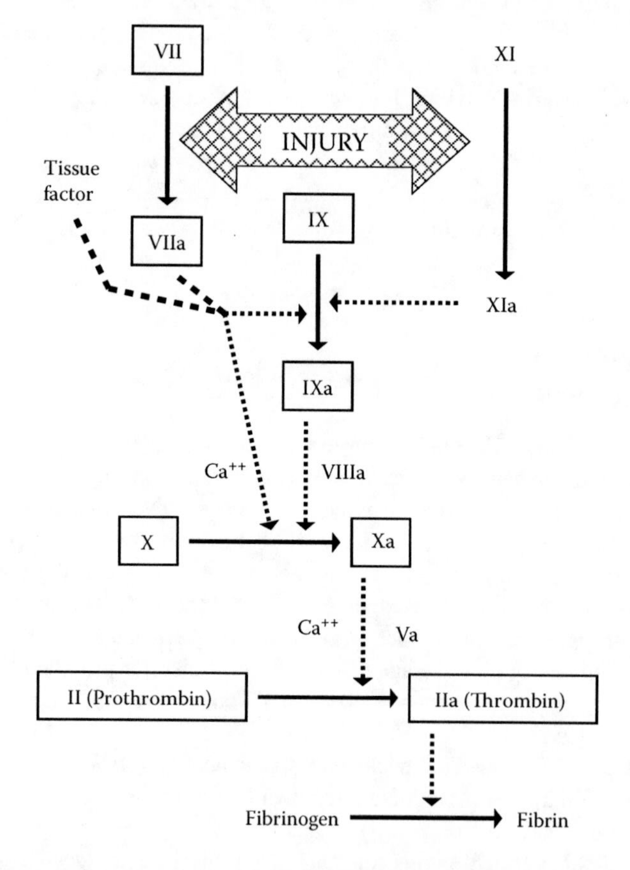

FIGURE 36.1 The coagulation cascade (simplified). Vascular injury results in activation of the coagulation cascade via activated factor XI (extrinsic pathway) and activated factor VII plus tissue factor (intrinsic pathway). These pathways converge to activate factor X, which in turn converts prothrombin to thrombin, which then catalyzes the conversion of circulating fibrinogen to fibrin, the constitutive protein of a clot. (Lower case 'a' represents the activated form of the factor. Factors in boxes are those dependent of vitamin K. Solid arrows indicate reactions, dotted ones indicate enzymes and cofactors).

catalyzes the activation of the next factor in the cascade, accelerating the process to the eventual production of fibrin. This cascade is schematically represented in Figure 36.1. The clotting factors are most commonly designated by Roman numerals with the presence of a lower case "a" indicating the activated enzymatic form.

36.3 VITAMIN K ANTAGONISTS

Most of the clotting factors are synthesized in the liver. Four of these (II, VII, IX, and X) undergo a gamma carboxylation step required to produce proteins that can be activated and participate in the cascade. If that gamma carboxylation step is missing or inadequate, the clotting factor that is produced is ineffective. The carboxylase enzyme responsible for this critical step requires reduced vitamin K as a cofactor. (Note that the term "reduced" refers to oxidation status, not quantitative amount.) It becomes apparent, then, that if supplies of reduced vitamin K are depleted, inactive clotting factors will be produced and blood coagulation will be impaired. (It should also be noted that the production of proteins C and S, factors that help restrain the clotting process, is also dependent on vitamin K.)

Warfarin exerts its anticoagulant properties by inhibiting the enzyme vitamin K oxide reductase. This enzyme catalyzes the reduction of oxidized vitamin K, allowing recycling of the vitamin K depleted by the activity of carboxylase. The result of warfarin therapy then is a decrease in the availability of reduced vitamin K. These pathways are illustrated in Figure 36.2. Because the enzyme inhibition is competitive, the level of anticoagulation is dependent upon the amount of warfarin present. This allows for adjustment of the clinical degree of anticoagulant effect by varying the dose of warfarin.

Mr. Carlson's dying cows perfectly illustrate this physiology and pharmacology. Sweet clover hay is excellent forage (and also a good source of vitamin K). However, when it is improperly cured, the VKA dicoumarol is produced. As long as the amount of dicoumarol in the hay is small enough, the remaining vitamin K in the hay controls the VKA effect, resulting in a minor or balanced anticoagulant effect. But when the VKA content is high enough, the capacity for synthesis of active clotting factors is overwhelmed, resulting in loss of blood clotting capability, hemorrhage, and dead cows (or rodents or people in the case of warfarin). This balance between the VKA effect of warfarin and the replenishment of supplies of reduced vitamin K is the essence of the major warfarin-nutrition interaction.

36.4 WARFARIN IN CLINICAL PRACTICE

In medical practice warfarin is used to produce a controlled, moderately anticoagulated state. Since the anticoagulant effect of warfarin is inhibition of the production of new clotting factors

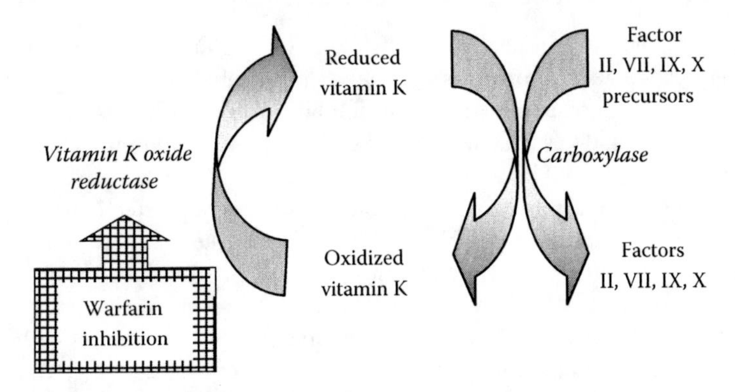

FIGURE 36.2 The effect of warfarin on clotting factor synthesis. The enzyme carboxylase catalyzes a crucial step in the synthesis of clotting factors II, VII, IX, and X. Carboxylase requires chemically reduced vitamin K as a cofactor. Warfarin inhibits the enzyme vitamin K oxide reductase that replenishes stores of reduced vitamin K. This in turn prevents the completion of the carboxylase step and leads to the production of inactive clotting factors. (From Ansell et al., *CHEST*, 133, 160S, 2008.)

TABLE 36.1
Key Points of Warfarin Therapy

- Warfarin is an anticoagulant drug used to treat or prevent abnormal blood clots in conditions such as deep vein thrombosis, pulmonary embolism, atrial fibrillation, and implanted prosthetic heart valves
- Warfarin exerts its anticoagulant effect by competitively inhibiting the availability of vitamin K, a required cofactor for synthesis of clotting factors II, VII, IX, and X
- The degree of anticoagulant effect must be closely monitored to avoid hemorrhage and recurrent blood clots
- The dynamic balance between warfarin dose and vitamin K intake requires consistent dietary vitamin K intake
- Vitamin K is useful as an antidote for excess warfarin effect but must be used judiciously to avoid total negation of anticoagulation
- Nutritional impairment is an important factor in the consideration of when anticoagulant therapy is no longer appropriate as patients approach the end of life

II, VII, IX, and X, that effect is not seen until previously synthesized factors are depleted. Because of this, initiation or change in warfarin dose will not produce a measurable effect for a few days and a stable level requires about a week. On the other hand, administration of excess vitamin K results in the prompt production of normal factors leading to some measurable reversal of the anticoagulant effect in several hours. Key points of warfarin therapy are summarized in Table 36.1.

The anticoagulant effect of warfarin is measured using the prothrombin time (PT). This is the time it takes the patient's plasma to clot after the cascade beginning with factor VII is activated by the addition of a thromboplastin (a substance that stimulates clotting). A normal PT is about 11–13 seconds. For most clinical uses of warfarin the safest balance between risk of clotting and risk of bleeding is achieved when the PT is two to three times normal. Because of variability among laboratories and reagents, this degree of measured anticoagulant effect is now reported as the ratio of the patient's measured PT to the normal PT, adjusted by a factor reflecting the potency of the thromboplastin used by the laboratory. This final result is called the International Normalized Ratio (INR) and is the standard reporting format worldwide. The target INR for most patients on warfarin is somewhere between 2 and 3.5, depending on the indication for anticoagulation and individual patient characteristics (Ansell et al. 2008).

36.5 WARFARIN INDICATIONS AND CAUTIONS

Common indications for warfarin therapy are listed in Table 36.2. For venous thromboembolism (VTE), including deep venous thrombosis and pulmonary embolism, anticoagulation is initiated after a clot has occurred. Here, therapy serves to inhibit further clotting, allowing the body's own clot-dissolving processes and vascular wall healing to occur. Most commonly, warfarin therapy is continued for several months and then stopped.

For other conditions like atrial fibrillation or the presence of a prosthetic heart valve, warfarin is used to prevent the formation of a clot. When therapy is indicated in these situations it is usually continued for most or all of the patient's remaining life.

Because the anticoagulant effect of warfarin is the result of a dynamic balance with the patient's intake of vitamin K and because numerous drugs and other factors can interact with warfarin, careful and frequent laboratory monitoring is required. Too little effect risks the development of new blood clots and too much effect risks bleeding, even catastrophic hemorrhage. For example the risk of intracranial hemorrhage increases dramatically as the INR climbs above 4.5 (Berwaerts and Webster 2000). In addition there is evidence that the risk of major bleeding develops rapidly after overanticoagulation (Kucher et al. 2004). An American study of patients aged 65 or older demonstrated that warfarin is the most common agent to produce an adverse reaction leading to a visit to

TABLE 36.2
Common Indications for Warfarin Therapy

Primary prevention
Prevention of embolic stroke and other arterial emboli
- Atrial fibrillation
- Prosthetic heart valve
- After myocardial infarction

Prevention of arterial thrombosis
- Carotid artery disease
- Coronary artery disease
- Endovascular stents

Prevention of thrombosis on intravascular catheters

Secondary prevention
Management of venous thromboembolism
- Deep venous thrombosis
- Pulmonary embolism
- Hypercoagulable states

an emergency department, with some 30,000 such encounters annually (Budnitz et al. 2007). This illustrates that the patient-specific and public health implications of getting the warfarin-vitamin K balance right are major.

36.6 VITAMIN K

Vitamin K (phylloquinone) is found in high concentrations in green leafy vegetables. A summary of key features of Vitamin K are is found in Table 36.3. The United States Dietary Reference Intake (DRI) of vitamin K in adults is 90–120 μg, dependent on age and gender. The vitamin K content of various foods is widely available in published resources; some examples are presented in Table 36.4. The dynamic balance described above between vitamin K and its antagonists like warfarin implies that dietary intake of vitamin K needs to be fairly consistent. Patients should not necessarily be counseled to consume or avoid vitamin K-containing foods, but to eat a reasonably consistent amount. Fluctuation in vitamin K intake can lead to fluctuation in degree of anticoagulation.

Commercially formulated nutritional support products generally provide DRI amounts of vitamin K if used as total nutrition. Herbal remedies, over-the-counter vitamins, and other nutritional supplements are frequently used by patients and can be an additional source of vitamin K. All of these sources need to be considered when evaluating the risk of a significant warfarin-dietary vitamin K interaction and also in providing education to patients on VKA therapy.

Consistent dietary intake of vitamin K, as well as many other nutrients, can be difficult to achieve for many persons with serious illness and for those approaching the end of life. As has been described elsewhere in this volume, anorexia, nausea, disorders of taste and smell, and other

TABLE 36.3
Key Features of Vitamin K

- Vitamin K (phylloquinone) is a fat-soluble vitamin found in highest concentrations in green leafy vegetables
- The Dietary Reference Intake of vitamin K for adults is 90–120 μg daily
- Nutritional support products and herbal supplements need to be included in evaluating vitamin K intake
- Patients on warfarin require consistent vitamin K intake to help prevent complications

TABLE 36.4
Vitamin K (Phylloquinone) Content of Selected Foods

Food	Vitamin K Content (μg)
Cooked spinach	889
Cooked collards	836
Cooked dandelion greens	579
Cooked broccoli	220
Cooked Brussels sprouts	218
Raw onions	207
Green leaf lettuce (raw)	97
Stewed prunes	65
Cooked okra	64
Raw cabbage	48
Cooked peas	40
Canned pumpkin	39
Canned tomato paste	30
Cooked snap green beans	20
Home-prepared mashed potatoes	13

Source: U.S. Department of Agriculture, Agricultural Research Service. 2009. USDA National Nutrient Database for Standard Reference, Release 22. Nutrient Data Laboratory Home Page, http://www.ars.udsa.gov/ba/bhnrc/ndl.

inhibitors of normal nutrition are common in this population. This impaired nutrition along with the frailty, comorbidities, and frequent complex drug regimens common in these patients increase risk of warfarin anticoagulation. Stopping anticoagulant therapy can often be the safest intervention (Spiess 2009).

36.7 VITAMIN K AS A THERAPEUTIC AGENT

Because the effect of warfarin and the supply of Vitamin K are in dynamic competition, vitamin K is useful as a clinical antidote for overanticoagulation. Since the effect of vitamin K takes several hours to appear, the patient who is actively bleeding requires replacement of clotting factors by transfusion of fresh frozen plasma in addition to vitamin K replacement. However, for the patient with excess VKA effect and no active bleeding, vitamin K can usually be used alone.

As large doses of vitamin K negate warfarin's anticoagulant effect, it is imperative that therapeutic vitamin K be used judiciously. Recommendations vary on when to administer therapeutic vitamin K and how much to use. Guideline consensus and randomized controlled trials suggest that if the INR is less than 9–10, no vitamin K is required as long as the warfarin is maintained until the appropriate anticoagulant balance is reestablished. For a more prolonged INR, a dose of 2.5–5 mg of oral vitamin K should be added (Ansell et al. 2008; Crowther et al. 2009).

Another therapeutic use of vitamin K in patients on chronic warfarin therapy is in the management of persistently unstable INR. While variability in degree of anticoagulation is often caused by lack of constant adherence to the VKA dosage, patients who have a relatively poor dietary intake of vitamin K may also demonstrate exaggerated variability. The daily administration of a modest dose (100–200 μg) of vitamin K can create a less volatile anticoagulation pattern (Ansell et al. 2008).

36.8 NON-VITAMIN K WARFARIN-NUTRITION INTERACTIONS

There have also been reported interactions between warfarin and nutrition unrelated to vitamin K. Foods that probably potentiate warfarin's effect include fish oil, mango, and grapefruit juice. Conversely, soy milk and large amounts of avocado can inhibit warfarin. The herbal supplements boldo-fenugreek, quilinggao, danshen, dong quai, *Lycium barbarum* L., and PC-SPES probably exaggerate the anticoagulant effect of warfarin, while ginseng can produce a negative interaction (Holbrook et al. 2005).

The gastrointestinal absorption of warfarin is unaffected by food. There is a risk, however, that proteins in some commercial enteral nutritional formulations may bind to warfarin. Some clinicians recommend avoiding enteral nutritional administration within an hour of a warfarin dose (Wohlt et al. 2009).

36.9 APPLICATION TO OTHER AREAS OF TERMINAL OR PALLIATIVE CARE

Patients in hospice and palliative care programs are frequently receiving numerous medications. Warfarin commonly interacts with many of these medications. Management of the warfarin-vitamin K interaction avoids one of the critical risks of this polypharmacy.

Another issue in patients with progressive debility, especially as nutritional intake becomes increasingly impaired, is identification of the point at which preventative measures such as anticoagulation are no longer consistent with the goals of care.

36.10 GUIDELINES

Patients being treated with warfarin require a reasonably consistent intake of vitamin K. Dietitians involved in the care of these patients need to be accurately informed as to the vitamin K content of foods and nutritional supplements and to appropriately educate them on the impact their dietary intake has on their anticoagulant therapy. This becomes particularly challenging with the nutritional impairment commonly seen near the end of life.

ETHICAL ISSUES

The primary ethical issue presented by the warfarin-nutrition interaction is minimizing the risk of warfarin therapy (nonmaleficence) while maintaining the benefits of therapy (beneficence).

SUMMARY POINTS

- Until safer effective oral anticoagulants are developed, warfarin will remain an important and commonly used drug for patients in hospice and palliative care.
- Warfarin exerts its anticoagulant effect by depleting the availability of reduced vitamin K, a required cofactor in the synthesis of clotting factors II, VII, IX, and X.
- The dynamic balance between warfarin's anticoagulant effect and stores of vitamin K is the focal point of warfarin-nutrition interactions.
- As long as warfarin therapy remains appropriate for the patient's goals of care, dietary intake of vitamin K should be consistent to avoid over- or under-anticoagulation, maximizing benefit and minimizing risk. The lessons of Mr. Carlson's cows should not be forgotten.

ACKNOWLEDGMENTS

I would like to thank Janice Scheufler, Leslie Griffith, and Patricia Spiess for their invaluable insights and criticisms.

LIST OF ABBREVIATIONS

DRI Dietary reference intake
INR International normalized ratio
PT Prothrombin Time
VKA Vitamin K antagonist
VTE Venous thromboembolism

REFERENCES

Ansell, J., J. Hirsh, E. Hylek, A. Jacobson, M. Crowther, and G. Palareti. 2008. Pharmacology and management of the vitamin K antagonists: American college of chest physicians evidence-based clinical practice guidelines (8th Edition). *CHEST* 133:160S–98S.

Berwaerts, J., and J. Webster. 2000. Analysis of risk factors involved in oral-anticoagulant-related intracranial haemorrhages. *Q J Med* 93:513–21.

Budnitz, D., N. Shehab, S. R. Kegler, and C. L. Richards. 2007. Medication use leading to emergency department visits for adverse drug events in older adults. *Ann Intern Med* 147:755–65.

Crowther, M. A., W. Ageno, D. Garcia, L. Wang, D. M. Witt, N. P. Clark, M. D. Blostein, et al. 2009. Oral Vitamin K versus placebo to correct excessive anticoagulation in patients receiving warfarin: A randomized trial. *Ann Intern Med* 150:293–300.

Holbrook, A. M., J. A. Pereira, R. Labiris, H. McDonald, J. D. Douhetis, M. Crowther, and P. S. Wells. 2005. Systematic overview of warfarin and its drug and food interactions. *Arch Intern Med* 165:1095–106.

Kucher, N. S., S. Connolly, J. A. Beckman, L. H. Cheng, K. V. Tsilimingras, J. Panikos, and S. Z. Goldhaber. 2004. International normalized ratio increase before warfarin-associated hemorrhage: Brief and subtle. *Arch Intern Med* 164:2176–79.

Link, K. P. 1959. The discovery of dicumarol and its sequels. *Circulation* 19:97–107.

Spiess, J. L. 2009. Can I stop the warfarin? A review of the risks and benefits of discontinuing anticoagulation. *J Pall Med* 12:83–87.

Wohlt, P. D., L. Zheng, S. Gunderson, S. A. Balzar, B. D. Johnson, and J. T. Fish. 2009. Recommendations for the use of medications with continuous enteral nutrition. *Am J Health-Syst Pharm* 66:1458–67.

Index

D

O

P

U

V

W

Z